D0214688

FRONTIERS IN NUTRITIONAL SCIENCE

This series of books addresses a wide range of topics in nutritional science. The books are aimed at advanced undergraduate and graduate students, researchers, university teachers, policy makers and nutrition and health professionals. They offer original syntheses of knowledge, providing a fresh perspective on key topics in nutritional science. Each title is written by a single author or by groups of authors who are acknowledged experts in their field. Titles include aspects of molecular, cellular and whole body nutrition and cover humans and wild, captive and domesticated animals. Basic nutritional science, clinical nutrition and public health nutrition are each addressed by titles in the series.

Editor in Chief
P.C. Calder, University of Southampton, UK

Editorial Board
A. Bell, Cornell University, Ithaca, New York, USA
F. Kok, Wageningen University, The Netherlands
A. Lichtenstein, Tufts University, Massachusetts, USA
I. Ortigues-Marty, INRA, Thiex, France
P. Yaqoob, University of Reading, UK
K. Younger, Dublin Institute of Technology, Ireland

Titles available
1. Nutrition and Immune Function
   Edited by P.C. Calder, C.J. Field and H.S. Gill

616.079
N976i

NUTRITION AND IMMUNE FUNCTION

Edited by

Philip C. Calder
University of Southampton, UK

Catherine J. Field
University of Alberta, Canada

and

Harsharnjit S. Gill
Massey University, New Zealand

CABI *Publishing*
in association with
The Nutrition Society

CABI *Publishing* is a division of CAB *International*

CABI Publishing
CAB International
Wallingford
Oxon OX10 8DE
UK

CABI Publishing
10 E 40th Street
Suite 3203
New York, NY 10016
USA

Tel: +44 (0)1491 832111
Fax: +44 (0)1491 833508
E-mail: cabi@cabi.org
Web site: www.cabi-publishing.org

Tel: +1 212 481 7018
Fax: +1 212 686 7993
E-mail: cabi-nao@cabi.org

© CAB *International* 2002. All rights reserved. No part of this publication may be reproduced in any form or by any means, electronically, mechanically, by photocopying, recording or otherwise, without the prior permission of the copyright owners.

A catalogue record for this book is available from the British Library, London, UK.

Library of Congress Cataloging-in-Publication Data
Nutrition and immune function / edited by Philip C. Calder.
        p. cm. -- (Frontiers in nutritional science ; no. 1)
Includes bibliographical references and index.
        ISBN 0-85199-583-7
    1. Immune system. 2. Nutrition. 3. Natural immunity. 4. Dietary supplements. I. Calder, Philip C. II. Series.
        QR182 .N88 2002
        616.07'9--dc21

                                                        2002004470

ISBN 0 85199 583 7

Typeset in Souvenir Light by Columns Design Ltd, Reading
Printed and bound in the UK by Biddles Ltd, Guildford and King's Lynn

Contents

Contributors

J.R. Arthur, *Division of Cell Integrity, Rowett Research Institute, Bucksburn, Aberdeen AB21 9SB, UK.*

B.S. Baliga, *Department of Pediatrics, College of Medicine, University of South Alabama, 2451 Fillingim Street, Mobile, AL 36617, USA.*

G.J. Beckett, *Department of Clinical Biochemistry, University of Edinburgh, Lauriston Building, Royal Infirmary of Edinburgh, Edinburgh EH3 9YW, UK.*

P. Brandtzaeg, *Laboratory for Immunohistochemistry and Immunopathology (LIIPAT), Institute of Pathology, University of Oslo, Rikshospitalet, N-0027 Oslo, Norway.*

P.C. Calder, *Institute of Human Nutrition, School of Medicine, University of Southampton, Bassett Crescent East, Southampton SO16 7PX, UK.*

R.K. Chandra, *Janeway Child Health Centre, Room 2J740, 300 Prince Philip Drive, St John's, Newfoundland, Canada A1B 3V6.*

M.L. Cross, *Institute of Food, Nutrition and Human Health, Massey University, Palmerston North, New Zealand.*

S. Cunningham-Rundles, *Immunology Research Laboratory, Division of Hematology and Oncology, Department of Pediatrics, New York Presbyterian Hospital, Cornell University Weill Medical College, 1300 York Avenue, New York, NY 10021, USA.*

J.M. Daly, *Department of Surgery, New York Presbyterian Hospital, Weill Medical College of Cornell University and 525 East 68th Street, New York, NY 10021, USA.*

G. Devereux, *Aberdeen Royal Infirmary, Foresterhill, Aberdeen AB25 2ZD, UK.*

M.D. Duff, *Department of Surgery, New York Presbyterian Hospital, Weill Medical College of Cornell University and 525 East 68th Street, New York, NY 10021, USA.*

C.J. Field, *Nutrition and Metabolism Research Group, Department of Agricultural, Food and Nutritional Science, 4–10 Agriculture Forestry Centre, University of Alberta, Edmonton, Canada T6G 2P5.*

H.S. Gill, *Institute of Food, Nutrition and Human Health, Massey University, Palmerston North, New Zealand.*

R.F. Grimble, *Institute of Human Nutrition, School of Medicine, University of Southampton, Bassett Crescent East, Southampton SO16 7PX, UK.*

D.A. Hughes, *Nutrition and Consumer Science Division, Institute of Food Research, Norwich Research Park, Norwich NR4 7UA, UK.*

S. Kuvibidila, *Division of Hematology/Oncology, Department of Pediatrics, Louisiana State University Health Sciences Center, Box T8-1, 1542 Tulane Avenue, New Orleans, LA 70112, USA.*

B. Lesourd, *Département de Gérontologie Clinique, Hôpital Nord du CHU de Clermont-Ferrand, BP 56, 63118 Cébazat, France.*

R.C. McKenzie, *Department of Medical and Radiological Sciences, University of Edinburgh, Lauriston Building, Royal Infirmary of Edinburgh, Edinburgh EH3 9YW, UK.* Corresponding address: *Section of Dermatology, Lauriston Building, Royal Infirmary of Edinburgh, Edinburgh EH3 9YW, UK.*

L. Mazari, *Département de Gérontologie Clinique, Hôpital Nord du CHU de Clermont-Ferrand, BP 56, 63118 Cébazat, France.*

S.M. Miller, *Department of Clinical Biochemistry, University of Edinburgh, Lauriston Building, Royal Infirmary of Edinburgh, Edinburgh EH3 9YW, UK.*

P. Newsholme, *Department of Biochemistry, Conway Institute of Biomolecular and Biomedical Research, University College Dublin, Belfield, Dublin 4, Republic of Ireland.*

E. Opara, *School of Life Sciences, Kingston University and Faculty of Health and Social Care Sciences, St George's Hospital Medical School, Penrhyn Road, Kingston upon Thames, Surrey KT1 2EE, UK.*

B.K. Pedersen, *Copenhagen Muscle Research Centre and Department of Infectious Diseases, Rigshospitalet, University of Copenhagen, Tagensvej 20, 2200 Copenhagen N, Denmark.*

E.W. Petersen, *Copenhagen Muscle Research Centre and Department of Infectious Diseases, Rigshospitalet, University of Copenhagen, Tagensvej 20, 2200 Copenhagen N, Denmark.*

A.S. Prasad, *Division of Hematology and Oncology, Department of Internal Medicine, Wayne State University School of Medicine, 4201 St Antoine, Detroit, MI 48201, USA.*

T.S. Rafferty, *Department of Medical and Radiological Sciences, University of Edinburgh, Lauriston Building, Royal Infirmary of Edinburgh, Edinburgh EH3 9YW, UK.*

A. Raynaud-Simon, *Département de Gérontologie Clinique, Hôpital Nord du CHU de Clermont-Ferrand, BP 56, 63118 Cébazat, France.*

R.D. Semba, *Department of Opthalmology, Johns Hopkins University School of Medicine, Baltimore, MD 21205, USA.* Correspondence address: *550 North Broadway, Suite 700, Baltimore, MD 21205, USA.*

A. Tomkins, *Centre for International Child Health, Institute of Child Health, 30 Guilford Street, London WC1N 1EH, UK.*

Preface

'This fortress built by Nature for herself
Against infection and hand of war'

(*The Tragedy of King Richard II*, Act II, Scene I, lines 43 and 44,
William Shakespeare)

It has been recognized for many years that states of nutrient deficiency are associated with an impaired immune response and with increased susceptibility to infectious disease. In turn, infection can affect the status of several nutrients, thus setting up a vicious circle of under nutrition, compromised immune function and infection. Thus, the focus of much of the research into nutrition, infection and immunity has been related to identifying the effects of nutrient deficiencies upon components of the immune response (often using animal models) and, importantly, upon attempts to reduce the occurrence and severity of infectious diseases (often in human settings). Although it is often considered that the problems of under nutrition relate mainly to the developing world, they exist in developed countries, especially among the elderly, individuals with eating disorders, alcoholics, patients with certain diseases and premature and small-for-gestational-age babies. Thus, immunological problems in these groups probably relate, at least in part, to nutrient status. In addition, many diseases that exist among the apparently well nourished have a strong immunological component and it is now recognized that at least some of these diseases relate to diet and that their course may be modified by specific changes in nutrient supply. Examples of these diseases include rheumatoid arthritis, Crohn's disease and atopic diseases. Furthermore, it is now recognized that atherosclerosis, a disease strongly influenced by diet, has an immunological component. Thus, understanding the interaction between nutrition and immune function is fundamental to understanding the development of a multitude of communicable and non-communicable diseases and will offer preventive and therapeutic opportunities to control the incidence and severity of those diseases. It is also now recognized that immune dysfunction plays a role in the events that follow trauma, burns or major surgery, and which, in some patients, can lead to organ failure and death. Thus, understanding the interaction between nutrition and immune function is fundamental in designing therapies to control the severity of these aberrant responses and to improve patient outcome.

The aim of this book is to provide a state of the art description of the interaction between nutrition and immunity, with an emphasis on the mechanism(s) of action of the nutrients concerned and the impact on human health. The book is divided into three parts.

Part 1 contains two chapters. The first is an overview of the immune system, its components and the way in which it functions and regulates its activities. The second is a description, using examples from the recent literature, of the methodological approaches that can be used to investigate the impact of altered nutrient supply on immune outcomes.

Part 2 contains 11 chapters. The first of these is devoted to the immunological effects of protein–energy malnutrition and of intrauterine growth retardation. Each of a further nine chapters is devoted to a specific nutrient or a family of nutrients: fatty acids, arginine, glutamine, sulphur amino acids, vitamin A, antioxidant vitamins (vitamins C and E and β-carotene), zinc, iron and selenium are all featured. The final chapter in this section deals with probiotics, an emerging area of great interest.

Part 3 contains five chapters. Rather than taking a nutrient-led approach these deal with changes in immune competence through the life cycle and with how nutrition affects these. The development of immunity in early life and the role of breast-feeding are covered in one chapter. A later chapter describes the current understanding of the impact of ageing on immune competence and how nutrient status plays a role in accelerating or delaying this ageing process. In between these two chapters are chapters on food allergy and on the influence of exercise on immune function. The final chapter tackles the public health implications of our increased understanding of the interaction between nutrition and immune function and poses important questions about how we can harness our knowledge for greater benefit.

Each chapter of this book includes an extensive reference list, which will guide the reader who wishes to seek more detailed information.

> The true remedy for all diseases is Nature's remedy. Nature and Science are at one … Nature has provided, in the white corpuscles as you call them – in the phagocytes as we call them – a natural means of devouring and destroying all disease germs. There is at bottom only one genuinely scientific treatment for all diseases, and that is to stimulate the phagocytes. Stimulate the phagocytes… The phagocytes are stimulated; they devour the disease; and the patient recovers.

The Doctor's Dilemma, Bernard Shaw

P.C. Calder, C.J. Field and H.S. Gill
Editors
December 2001

1 The Immune System: an Overview

GRAHAM DEVEREUX

Aberdeen Royal Infirmary, Foresterhill, Aberdeen AB25 2ZD, UK

Introduction

To parasitic microorganisms, the human body represents an extremely attractive environment and source of nutrients. Consequently, we live under the constant threat of overwhelming attack by viruses, bacteria and parasites. Microorganisms evolve more rapidly than humans, so that the nature of the microbiological threat to humans is changing as exposure to new or variant organisms occurs. To combat this potentially devastating threat, evolution has provided humans with a highly sophisticated, flexible and potent immune system, which is able to protect humans against rapidly evolving microorganisms. The critical protective function of the immune system becomes apparent when it fails. The inherited and acquired immunodeficiency states are characterized by increased susceptibility to all infections, including those organisms not normally considered to be pathogenic.

The immune system is a two-edged sword: the extremely potent and toxic biological effector mechanisms of the immune system can destroy not only threatening microorganisms but also body tissues. Usually the tissue destruction and inflammation associated with the eradication of a microbiological threat are acceptable and functionally insignificant. However, in several human diseases, the immunologically associated tissue destruction and inflammation are harmful, e.g. tuberculosis, fulminant hepatitis and meningitis, and, although this may be advantageous to the species as a whole, the effect on the individual may be devastating. It is because of their potential to destroy tissues that the effector mechanisms of the immune system are very tightly regulated. Failure of these regulatory mechanisms results in the full might of the immune system being inappropriately directed against body tissues and the development of autoimmune diseases, such as rheumatoid arthritis, systemic lupus erythematosus (SLE), myasthenia gravis and multiple sclerosis. If immune responses are directed against innocuous targets, such as allergens or transplanted

© CAB *International* 2002. *Nutrition and Immune Function*
(eds P.C. Calder, C.J. Field and H.S. Gill)

organs, the resulting immunologically mediated tissue damage and inflammation are the basis of allergy and transplant rejection. The immune response to
microorganisms is divided into two general systems: innate (natural) immunity
and adaptive (specific, acquired) immunity.

Innate Immunity (Medzhitov and Janeway, 1997)

Innate immunity comprises physical barriers, soluble factors and phagocytic
cells, which can be considered to provide an immediate first line of defence
against invading microorganisms. Innate immunity is encoded in the germline, it
is very similar among normal individuals and there is no memory effect, with re-
exposure to the same pathogen eliciting the same response. Innate immunity is
directed against molecular structures of microorganisms that are essential for
microbial survival, present in many types of microorganisms and unique to
pathogenic microorganisms, e.g. bacterial lipopolysaccharides and teichoic
acids. The major cells of innate immunity are phagocytic macrophages and neutrophils, which possess surface receptors specific for common bacterial surface
molecules. Engagement of these receptors triggers phagocytosis and destruction
of the microorganism. Although pathogenic microorganisms have evolved
mechanisms to evade the innate immune response, e.g. bacterial capsules, they
are usually eliminated by the adaptive immune response, which is able to mount
an appropriate neutralizing response directed specifically against the invading
microorganism. Although innate immunity is inflexible, it provides a very rapid
first line of defence until the more powerful and flexible adaptive immune
response takes effect. The innate and adaptive immune systems are not independent; the innate immune response probably influences the character of the
adaptive response and the effector arm of the adaptive response harnesses
innate effector mechanisms, such as phagocytes (Fearon and Locksley, 1996).

Adaptive Immunity (Huston, 1997)

Cells and tissues involved

It is the functional properties of B lymphocytes (B-cells) and T lymphocytes
(T-cells) that enable the adaptive immune response to be extremely powerful
and yet, at the same time, regulated and flexible. Lymphocytes originate in the
bone marrow from a common lymphoid stem cell. Further development and
maturation of B- and T-cells occur in the bone marrow and thymus, respectively. Mature T- and B-cells enter the bloodstream; specific receptors enable
adherence to capillary endothelial cells and migration into peripheral lymphoid
organs. These comprise the lymph nodes, spleen, bronchial-associated lymphoid tissue, mucosa-associated lymphoid tissue and gut-associated lymphoid
tissues (tonsils, adenoids, appendix and the Peyer's patches of the small intestine). Peripheral lymphoid organs are highly anatomically and functionally
organized to facilitate interactions between migrating lymphocytes and antigens

transported actively (by antigen-presenting cells) or passively (in lymph) to the peripheral lymphoid organs from the tissues. Lymphocytes that do not encounter antigen re-enter the bloodstream by way of efferent lymphatics and the thoracic duct. The functional consequence of this T- and B-cell circulation is that all of the body tissues are under continuous immunological surveillance for invading pathogens.

Clonal expansion of lymphocytes

Each T- and B-cell bears surface receptors with a single antigenic specificity, but the specificity of each individual lymphocyte is different. The population of T- and B-cells in a human is able to recognize an estimated 10^{11} different antigens. This huge receptor repertoire is generated during lymphocyte development by the random rearrangement of a limited number of receptor genes (Fanning *et al.*, 1996). Although the immune system is able to recognize a huge number of antigens, any single antigen is recognized by relatively few lymphocytes, typically 1 in 1,000,000; consequently, there are not enough lymphocytes to immediately eliminate an invading microorganism. When a lymphocyte antigen receptor engages its complementary antigen, the lymphocyte ceases migration, enlarges and rapidly proliferates so that, within 3–5 days, there are a large number of effector cells, each specific for the initiating antigen. This antigen-driven clonal expansion accounts for the characteristic delay of several days before adaptive immune responses become effective. Some of the effector cells generated by clonal expansion are very long-living and are the basis of the immunological memory that is characteristic of adaptive immunity. Functionally, immunological memory enables a more rapid and effective immune response upon re-exposure to microorganisms. In contrast to innate immunity, the antigen specificities of adaptive immunity reflect the individual's lifetime exposure to infectious agents and will consequently differ between individuals.

B-cells, immunoglobulins and humoral immunity

Protection against certain infections can be transferred by serum. This is called humoral immunity and is mediated by circulating antibodies, also known as immunoglobulins (Ig). The cell surface of B-cells incorporates the membrane-bound form of immunoglobulin, which functions as an antigen-specific receptor. Engagement of surface Ig by complementary antigen initiates B-cell proliferation, with the majority of the resulting cells transforming into plasma cells secreting large amounts of antibody with the same specificity as the progenitor B-cell surface Ig receptor.

Structure of immunoglobulins (Huston, 1997)

The general structural features of antibodies can be demonstrated by immunoglobulin G (IgG) (molecular weight 150 kDa), which comprises two identical heavy chains (50 kDa each) and two identical light chains (25 kDa each). Each of the two heavy chains is linked to the other and to a light chain by disulphide bonds, giving a roughly Y-shaped molecule (Fig. 1.1). Each immunoglobulin molecule possesses two antigen-binding (Fab) sites, each with the same specificity situated at the amino ends of the light and heavy chains. The Fab segments are divided into a variable (V) and a constant (C) region and the structural diversity of the V regions produces the diversity of antibody specificity. There are five main types of heavy chain, μ, δ, γ, α and ϵ, which confer differing functional properties between the five major classes (isotypes) of immunoglobulin, namely IgM, IgD, IgG, IgA and IgE, respectively. The functional activity of antibodies resides at the carboxyl-terminal (Fc) region of the heavy chains.

Immunoglobulin isotypes

The antigen specificity of antibodies is mediated by the two antigen-binding sites, while the differing Fc regions of the various immunoglobulin isotypes engage differing effector mechanisms. Monomeric IgM and IgD act as B-cell surface antigen-specific receptors. The affinity of each IgM antigen-binding site tends to be low; however, IgM in serum usually polymerizes into a pentamer with ten antigen-binding sites, which give the antibody high binding strength.

IgM dominates the initial humoral immune response; however, IgG and IgA predominate later, although IgE is prominent during an allergic response. This process is known as isotype switching and is the consequence of DNA

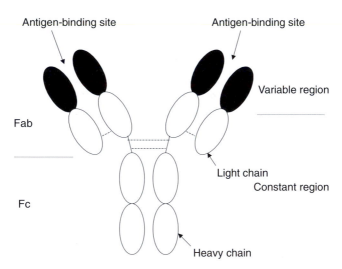

Fig. 1.1. Schematic representation of an IgG molecule. The two domains of each of the two light chains are termed V_L and C_L. The four domains of each of the two heavy chains are termed V_H, C_H1, C_H2 and C_H3. The amino terminal (dark) domain of each chain is the variable region and it is the tips of these regions that form the two antigen-binding sites of the molecule.

rearrangements in the genes encoding for the C (but not the V) regions of the heavy chains (Stavnezer, 1996). Isotype switching results in differing classes of antibodies with differing functional properties, although antigen specificity remains constant. Isotype switching is dependent on T-cells and their secretion of cytokines, with interleukin-4 (IL-4) inducing B-cell switching to IgE; this is antagonized by interferon-γ (IFN-γ) (Pene *et al.*, 1988). Switching to IgA is promoted by transforming growth factor-β (TGF-β), in combination with IL-10 (Defrance *et al.*, 1992). In addition to isotype switching, as the humoral immune response matures, point mutations in the immunoglobulin V-region genes occur. A T-cell-dependent process, known as affinity maturation, selects those B-cells with point mutations producing antibodies with an increased affinity for the stimulating antigen. Consequently, as the humoral immune response progresses, the affinity and specificity of the antibodies increase and the resulting memory cells provide highly effective protection against reinfection by the same microorganism (Neuberger and Milstein, 1995).

IgG antibodies are monomeric and are further subdivided into IgG_1, IgG_2, IgG_3 and IgG_4, with IgG_1 being found in the greatest quantities in serum. IgG_1 and IgG_3 are transferred across the placenta to the fetus. IgA circulates in the bloodstream but, of more functional importance, IgA is secreted across mucous membranes and is found in intestinal and bronchial secretions, tears and breast milk. Circulating IgA is monomeric, while secreted IgA polymerizes into dimers; polymerization is required for transport across epithelia. IgA is subdivided into IgA_1 and IgA_2. IgE is the principal antibody isotype involved in the immune response to parasites and in allergic reactions. The ϵ heavy chains possess an extra constant heavy-chain (C_H) domain and the Fc component binds with high affinity to the FcϵR1 receptor found on the surface membranes of mast cells, basophils and activated eosinophils.

Effector functions of immunoglobulins

The humoral arm of the adaptive immune responses is particularly effective against extracellular microorganisms and their toxins. Antibodies bind to functionally critical antigenic sites on soluble toxins and to the surface antigens of extracellular microorganisms. Such binding effectively neutralizes toxins and microorganisms by preventing binding to host-cell surface molecules. Antibodies bound to bacteria are also able to activate a series of plasma proteins, known as complement, to produce molecules that are chemotactic for phagocytes, promote phagocytosis and can also directly destroy bacteria (Lambris *et al.*, 1999).

Antibodies bind to bacteria by the amino-terminal antigen-binding sites, leaving the Fc component of the antibody exposed. Engagement of these exposed Fc fragments by surface Fc receptors on phagocytic cells induces phagocytosis and destruction of the coated bacterium; this process is known as opsonization. Macrophages and neutrophils possess IgM- and IgG-specific Fc receptors, while eosinophils possess IgE-specific Fc receptors. Phagocytes form part of the innate immune system and possess very limited antigen-specific receptors. Opsonizing antibodies enable phagocytes to recognize a wide range of antigens by effectively converting an antigen to an Fc segment that is easily recognized by phagocytes that are otherwise unable to engage and destroy the bacteria.

Antibodies are mainly directed against extracellular pathogens; however, they can be effective against virally infected cells that express viral antigens on their surfaces. These exposed viral antigens are bound by antigen-specific antibodies and the infected cell is destroyed by natural killer (NK) cells. NK cells are large granular lymphocytes, defined by the absence of surface immunoglobulin or T-cell receptors and the presence of Fcγ receptors. NK cells do not undergo clonal expansion; instead, they provide innate cytotoxic immune responses directed against virally infected cells, although they can interact with the adaptive immune response as outlined above (Fearon and Locksley, 1996).

T-cells and cell-mediated immunity

Antibodies are highly effective against extracellular pathogens, but they have very limited potency against intracellular pathogens, such as viruses and certain bacteria. T-cells, however, are particularly effective against intracellular pathogens, because of their ability to identify infected cells and then mount and coordinate an effective cell mediated immune response.

The T-cell receptor

Each T-cell possesses approximately 30,000 antigen-specific T-cell receptor (TCR) molecules on its surface, each with the same antigen specificity. Unlike B-cell immunuoglobulin molecules, TCR is always surface-bound, is not secreted and does not undergo any form of isotype switching or somatic hypermutation. The TCR (Fig. 1.2) comprises two transmembrane glycoprotein chains, linked by a disulphide bond. A single α and a single β chain associate to form the majority (90%) of TCRs. However, 10% of T-cell TCRs are composed of a single γ chain and a single δ chain. The true functional significance of $\alpha\beta$ and $\gamma\delta$ T-cells is unknown. Each TCR traverses the T-cell membrane, and the external part of each TCR chain consists of a V and a C domain, with the V region being highly polymorphic, and the single antigen-binding site is formed by the apposition of the two amino-terminal V regions. TCR antigen-specificity diversity is generated during T-cell maturation by random rearrangement of gene segments encoding the TCR Vα and Vβ regions. Rearrangement of the genes encoding the $\alpha\beta$ TCR produces an estimated 10^{15} variants, each with a different antigen specificity; $\gamma\delta$ chain diversity is even greater, with an estimated 10^{18} specificities. In contrast to B-cells, T-cells are only able to recognize antigens displayed on cell surfaces. Infection of a cell by an intracellular pathogen is signalled by the surface expression of pathogen-derived peptide fragments, expressed in conjunction with glycoproteins encoded by the major histocompatibility complex (MHC). It is the combination of pathogen peptide fragment bound to MHC molecule that is recognized by T-cells (Fremont *et al.*, 1996).

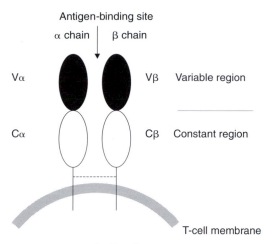

Fig. 1.2. Schematic representation of a T-cell-receptor molecule. Each of the constituent α and β chains comprises a V and a C domain. The apposition of the two V (dark) domains forms the antigen-binding site of the molecule. The two chains are linked by a disulphide bond and anchored in the T-cell surface membrane.

The MHC (Germain, 1994; Huston, 1997)

The MHC is a large complex of genes that encode the major histocompatibility glycoproteins. These large cell-surface glycoproteins are present in some form on every nucleated cell and there are two structural variants (MHC class I and MHC class II). The MHC was originally identified and characterized by its profound influence on the rejection or acceptance of transplanted organs. The MHC is the molecular basis by which T-cells recognize intracellular pathogens in order to initiate or effect an immune response.

An MHC class I molecule (Fig. 1.3) consists of a highly polymorphic 44 kDa α chain that is non-covalently associated with a smaller non-polymorphic 12 kDa β_2-microglobulin chain. The α chain spans the cell membrane and forms a cleft into which the pathogen-derived peptide fragment is inserted during assembly of the MHC molecule. An MHC class II molecule comprises a 34 kDa α chain and a 29 kDa β chain; both span the cell membrane (Fig. 1.4). Each chain is divided into two domains, with association of the α_1 and β_1 domains forming an open-ended peptide-binding cleft into which a processed antigen peptide fragment is incorporated. MHC class I molecules bind peptides of eight to ten amino acids that originate from pathogen proteins synthesized within the cell cytosol, typically from viruses and certain bacteria. MHC class II molecules bind peptides derived from pathogens that have been phagocytosed by macrophages or endocytosed by antigen-presenting cells' such as macrophages, B-cells and professional antigen-presenting cells. MHC–pathogen–peptide complexes are very stable and are expressed on the cell surface, ready for recognition by a T-cell with TCRs specific for the peptide–MHC complex; this is known as MHC restriction.

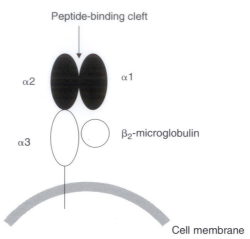

Peptide-binding cleft

Fig. 1.3. Schematic representation of an MHC class I molecule. A single α chain is composed of three domains, α1, α2 and α3, and the apposition of the α1 and α2 domains forms the peptide-binding cleft. The α chain is non-covalently associated with a smaller non-polymorphic protein β_2-microglobulin.

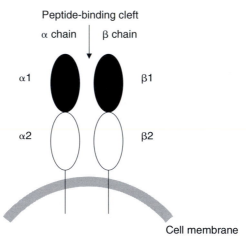

Fig. 1.4. Schematic representation of an MHC class II molecule. Each of the constituent α and β chains comprises two domains. Apposition of the α1 and β1 domains forms the peptide-binding cleft.

T-cells expressing the CD8 antigen recognize peptides complexed with MHC class I molecules, which are expressed by all nucleated cells. The CD8 antigen is a surface molecule that acts as a co-receptor by simultaneously binding to the TCR and the MHC class I α_3 domain. MHC class II–peptide complexes are recognized by T-cells expressing the CD4 antigen, which acts as a co-receptor (like CD8) by binding to the β_2 domain of the MHC class II molecules already bound by TCR. In humans, approximately one-third of peripheral blood T-cells are CD8, two-thirds are CD4 and approximately 5–10% are CD4– CD8–, the functions of which are unclear.

The structure of the peptide-binding cleft determines the peptide-binding specificity of an MHC molecule, such that it binds to peptides with a broadly similar structure. There are several genetic organizational features of the MHC that result in nucleated cells expressing a highly polymorphic set of MHC molecules, each with differing peptide-binding specificities. The polymorphic nature of the MHC is the consequence of the MHC being formed by three major class I genes designated human leucocyte antigen (HLA)-A, HLA-B and HLA-C, and three main class II genes, HLA-DP, HLA-DQ and HLA-DR; each of these loci is highly polymorphic. Furthermore, most individuals are heterozygous for MHC genes and there is co-dominant expression of the antigens coded by the maternally and paternally derived loci. Consequently, nearly all individuals express six class I and ten class II molecules, each with differing specificities. During an infection, it is highly likely that the proteins of a pathogen include peptide sequences that are recognized and presented to T-cells by at least one MHC molecule. The general explanation for MHC polymorphism is that it is an evolutionary response to pathogenic diversity, enabling the immune systems of individuals to respond to a wide range of existing and evolving pathogens. MHC polymorphism results in individuals with differing immunological capabilities to combat an individual pathogen, but on a population scale it is highly unlikely that any individual pathogen will be able to evade the immune system of every individual.

The generation of effector T-cells (Janeway and Bottomly, 1994)

Activation of a T-cell is a complex, tightly regulated process. This is necessary in order to ensure that T-cell activation is directed only against pathogens and not against body tissues. Furthermore, increased complexity decreases the likelihood that a microorganism can evolve mechanisms to subvert T-cell activation. T-cell activation takes place in the peripheral lymphoid organs. However, before this can occur, antigen is processed and presented in association with MHC molecules, and the antigen is then transported from the site of infection to the peripheral lymphoid organs and presented to T-cells. The processing, transportation and presentation of antigen are performed by antigen-presenting cells, the most important and efficient of which are dendritic cells. Dendritic cells are mandatory for the initiation of a primary immune response against a new pathogen, although both dendritic cells and non-professional antigen-presenting cells, such as macrophages and B-cells, are able to initiate secondary (memory) responses against reinfecting organisms.

Dendritic cells (Banchereau and Steinman, 1998)

These are generated in the bone marrow but are subsequently widely distributed throughout the tissues, typically in association with epithelial surfaces. When viewed by phase-contrast microscopy, dendritic cells extend long, delicate, motile processes in all directions. In peripheral tissues, so-called 'immature' dendritic cells have poor T-cell stimulatory activity. Instead, they act as sentinels, constantly sampling the surrounding tissues for pathogens. Immature dendritic cells accumulate foreign antigens in their surroundings by macropinocytosis of soluble antigens and phagocytosis of particulate antigens and microorganisms. These processes are so efficient that dendritic cells can initiate immune responses with pico- and nanomolar concentrations of antigens, compared with the micromolar concentrations required by non-professional antigen-presenting cells, such as B-cells and macrophages.

After a dendritic cell captures a pathogen-associated antigen, its sampling function declines and, instead, it starts to process pathogenic antigens and present them in association with MHC molecules on its cell surface. Endocytosed antigens are presented in association with MHC class II molecules, while endogenously produced antigen, e.g. from a virus infecting the dendritic cell, is presented in association with MHC class I molecules. Dendritic cells are able to process and present, in a class I-restricted manner, antigens that do not enter the cytosolic compartment, e.g. viruses unable to infect dendritic cells. However, the mechanism for this is unclear. As antigens are processed and expressed, dendritic cells up-regulate surface expression of T-cell co-stimulatory molecules, such as CD40 and B7. Dendritic-cell maturation is also associated with secretion of cytokines and chemotactic cytokines (chemokines), which recruit macrophages, granulocytes, NK cells and more dendritic cells to counter the invading pathogen.

After processing and presenting antigen, dendritic cells bearing processed antigen migrate from the site of infection to the T-cell areas of local lymph nodes. There migration stops and they interact with T- and B-cells to initiate an immune response. Mature dendritic cells are extremely potent activators of T-cells, with a single dendritic cell being able to activate 100–3000 T-cells. This is because of the high density of MHC, co-stimulatory and adhesion molecules expressed by dendritic cells and the secretion of cytokines that profoundly influence T-cells, e.g. IL-12.

Dendritic–T-cell interactions

As T-cells circulate around the body, they pass through the peripheral lymphoid organs, where they transiently adhere to antigen-presenting cells. Contact is made with many thousands of dendritic cells every day. This enables T-cells to 'sample' the many MHC–peptide complexes on the surface of the antigen-presenting cells. Rarely, a circulating T-cell will possess TCRs that conform to the peptide–MHC complex. Binding of the TCR and peptide–MHC complex induces conformational changes in adhesion molecules that increase the interaction between the antigen-presenting cell and the T-cell and keep the T-cell and its progeny in close proximity to the source of their stimulation. T-cell activation is not induced solely by ligation of a TCR, CD4 or CD8 co-receptor with a specific MHC–peptide complex. T-cell proliferation requires a further stimulus from the antigen-presenting cell and this is provided by the antigen-presenting cell surface glycoproteins B7.1 (CD80) and B7.2 (CD86) binding to their receptor (CD28) present on the T-cell. Typically, a TCR binding to an MHC–peptide complex in the absence of co-stimulation leads to T-cell anergy (unresponsiveness) or apoptosis.

Clonal expansion and differentiation of T-cells into effector cells

Antigen-specific and co-stimulatory interaction between T-cell and antigen-presenting cell triggers T-cell proliferation. After a few days, thousands of T-cell progeny emerge from the peripheral lymphoid organs and localize to the areas of infection or inflammation. Each of these effector T-cells possesses the same antigen specificity as the parent T-cell and they are now available to counteract the stimulating pathogen. These effector T-cells differ from the parent T-cell, because they do not require the co-stimulation provided by antigen-presenting cells; therefore, further encounters by effector T-cells with their specific antigen results in immunological attack. The nature of immunological attack depends on the effector T-cell CD4/CD8 status.

Effector CD8 T-cells

Effector CD8 T-cells (also known as cytotoxic T-cells) play a vital role in counteracting viral infections (Fig. 1.5), which are intracellular and almost completely hidden from the humoral immune response. Effector CD8 T-cells are

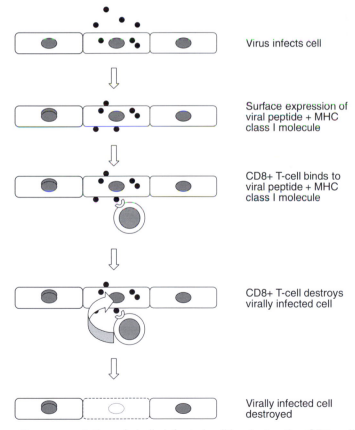

Virus infects cell

Surface expression of viral peptide + MHC class I molecule

CD8+ T-cell binds to viral peptide + MHC class I molecule

CD8+ T-cell destroys virally infected cell

Virally infected cell destroyed

Fig. 1.5. Schematic representation of virally infected cell by destruction CD8+ effector T-cell.

induced by antigen-presenting cell presentation of MHC class I–peptide complexes to CD8 T-cells. The anti-viral activity of CD8 cytotoxic T-cells depends on the ability of virally infected cells to signal their corrupted state by the cell-surface expression of viral peptide sequences in association with MHC class I molecules. It is these MHC–peptide complexes that are recognized by CD8 TCRs and trigger immunological attack by the CD8 T-cell. It is the interaction between CD8 T-cell and infected cell that enables precise destruction of infected cells and preservation of uninfected cells. After migrating to a site of viral infection, CD8 cytotoxic T-cells sample cell surfaces. If the CD8 T-cell adheres to and identifies an infected cell, the corrupted cell is destroyed by directed localized secretion of cytotoxic enzymes (perforin and granzymes) by the CD8 cell. This effectively neutralizes the viruses infecting the cell. Other anti-viral properties of CD8 cytotoxic T-cells include the secretion of the anti-viral cytokine IFN-γ and expression of Fas ligand (CD95L), which induces apoptosis in target cells bearing the Fas (CD95) receptor protein. Clearly, if control of this extremely destructive but precise process is lost and CD8 T-cells start destroying 'self' cells, the consequences are potentially catastrophic. Such a breakdown in control is probably the basis of the immunological destruction of insulin-secreting β cells of the pancreatic islets, resulting in type I (insulin-dependent) diabetes mellitus.

Effector CD4 T-cells

Although CD8 effector T-cells are of major importance in the defence against viruses, they are ineffective in eliminating certain intracellular bacteria, fungi and parasites that are not neutralized by destruction of their host cell. These micro-organisms are also resistant to the humoral immune response. These particularly resistant organisms are neutralized by effector CD4 T-cells, which are generated by MHC class II-restricted presentation of peptide by antigen-presenting cells. Effector CD4 T-cells are more commonly known as T-helper (Th) cells.

Th-cells and macrophages (Stout and Bottomly, 1989)

Macrophages usually destroy phagocytosed microorganisms. However, certain pathogens (e.g. *Mycobacteria*, *Leishmania* and *Pneumocystis*) have evolved mechanisms that resist macrophage destruction. After directed migration of Th-cells to the site of infection, Th-cells sample the peptide–MHC class II surface-molecular repertoire of adjacent cells. Macrophage activation occurs if the surface-expressed peptide–MHC class II is recognized by a Th-cell possessing the complementary TCR. This macrophage–Th-cell interaction alone is insufficient to activate the macrophage, and two further signals are required (Fig. 1.6). The first is IFN-γ; this is usually secreted by the engaged Th-cell, but other sources of IFN-γ are also important, e.g. CD8 cytotoxic T-cells. The second signal sensitizes the macrophage to IFN-γ and this second signal can also be provided by Th-cells, which express surface CD40 ligand molecules; these interact with macrophage surface CD40 molecules.

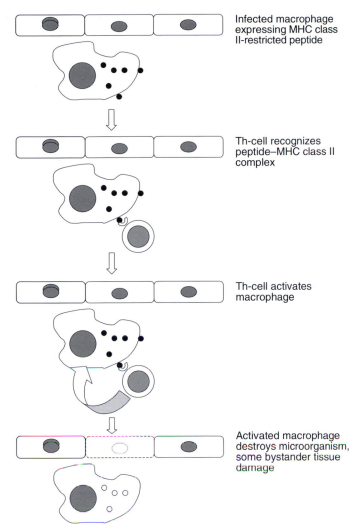

Infected macrophage expressing MHC class II-restricted peptide

Th-cell recognizes peptide–MHC class II complex

Th-cell activates macrophage

Activated macrophage destroys microorganism, some bystander tissue damage

Fig. 1.6. Schematic representation of Th-cell activation of macrophage infected with resistant microorganism.

Clearly, Th-cells are extremely potent antigen-specific macrophage activators, because they provide both the IFN-γ and the CD40 signals required for macrophage activation. Th-cell-induced activation greatly enhances macrophage antimicrobial and antigen-presenting capacity. The increased antimicrobial capacity of activated macrophages in part derives from the following:

1. Increased efficiency of lysosome fusion with microbe-containing phagosomes.
2. Increased synthesis of antimicrobial proteases and peptides, such as defensins.

3. Induction of the respiratory burst produces extremely microbiocidal products, such as the superoxide anion ($O_2^-\cdot$), singlet oxygen ($^1O_2$), the hydroxyl radical ($OH\cdot$), and hydrogen peroxide (H_2O_2).
4. Production of the reactive nitrogen metabolite nitric oxide (NO) is increased by activation of the enzyme inducible NO synthase (iNOS).

Macrophage activation is associated with the release of anti-microbial mediators that are not only toxic to microorganisms but also extremely toxic to host cells, resulting in host tissue damage. If macrophages constitutively remained in this activated state, massive tissue damage would occur. Therefore, macrophage activation is tightly regulated and extremely pathogen-specific. The control and antigen specificity of macrophage activation is provided by antigen-specific Th-cells. Thus the price paid by the host, in terms of tissue damage, in order to destroy these difficult invading intracellular organisms is minimized.

Th-cells and B-cells

Certain bacterial-associated antigens can elicit a T-cell-independent B-cell response (Mond *et al.*, 1995). These thymus-independent (TI) antigens tend to have highly repetitive epitopes, which enable extensive cross-linking of surface immunoglobulin molecules, resulting in B-cell activation. Typical bacterial TI antigens are capsular polysaccharides, lipopolysaccharides and polymeric proteins. T-cell-independent B-cell responses provide a rapid specific response directed against bacteria possessing anti-phagocytic polysaccharide capsules, e.g. *Streptococcus pneumoniae*.

In general, B-cell activation requires signals from two sources; the first arises from the binding of B-cell surface-bound IgM/D to the complementary microorganism surface epitope and the second is Th-cell-derived (Fig. 1.7). This Th-cell facilitation of B-cell activation is essential for full expression of the humoral immune response, particularly isotype switching, affinity maturation and the efficient development of memory B-cells. To enable Th-cell facilitation of B-cell activation, B-cells are able to internalize antigen–immunoglobulin complexes and then express the resulting pathogen peptide sequences in an MHC class II-restricted fashion on the B-cell surface. It is these peptide–MHC class II complexes that are recognized by the Th-cell. It is essential that the peptide sequences recognized by the Th-cell originate from the antigen recognized by the B-cell. This process of linked recognition means that the B-cell and the Th-cell respond to different epitopes; however, the epitopes originate from the same antigen. Typically, the B-cell recognizes a surface epitope and the Th-cell possibly an internal peptide sequence.

The second signal provided by the Th-cell to enable B-cell activation takes the form of secreted and cell-bound signals. Effector Th-cells express surface CD40 ligand and this binds to B-cell surface CD40. Th-cell cytokine secretion is also critical in B-cell activation and maturation. Once activated, B-cells undergo clonal expansion and differentiation into immunoglobulin-secreting plasma cells, each secreting immunoglobulin isotypes with the same antigen specificity

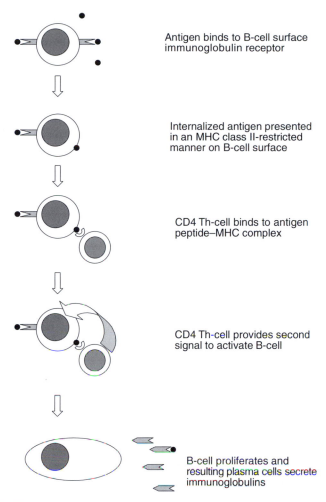

Antigen binds to B-cell surface
immunoglobulin receptor

Internalized antigen presented
in an MHC class II-restricted
manner on B-cell surface

CD4 Th-cell binds to antigen
peptide–MHC complex

CD4 Th-cell provides second
signal to activate B-cell

B-cell proliferates and
resulting plasma cells secrete
immunoglobulins

Fig. 1.7. Schematic representation of Th-cell-dependent B-cell activation through linked
recognition of a pathogen antigen.

as the parent B-cell. Although plasma cells tend to localize to lymph nodes and
bone marrow, their anti-microbial actions are widespread because of the extensive distribution of their secreted immunoglobulins.

Although macrophages and B-cells are critically dependent on Th-cells,
clinical and experimental observations suggest that there is selective utilization
of these cells during immune responses. Some CD4 Th-cell-mediated responses
are predominantly antibody-based, while others are macrophage-dependent.
For example, healing tuberculoid leprosy is associated with strong macrophage-
mediated immunity with low antibody levels, whereas non-healing lepromatous
leprosy is associated with high (but ineffective) antibody levels, weak
macrophage-based effector responses and uncontrolled proliferation of
microorganisms. The discovery that Th-cells are functionally diverse has helped
in the understanding of these observations.

Th-cell functional diversity (Abbas *et al.*, 1996; Mosmann and Sad, 1996)

The ability of CD4 Th-cells to initiate immune responses with differing effector mechanisms was clarified by a demonstration by Mosmann and Coffman (1989) that murine CD4 T-cell clones could be categorized into two broad functional groups, Th1 and Th2, depending on their secreted cytokines. Th1 cells secrete IFN-γ, IL-2 and tumour necrosis factor β (TNF-β), while Th2 cells secrete IL-4, IL-5, IL-6, IL-9, IL-10 and IL-13. Human Th1 and Th2 secretory cytokine patterns are similar to the murine model, although the synthesis of IL-2, IL-6, IL-10 and IL-13 is not so tightly restricted to a single subset. Additionally, however, individual human Th-cells can secrete both Th1 and Th2 cytokines and these are commonly known as Th0 cells. Human Th-cells appear to form a continuum, with some extremely polarized cells secreting either typically Th1 or Th2 cytokines but the majority are Th0 cells, secreting a mixture of Th1 and Th2 cytokines. The subdivision of Th-cells is complicated further by the recognition that some Th2 cells secrete the suppressive regulatory cytokine TGF-β, with some authorities terming these cells Th3. In recent years, it has become apparent that the Th1/Th2 subdivision is overly simple, but the concept of the functional dichotomy of Th1/Th2 is extremely useful in aiding the understanding of immune responses.

Th1 and Th2 cytokines have important effector and Th-cell regulatory functions (Fig. 1.8). Th1 and Th2 cytokines augment Th-cell differentiation in favour of the secreting subset, i.e. Th1 cytokines promote differentiation towards the Th1 phenotype and Th2 cytokines towards the Th2 phenotype. In addition, Th cytokines inhibit Th-cell differentiation towards the reciprocal phenotype, i.e. Th1 cytokines inhibit differentiation towards the Th2 phenotype and Th2 cytokines antagonize development of Th1 cells. The consequence of this self-amplification and mutual antagonism of the reciprocal phenotype is that, once a Th-cell-mediated immune response deviates towards either the Th1 or Th2 phenotype, the Th-cell response becomes increasingly polarized towards that phenotype.

Factors affecting Th1/Th2 differentiation

CD8 T-cells are predestined to mature into cytotoxic T-cells. However, Th1 and Th2 cells develop from a common CD4 T-cell precursor. Differentiation of precursor Th-cells is determined by genetic and environmental factors influential at the time of T-cell antigen recognition. Several factors influencing Th1/Th2 polarization have been proposed and demonstrated, but the most potent factor is the local cytokine milieu present at the time of T-cell activation.

The most potent cytokine promoting development of the Th1 phenotype is IL-12 in the absence of IL-4 (Trinchieri and Gerosa, 1996). Macrophages and professional antigen-presenting cells, such as dendritic cells, secrete IL-12 in response to bacteria, bacterial products and intracellular parasites. IL-12 is extremely potent in promoting Th1-biased differentiation by direct influences on the Th-cells. The most potent Th2-promoting stimulus is IL-4 in the absence of IFN-γ, but the initial source of polarizing IL-4 is not established (Ricci *et al.*,

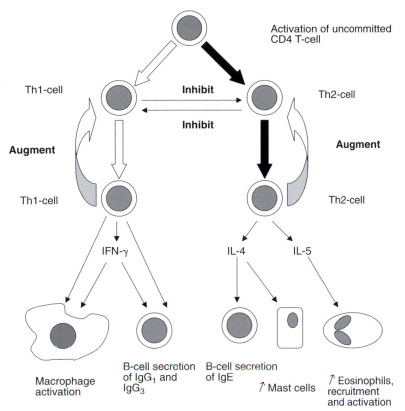

Fig. 1.8. Schematic representation of CD4 Th-cell differentiation into Th1 or Th2 cells. Th1 differentiation leads to macrophage activation and the secretion of opsonizing IgG. Th2 differentiation results in IgE secretion, mastocytosis and eosinophilia.

1997). Environmental and/or genetic factors may induce IL-4 secretion during activation of CD4 cells; a small specialized subset of CD4 T-cells known as CD4 NK1.1 secrete IL-4 on stimulation, and antigen presentation by B-cells can stimulate Th2 differentiation (Mason, 1996).

Although the cytokine microenvironment is the most potent determinant of Th1/Th2 polarization, Th1/Th2 differentiation is also influenced by complex interactions between antigen dose, TCR and MHC antigen affinities. Influential antigenic properties include the nature of the antigen, with viruses and bacteria favouring Th1 differentiation and helminths Th2. Th2 differentiation appears to be promoted by the small, highly soluble proteins characteristic of allergens. Some important allergens (house dust-mite allergen *Der p1*, subtilisin and papain) are proteases, and it is suggested that this favours Th2 differentiation, because helminths secrete proteases to aid tissue penetration. It is apparent that many factors influence Th1/Th2 differentiation, but it is highly unlikely that any single criterion is the sole determinant of Th-cell differentiation, because this would be quickly perverted by rapidly evolving pathogens. The complex matrix of factors that eventually determine Th0, Th1 or Th2 polarization is probably an immunological evolutionary adaptation to reduce the scope for pathogen interference.

Effector mechanisms of Th1-mediated immunity

Th1 cells appear to be critical in effecting an antigen-specific phagocytic-mediated defence against microorganisms, principally bacteria, fungi and some parasites. If, however, Th1-biased immunity is directed against self-antigens, extensive tissue destruction and autoimmune disease may ensue. Common autoimmune diseases resulting from inappropriate Th1 responses include autoimmune haemolytic anaemia, autoimmune thrombocytopenic purpura, Goodpasture's syndrome, type I insulin-dependent diabetes mellitus, rheumatoid arthritis and multiple sclerosis. Disease may also ensue if a Th1-biased immune response is inappropriately directed against innocuous antigens, such as occurs in coeliac disease.

The effector mechanisms of Th1-biased immune responses include activation of macrophages that have phagocytosed microorganisms normally resistant to lysosomal destruction. Th1 cytokines direct isotype switching of B-cells towards IgG production. In mice, Th1 cytokines promote secretion of the opsonizing antibodies IgG_{2a} and IgG_3; in humans, the equivalent IgG subtypes are probably IgG_1 and IgG_3. These opsonizing antibodies bind to microorganisms and promote their phagocytosis by macrophages and neutrophils, because of their affinity for phagocytes possessing Fcγ receptors and their ability to activate components of complement. Th1 cytokines also mobilize and localize appropriate phagocytic cells to sites of infection. IL-3 and granulocyte–macrophage colony-stimulating factor (GM-CSF) promote bone-marrow stem-cell proliferation and differentiation and the generation of large numbers of phagocytes. Localization of these phagocytes to sites of infection is achieved by Th1-cell secretion of TNF-α and TNF-β and chemokines that alter the adhesive properties of local endothelial cells and act as chemotactic agents. Therefore, in an elegantly efficient, controlled and microorganism-specific manner, Th1-biased Th-cells secrete cytokines that not only promote Th1 differentiation and inhibit Th2 development but also induce a complex package of biological responses directed towards the phagocytic destruction of invading microorganisms.

Effector mechanisms of Th2-mediated immunity

Th2-biased immune responses are believed to be important in the immune responses against helminth infections. If, however, Th2-biased immune responses are inappropriately directed against innocuous antigens, such as allergens, tissue damage and inflammation may ensue. These inappropriate Th2 responses underlie asthma, eczema, hay fever and some food allergies.

Th2 cytokines induce the isotype switching of B-cells to the synthesis of IgE. They also promote the growth, differentiation and release of mast cells and eosinophils from the bone marrow. Eosinophils are directed towards sites of helminth infection and allergy by chemokines, such as eotaxin, which are released by Th-cells. Th2 cytokines also activate eosinophils. In a situation analogous to Th1-biased responses, Th2-biased Th-cells induce a package of biological responses that are characteristic of allergy and helminth infection, namely, high levels of circulating IgE, mastocytosis and tissue eosinophilia.

Summary

The immune system has evolved to combat the constant threat of tissue invasion by microorganisms. If, however, the immune system is directed against innocuous antigens or tissue antigens, the same immune responses that are vital for defence against microorganisms can result in autoimmune disease and allergy. The adaptive immune response is reliant on the properties of B- and T-cells that enable the response to be powerful, flexible and antigen-specific and exhibit immunological memory. B-cells secrete antibodies that are effective against extracellular bacteria and their toxins, whereas CD8 T-cells are adept at neutralizing virally infected cells. CD4 T-cells, also known as Th-cells, do not directly neutralize invading pathogens; instead, they interact with other cells (e.g. macrophages and B-cells) to direct a coordinated, antigen-specific immune response against microorganisms. CD4 Th-cell differentiation can be usefully considered to be either Th1- or Th2-biased. Th1-biased immune responses are characterized by IgG production and macrophage activation; such a response is vital for defence against extra/intracellular bacteria, fungi and some parasites. Conversely, inappropriate Th1-biased immune responses underlie autoimmune diseases. Th2-biased immune responses are characterized by IgE secretion, mastocytosis and eosinophilia, and, although useful in eliminating helminth infestations, such responses underlie the allergic diseases of asthma, eczema and hay fever.

This chapter is an attempt to provide an outline of the immune system; inevitably space constraints have necessitated oversimplification and the omission of some aspects. The major aspects of the immune system have been covered but if readers require further detail, they should consult one of the many readily available large immunological textbooks.

References

Abbas, A.K., Murphy, K.M. and Sher, A. (1996) Functional diversity of helper T lymphocytes. *Nature* 383, 787–793.

Banchereau, J. and Steinman, R.M. (1998) Dendritic cells and the control of immunity. *Nature* 392, 245–252.

Defrance, T., Vanbervliet, B., Briere, F., Durand, I., Rousset, F. and Banchereau, J. (1992) Interleukin-10 and transforming growth factor beta cooperate to induce anti-CD40 activated naive human B-cells to secrete immunoglobulin A. *Journal of Experimental Medicine* 175, 671–682.

Fanning, L.J., Connor, A.M. and Wu, G.E. (1996) Development of the immunoglobulin repertoire. *Clinical Immunology and Immunopathology* 79, 1–14.

Fearon, D.T. and Locksley, R.M. (1996) The instructive role of innate immunity in the acquired immune response. *Science* 272, 50–53.

Fremont, D.H., Rees, W.A. and Kozono, H. (1996) Biophysical studies of T-cell receptors and their ligands. *Current Opinion in Immunology* 8, 93–100.

Germain, R.N. (1994) MHC-dependent antigen processing and peptide presentation: providing ligands for T lymphocyte activation. *Cell* 76, 287–299.

Huston, D.P. (1997) The biology of the immune system. *Journal of the American Medical Association* 278, 1804–1814.

Janeway, C.A. and Bottomly, K. (1994) Signals and signs for lymphocyte responses. *Cell* 76, 275–285.

Lambris, J.D., Reid, K.B.M. and Volanakis, J.E. (1999) The evolution, structure, biology and pathophysiology of complement. *Immunology Today* 20, 207–211.

Mason, D. (1996) The role of B-cells in the programming of T-cells for IL-4 synthesis. *Journal of Experimental Medicine* 183, 717–719.

Medzhitov, R. and Janeway, C.A. (1997) Innate immunity: the virtues of a nonclonal system of recognition. *Cell* 91, 295–298.

Mond, J.J., Lees, A. and Snapper, C.M. (1995) T-cell independent antigens type 2. *Annual Review of Immunology* 13, 655–692.

Mosmann, T.R. and Coffman, R.L. (1989) Th1 and Th2 cells: different patterns of lymphokine secretion lead to different functional properties. *Annual Review of Immunology* 7, 145–173.

Mosmann, T.R. and Sad, S. (1996) The expanding universe of T-cell subsets: Th1, Th2 and more. *Immunology Today* 17, 139–145.

Neuberger, M.S. and Milstein, C. (1995) Somatic hypermutation. *Current Opinion in Immunology* 7, 248–254.

Pene, J., Rousett, F., Briere, F., Bonnefoy, J.Y. and de Vries, J.E. (1988) IgE by normal human lymphocytes is induced by interleukin-4 and suppressed by interferons gamma and alpha and prostaglandin E2. *Proceedings of the National Academy of Sciences of the USA* 85, 6880–6884.

Ricci, M., Matucc, A. and Rossi, O. (1997) Source of IL-4 able to induce the development of TH2 like cells. *Clinical and Experimental Allergy* 27, 488–500.

Stavnezer, J. (1996) Immunoglobulin class switching. *Current Opinion in Immunology* 8, 199–205.

Stout, R. and Bottomly, K. (1989) Antigen-specific activation of effector macrophages by interferon-γ producing (Th1) T-cell clones: failure of IL-4 producing (Th2) T-cell clones to activate effector functions in macrophages. *Journal of Immunology* 142, 760–768.

Trinchieri, G. and Gerosa, F. (1996) Immunoregulation by interleukin-12. *Journal of Leukocyte Biology* 59, 505–511.

2 Evaluation of the Effects of Nutrients on Immune Function

SUSANNA CUNNINGHAM-RUNDLES

Immunology Research Laboratory, Division of Hematology and Oncology, Department of Pediatrics, New York Presbyterian Hospital, Cornell University Weill Medical College, 1300 York Avenue, New York, NY 10021, USA

Introduction and Overview

Nutrients are primary factors in the regulation of the human immune response. Both macronutrients and micronutrients derived from the diet affect immune-system function through actions at several levels in the gastrointestinal tract, thymus, spleen, regional lymph nodes and immune cells of the circulating blood (Chandra, 1997; Cunningham-Rundles and Lin, 1998; Wallace *et al.*, 2000; Cunningham-Rundles, 2001). Effects at one level may be opposed or modified at another level. Thus, the development of an experimental approach capable of revealing critical interactions requires study of more than one aspect of immune function (Cunningham-Rundles, 1993; Muga and Grider, 1999; Beisel, 2000). The effect of any single nutrient is dependent upon concentration, interactions with other key nutrients, host genetic expression and internal environmental conditions. In situations of nutrient imbalance, duration of the altered condition and age of the host are also often critical factors (Cunningham-Rundles and Cervia, 1996; Hirve and Ganatra, 1997; Miles *et al.*, 2001).

Nutrients affect specific immune–cell types differently through influencing intrinsic cell function and by influencing cell–cell interactions. Much of the critical action appears to occur in the local microenvironment during the response to antigen. Classically, the immune system has been considered as an operational duality divided into an innate system, mediating immune reactions that do not functionally change with re-exposure to signal, and an adaptive immune system, which is capable of developing the response to antigen encounter and evolving with re-exposure. Adaptive immunity has been further characterized according to cell type, as the response of bone-marrow-derived B-cells of the humoral immune system and thymus-derived T-cells of the cellular immune system. This rather static picture of compartmentalized function is changing. Now, it is increasingly clear that significant T-cell differentiation does occur independently of the thymus – for example, in the gastrointestinal tract. Current studies also show that the innate immune system, mediated by such cells as natural killer (NK) and NK T-cells, monocytes and dendritic cells, influences the nature of cytokine production by the adaptive immune system. This occurs through secretion of cytokines by innate immune cells into the microenvironment (Doherty *et al.*, 1999; Garcia *et al.*, 1999; see also Devereux, Chapter 1, this volume). The effect of the microenvironment is to drive the immune response towards either a T-helper type 1 (Th1) or a T-helper type 2 (Th2) response (see Devereux, Chapter 1, this volume). Micronutrients, such as trace elements and vitamins, are present in the local environment and have important regulatory effects on adaptive immune-cell function. For example, the trace element zinc supports a Th1 response, whereas vitamin A appears to produce a Th2 response (Frankenburg *et al.*, 1998; Shankar and Prasad, 1998). Thus the new immunology provides a more fluid representation of a potentially evolving process that presents as a defined pattern according to an environmental dynamic rather than a static programme that is derived from fixed cellular characteristics. The basic elements are shown in Fig. 2.1.

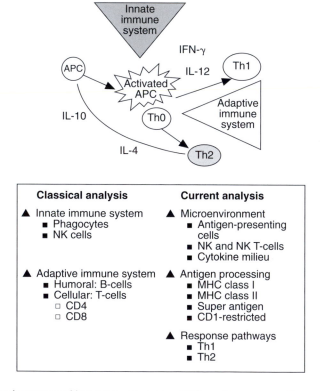

Fig. 2.1. Microenvironment of immune response. APC, antigen-presenting cell; IFN-γ, interferon-γ; IL, interleukin; MHC, major histocompatibility complex.

Age of the host or developmental stage is often a critical variable. Antigen-specific humoral and cellular immunity are central to the adaptive immune response generated in the adult host. In contrast, neonates and infants rely primarily on innate immunity, specifically complement, maternal antibody, circulating mediators of the inflammatory response and phagocytes (see Brandtzaeg, Chapter 14, this volume). However, many of the components of innate immunity are not as functional in young children as in adults (Insoft *et al.*, 1996; see also Chapter 14). Encounters with potential pathogens, such as parasitic infections or viruses, may easily compromise these resources. Study of this permits a glimpse of how the naive immune system copes with the sudden influx of signals, new antigens and potential pathogens. When malnutrition is present, the overall development and expression of the immune response are significantly impaired (Cunningham-Rundles *et al.*, 2000, 2002; see Chandra, Chapter 3, this volume). Similarly, the ageing process affects nutrient needs and the immune response in an interactive fashion. The effect of ageing on the response to immunization and the enhancing effects of micronutrients are well known (Lesourd, 1997; Pallast *et al.*, 1999; see Lesourd *et al.*, Chapter 17, this volume). In addition, there are fundamental age-related changes, which may reflect inflammatory processes (see Chapter 17), such as the report that plasma levels of certain adhesion molecules increase with age and appear to influence the impact of dietary fish oil supplementation (Miles *et al.*, 2001).

Assessment of how nutrients may interact in human immune function is a complex undertaking, more difficult than the assay of the response to a specific antigen of interest – for example, the serological antibody response to a virus. In the latter case, it is usually possible to know what level of response correlates with protection. Because of the great specificity and sensitivity of this information, some of the best data regarding nutrient interaction with the human immune system have been based on the use of response to specific pathogens as the point of reference. However, extrapolation from specific settings may be hazardous. It is seldom clear that immune deficiencies *in vitro* will predict immune deficiency *in vivo*. Therefore, investigators often seek to strengthen inferences by inclusion of *in vivo* tests, such as delayed-type hypersensitivity measured by skin testing, and by assessment of the humoral immune response through assay of specific antibodies arising in response to primary or secondary (booster) immunization. Consistency of an altered immune response in the absence of acute clinical presentation continues to serve as the benchmark indicator of a putative intrinsic immune defect. By analogy, repeated studies in the absence of the acute clinical process are crucial for the study of immune changes secondary to chronic malnutrition.

General assessment of the anatomy of the immune system in humans includes measurement of serum immunoglobulins and complement and the evaluation of lymphocyte subsets by immunophenotyping. Analytical studies require selection among a wide range of tests that measure immune function *in vitro* or *ex vivo* as a reflection of the immune response *in vivo* (Kramer and Burri, 1997; Jaye *et al.*, 1998; Cunningham-Rundles, 1999; Bergquist *et al.*, 2000). A basic panel of tests is also required to reveal how the overall balance of the immune system has been affected. Immune studies are often based on limited studies of immune-cell subsets, serum or plasma concentrations of cytokines or the functional response of mononuclear cells cultured in highly standardized systems, using a chosen stimulus and often a single end-point. Newer methods have made it possible to assess differentiation in antigen expression on peripheral-blood mononuclear cells in response to activation, to study early events in the activation pathway and to analyse gene activation.

The development of cytokine biology has provided a critical means of clarifying the fundamental impact of nutrients on immune response. In general, nutrients appear to affect the immune system most profoundly through regulatory mechanisms affecting the expression and production of cytokines (e.g. Savendahl and Underwood, 1997; Rink and Kirchner, 2000). Since the type of cytokine pattern produced is crucial for the response to infectious pathogens, serious nutrient imbalance will ultimately compromise the development of the future immune response. However, while malnutrition promotes susceptibility to pathogens, even subclinical infections directly affect nutrient intake and metabolism. Severe, acute infection will have a very strong impact. The fact that cytokine production during the acute-phase response to generalized sepsis can lead to loss of lean tissue and body fat is well known (Lin *et al.*, 1998). Interestingly, this cascade of events can be altered by nutritional intervention (Jeevanandam *et al.*, 1999). Immune deficiency and susceptibility to infection are often directly linked with malnutrition, which was the leading cause of acquired immune deficiency before the appearance of the human immunodeficiency virus (HIV). Malnutrition is also a major factor contributing to the progression of HIV infection, especially in less developed countries. Since malnutrition and HIV affect the host in similar ways, the combination is particularly devastating. Many of the infections observed in human protein–energy malnutrition (PEM), such as tuberculosis, herpes, *Pneumocystis carinii* pneumonia and measles, are caused by intracellular pathogens, indicating that the cellular immune system is particularly affected (Keusch, 1993; see Chandra, Chapter 3, this volume).

While the effects of infection and malnutrition on the immune response are interactive, the effects of each upon immune response are also independent. A recent examination by Mishra *et al.* (1998) of graded PEM in children in relationship to tuberculosis infection and response to a skin-test anergy panel, including purified protein derivative of *M. tuberculosis* (PPD), has shown that impaired cellular immunity was observable in all grades of malnutrition, except for response to PPD in grade I, and that infection did not affect this.

Differentiation of lymphocyte subpopulations is also directly affected by malnutrition. Studies show that T-cells from children with severe PEM are immature, compared with those from well-nourished children, and that the degree of immaturity is directly associated with thymic involution, as measured by echo radiography (Parent *et al.*, 1994). While nutritional repletion affected anthropometric measures within 1 month, regrowth of the thymus took longer (Chevalier *et al.*, 1996, 1998). The long-term consequences of slow thymic regrowth are unknown. These studies underscore the importance of longitudinal studies.

Response to certain pathogens may actually be enhanced in some states of malnutrition. Genton *et al.* (1998) assessed the incidence of malaria in children in Papua New Guinea, and found that increased height-for-weight at baseline (an indicator of a better nutritional state) predicted susceptibility to malaria during the year of study and that the lymphocyte response to malarial antigens was lower among the less wasted children. Furthermore, cytokine production towards malarial antigens was greater among malnourished children, suggesting that a favourable cytokine regulatory shift might be the basis of improved response among stunted, but not wasted, children. Stunting has often been considered as an adaptive and partially protective host response to prolonged nutrient deprivation. Rikimaru *et al.* (1998) evaluated lymphocyte subpopulations and immunoglobulins among healthy children and children with kwashiorkor, marasmus and marasmic kwashiorkor in Ghana. Interestingly, immunoglobulin A (IgA) and C4 were higher, whereas C3 and relative B-cell percentage were lower, in the severely malnourished groups. These studies demonstrate the advantages of using linked measurements to develop a full immunological profile.

In summary, the study of nutrient immune interaction requires consideration of the setting and a design that includes evaluation of possible complementary effects at more than one level. Longitudinal studies are often useful and permit assessment of the evolution of the immune response and characterization of downstream effects, which may modulate outcome.

Evaluation of Human Immune Response

Until recently, methods for evaluating the human immune system were derived largely from experimental approaches designed to analyse deficits in host defence in specific clinical settings. With the advent of molecular approaches, immune function has been studied more directly and has led to clarification of specific pathways. As a result, the molecular basis of primary and acquired immune deficiency syndromes is better understood. In addition, the development of vaccines and the study of the natural response to infectious exposure have expanded exponentially in the wake of the HIV crisis, leading to the development of increasingly targeted methods of measuring the immune response. While assessment of the humoral immune response at the level of specific antibody is now well standardized and often routine, evaluation of the complex interactions that are needed to produce specific antibody and the idiotypic interactions that govern this remains a specialized research endeavour. The study of the cellular immune response as a whole continues to remain largely a research activity, although this is beginning to change. This discussion will focus on methods that have been applied to the study of nutrients, and will include approaches that have led to new discoveries in other areas.

The most widely applied methods of evaluating T lymphocyte activation have used peripheral-blood mononuclear cells, isolated by density-gradient centrifugation and cultured with plant lectins (mitogens), or bacterial or viral activators, or antigens, which elicit a secondary response that depends upon prior priming or natural exposure *in vitro* (Paxton *et al.*, 2001). The typical mononuclear-cell culture contains a mixture of T-cells, B-cells and monocytes. After several days in culture, the cells are pulse-labelled with a radioactive precursor (usually thymidine), and incorporation is measured by assessing incorporation into DNA. The amount of incorporated tracer is closely related to the amount of DNA synthesis and ensuing cell division. The use of whole blood diluted and cultured in the presence of activators also provides an index of mononuclear-cell response but is fundamentally different, since the concentration of cells is not standardized, as it is when mononuclear cells are isolated from whole blood. However, the advantage of this kind of *ex vivo* test is that plasma proteins and soluble factors present in blood are not removed (Sottong *et al.*, 2000). Further, the interrelationships among cell types are preserved.

The development of monoclonal antibodies directed against cell-surface determinants has evolved from the detection of lymphocyte-subset differentiation antigens defining T-cells, B-cells and NK cells to the elucidation of critical receptors, such as cytokine and growth-factor receptors, as well as many molecules involved in the activation, differentiation and dissemination of immune response. These methods are applicable to a wide range of studies (Cunningham-Rundles, 1998). Examples include monoclonal antibodies recognizing intracellular cytokines, adhesion molecules and early surface markers produced in response to antigen. Flow cytometry provides a means of studying lymphocyte-subset activation without resort to the use of radioactive tracers. In the following section, examples from current work will be discussed.

Overall design

Nutrition research offers a very interesting and potentially novel way to study the human immune system, and provides an important counterpart to the study of the immune response in primary or secondary immune deficiency where infection, autoimmunity or malignancy are manifest at clinical presentation. While it is clear that there is substantial variation in the normal immune response, the basis of this difference, whether genetic or environmental, remains to be determined. Fundamental studies are needed to determine how nutrient status may influence the development and expression of host genes involved in the immune response. Bendich (1995) has proposed that tests of immune function should be considered in determining the recommended daily allowance (RDA) of certain nutrients, since the levels of several micronutrients needed to support optimal immune function are often higher than those levels needed to qualify as clinical nutrient deficiency, which are usually defined in association with secondary clinical presentation. While there is good evidence that reduced immune function as measured *in vitro* or *ex vivo* is linked to risk of infection or to the development of tumours *in vivo*, tests of immune function are not specific for specific nutrients. A valid test of the effect of nutrient deficiency on immune function would probably require that repletion be proved to correct the defect induced by depletion. This has been achieved for zinc by Prasad (2000), who has demonstrated that experimental human zinc depletion by dietary means leads to reduced levels of Th1 cytokines.

Evidence that nutrients have direct effects on human host defence has come mainly from clinical observations and field studies in settings of severe or chronic nutrient deficiency. These investigations are often complicated by host environmental factors or by exposure to toxins, carcinogens, pathogens or endemic infection (Blot *et al.*, 1993; Zhang *et al.*, 1995; Giuliano *et al.*, 1997; Dai and Walker, 1999). While many studies have described interesting and potentially critical associations, few have identified causal relationships. No single investigational design is necessarily capable of revealing the causal links that govern these intricate relationships.

The choice of study population is fundamental and this directly affects the kinds of controls that are needed. Laboratory controls are highly informative for internal technical quality if run in parallel with subject studies. In some cases, this can be achieved by using aliquots of frozen cells from the same donor, but this has the disadvantage of not providing information concerning the normal range. Parallel controls should include fresh samples from subjects matched for age, sex and clinical status. Longitudinal studies may be crucial and, in some cases, may enable the use of each subject as his/her own control.

When the study design is observational and a nutrient or immune abnormality is known or suspected, study of other potentially related immune-function variables becomes critical. For example, both Th1 and Th2 cytokines should be measured when a Th1 deficiency is suspected. In the context of intervention studies, reliable data can be obtained using different designs, such as placebo-controlled, double-blind and crossover. Inferences may also be drawn from some single-arm studies with unambiguous and quantifiable endpoints. In some cases, it has been possible to use experimental depletion and repletion of the same study group. In other cases, lingering effects have blurred distinctions. For greater stringency, it may be necessary to include several repletion arms at graded doses and to follow changes for a length of time, since the immune system often shows a transient rebound effect that is not seen at later time points. It is also essential to measure other nutrient levels that are positively or negatively regulated by the nutrient under study.

Experimental approach

Immune activators

Immune activation requires a signal when circulating blood is used as the cell source, since the peripheral-blood lymphocyte is a resting cell. This signal is often a plant lectin, or another signal, such as certain divalent cations, calcium ionophores or surface-reactive molecules, including monoclonal antibodies to CD3, which provide a non-antigenic stimulus that activates T lymphocytes independently of antigenic history. Impaired response to mitogens in human settings of PEM may or may not be accompanied by loss of response to pathogens. Examples include the study of response to PPD in malnourished children at risk of tuberculosis and the effect of stunting on the response to malarial antigens (discussed above). It is well known that infections with even relatively non-pathogenic viruses, such as measles, are often fatal in children with PEM, because measles-virus infection causes a serious but usually transient suppression of the cellular immune response (Schlender *et al.*, 1996; Ito *et al.*, 1997), which, in the malnourished host, may continue to prevent immune clearance. Longitudinal studies are often essential to demonstrate long-term effects, such as the lingering effect of vitamin A deficiency, which increases mortality from infections (West *et al.*, 1999). Current studies suggest that the specificity of the response, defined as a Th1 or Th2 cytokine-pattern, to a specific microbe is critically associated with host defence. Study designs that incorporate antigens that are actually being encountered at the time of study or that focus on the type of cytokine production may therefore provide important and unique information.

Selection of methodology

Good study design is based on the formulation of a clear question that addresses a critical issue. Table 2.1 illustrates how the integration of the study design with a well-chosen methodology can lead to informative results in different areas of research. A balance of human and experimental animal-model studies is presented, since development of this field has depended upon both.

The study of whole foods, fats and certain micronutrients and how these could influence immune function is currently under development. Fundamental observation of human PEM has shown that generalized malnutrition leads to impaired immune response and susceptibility to infection (see Chandra, Chapter 3, this volume). However, direct examination of how dietary intake of any particular nutrient affects the immune response is a complex undertaking. Table 2.1 includes four studies on dietary intake. Labeta *et al.* (2000) addressed the fundamental question of how human milk might activate the neonatal immune system by molecular mimicry through the isolation and sequencing of a relevant polypeptide. Fawzi *et al.* (2000) focused on how a whole food, specifically tomatoes, may protect against morbidity and mortality, an idea that has come from studies implicating antioxidants as improving immune function (see Hughes, Chapter 9, this volume). The relationship held true even with correction for total vitamin A level (Fawzi *et al.*, 2000). The strength of this study is derived from the large scale – more than 28,000 infants studied – and the careful surveys conducted, combined with excellent statistical analysis.

When stress is added to the equation, the nutrient requirements for immune response are further altered, and development of hypotheses often requires more than one approach. For example, there are extensive observations showing that total parenteral nutrition suppresses immune response in the surgical patient and related studies showing that glutamine becomes a conditional essential amino acid during metabolic stress (Calder and Yaqoob, 1999; O'Flaherty and Bouchier-Hayes, 1999; see also Calder and Newsholme, Chapter 6, this volume). These observations have led to the discovery that nutrients provide an essential stimulus for the induction, differentiation and maintenance of the mucosal immune system. Lack of enteral dietary intake

Table 2.1. Experimental approach to nutrient–immune function interaction.

Study	Design	Methods	Findings	Reference
Effect of glutamine on mucosal immunity	Randomized study; groups of rats given food, total parenteral nutrition (TPN) or isocaloric/isonitrogenous TPN with 2% glutamine	Respiratory tract and intestinal washings obtained for IgA and Th2 cytokines measured	TPN decreased IgA, IL-4 and IL-10; supplementation with 2% glutamine enhanced levels of IgA and Th2 cytokines	Kudsk et al. (2000)
Effect of gene for haemochromatosis (HFE) on iron metabolism and immunity	Deletion of HFE α1 and α2 putative ligand-binding domains in vivo	HFE-deficient animals were analysed for a comprehensive set of metabolic and immune parameters	Plasma iron, transferrin saturation and hepatic iron were increased – traceable to augmented duodenal iron absorption; no obvious effect on immune system	Bahram et al. (1999)
Dietary fats and immune response	Mice fed high-fat (saturated, n-6 or n-3) or low-fat diet	Fatty-acid composition, spleen lymphocyte proliferation, Th1 and Th2 cytokine profile of spleen cells measured	Polyunsaturated but not saturated fatty acids decreased Th1 cytokine production; little effect on Th2 cytokines; effect shown at level of mRNA	Wallace et al. (2001)
Innate immunity to bacteria after birth	Identification of bacterial-type pattern in human milk protein	Isolation of human milk polypeptide – studied by mass spectrometry and sequencing	Confirmed protein to be a soluble form of the bacterial pattern-recognition receptor CD14 (sCD14)	Labeta et al. (2000)
Tomato intake and morbidity/mortality	Large-scale longitudinal study of infants in Sudan	Morbidity/mortality from diarrhoeal/respiratory disease and intake of tomatoes during previous 2–3 days	Intake linked to reduced mortality after adjustment for total vitamin A intake, inversely correlated with diarrhoeal incidence, respiratory infection	Fawzi et al. (2000)
Risk of mortality in selenium-deficient HIV+ children	Perinatally exposed children enrolled over a 3-month period studied for 5 years	CD4 cell count and nutritional status were studied; regression models were used to test relationship to survival	Low plasma selenium and CD4+ T-cell number below 200 linked independently with mortality	Campa et al. (1999)

IL4, interleukin; IgA, immunoglobulin A.

impairs mucosal IgA and secretory-component production, the number of IgA-containing cells and the level of IgG and promotes mucosal growth (Heel et al., 1998; Kudsk et al., 2000). Even foods such as indigestible saccharides can have a stimulating effect upon the immune system (Kudoh et al., 1998). The study of Kudsk et al. (2000), included in Table 2.1, has added significantly to this field, showing specific differences among animals fed on laboratory food, by total parenteral nutrition and by parenteral nutrition supplemented with glutamine on the pattern of cytokine and IgA production. Loss of nutrient stimulation led to loss of total lymphocyte number in Peyer's patches, in the intraepithelial layer and in the lamina propria, a reduced CD4+ T-cell to CD8+ T-cell ratio and a reduced intestinal level of IgA (Kudsk et al., 2000). Furthermore, lack of enteral nutrition may signal increased neutrophil recruitment through up-regulation of the intercellular adhesion molecule 1 (ICAM-1), causing increased leucocyte binding in the intestine (Fukatsu et al., 1999). These studies indicate how the immune response during stress may be modulated experimentally by specific amino acids in the diet.

The study of lipids provides great challenges for study design, since incorporation into membranes, as well as direct effects on metabolic pathways, must be considered. There is increasing evidence that increase in fat intake may impair immune function, as well as leading to obesity (Nieman et al., 1996). A relationship between fat intake and cancer risk has been indicated (Risch et al., 1994), but the mechanisms remain unclear. Recent data demonstrate that the fatty-acid composition of cellular membranes can cause immune perturbation. Mechanisms of action include modulation of adhesion-molecule expression (Miles et al., 2000) and are apparently related to specific fatty-acid composition. The activation state of the cell is a determining factor in how fatty acids affect the immune response (Wallace et al., 2000). This topic has been addressed by Wallace et al. (2001) in a thorough study in which mice were fed low-fat diets or high-fat diets, containing either saturated or unsaturated fats. Both n-3 and n-6 polyunsaturated fatty acids were used, permitting distinction of their effects on cytokine production. Data showed that n-3 fatty acids were strongly suppressive of Th1 cytokines (see also Calder and Field, Chapter 4, this volume). This classic feeding study included measurement of fatty-acid incorporation, cytokine secretion and cytokine mRNA production.

Other work has shown how emerging information about the human genome may be used to study basic mechanisms. For example, the discovery of the gene HFE has revealed that the molecular basis of hereditary haemochromatosis, which involves increased iron uptake from the gastrointestinal tract, can be attributed to homozygous inheritance of one mutation (Feder et al., 1998; Gross et al., 1998). HFE regulates the metabolism and distribution of iron by affecting the binding of iron to transferrin, is a major histocompatibility complex (MHC) class I protein and is also non-covalently associated with β_2-microglobulin (β_2m). The significance of this physical association is unclear. Excess iron has been observed in association with loss of CD8+ T lymphocytes in the β_2m-knockout mouse. CD8+ T-cells are also reduced in a subgroup of haemochromatosis patients who show an increased rate of iron loading (Porto et al., 1997). The low-CD8 phenotype is also observed in a subset of patients with transfusion-related iron overload (Cunningham-Rundles *et al.*, 2000). Interestingly, studies in compound mutant mice lacking both HFE and β_2m have shown that more iron was deposited in various tissues than was observed in mice with either mutation alone (Levy *et al.*, 2000). However, studies in genetic-deletion models (e.g. the work of Bahram *et al.*, 1999) indicate that the basis of a putative link between immune function and iron handling remains unresolved.

Good study design is critically important for studies in complex settings, such as HIV infection, where nutrient imbalance is fundamentally linked to infection but hard to study in a clear-cut manner. Weight loss is a common occurrence in general chronic viral illness and, in the case of HIV infection, can evolve into a wasting condition, which may become intractable with failure of antiretroviral therapy. Infection-induced malnutrition, as discussed above, is primarily cytokine-mediated and is associated with the acute-phase response. This is accompanied by multiple effects on metabolism, such as altered fluxes of iron and zinc and loss of nitrogen, potassium, magnesium, phosphate, zinc and vitamins. This process is accompanied by retention of salt and water. Malnutrition may also present during the asymptomatic phase of HIV infection (Niyongabo *et al.*, 1997; Peters *et al.*, 1998). Many studies have shown that micronutrient status is profoundly affected in HIV infection, but the aetiological significance of these changes has been difficult to demonstrate (Cunningham-Rundles, 2000). Therefore, the work of Campa *et al.* (1999), included in Table 2.1, has provided an important advance. Using careful longitudinal studies and good statistical design, this group was able to establish that selenium deficiency in children with acquired immune deficiency syndrome (AIDS) was independently associated with mortality.

Immune assessment

New assay methods have enabled the design of experiments addressing different stages involved in immune-cell activation and the study of effects on signalling pathways, which may then lead to the characterization of causal relationships. Table 2.2 outlines some of the types of methods currently in use. Most investigations begin with a general assessment of how a nutrient or altered nutritional state affects the general parameters of the immune system, immune-cell subsets and function. Measurement of changes in frequency and number of circulating lymphocyte subpopulations in the course of observation or dietary intervention is now accepted as a useful and widely comparable procedure, but attention must be given to the issue of controls This analysis should include standardized performance of immunophenotyping, using correction for purity of the gating region, quantitative recovery of the cell type and positive identification of cellular subsets. For human studies, a complete blood count and differential are needed to quantify effects on absolute numbers of cells. Although there is frequently a limitation on blood to be drawn for nutritional studies, it is essential that the baseline evaluation includes parallel studies providing a complete blood count, haematological analysis of haemoglobin, haematocrit, etc., on an aliquot of the same specimen of blood.

Table 2.2. Assessment of functional immune response.

Assay	Function	Determinant of specificity	Principle	Methods
Early activation event	Response to signal	Signal, identity of responder cell	Biochemical or monoclonal antibody assay or gene activation of responder cell	ATP production Flow-cytometric assay of CD69 up-regulation mRNA
Proliferation: magnitude of cellular response to signal	Cell division	Signal, cell population, culture conditions	Radioisotopic tracer incorporation measures DNA synthesis after cell culture with activator; DNA-binding dyes	Microtitre culture Whole blood Mononuclear cells isolated by density gradient Purified cell populations
Cytokine response Cytokine pattern	Specific cytokine Th1/Th2 response to signal	Reagent specificity, identity of producer cell	ELISA and ELISPOT use antibody/antigen; intracellular cytokine use monoclonal antibodies	ELISA: cytokine level ELISPOT can identify secreting-cell frequency Intracellular detection can identify producer cell
Immune-cell subsets	Subpopulation analysis	Monoclonal antibody and accuracy of the gating strategy	Monoclonal antibodies coupled to fluorochromes	Flow cytometry
Antigen-specific cells	Functional response	Specificity depends on signal and detection system	Detection of interferon secretion as enzyme-labelled antibody reaction, specific activation	ELISPOT Flow-cytometric detection of activated cell ATP production by specific cells
Antibody secretion	Antibody-secreting cell	Antigen/antibody – may require antigenic stimulation	Recombinant antigens, monoclonal antibody, limiting-dilution methods	ELISA RIA ELISPOT
Cytotoxicity	Specific and non-specific target-cell killing	Depends upon target and effector cell	Specificity of target-cell killing, relative strength/restriction measured	Chromium release ELISPOT Flow cytometry

ELISA, enzyme-linked immunosorbent assay; ELISPOT, enzyme linked immune spot; RIA, radioimmune assay.

In addition to assessment of relative percentages of T-cells, B-cells and NK cells, immunophenotyping for activation-antigen expression (e.g. CD69), coexpression of critical molecules involved in cell–cell interaction (e.g. CD28), T-cell receptor (TCR) changes and percentages of naive and memory cells may be informative. Functional studies should be carried out on fresh anticoagulated blood whenever possible (or blood stored at room temperature in the dark for under 24 h) before mononuclear cells are isolated. When blood is being sent by air or transported to a distant laboratory, it is extremely important to include a control specimen drawn in parallel to serve as an internal standard for the shipping process. In addition, the type of tube chosen to draw the blood is important. Lithium heparin- or ethylenediamine tetra-acetic acid (EDTA)-containing tubes cannot be used for functional studies. Sodium heparin (preservative-free) or acid citrate dextrose (ACD) tubes should be used and consistency of tube type is important. There may be differences between venous and arterial blood. The question of when the blood should be drawn is important. In general, most data have been obtained with blood drawn in the morning and there are circadian effects on hormones and immune-cell phenotypes that may influence results. When this cannot be done, it is helpful to continue to maintain a uniformity of drawing time for an individual subject or group. Concurrent control blood must be drawn to ensure that technical performance standards are met. It is important that positive and negative (normal range and abnormal range) controls be included. Double-baseline studies – as a minimum, before and after intervention is undertaken – are recommended.

Studies of immune function usually start with a general assessment of mononuclear response *in vitro* to a mitogen, to another non-specific activator or to antigen, as discussed above. These methods are generally based on assay of cell division at the peak of response following microtitre plate culture for several days. Culture methods profoundly affect results, and conditions need to be optimized according to the kinetics of the response. Responses measured under most conditions favour T-cell proliferation, as the T-cell is the most prevalent lymphocyte in peripheral blood. The elicited composite response is highly quantitative when radioactive tracers – usually thymidine – are used. Recently, whole-blood methodology has been introduced as an alternative *ex vivo* method that can reflect potential response *in vivo* (Sottong *et al.*, 2000); this method correlates with the level of DNA synthesis found when isolated mononuclear cells are cultured under optimal standard conditions. Comparative studies have also shown that there is a significant correlation between the whole-blood method and isolated mononuclear cells for cytokine production (Yaqoob *et al.*, 1999). Some laboratories have replaced thymidine incorporation assays with a combination of cell-surface marker-induction assays and a measurement of the percentage of cells in various phases of the cell cycle following activation. Dyes have been developed that stably integrate into the membranes of live lymphocytes, such that, with each successive division, the amount of dye per cell is decreased. Fluorescence can be used to measure the number of cell divisions. Other assays based on whole blood measure early responses of cells selected through adherence to magnetic beads to which monoclonal antibodies recognizing cells of particular interest are attached. Assessment is achieved by an assay of adenosine triphosphate (ATP) production by the luciferin/luciferase reaction (Sottong et al., 2000). Assays such as this may provide accurate assessment of in vivo response in vitro. This method may be combined with a quantitative measure of specific lymphocyte subsets by flow cytometry for examination of response per cell.

Other approaches use measurement of cytokine response, receptor up-regulation or activation antigen to assess initial immune response, rather than the secondary response of cells recruited in the amplified reaction. Also, in vivo regulation of the immune response can be assessed through evaluation of unstimulated levels of secreted products when the producer-cell source of these products and normal levels are known. Methods measuring early events in T lymphocyte activation may or may not correlate with cell division, since cell division is only one aspect of the immune response. One of the earliest events that occurs following T-cell activation is the rapid increase in intracellular free calcium. This is followed by a change in pH and changes in the membrane potential. All of these effects can be measured by flow cytometry, using functional probes. Following T-cell activation via CD3/TCR or via CD2 (the alternate T-cell activation pathway), the first measurable surface marker induced is CD69. This marker is a disulphide-linked homodimer that is present on 20–30% of normal thymocytes, but which is not expressed on resting peripheral-blood lymphocytes. CD69 reaches peak levels within 18–24 h and declines if the stimulus is removed. Using flow cytometry, it is possible to measure increase in CD69 expression on specific lymphocyte subsets. It is apparent that CD69 induction is not part of the pathway leading to cell division, as induction of CD69 can occur without subsequent cell proliferation. A good way to measure CD69 expression is to consider the relative expression of this marker on the subpopulation of interest, as this removes the confounding effect of subpopulation size. Other cell-surface markers appear on activated T-cells at variable times following activation, including CD25 (the α chain of the interleukin-2 (IL-2) receptor) and the transferrin receptor CD71 (both within 24–48 h) and human leucocyte antigen (HLA)-DR (after 48 h).

Finally, statistical evaluation is crucial to all of the studies described here. This includes evaluation of both the internal and the study-group controls. Studies of certain types may be suitable for the collection and banking of specimens prior to assay, such as cytokine supernatants. This may be helpful in giving a homogeneous data set with a low coefficient of variation, as long as controls and experimental specimens are run simultaneously. Good design is often based on internal cross-checks, which can be developed from the working hypothesis and which allow for different elements in the same pathway to be considered.

In summary, the emerging field of nutritional immunology has benefited from the evolution of cellular and molecular immunology. New approaches have provided a strong foundation for experimental design and offer a choice of analytical methods for approaching hypothesis testing. The key to any specific investigation is the identification of clear questions and the choice of relevant and practical methods. These methods then need to be tested in a pilot study, before launching the investigation. The use of an integrated design, including biostatistical considerations and complementary assays, is important in the development of meaningful data and of critical knowledge.

References

Bahram, S., Gilfillan, S., Kuhn, L., Moret, R., Schulze, J., Lebeau, A. and Schumann, K. (1999) Experimental hemochromatosis due to MHC class I HFE deficiency: immune status and iron metabolism. *Proceedings of the National Academy of Sciences of the USA* 23, 13312–13317.

Beisel, W.R. (2000) Interactions between nutrition and infection. In: Strickland, G.T. (ed.) *Hunter's Tropical Medicine and Emerging Infectious Diseases*, 8th edn. W.B. Saunders, Philadelphia, pp. 967–968.

Bendich, A. (1995) Immunology functions to assess nutrient requirements. *Journal of Nutritional Immunology* 3, 47–56.

Bergquist, C., Mattsson-Rydberg, A., Lonroth, H. and Svennerholm, A. (2000) Development of a new method for the determination of immune responses in the human stomach. *Journal of Immunological Methods* 234, 51–59.

Blot, W.J., Li, J.Y., Taylor, P.R., Guo, W., Dawsey, S., Wang, G.Q., Yang, C.S., Zheng, S.F., Gail, M., Li, G.Y., Yu, Y., Liu, B., Tangrea, J., Sun, Y., Liu, F., Fraumeni, J.F., Jr, Zhang, Y.H. and Li, B. (1993) Nutrition intervention trials in Linxian, China: supplementation with specific vitamin/mineral combinations, cancer incidence, and disease specific mortality in the general population. *Journal of the National Cancer Institute* 85,1483–1491.

Calder, P.C. and Yaqoob, P. (1999) Glutamine and the immune system. *Amino Acids* 17, 227–241.

Campa, A., Shor-Posner, G., Indacochea, F., Zhang, G., Lai, H., Asthana, D., Scott, G.B. and Baum, M.K. (1999) Mortality risk in selenium-deficient HIV-positive children. *Journal of Acquired Immune Deficiency Syndrome and Human Retrovirology* 20, 508–513.

Chandra, R.K. (1997) Nutrition and the immune system: an introduction. *American Journal of Clinical Nutrition* 66, S460–S463.

Chevalier, P., Sevilla, R., Zalles, L., Sejas, E., Belmonte, G., Parent, G. and Jambon, B. (1996) Immuno-nutritional recovery of children with severe malnutrition. *Santé* 6, 201–208.

Chevalier, P., Sevilla, R., Sejas, E., Zalles, L., Belmonte, G. and Parent, G. (1998) Immune recovery of malnourished children takes longer than nutritional recovery: implications for treatment and discharge. *Journal of Tropical Pediatrics* 44, 304–307.

Cunningham-Rundles, S. (ed.) (1993) *Nutrient Modulation of Immune Response.* Marcel Dekker, New York.

Cunningham-Rundles, S. (1998) Analytical methods for evaluation of nutrient intervention. *Nutrition Reviews* 56, S27-S37.

Cunningham-Rundles, S. (1999) Issues in assessment of human immune function. In: *Military Strategies for Sustainment of Nutrition and Immune Function in the Field.* Institute of Medicine, National Academy Press, Washington, DC, pp. 235–248.

Cunningham-Rundles, S. (2000) Trace elements and minerals in HIV infection and AIDS: implications for host defence. In: Bogden, J.D. and Kelvay, L.M. (eds) *The Clinical Nutrition of the Essential Trace Elements and Minerals.* Humana Press, Washington, DC, pp. 333–351.

Cunningham-Rundles, S. (2001) Nutrition and the mucosal immune system. *Current Opinion in Gastroenterology* 17, 171–176.

Cunningham-Rundles, S. and Cervia, J.S. (1996) Malnutrition and host defense. In: Walker, W.A. and Watkins, J.B. (eds) *Nutrition in Pediatrics: Basic Science and Clinical Application*, 2nd edn. B.C. Decker, Hamilton, Ontario, pp. 295–307.

Cunningham-Rundles, S. and Lin, D.H. (1998) Nutrition and the immune system of the gut. *Journal of Nutrition* 14, 573–579.

Cunningham-Rundles, S., Giardina, P., Grady, R., Califano, C., McKenzie, P. and DeSousa, M. (2000) Immune response in iron overload: implications for host defence. *Journal of Infectious Disease* 182, s115–s121.

Cunningham-Rundles, S., McNeely, D. and Ananworanich, J. (2002) Immune response in malnutrition. In: Stiehm, E.R., Ochs, H.D. and Winkelsten, J.A. (eds) *Immunologic Disorders in Infants and Children*, 5th edn. W.B. Saunders, Philadelphia (in press).

Dai, D. and Walker, W.A. (1999) Protective nutrients and bacterial colonization in the immature human gut. *Advances in Pediatrics* 46, 353–382.

Doherty, D.G., Norris, S., Madrigal-Estebas, L., McEntee, G., Traynor, O., Hegarty, J.E. and O'Farrelly, C. (1999) The human liver contains multiple populations of NK cells, T-cells, and CD3+CD56+ natural T-cells with distinct cytotoxic activities and Th1, Th2, and Th0 cytokine secretion patterns. *Journal of Immunology* 15 (163), 2314–2321.

Fawzi, W., Herrera, M.G. and Nestel, P. (2000) Tomato intake in relation to mortality and morbidity among Sudanese children. *Journal of Nutrition* 130, 2537–2542.

Feder, J.N., Penny, D.M., Irrinki, A., Lee, V.K., Lebron, J.A., Watson, N., Tsuchihashi, Z., Sigal, E., Bjorkman, P.J. and Schatzman, R.C. (1998) The hemochromatosis gene product complexes with the transferrin receptor and lowers its affinity for ligand binding. *Proceedings of the National Academy of Sciences of the USA* 95, 1472–1477.

Frankenburg, S., Wang, X. and Milner, Y. (1998) Vitamin A inhibits cytokines produced by type 1 lymphocytes *in vitro*. *Cellular Immunology* 185, 75–81.

Fukatsu, K., Lundberg, A.H., Hanna, M.K., Wu, Y., Wilcox, H.G., Granger, D.N., Gaber, A.O. and Kudsk, K.A. (1999) Route of nutrition influences intercellular adhesion molecule-1 expression and neutrophil accumulation in intestine. *Archives of Surgery* 134, 1055–1060.

Garcia, V.E., Uyemura, K., Sieling, P.A., Ochoa, M.T., Morita, C.T., Okamura, H., Kurimoto, M., Rea, T.H. and Modlin, R.L. (1999) IL-18 promotes type 1 cytokine production from NK cells and T-cells in human intracellular infection. *Journal of Immunology* 15 (162), 6114–6121.

Genton, B., Al-Yaman, F., Ginny, M., Taraika, J. and Alpers, M.P. (1998) Relation of anthropometry to malaria morbidity and immunity in Papua New Guinean children. *American Journal of Clinical Nutrition* 68, 734–741.

Giuliano, A.R., Papenfuss, M., Nour, M., Canfield, L.M., Schneider, A. and Hatch, K. (1997) Antioxidant nutrients: associations with persistent human papillomavirus infection. *Cancer Epidemiology Biomarkers and Prevention* 6, 917–923.

Gross, C.N., Irrinki, A., Feder, J.N. and Enns, C.A. (1998) Co-trafficking of HFE, a non-classical major histocompatibility complex class I protein, with the transferrin receptor implies a role in intracellular iron regulation. *Journal of Biological Chemistry* 21, 22068–22074.

Heel, K.A., Kong, S.E., McCauley, R.D., Erber, W.N. and Hall, J. (1998) The effect of minimum luminal nutrition on mucosal cellularity and immunity of the gut. *Journal of Gastroenterology and Hepatology* 10, 1015–1019.

Hirve, S. and Ganatra, B. (1997) A prospective cohort study on the survival experience of under five children in rural western India. *Indian Pediatrics* 34, 995–1001.

Insoft, R.M., Sanderson, I.R. and Walker, W.A. (1996) Development of immune function in the intestine and its role in neonatal diseases. *Pediatric Clinics of North America* 43, 551–571.

Ito, M., Watanabe, M., Kamiya, H. and Sakurai, M. (1997) Changes in intracellular cytokine levels in lymphocytes induced by measles virus. *Clinical Immunology and Immunopathology* 83, 281–286.

Jaye, A., Magnusen, A.F., Sadiq, A.D., Corrah, T. and Whittle, H.C. (1998) *Ex vivo* analysis of cytotoxic T lymphocytes to measles antigens during infection and after vaccination in Gambian children. *Journal of Clinical Investigation* 102, 1969–1977.

Jeevanandam, M., Shahbazian, L.M. and Petersen, S.R. (1999) Proinflammatory cytokine production by mitogen-stimulated peripheral blood mononuclear cells (PBMCs) in trauma patients fed immune-enhancing enteral diets. *Nutrition* 15, 842–847.

Keusch, G.T. (1993) Malnutrition and the thymus gland. In: Cunningham-Rundles, S. (ed.) *Nutrient Modulation of Immune Response.* Marcel Dekker, New York, pp. 283–299.

Kramer, T.R. and Burri, B.J. (1997) Modulated mitogenic proliferative responsiveness of lymphocytes in whole-blood cultures after a low-carotene diet and mixed-carotenoid supplementation in women. *American Journal of Clinical Nutrition* 65, 871–875.

Kudoh, K., Shimizu, J., Wada, M., Takita, T., Kanke, Y. and Innami, S. (1998) Effect of indigestible saccharides on B lymphocyte response of intestinal mucosa and cecal fermentation in rats. *Journal of Nutritional Science and Vitaminology* 44, 103–112.

Kudsk, K.A., Wu, Y., Fukatsu, K., Zarzaur, B.L., Johnson, C.D., Wang, R. and Hanna, M.K. (2000) Glutamine-enriched total parenteral nutrition maintains intestinal interleukin-4 and mucosal immunoglobulin A levels. *Journal of Parenteral and Enteral Nutrition* 24, 270–274.

Labeta, M.O., Vidal, K., Nores, J.E., Arias, M., Vita, N., Morgan, B.P., Guillemot, J.C., Loyaux, D., Ferrara, P., Schmid, D., Affolter, M., Borysiewicz, L.K., Donnet-Hughes, A. and Schiffrin, E.J. (2000) Innate recognition of bacteria in human milk is mediated by a milk-derived highly expressed pattern recognition receptor, soluble CD14. *Journal of Experimental Medicine* 191, 1807–1812.

Lesourd, B.M. (1997) Nutrition and immunity in the elderly: modification of immune responses with nutritional treatments. *American Journal of Clinical Nutrition* 66, 478S-484S.

Levy, J.E., Montross, L.K. and Andrews, N.C. (2000) Genes that modify the hemochromatosis phenotype in mice. *Journal of Clinical Investigation* 105, 1209–1216.

Lin, E., Kotani, J.G. and Lowry, S.F. (1998) Nutritional modulation of immunity and the inflammatory response. *Nutrition* 14, 545–550.

Miles, E.A., Wallace, F.A. and Calder, P.C. (2000) Dietary fish oil reduces intercellular adhesion molecule 1 and scavenger receptor expression on murine macrophages. *Atherosclerosis* 152, 43–50.

Miles, E.A., Thies, F., Wallace, F.A., Powell, J.R., Hurst, T.L., Newsholme, E.A. and Calder, P.C. (2001) Influence of age and dietary fish oil on plasma soluble adhesion molecule concentrations. *Clinical Science* 100, 91–100.

Mishra, O.P., Agrawal, S., Ali, Z. and Usha (1998) Adenosine deaminase activity in protein–energy malnutrition. *Acta Paediatrica* 87, 1116–1119.

Muga, S.J. and Grider, A. (1999) Partial characterization of a human zinc-deficiency syndrome by differential display. *Biological Trace Element Research* 68, 1–12.

Nieman, D.C., Nehlsen-Cannarella, S.I., Henson, D.A., Butterworth, D.E., Fagoaga, O.R., Warren, B.J. and Rainwater, M.K. (1996) Immune response to obesity and moderate weight loss. *International Journal of Obesity and Related Metabolic Disorders* 20, 353–360.

Niyongabo, T., Bouchaud, O., Henzel, D., Melchior, J.C., Samb, B., Dazza, M.C., Ruggeri, C., Begue, J.C., Coulaud, J.P. and Larouze, B. (1997) Nutritional status of

HIV-seropositive subjects in an AIDS clinic in Paris. *European Journal of Clinical Nutrition* 51, 660–664.

O'Flaherty, L. and Bouchier-Hayes, D. (1999) Immunonutrition and surgical practice. *Proceedings of the Nutrition Society* 58, 831–837.

Pallast, E.G., Schouten, E.G., de Waart, F.G., Fonk, H.C., Doekes, G., von Blomberg, B.M. and Kok, F.J. (1999) Effect of 50- and 100-mg vitamin E supplements on cellular immune function in noninstitutionalized elderly persons. *American Journal of Clinical Nutrition* 69, 1273–1281.

Parent, G., Chevalier, P., Zalles, L., Sevilla, R., Bustos, M., Dhenin, J.M. and Jambon, B. (1994) *In vitro* lymphocyte-differentiating effects of thymulin (Zn-FTS) on lymphocyte subpopulations of severely malnourished children. *American Journal of Clinical Nutrition* 60, 274–278.

Paxton, H., Cunningham-Rundles, S. and O'Gorman, M.R.G. (2001) Laboratory evaluation of the cellular immune system. In: Henry, J.B. (ed.) *Clinical Diagnosis and Management by Laboratory Methods*, 20th edn. W.B. Saunders, Philadelphia, pp. 850–877.

Peters, V.B., Rosh, J.R., Mugrditchian, L., Birnbaum, A.H., Benkov, K.J., Hodes, D.S. and Le Leiko, N.S. (1998) Growth failure as the first expression of malnutrition in children with human immunodeficiency virus infection. *Mount Sinai Journal of Medicine* 65, 1–4.

Porto, G., Vicente, C., Teixeira, M.A., Martins, O., Cabeda, J.M., Lacerda, R., Goncalves, C., Fraga, J., Macedo, G., Silva, B.M., Alves, H., Justica, B. and de Sousa, M. (1997) Relative impact of HLA phenotype and CD4–CD8 ratios on the clinical expression of hemochromatosis. *Hepatology* 25, 397–402.

Prasad, A.S. (2000) Effects of zinc deficiency on Th1 and Th2 cytokine shifts. *Journal of Infectious Disease* 182 (Suppl. 1), S62–S68.

Rikimaru, T., Taniguchi, K., Yartey, J.E., Kennedy, D.O. and Nkrumah, F.K. (1998) Humoral and cell-mediated immunity in malnourished children in Ghana. *European Journal of Clinical Nutrition* 52, 344–350.

Rink, L. and Kirchner, H. (2000) Zinc-altered immune function and cytokine production. *Journal of Nutrition* 130, 1407S–1411S.

Risch, H.A., Jain, M., Marrett, L.D. and Howe, G.R. (1994) Dietary fat intake and risk of epithelial ovarian cancer. *Journal of the National Cancer Institute* 86, 1409–1415.

Savendahl, L. and Underwood, L.E. (1997) Decreased interleukin-2 production from cultured peripheral blood mononuclear cells in human acute starvation. *Journal of Clinical Endocrinology and Metabolism* 82, 1177–1180.

Schlender, J., Schnorr, J.J., Spielhoffer, P., Cathomen, T., Cattaneo, R., Billeter, M.A., ter Meulen, V. and Schneider-Schaulies, S. (1996) Interaction of measles virus glycoproteins with the surface of uninfected peripheral blood lymphocytes induces immunosuppression *in vitro*. *Proceedings of the National Academy of Sciences of the USA* 93, 13194–13199.

Shankar, A.H. and Prasad, A.S. (1998) Zinc and immune function: the biological basis of altered resistance to infection. *American Journal of Clinical Nutrition* 68, 447S–463S.

Sottong, P.R., Rosebrock, J.A., Britz, J.A. and Kramer, T.R. (2000) Measurement of T-lymphocyte responses in whole-blood cultures using newly synthesized DNA and ATP. *Clinical and Diagnostic Laboratory Immunology* 7, 307–311.

Wallace, F.A., Miles, E.A. and Calder, P.C. (2000) Activation state alters the effect of dietary fatty acids on pro-inflammatory mediator production by murine macrophages. *Cytokine* 12, 1374–1379.

Wallace, F.A., Miles, E.A., Evans, C., Stock, T.E., Yaqoob, P. and Calder, P.C. (2001) Dietary fatty acids influence the production of Th1- but not Th2-type cytokines. *Journal of Leukocyte Biology* 69, 449–457.

West, K.P., Jr, Katz, J., Khatry, S.K., Le Clerq, S.C., Pradhan, E.K., Shrestha, S.R., Connor, P.B., Dali, S.M., Christian, P., Pokhrel, R.P. and Sommer, A. (1999) Double blind, cluster randomised trial of low dose supplementation with vitamin A or beta carotene on mortality related to pregnancy in Nepal. The NNIPS-2 Study Group. *British Medical Journal* 318, 570–575.

Yaqoob, P., Newsholme, E.A. and Calder, P.C. (1999) Comparison of cytokine production in cultures of whole human blood and purified mononuclear cells. *Cytokine* 11, 600–605.

Zhang, Y.H., Kramer, T.R., Taylor, P.R., Li, J.Y., Blot, W.J., Brown, C.C., Guo, W., Dawsey, S.M. and Li, B. (1995) Possible immunologic involvement of antioxidants in cancer prevention. *American Journal of Clinical Nutrition* 62, 1477S-1482S.

3

Effect of Post-natal Protein Malnutrition and Intrauterine Growth Retardation on Immunity and Risk of Infection

RANJIT KUMAR CHANDRA*

Janeway Child Health Centre, Room 2J740, 300 Prince Philip Drive, St John's, Newfoundland, Canada A1B 3V6

Introduction

In spite of projections and plans announced by both politicians and professionals in the last 25 years, protein–energy malnutrition (PEM) continues to be widely prevalent, particularly in Asia and Africa. This is associated with considerable morbidity due to infectious illness. Work during the last 30 years has demonstrated the important pathogenetic role of impaired immune responses in the two-way interaction between malnutrition and infection. Similarly, intrauterine growth retardation (IUGR) resulting from a variety of maternal and fetal factors is associated with impaired immune responses and enhanced susceptibility to infection. Unlike the reversibility of reduced immunity in post-natal PEM, decreased immunity in small-for-gestational-age (SGA) infants is prolonged and may last for months, even years.

Protein–Energy Malnutrition

The clinical spectrum of PEM is somewhat varied, depending upon the age of occurrence, the concurrent presence of infection and the area of the world where it occurs. The same applies, to some extent, to the immunological effects of PEM.

From a historical perspective, it is useful to cite the clinical stimulus that led to the first comprehensive examination of the immune system in PEM (Chandra, 1972). Interest in nutrition–immune interactions was kindled by the story, with an unhappy ending, of a child. Eighteen-month-old Kamala was thin, her skin pale as wax and her lungs screaming for air. She wore a spectral

*Other affiliations: Memorial University of Newfoundland and World Health Organization Centre for Nutritional Immunology.

© CAB *International* 2002. *Nutrition and Immune Function*
(eds P.C. Calder, C.J. Field and H.S. Gill)

white death-mask in a frame of black hair. Her shrivelled body and swollen legs were typical of marasmic kwashiorkor, and she had an obvious fulminant infection. Lung aspirate revealed the opportunistic organism *Pneumocystis carinii*. Despite our best efforts, we lost the child. We speculated that malnutrition had robbed Kamala of her defences against infection and led to her premature demise. Against this background in 1969, I applied the available techniques to study the immunocompetence of undernourished children. To convey a sense of time, the discipline of immunology did not even involve the general use of terms such as cell-mediated immunity, lymphocyte subsets, immunoregulation and so on. In malnourished patients, we found a number of impaired immune responses, including delayed cutaneous hypersensitivity, lymphocyte-proliferation responses to mitogens, complement activity and secondary antibody responses to some antigens. These findings were soon confirmed by several investigators (Anon., 1987).

Any discussion of the effects of nutritional deficiencies on immune responses must be prefaced by emphasizing the complexities and heterogeneity of both clinical malnutrition and immune responses. The critical role of nutrition in modulation of immune responses is based on physiological considerations. The severity and extent of dysfunction caused by malnutrition in various organ systems depend on several factors, including the rate of cell proliferation, the amount and rate of protein synthesis and the role of individual nutrients in metabolic pathways. Lymphoid tissues are very vulnerable to marked involution as a result of nutritional deficiency. Many cells of the immune system are known to depend for their function on metabolic pathways that employ various nutrients as critical cofactors. Numerous enzymes require micronutrients.

The consistent impairment of immunity in PEM and the recognized increase in infections in patients with primary immunodeficiencies are compatible with the hypothesis that a depressed immune system in malnutrition enhances the risk and severity of infection. The work on children has now been extended to other age-groups and to other parts of the world, including the malnourished groups seen in hospitals and in underprivileged communities in industrialized affluent countries. For example, the cellular immune changes seen in young children with PEM in developing countries are replicated to a large extent in subjects with primary or secondary PEM in industrialized countries, such as those with anorexia nervosa (for a review, see Marcos *et al.*, 2001). It should be pointed out that malnutrition is a complex syndrome where several deficiencies exist simultaneously. Even in laboratory animals deprived of a single nutrient, the functional effects may be the consequence of changes in the absorption or body stores of other substances. Thus, what is observed in an undernourished individual is the sum of the contributions and responses of many components of the immune system that have been altered by one or more nutrient deficiencies.

The interaction between malnutrition and infection is bidirectional: one aggravates the other. Scrimshaw *et al.* (1968) proposed the interesting concept of synergism and antagonism between the host's nutritional status and the microbe's ability to produce disease; the direction of interaction is more often synergistic, namely, PEM increases the incidence, duration and severity of infectious illness.

Longitudinal prospective studies of infants have shown that reduction in various parameters of immunocompetence preceded clinical infection and growth faltering. Findings such as these suggest, first that altered immune responses are early functional indices of growth failure secondary to latent nutritional deficiency and, second, that episodes of infection worsen the child's nutritional state.

PEM has been documented to increase morbidity and mortality caused by diarrhoea and respiratory illness (James, 1972; Tomkins, 1981; Chandra, 1983a). The incidence of infectious diarrhoea is increased and there is a more profound and consistent effect on the duration of each episode. Victora *et al.* (1990) studied the synergism between nutritional status and hospital admissions due to diarrhoea and pneumonia in a cohort of 5914 live births in southern Brazil and found that malnutrition was a more important risk factor for pneumonia than for diarrhoea, whereas diarrhoea was a stronger predictor of malnutrition than was pneumonia, the association being strongest in the first 2 years of life. In rural India, there was a significant correlation between weight-for-height as an index of protein–energy status and risk of death from infectious disease (Chandra, 1983b).

The term 'nutritional thymectomy' has been used to dramatize the extensive reduction in the size and weight of the thymus that occurs with malnutrition (see Chandra and Newberne, 1977). Histologically, there is a loss of corticomedullary differentiation, there are fewer lymphoid cells and the Hassal bodies are enlarged, degenerated and, occasionally, calcified. These changes are easily differentiated from findings in primary immune deficiency, such as DiGeorge's syndrome. In the spleen, there is a loss of lymphoid cells around small blood vessels. In the lymph node, the thymus-dependent paracortical areas show depletion of lymphocytes.

The consistent adverse effects of PEM on cell-mediated immunity, production of cytokines, phagocyte function, the complement system and mucosal immunoglobulin A (IgA) antibody responses have been demonstrated in several studies in many countries. These observations have been reviewed several times (see Chandra and Newberne, 1977; Keusch *et al.*, 1983; Gershwin *et al.*, 1984; Watson, 1984; Chandra, 1992, 1996, 1999; Woodward, 2001).

In PEM, most of the host defence mechanisms are breached (Fig. 3.1). Delayed cutaneous hypersensitivity responses to both recall and new antigens are markedly depressed. It is not uncommon to have complete anergy to a battery of different antigens (Chandra, 1972). These changes are observed in moderate nutrient deficiencies as well (Kielmann *et al.*, 1976; McMurray *et al.*, 1981). Findings in patients with kwashiorkor are more striking compared with those in marasmus. There is a significant correlation between the cumulative diameter of induration response to five common antigens and the serum concentration of albumin, an index of visceral protein synthesis. Similarly, there is a significant correlation between the size of the delayed-hypersensitivity skin-test response and lean body mass (Fig. 3.2). The skin reactions are restored after appropriate nutritional therapy for several weeks or months.

The cellular and molecular reason for impaired skin responses lies in changes in the number and function of T lymphocyte subsets and macrophages

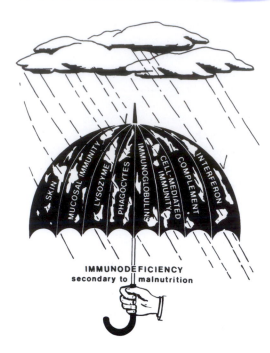

Fig. 3.1. In PEM, most of the host defence mechanisms are breached, allowing microbes to invade and produce clinical infections that are more severe and prolonged (copyright ARTS Biomedical Publishers 1981).

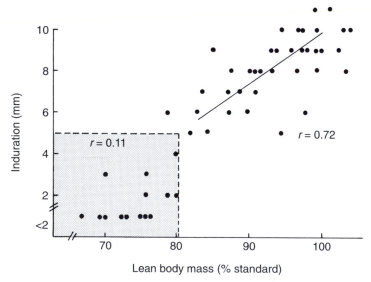

Fig. 3.2. Correlation between the diameter of maximum skin induration, in response to delayed hypersensitivity challenge, and lean body mass. Those with a negative response, defined as induration of less than 5 mm (shaded box), had a lean body mass of 80% of standard for age or less.

and the production of various cytokines. There is a significant reduction in the number of mature, fully differentiated T lymphocytes, which can be recognized by the classical technique of rosette formation or by the newer method of fluorescent labelling with monoclonal antibodies. The reduction in serum thymic-factor activity observed in primary PEM, including in adolescents with anorexia nervosa (Wade *et al.*, 1985), may underlie the impaired maturation of T lymphocytes. There is an increase in deoxynucleotidyl transferase activity in leucocytes (Chandra, 1983a), a feature of immaturity. The proportion of helper/inducer T lymphocytes, recognized by the presence of CD4+ antigen on the cell surface, is markedly decreased in PEM (Fig. 3.3; Chandra, 1983c). There is a moderate reduction in the number of suppressor/cytotoxic CD8+ cells. Thus the ratio CD4+/CD8+ is significantly decreased compared with that in well-nourished controls.

The proliferative response to mitogens and microbial antigens is decreased. The synthesis of DNA is reduced, especially when autologous patient's plasma is used in cell cultures. This may be the result of the presence of inhibitory factors, as well as deficiency of essential nutrients in the patient's plasma (Beatty and Dowdle, 1978). Another aspect of lymphocyte function that changes in PEM is the traffic and 'homing' pattern (Chandra, 1991a). For example, lymphocytes derived from mesenteric lymph nodes of immunized rodents normally revert back to the intestine in large numbers, whereas in malnutrition this homing is reduced.

Co-culture experiments have shown a reduction in the number of antibody-producing cells in malnutrition (Fig. 3.4) and in the amount of immunoglobulin secreted (Chandra, 1983c). These observations may reflect the amount of 'help' provided by T-cells, since the impairment is reversed when T-cells are derived from well-nourished controls.

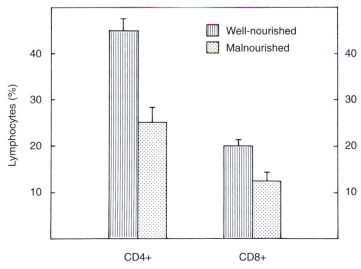

Fig. 3.3. The proportion of T lymphocyte subsets in children with PEM and well-nourished controls matched for age and gender. The CD4/CD8 ratio is decreased.

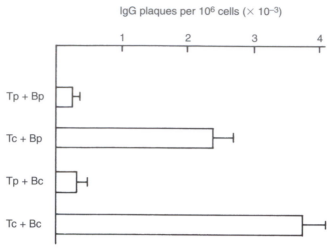

IgG plaques per 10^6 cells ($\times$ 10^{-3})

Fig. 3.4. Number of immunoglobulin (IgG)-producing cells in co-cultures of T and B lymphocytes. T lymphocytes (T) and B lymphocytes (B) from children with PEM (p) or well-nourished controls (c) were co-cultured and stimulated with pokeweed mitogen. IgG-forming cells were identified by rosetting with sheep red blood cells. (Data are from Chandra, 1983b.)

Serum antibody responses are generally intact in PEM, particularly when antigens are administered with an adjuvant or in the case of those materials that do not evoke a T-cell response. Rarely, the antibody response to organisms such as *Salmonella typhi* and influenza virus (Fig. 3.5) may be decreased. However, before an impaired antibody response can be attributed to nutritional deficiency, infection as a confounding factor must be ruled out. Antibody affinity is decreased in patients who are malnourished (Fig. 3.5; Chandra *et al.*, 1984). This may provide an explanation for a higher frequency of antigen–antibody complexes found in such patients. As opposed to serum antibody responses, secretory IgA antibody levels after deliberate immunization with viral vaccines are decreased (Chandra, 1975a); there is a selective reduction in secretory IgA levels. This may have several clinical implications, including the increased frequency of septicaemia commonly observed in undernourished children.

The production of several cytokines, particularly interleukin-2 and interferon-γ, is decreased in PEM (Chandra, 1992). Moreover, PEM alters the ability of T lymphocytes to respond appropriately to cytokines (Hoffman-Goetz *et al.*, 1984).

Phagocytic function is deranged in PEM. Chemotactic migration of phagocytes is slower and less efficient (Chandra *et al.*, 1976). In the presence of control serum that provides the normal concentrations and activity of various opsonins, phagocytes are able to ingest particles such as bacteria (Seth and Chandra, 1972). However, the next steps of metabolic activation – discharge of digestive enzymes into phagolysosomes, and microbial killing – are reduced (Seth and Chandra, 1972).

Many components of the complement system are reduced in concentration and activity in PEM (Chandra, 1975b; Haller *et al.*, 1978). The most affected are complement C3, C5 and factor B. Total haemolytic activity is decreased. These changes affect the opsonic activity that facilitates phagocytosis.

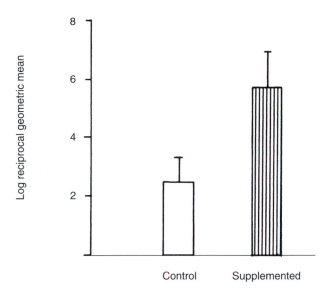

Fig. 3.5. Antibody response to influenza virus vaccine in the elderly given a nutritional supplement and in controls on a placebo.

There is very little work on the effect of malnutrition on the integrity of physical barriers, quality of mucus or several other innate immune defences. However, lysozyme levels are decreased, largely as a result of reduced production by monocytes and neutrophils, but also due to increased excretion in the urine (Chandra *et al.*, 1977a). Adherence of bacteria to epithelial cells is a first step before invasion and infection can occur. The number of bacteria adhering to respiratory epithelial cells is increased in PEM (Fig. 3.6; Chandra and Gupta, 1991). Work in laboratory-animal models of PEM has demonstrated a reduction in ciliary movement, particularly in the presence of mucosal infection (Fig. 3.7).

Intrauterine Growth Retardation

There is much clinical evidence that neonates have suboptimal immune responses and are susceptible to infection. When growth retardation and nutritional deficiency complicate the picture, as in low-birth-weight (LBW) infants, impairment of immunocompetence and risk of infection are more marked and longer-lasting (Chandra, 1991b). This results in higher morbidity (Ashworth, 2001; Table 3.1), enhanced occurrence of admission to hospital and increased mortality (Ashworth, 2001; Table 3.2).

The worldwide incidence of LBW, defined as a weight less than 2500 g, varies considerably from one population group to another, from 8% in some industrialized countries to 41% in some developing countries of Africa. In the former, the majority are preterm appropriate for gestational age (AGA), whereas, in the latter, the majority are SGA. The aetiology of fetal growth retardation includes maternal malnutrition.

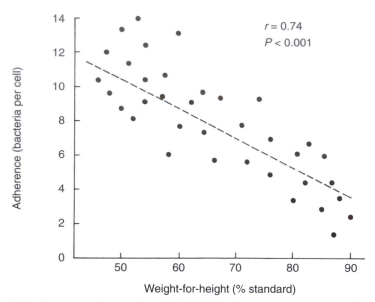

Fig. 3.6. Correlation between the number of *Klebsiella* adhering to tracheal epithelial cells and nutritional status, assessed by weight-for-height.

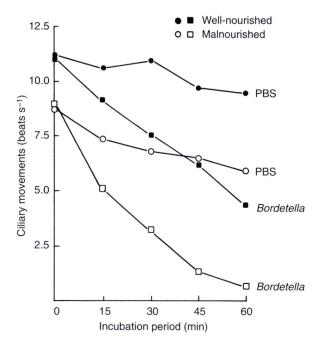

Fig. 3.7. Movement of tracheal-cell cilia in dogs with PEM and well-nourished controls. The experiment was run with phosphate-buffered saline (PBS) and after infection with *Bordetella* sp.

Table 3.1. Low birth weight and risk of mortality.

Country	Design	Gestation	Age (months)	Sample size (deaths)	Birth weight (g)	Risk ratio (95% CI)	Outcome
Brazil	Cohort	Term	0–6	393 (12)	3000–3499	1.0	All causes
					1500–2499	10.2 (2.2–46.7)	
						6.6[a] (1.4–31.2)	
India	Cohort	Term	0–11	4,590 (213)	≥ 2500	1.0	All causes
					2000–2499	2.6	
India	Cohort	Term	0–11	4,220 (362)	≥ 2500	1.0	All causes
					< 2500	1.7	
Guatemala	Cohort	Term	0–11	385 (24)	≥ 2500	1.0	All causes
					< 2500	1.7	
Indonesia	Cohort	Term + preterm	12–47	(39)		1.8	All causes
			0–11	687 (83)	≥ 2500	1.0	
					< 2500	3.4	
Nigeria	Cohort	Term + preterm	0–11	4,334 (133)	> 2500	1.0	All causes
					⩽ 2500	5.8	
Brazil	Cohort	Term + preterm	0–11	5,914 (215)	≥ 2500	1.0	All causes
					< 2500	11.0 (8.7–14.4)	
						6.7 (3.0–14.9)	ARI
						2.5 (0.9–6.7)	Diarrhoea
						2.9 (1.0–8.3)	Other infections
						3.3	All causes
Brazil	Case–control	Term + preterm	12–59	(29)	≥ 2500	1.0	ARI
			0.25–11	1,070 (357)	1500–2499	1.9[a] (1.1–3.6)[b]	
						2.0[a] (1.1–3.6)[b]	Diarrhoea
						5.0[a] (1.3–18.6)[b]	Other infections
						2.3[a] (1.6–3.4)[b]	All infections
India	Cohort	Term + preterm	0–11	659 (19)	≥ 2500	1.0	ARI
					< 2500	8.0	
UK	Cohort	Term + preterm	1–50	5,522 (40)	≥ 2500	1.0	Bronchitis + pneumonia
					< 2500	3.6	
USA	Cohort	Term + preterm	1–11	51,931 (371)	≥ 2500	1.0	Infectious disease
					< 2500	2.4 (1.4–4.0)	
					1500–2499	2.5 (1.3–4.5)	
USA	Cohort	Term + preterm	12–84	(258)	≥ 2500	1.0	Diarrhoea
			1–11	193,733 (93)	< 2500	7.1	

[a] Adjusted for confounders.
[b] 90% confidence intervals.
CI, confidence interval; ARI, acute respiratory infections.
See Ashworth (2001) for references.

Table 3.2. Low birth weight and risk of morbidity.

Country	Design	Gestation	Age (months)	Sample size	Birth weight (g)	Risk ratio (95% CI)	Outcome
Ethiopia	Cohort	Term	3–40	201	≥ 2500 < 2500	1.0 1.5 (1.1–2.1)	All infections
Brazil	Cohort	Term	0–6	393	3000–3499 1500–2499	1.0 1.3[a] (1.1–1.6)	Diarrhoea
India	Cohort	Term	0–3	152	≥ 2500 1500–2499	1.0 2.4 3.6	Diarrhoea ALRI
Guatemala	Cohort	Term	2 days–3 months	267	≥ 2500 < 2500	1.0 3.0	Mostly sepsis and ALRI
Papua New Guinea	Cohort	Term + preterm	0–17 18–35 36–59	400	≥ 2500 < 2500	1.0 1.7[a] (1.4–2.1) 1.4[a] (1.0–1.9) 1.2[a] (0.5–1.8)	Diarrhoea
Brazil	Case–control	Term + preterm	0–23	1300	≥ 2500 2000–2499 < 2000	1.0 1.4 3.2[a] (1.1 to 8.9)	Pneumonia
India	Cohort	Term + preterm	0–11	659	≥ 2500 < 2500	1.0 1.2	ARI
Uruguay	Cohort	Term + preterm	0–35	166	≥ 2500 < 2500	1.0 0.9 (0.7–1.2)	ARI
UK	Cohort	Term + preterm	0–23	690	≥ 2500 2300–2499 2000–2299 < 2000	1.0 1.2 1.6 3.5	ALRI

[a]Adjusted for confounders.
ARI, acute respiratory-tract infection; CI, confidence interval; ALRI, acute lower respiratory-tract infection.
See Ashworth (2001) for references.

LBW is associated with higher mortality. Whereas the total proportion of infants who die or are handicapped is similar in AGA and SGA groups, the former are at a higher risk of death in the immediate post-natal period, whereas the latter are at a higher risk of morbidity in the first year of life (Chandra, 1984). Infection is one of the recognized causes of increased illness in SGA infants. Upper and lower respiratory-tract infections are three times more frequent in SGA infants compared with AGA infants (Chandra, 1984). It appears that the morbidity pattern in the former group shows a bimodal distribution; about two-thirds exhibit a near-normal rate of illness, comparable to that of healthy full-term infants, whereas one-third have an increased illness rate – almost three times that of the full-term infants (Chandra, 1984). The SGA group is also at risk of developing infection with opportunistic microorganisms, such as *P. carinii*, as observed in post-natal malnutrition (Chandra, 1984).

SGA infants show atrophy of the thymus and prolonged impairment of cell-mediated immunity (Chandra, 1975c; Moscatelli *et al.*, 1976). Delayed cutaneous hypersensitivity to a variety of microbial recall antigens, as well as to the strong chemical sensitizer 2,4-dinitrochlorobenzene, is impaired. Serum thymic-factor activity is lower in SGA infants tested at 1 month of age or later. In contrast to AGA LBW infants, who recover immunologically by about 2–3 months of age, SGA infants continue to exhibit impaired cell-mediated immune responses for several months or even years (Chandra *et al.*, 1977b; Chandra, 1980). This is particularly true of those infants whose weight-for-height is less than 80% of standard. The prolonged immunosuppression in some SGA infants correlates with clinical experience of infectious illness (Chandra, 1991b) and thus may have considerable biological significance. In animal models of intrauterine nutritional deficiency, PEM results in reduced immune responses in the offspring (Chandra, 1975d).

Phagocyte function is deranged in LBW infants (Chandra, 1975c). There is a slight reduction in ingestion of particulate matter and a significant reduction in both metabolic activity and bactericidal capacity.

IgG from the mother, acquired through placental transfer, is the principal immunoglobulin in cord blood. The half-life of IgG is 21 days and thus all infants show physiological hypoimmunoglobulinaemia between 3 and 5 months of age. This is pronounced and prolonged in LBW infants (Chandra, 1975c), since their level of IgG at birth is significantly lower compared with that of full-term infants. There is a progressive rise in IgG concentration with gestational age and birth weight, especially in infants below 2500 g. All four subclasses of IgG are detected in fetal sera as early as 16 weeks of gestation, the bulk being IgG_1 (Chandra, 1988). In SGA LBW infants, the cord-blood level of IgG_1 is reduced much more than that of other subclasses (Chandra, 1988). Thus the infant : maternal ratio is significantly low for IgG_1 but not for IgG_2. The number of immunoglobulin-producing cells and the amount of immunoglobulin secreted are decreased in SGA infants who are symptomatic, i.e. those who have recurrent infection (Chandra, 1986). In the second year of life, SGA infants show a marked reduction in IgG_2 levels and often show infections with organisms that have a polysaccharide capsule.

In preterm infants with a birth weight between 1800 and 2200 g, moderate oral zinc supplementation accelerates immunological recovery (Chandra, 1991a). In SGA infants, zinc supplements given from birth to 6 months of age improve immune responses and reduce mortality from diarrhoea and respiratory illness. A micronutrient supplement is more beneficial (Chandra, 2001).

Clinical Application and Intervention Strategies

The interactions between nutrition, the immune system and infection have much clinical and public health significance (Chandra, 1992). The fact that changes in immune responses occur early in the course of nutritional deficiency has led to the suggestion that immunocompetence can be used as a sensitive functional indicator of nutritional status. In patients with obvious primary or secondary malnutrition, the number of T lymphocytes is a useful measure of response to supplementation therapy. Anergy and other immunological changes correlate with poor outcome, in both medical and surgical patients, if impaired immunity is considered in association with hypoalbuminaemia (Chandra, 1983a,b,c). Opportunist infections occur more frequently among those patients with cancer who are also malnourished. The incidence of complicating infections can be reduced if appropriate preventive and therapeutic nutritional management is carried out in patients with leukaemia. It has been postulated that nutritional deficiency may influence the biological gradient and natural history of human immunodeficiency virus (HIV) infection (Jain and Chandra, 1984). Recent surveys indicate that attention to the nutritional needs of the HIV-infected individual is an important part of the overall management of this life-threatening infection (Subcommittee on Nutrition, 2001). Response to immunization is modulated by the nutritional status of the host, and the protective efficacy of vaccines may be suboptimal in the undernourished individual (Chandra, 1972). Finally, immune responses can be used to define safe upper and lower limits of nutrient intake.

We are now able to outline intervention strategies that will reduce the incidence and adverse health impact of both PEM and infection (Chandra, 1992). We have much of the knowledge needed to improve health; this needs to be supported by political commitment and effective management (see also Tomkins, Chapter 18, this volume). The preventive and intervention measures discussed below are well within the combined resources of the world. Even within the health sector, there are glaring anomalies. We must assign priorities and implement methods to prevent and control contributors to morbidity and mortality.

The major intervention strategies and their relative importance in tackling the twin problems of malnutrition and infection are shown in Fig. 3.8. Improvement in socio-economic status and education and ensuring the availability of sufficient food to every individual will most certainly eliminate much of malnutrition and infection, the two diseases of poverty. Health and self-limitation of family size will usually follow these measures. There is a negative correlation between rates of adult female literacy and infant mortality.

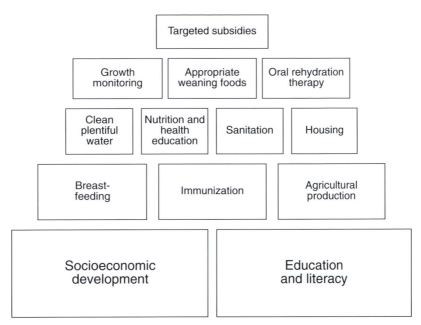

Fig. 3.8. Intervention strategies to deal with the conjugate problem of malnutrition and infection. The importance of each measure is indicated by the size of letters. (Copyright ARTS Biomedical Publishers 1990.)

Promotion of breast-feeding should be continued. The anti-infective prop-erties of human milk are well known and depend in part upon various cellular and soluble factors, as well as its buffering capacity and several antigen-non-specific protective factors (see also Brandtzaeg, Chapter 14, this volume). Secretory IgA antibodies against a variety of common pathogens have been found in human milk and correlate negatively with morbidity due to specific diseases, such as cholera (Chandra, 1992). The protective effect is particularly dramatic in underprivileged communities with poor sanitation, inadequate housing and contaminated food and water. Furthermore, breast-feeding con-tributes to birth spacing, an important factor in both maternal and child health.

More effective immunization programmes against the common communi-cable diseases are required for the majority of the susceptible population. There are still a large number of children in developing countries who die from or are disabled by preventable infectious diseases. Immunization programmes should include universal coverage of all the population at risk. Moreover, there is a need to develop new vaccines, such as those for malaria, *Shigella* and *Pneumococcus*, and to improve the quality of those against typhoid, cholera and tuberculosis. In addition, new methods of vaccine preparation, such as genetic recombination, subunit antigens, synthetic-peptide antigens, anti-idio-types and host-cell receptor-specific vaccines, show great promise. It would be ideal to have a single, stable, efficacious, inexpensive vaccine containing immu-nizing antigens for several infections, which can be given at birth, be easy to administer and have no serious adverse effects.

Other useful preventive measures include the availability of plentiful clean water and improved sanitation and housing. The early and adequate management of diarrhoea and respiratory infections using oral rehydration solution and antibiotics, respectively, has already proved useful and found applicability worldwide. The early detection of growth faltering, using simple weight and height charts, together with subsequent dietary advice, will reduce the prevalence and severity of malnutrition and its adverse consequences. Lastly, targeted subsidies during times of acute need, such as in famines and wars, and massive campaigns to eliminate specific nutrient deficiencies, such as those of vitamin A, iron and iodine, are justified.

References

Anon. (1987) This week's citation classic. *Current Contents* 30, 15.

Ashworth, A. (2001) Low birth weight infants, infection and immunity. In: Suskind, R.M. and Tontisirin, K. (eds) *Nutrition, Immunity and Infection in Infants and Children.* Lippincott Williams and Wilkins, Philadelphia, pp. 121–131.

Beatty, D.W. and Dowdle, E.B. (1978) The effects of kwashiorkor serum on lymphocyte transformation *in vitro*. *Clinical and Experimental Immunology* 32, 134–143.

Chandra, R.K. (1972) Immunocompetence in undernutrition. *Journal of Pediatrics* 81, 1194–1200.

Chandra, R.K. (1975a) Reduced secretory antibody response to live attenuated measles and polio virus vaccines in malnourished children. *British Medical Journal* 2, 583–585.

Chandra, R.K. (1975b) Serum complement and immunoglobulin in malnutrition. *Archives of Diseases of Childhood* 50, 225–259.

Chandra, R.K. (1975c) Fetal malnutrition and postnatal immunocompetence. *American Journal of Diseases of Childhood* 125, 450–455.

Chandra, R.K. (1975d) Antibody formation in first and generation offspring of nutritionally deprived rats. *Science* 190, 289–290.

Chandra, R.K. (1980) Serum thymic hormone activity and cell-mediated immunity in healthy neonates, preterm infants and small-for-gestational age infants. *Pediatrics* 67, 407–411.

Chandra, R.K. (1983a) The nutrition–immunity–infection nexus: the enumeration and functional assessment of lymphocyte subsets in nutritional deficiency. *Nutrition Research* 3, 605–615.

Chandra, R.K. (1983b) Nutrition, immunity and infection: present knowledge and future directions. *Lancet* i, 688–691.

Chandra, R.K. (1983c) Numerical and functional deficiency in T helper cells in protein–energy malnutrition. *Clinical and Experimental Immunology* 51, 126–132.

Chandra, R.K. (1984) Influence of nutrition–immunity axis on perinatal infections. In: Ogra, P.L. (ed.) *Neonatal Infections: Nutritional and Immunologic Interactions.* Grune and Stratton, Orlando, Florida, pp. 229–245.

Chandra, R.K. (1986) Serum levels and synthesis of IgG subclasses in small-for-gestation low birth weight infants and in patients with selective IgA deficiency. In: Hanson, L.A., Soderstrom, T. and Oxelius, V.-A. (eds) *Immunoglobulin Subclass Deficiencies.* Karger, Basle, pp. 90–99.

Chandra, R.K. (1988) Concentrations and production of IgG subclasses in preterm and small-for-gestation low birth weight infants. In: Skvaril, F., Morell, A. and Perret, B.

(eds) *Clinical Aspects of IgG Subclasses and Therapeutic Implications*. Karger, Basle, pp. 156–159.

Chandra, R.K. (1991a) 1990 McCollum Award lecture. Nutrition and immunity: lessons from the past and new insights into the future. *American Journal of Clinical Nutrition* 53, 1087–1101.

Chandra, R.K. (1991b) Interactions between early nutrition and the immune system. *Ciba Foundation Symposium* 156, 72–92.

Chandra, R.K. (ed.) (1992) *Nutrition and Immunology*. ARTS Biomedical, St John's.

Chandra, R.K. (1996) Nutrition, immunity and infection: from basic knowledge of dietary manipulation of immune responses to practical application of ameliorating suffering and improving survival. *Proceedings of the National Academy of Sciences of the USA* 93, 14304–14307.

Chandra, R.K. (1999) Nutrition and immunology; from the clinic to cellular biology and back again. *Proceedings of the Nutrition Society* 58, 681–683.

Chandra, R.K. (2001) Iron-zinc, immune responses, and infection. In: Suskind, R.M. and Tontisirin, K. (eds) *Nutrition, Immunity and Infection in Infants and Children*. Lippincott, Williams and Wilkins, Philadelphia, pp. 201–212.

Chandra, R.K. and Gupta, S.P. (1991) Increased bacterial adherence to respiratory epithelial cells in protein–energy malnutrition. *Immunology and Infectious Disease* 1, 55–57.

Chandra, R.K. and Newberne, P.M. (1977) *Nutrition, Immunity and Infection – Mechanisms of Interactions*. Plenum Press, New York.

Chandra, R.K., Chandra, S. and Ghai, O.P. (1976) Chemotaxis, random mobility and mobilization of polymorphonuclear leucocytes in malnutrition. *Journal of Clinical Pathology* 29, 224–227.

Chandra, R.K., Chandra, S., Khalil, N., Howse, D. and Kutty, K.M. (1977a) Lysozyme (muramidase) activity in plasma, neutrophils and urine in malnutrition and infection. In: Suskind, R.M. (ed.) *Malnutrition and the Immune Response*. Raven Press, New York, pp. 407–409.

Chandra, R.K., Ali, S., Kutty, K.M. and Chandra, S. (1977b) Thymus-dependent lymphocytes and delayed hypersensitivity in low birth weight infants. *Biology of the Neonate* 31, 15–18.

Chandra, R.K., Chandra, S. and Gupta, S. (1984) Antibody affinity and immune complexes after immunization with tetanus toxoid in protein–energy malnutrition. *American Journal of Clinical Nutrition* 40, 131–134.

Gershwin, M.B., Beach, R.S. and Hurley, L.S. (1984) *Nutrition and Immunity*. Academic Press, New York.

Haller, L., Zubler, R.H. and Lambert, P.H. (1978) Plasma levels of complement components and complement hemolytic activity in protein–energy malnutrition. *Clinical and Experimental Immunology* 34, 248–254.

Hoffman-Goetz, L., Bell, R.C. and Deir, R. (1984) Effect of protein malnutrition and interleukin-1 on *in vitro* rabbit lymphocyte mitogenesis. *Nutrition Research* 7, 769–780.

Jain, V.K. and Chandra, R.K. (1984) Does nutritional deficiency predispose to acquired immune deficiency syndrome? *Nutrition Research* 4, 537–543.

James, J.W. (1972) Longitudinal study of the morbidity of diarrheal and respiratory infections in malnourished children. *American Journal of Clinical Nutrition* 25, 690–694.

Keusch, G.T., Wilson, C.S. and Waksal, S.D. (1983) Nutrition, host defences, and the lymphoid system. *Archives of Host Defence Mechanisms* 2, 275–359.

Kielmann, A.A., Uberoi, I.S., Chandra, R.K. and Mehra, V.L. (1976) The effect of nutrition status on immune capacity and immune responses in preschool children in a rural community in India. *Bulletin of the World Health Organisation* 54, 477–483.

McMurray, D.N., Loomis, S.A., Casazza, L.J., Rey, H. and Miranda, R. (1981) Development of impaired cell-mediated immunity in mild and moderate malnutrition. *American Journal of Clinical Nutrition* 34, 68–77.

Marcos, A., Montero, A., Lopez-Varela, S. and Morande, G. (2001) Eating disorders (obesity, anorexia nervosa, bullemia nervosa), immunity and infection. In: Suskind, R.M. and Tontisirin, K. (eds) *Nutrition, Immunity and Infection in Infants and Children*. Lippincott, Williams and Wilkins, Philadelphia, pp. 243–258.

Moscatelli, P., Bricarelli, F.G., Piccinini, A., Tomatis, C. and Dufour, M. (1976) Defective immunocompetence in fetal malnutrition. *Helvetica Paediatrica Acta* 31, 241–247.

Scrimshaw, N.S., Taylor, C.E. and Gordon, J.E. (1968) *Interactions of Nutrition and Infection*. World Health Organization, Geneva.

Seth, V. and Chandra, R.K. (1972) Opsonic activity, phagocytosis and intracellular bactericidal capacity of polymorphs in undernutrition. *Archives of Diseases of Childhood* 47, 282–284.

Subcommittee on Nutrition (2001) *Nutrition and HIV/AIDS*. Policy Paper No. 20, World Health Organization, Geneva.

Tomkins, A. (1981) Nutritional status and severity of diarrhoea among pre-school children in rural Nigeria. *Lancet* i, 860–862.

Victora, C.G., Barros, F.C., Kirkwood, B.R. and Vaughan, J.P. (1990) Pneumonia, diarrhoea, and growth in the first 4 y of life: a longitudinal study of 5914 urban Brazilian children. *American Journal of Clinical Nutrition* 52, 391–396.

Wade, S., Bleiberg, F.K., Mosse, A., Lubetzki, J., Flavigny, H., Chapius, P., Roche, D., Lemonnier, D. and Dardenne, M. (1985) Thymulin (Zn-facteur thymique serique) activity in anorexia nervosa patients. *American Journal of Clinical Nutrition* 41, 275–280.

Watson, R.R. (ed.) (1984) *Nutrition, Disease Resistance, and Immune Function*. Marcel Dekker, New York.

Woodward, B. (2001) The effect of protein-energy malnutrition on immune competence. In: Suskind, R.M. and Tontisirin, K. (eds) *Nutrition, Immunity and Infection in Infants and Children*. Lippincott, Williams and Wilkins, Philadelphia, pp. 89–116.

4 Fatty Acids, Inflammation and Immunity

PHILIP C. CALDER[1] AND CATHERINE J. FIELD[2]

[1]*Institute of Human Nutrition, School of Medicine, University of Southampton, Bassett Crescent East, Southampton SO16 7PX, UK;* [2]*Nutrition and Metabolism Research Group, Department of Agricultural, Food and Nutritional Science, 4–10 Agriculture Forestry Centre, University of Alberta, Edmonton, Canada T6G 2P5*

Introduction

In Western countries, an adult eats, on average, 75–150 g of fat each day and fat contributes 30–45% of dietary energy. By far the most important component of dietary fat in quantitative terms is triacylglycerol, which, in most diets, constitutes > 95% of dietary fat. Each triacylglycerol molecule is composed of three fatty acids esterified to a glycerol backbone. Thus, fatty acids are major constituents of dietary fat. In recent years, it has become clear that fatty acids, especially polyunsaturated long-chain fatty acids (PUFAs), are important regulators of numerous cellular functions, including those related to inflammation and immunity. Interest in the effects of fatty acids upon inflammation and immunity has intensified during the past two decades. The influence of various fatty acids on the functional responses of cells of the immune system has been examined in numerous *in vitro* studies and in animal feeding models and human intervention studies. The effects of linoleic acid and the n-3 PUFAs found in fish oil have been most extensively investigated. There is now convincing evidence that the type of fat in the diet has a major impact on inflammation and other aspects of immune function, and this has formed the basis for interventions with fish oil in diseases characterized by immune dysfunction. This chapter will describe the nature of the fatty acids available in the human diet, the influence of different types of fatty acids on inflammation and immune function, the mechanisms by which fatty acids might exert their effects and the potential applications of those effects. However, it is not possible in this chapter to review the breadth of information available. The reader is referred to recent detailed reviews of the many aspects of fatty acids, inflammation and immunity in health and disease (Kinsella *et al.*, 1990; Kelley and Daudu, 1993; Blok *et al.*, 1996; Calder, 1996, 1997, 1998a, b, c, 2001a, b, c; Alexander, 1998; Fernandes *et al.*, 1998; Grimble, 1998; Harbige, 1998; Hughes, 1998; Miles and Calder, 1998; Sperling, 1998; Wu and Meydani, 1998; Yaqoob, 1998a, b; de Pablo and Alvarezda Cienfuegos, 2000; James *et al.*, 2000; Field *et al.*, 2001; Calder *et al.*, 2002).

© CAB *International* 2002. *Nutrition and Immune Function*
(eds P.C. Calder, C.J. Field and H.S. Gill)

Nomenclature, Synthesis and Dietary Sources of Fatty Acids

Because of the wide range of foods consumed, the human diet contains a great variety of fatty acids. The most abundant fatty acids have straight chains of an even number of carbon atoms. The chain lengths vary from four (e.g. in milk) to 30 (e.g. in some fish oils) and may contain double bonds (unsaturated fatty acids) (Fig. 4.1). It is the nature of the constituent fatty acids (their chain length and degree of unsaturation) that gives a fat its physical properties. Fatty acids are often referred to by their common names, but are more correctly identified by a systematic nomenclature (Table 4.1). This nomenclature indicates the number of carbon atoms and the number and position of double (unsaturated) bonds in the chain (see Fig. 4.1). It is the position of the first double bond in the hydrocarbon chain that is indicated by the n-7, n-9, n-6 or n-3 part of the shorthand notation for a fatty acid. Note that n-6 and n-3 are sometimes referred to as omega-6 and omega-3.

Mammalian cells are able to synthesize (from non-fat precursors) saturated fatty acids and unsaturated fatty acids of the n-9 and n-7 series but lack the delta-12 and delta-15 desaturase enzymes (found in most plants) for insertion of a double bond at the n-6 or n-3 position (Figs 4.1 and 4.2). Thus, mammalian cells cannot synthesize n-6 or n-3 PUFAs *de novo*. The n-6 and n-3 fatty acids are essential substrates for many of the major regulatory lipids in the body and, as they cannot be synthesized in the body, the body must obtain them from the diet. The commonly consumed PUFAs are linoleic acid (18:2n-6) and α-linolenic acid (18:3n-3). Once consumed, these fatty acids can be converted to the longer-chain, more unsaturated derivatives (Fig. 4.2). Thus linoleic acid is converted via γ-linolenic (18:3n-6) and dihomo-γ-linolenic

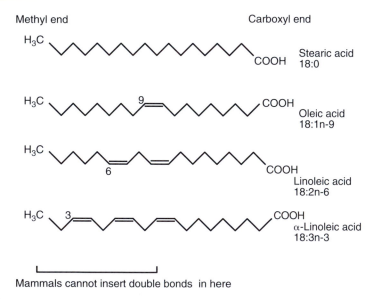

Fig. 4.1. Structure of some fatty acids.

Table 4.1. Fatty acid nomenclature and sources.

Systematic name	Trivial name	Shorthand notation	Sources
Decanoic	Capric	10:0	*De novo* synthesis; coconut oil
Dodecanoic	Lauric	12:0	*De novo* synthesis; coconut oil
Tetradecanoic	Myristic	14:0	*De novo* synthesis; milk
Hexadecanoic	Palmitic	16:0	*De novo* synthesis; milk; eggs; animal fats; meat; cocoa butter; palm oil (other vegetable oils contain lesser amounts); fish oils
Octadecanoic	Stearic	18:0	*De novo* synthesis; milk; eggs; animal fats; meat; cocoa butter
9-Hexadecenoic	Palmitoleic	16:1n-7	Desaturation of palmitic acid; fish oils
9-Octadecenoic	Oleic	18:1n-9	Desaturation of stearic acid; milk; eggs; animal fats; meat; cocoa butter; most vegetable oils, especially olive oil
9,12-Octadecadienoic	Linoleic	18:2n-6	Cannot be synthesized in mammals; some milks; eggs; animal fats; meat; most vegetable oils, especially maize, sunflower, safflower and soybean oils; green leaves
9,12,15-Octadecatrienoic	α-Linolenic	18:3n-3	Cannot be synthesized in mammals; green leaves; some vegetable oils, especially rapeseed, soybean and linseed oils
6,9,12-Octadecatrienoic	γ-Linolenic	18:3n-6	Synthesized from linoleic acid; borage and evening primrose oils
11,14,17-Eicosatrienoic	Mead	20:3n-9	Synthesized from oleic acid; indicator of essential fatty acid deficiency
8,11,14-Eicosatrienoic	Dihomo-γ-linolenic	20:3n-6	Synthesized from γ-linolenic acid
5,8,11,14-Eicosatetraenoic	Arachidonic	20:4n-6	Synthesized from linoleic acid via γ-linolenic and dihomo-γ-linolenic acids; meat
5,8,11,14,17-Eicosapentaenoic	Eicosapentaenoic	20:5n-3	Synthesized from α-linolenic acid; fish oils
7,10,13,16,19-Docosapentaenoic	Docosapentaenoic	22:5n-3	Synthesized from α-linolenic acid via eicosapentaenoic acid
4,7,10,13,16,19-Docosahexaenoic	Docosahexaenoic	22:6n-3	Synthesized from α-linolenic acid via eicosapentaenoic acid; fish oils

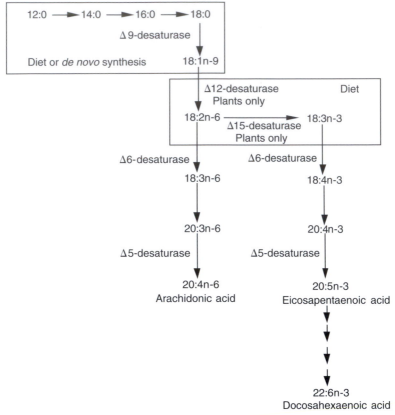

Fig. 4.2. Outline of the pathway of biosynthesis of polyunsaturated fatty acids.

(20:3n-6) acids to arachidonic acid (20:4n-6) (Fig. 4.2). Likewise, α-linolenic acid is converted to eicosapentaenoic acid (EPA) (20:5n-3) (Fig. 4.2). There is some controversy about the extent to which docosahexaenoic acid (DHA) (22:6n-3) can be synthesized from EPA in humans.

In the past 40 years, the absolute consumption of saturated fatty acids in Western diets has declined. For example, in the UK saturated fatty acid intake has declined by 40% since 1970, while the consumption of monounsaturated fatty acids has declined by 30% (Department of Health, 1994). The consumption of PUFAs increased by 25% over this period of time (Department of Health, 1994). This was largely the result of increased consumption of linoleic acid, which became generally available in margarines and cooking oils. This has also resulted in an alteration in the amounts of n-6 and n-3 PUFAs consumed, with the n-6 to n-3 PUFA ratio of the diet increasing. According to the UK Adult Survey conducted in 1986, the daily diet of the average adult male in the UK contains 42 g saturated fatty acids, 31 g monounsaturated fatty acids (mainly oleic acid) and 15.8 g PUFAs (Department of Health, 1994). The main PUFA in the diet is linoleic acid (intake is approximately 14 g day^{-1} for adult males), with α-linolenic acid contributing approximately 2 g day^{-1} (British

Nutrition Foundation, 1999). Adult females show a similar pattern of fatty-acid consumption to that of males, but the absolute amounts of each type of fatty acid consumed are about 70% of those consumed by males. Fat intakes are similar in North America to those in the UK, with the exception that the intake of n-3 fatty acids may be even lower (Kennedy *et al.*, 1999; Cavadini *et al.*, 2000). Longer-chain PUFAs are consumed in lower amounts than are linoleic and α-linolenic acids. Estimates of the intake of arachidonic acid intakes in Western populations vary between 50 and 300 mg day^{-1} for adults (Sinclair and O'Dea, 1993; Jonnalagadda *et al.*, 1995; Mann *et al.*, 1995). EPA and DHA are found in high quantities in many marine (e.g. herring, mackerel, fresh (i.e. not tinned) tuna, sardines) oils and in the oils extracted from the livers of fish that live in warmer waters (e.g. cod). EPA and DHA comprise 20–30% of the fatty acids in a typical preparation of fish oil, which means that a 1 g fish oil capsule can provide 200–300 mg of EPA plus DHA. In the absence of oily fish or fish oil consumption, α-linolenic acid is the main dietary n-3 PUFA. Average intake of the long-chain n-3 PUFAs in the UK is estimated at 250 mg day^{-1} (British Nutrition Foundation, 1999).

Fatty Acids and the Innate Immune System

Amount of fat in the diet and innate immune function

Several studies have compared the effects of feeding laboratory animals low- and high-fat diets on innate immune responses, such as natural killer cell activity. Most studies have found that high-fat diets result in diminished innate immune responses (for references, see Calder, 1998a), but the precise effect depends upon the exact level of fat used in the high-fat diet and its source. Human natural killer cell activity was significantly increased by a reduction in fat intake to less than 30% of energy (Barone *et al.*, 1989; Hebert *et al.*, 1990).

Linoleic and α-linolenic acids and innate immune function

Feeding rats or mice diets deficient in n-6 or n-3 fatty acids decreased neutrophil chemotaxis and macrophage-mediated phagocytic and cytotoxic activity, as compared with animals fed diets containing adequate amounts of these fatty acids (for references, see Kelley and Daudu, 1993). Thus, the immunological effects of essential fatty-acid deficiencies on innate immune responses are similar to the effects of other essential nutrient deficiencies. However, again as seen with other essential nutrients, an excess of essential fatty acids can impair aspects of the innate immune response. Animal studies have reported lower natural killer cell activity following the feeding of high fat including oils rich in linoleic acid (maize, sunflower or safflower oil) or in α-linolenic acid (e.g. linseed (flaxseed) oil), when compared with feeding high-saturated-fat diets (for references, see Kelley and Daudu, 1993; Calder, 1998a, b). These data suggest that a very high intake of linoleic or α-linolenic acid, compared with saturated fatty acids, has the potential to suppress natural killer cell activity. However, in humans, increasing linoleic acid intake by 6 g day^{-1} did not affect natural killer cell activity or the production of cytokines (interleukin (IL)-1β, tumour necrosis factor (TNF)-α) by monocytes (Yaqoob et al., 2000). Furthermore, increasing α-linolenic acid intake by 2 or 4 g day^{-1} (less than usually fed in animal studies) did not affect natural killer cell activity or the production of TNF-α, IL-1β or IL-6 by monocytes (Thies et al., 2001a, b), neutrophil respiratory burst (Healy et al., 2000; Thies et al., 2001b) or monocyte respiratory burst (Thies et al., 2001b). This suggests that the amount of essential fatty acids that humans could potentially consume in the habitual diet is not sufficient to negatively influence innate immunity. However, feeding a high dose of α-linolenic acid (approx. 15 g day^{-1}) was reported to decrease IL-1 and TNF production by human monocytes (Caughey et al., 1996).

EPA and DHA and innate immune function

Animal studies

There are many published animal studies investigating the effects of fish oil on aspects of inflammation and innate immunity. Most of these studies indicate that feeding high amounts of fish oil decreases a wide range of responses. However, not all studies agree with this generalization. Animal studies are often designed to demonstrate effects and to identify potential mechanisms and so result in the use of diets that differ markedly from human diets in both the level and the type of fat. Additional reasons for apparent contradictions in this literature might relate to the species of animal studied, the comparison being made (e.g. to a low-fat diet or to another high-fat diet; to saturated fat or to a diet high in n-6 PUFAs), the amount of vitamin E in the diets and the conditions used for ex vivo cell-culture experiments.

Feeding fish oil to laboratory animals has been reported to decrease macrophage functions, including generation of reactive oxygen species and production of TNF-α, IL-1 and IL-6 (e.g. Billiar et al., 1988; Hubbard et al., 1991; Renier et al., 1993). Fish oil, compared with other fat sources, resulted in lower concentrations of TNF-α, IL-1β and IL-6 in the bloodstream after endotoxin injection or burns (e.g. Hayashi et al., 1998; Sadeghi et al., 1999). Thus, these studies support the idea that fish oil has anti-inflammatory effects. There are, however, opposing studies. For example, Somers et al. (1989) reported that cultured peritoneal macrophages from mice fed fish-oil-supplemented diets exhibited higher TNF-α activity after endotoxin stimulation than did macrophages from mice fed a diet high in linoleic acid.

Animal feeding studies indicate that feeding high levels of fish oil decreases natural killer cell activity (e.g. Meydani et al., 1988; Yaqoob et al., 1994a), while lower levels (e.g. EPA plus DHA fed at less than 5% w/w of the diet) are reported to enhance this activity (Brouard and Pascaud, 1993; Robinson and Field, 1998). This effect may also be fatty-acid-specific, as a recent study reported that relatively low levels (4.4% of fatty acids; 1.7% of energy) of dietary EPA (but not DHA) inhibit rat natural killer cell activity (Peterson et al., 1998).

Human studies

Human studies have generally fed proportionately less fish oil than the amount provided in most animal studies. Nevertheless, a number of studies in healthy humans reveal significant immunomodulatory effects of long-chain n-3 PUFAs. Providing more than 2.3 g EPA plus DHA day^{-1} (and in some studies up to 14.5 g day^{-1}) has been reported to decrease chemotaxis and superoxide production by neutrophils (Lee *et al.*, 1985; Schmidt *et al.*, 1989, 1992; Luostarinen *et al.*, 1992; Sperling *et al.*, 1993) and by monocytes (Endres *et al.*, 1989; Schmidt *et al.*, 1989, 1992; Fisher *et al.*, 1990). Daily consumption of more than 2.4 g EPA plus DHA day^{-1} has been shown in some studies to decrease production of TNF, IL-1 and IL-6 by mononuclear cells (Endres *et al.*, 1989; Meydani *et al.*, 1991; Gallai *et al.*, 1993; Caughey *et al.*, 1996). Similarly, adding oily fish (providing 1.2 g EPA plus DHA day^{-1}) to a low-fat diet resulted in decreased production of TNF, IL-1 and IL-6 (Meydani *et al.*, 1993). Parenteral nutrition supplemented with fish oil decreased serum TNF-α and IL-6 concentrations in patients following major abdominal surgery, compared with n-6 fatty-acid-rich parenteral nutrition (Wachtler *et al.*, 1997). In contrast to these observations, a number of studies that provided from 0.55 g to 3.4 g EPA plus DHA day^{-1} failed to demonstrate an effect on neutrophil chemotaxis, neutrophil or monocyte respiratory burst or the production of TNF, IL-1 and IL-6 (Molvig *et al.*, 1991; Cooper *et al.*, 1993; Schmidt *et al.*, 1996; Blok *et al.*, 1997; Healy *et al.*, 2000; Yaqoob *et al.*, 2000; Thies *et al.*, 2001b).

Thus, studies in animals and humans have demonstrated that high levels of fish oil or its component n-3 PUFAs in the diet exert potent anti-inflammatory effects, particularly decreasing neutrophil and monocyte chemotaxis, superoxide production and production of pro-inflammatory cytokines. Reduced production of pro-inflammatory mediators may be beneficial in diseases characterized by excess production of these mediators (see later sections). On the other hand, these effects may compromise immune function in healthy and immune-compromised individuals. The effects of these lipids are probably dose-dependent (and disease-specific), as studies providing more modest amounts of long-chain n-3 PUFAs have not consistently demonstrated these effects on the innate immune system.

Fatty Acids and the Acquired Immune System

Amount of fat in the diet and acquired immune function

A number of studies have compared the effects of feeding laboratory animals low- and high-fat diets (usually high in saturated fat) upon lymphocytes. These studies have concluded that high-fat diets are associated with suppressed T-cell proliferation (for references, see Calder, 1998a). This conclusion is supported by studies in humans that showed significantly enhanced lymphocyte proliferation in response to mitogens if healthy subjects were fed a diet where fat contributed 25% of energy (Kelley *et al.*, 1989, 1992).

Linoleic and α-linolenic acids and acquired immune function

Essential fatty-acid deficiency is reported to decrease thymus and spleen weight and suppress cell-mediated immune responses and antibody production (for references, see Kelley and Daudu, 1993; Calder 1998a). However, a large number of studies in rats, mice, rabbits, chickens and monkeys have reported lower mitogen-stimulated lymphocyte proliferation and antibody production following the feeding of diets rich in linoleic acid (maize, sunflower or safflower oils), compared with feeding high-fat diets rich in saturated fatty acids (for references, see Kelley and Daudu, 1993; Calder, 1998a, b). These data suggest that linoleic acid has the potential to suppress acquired immune function. However, no difference in blood lymphocyte proliferation, circulating immunoglobulins or the delayed-type hypersensitivity response was seen in volunteers consuming low-fat diets (25% energy as fat) that were rich (12.9% of energy) or poor (3.5% of energy) in linoleic acid (Kelley et al., 1989, 1992). Furthermore, increasing linoleic acid intake by 6 g day^{-1} did not affect blood lymphocyte proliferation or the production of a range of cytokines by lymphocytes (Yaqoob et al., 2000). Again, the reason for the apparent discrepancy between animal and human studies most probably relates to the amount of linoleic acid in the diets studied.

Similarly to linoleic acid, feeding rodents diets containing very high levels of α-linolenic acid (linseed oil) is reported to decrease lymphocyte proliferation (e.g. Marshall and Johnston, 1985; Jeffery et al., 1996). The precise effect of α-linolenic acid on lymphocyte function appears to depend on both the level of the fatty acid and the total PUFA content of the diet (Jeffery et al., 1997). Feeding linseed oil (providing about 15 g α-linolenic acid day^{-1}) as part of a low-fat diet (total fat provided 29% energy) for 6 weeks resulted in significant decreases in human blood lymphocyte proliferation and in the delayed-type hypersensitivity response (Kelley et al., 1991). Thus, as was the case for linoleic acid, it appears that both a deficiency and an excess of α-linolenic acid can lead to suppressed immune function. However, increasing α-linolenic acid consumption by 2 g day^{-1} in healthy humans did not affect lymphocyte proliferation or the production of a range of cytokines by lymphocytes (Thies et al., 2001c), suggesting a limited immunological impact of a more moderate increase in α-linolenic acid intake.

EPA and DHA and acquired immune function

Animal studies

Studies in rabbits, chickens, rats and mice have clearly demonstrated that long-chain n-3 PUFAs can inhibit lymphocyte proliferation, IL-2 and interferon (IFN)-γ production, delayed-type hypersensitivity and antigen presentation, as compared with diets rich in lard, or hydrogenated coconut, safflower, maize or linseed oils (e.g. Fujikawa et al., 1992; Yaqoob et al., 1994b; Sanderson et al., 1995, 1997; Byleveld et al., 1999; Wallace et al., 2001).

The addition of either EPA or DHA to a diet was demonstrated to suppress T-cell proliferation in rats (Peterson *et al.*, 1998) and mice (Jolly *et al.*, 1997). Although mechanistically important, the physiological importance of many of the animal studies in this area is not clear, as the diets used to identify the effects of long-chain n-3 PUFAs often contain very high amounts of these fatty acids and very low amounts of linoleic acid. Indeed, in contrast to many other studies, adding EPA and DHA at 5% by weight in both a high- and low-PUFA diet improved rat lymphocyte responses, measured as activation-marker expression and cytokine production (Robinson and Field, 1998; Robinson *et al.*, 2001).

Human studies

Human studies have generally provided less fish oil (as a proportion of fat or energy) in the diet than the amount fed in most studies in animals. Despite this, data from studies investigating the influence of fish oil on human lymphocyte functions are also conflicting. Supplementation of the diet of healthy human volunteers with fish oil providing 2.4 g EPA plus DHA day^{-1} resulted in decreased proliferation of lymphocytes from older women (aged 51–68 years) but not young women (aged 21–33 years) and decreased IL-2 production (Meydani *et al.*, 1991). Molvig *et al.* (1991) reported decreased lymphocyte proliferation after providing 1.7 or 3.4 g EPA plus DHA day^{-1} to men, while Gallai *et al.* (1993) reported that 5.2 g EPA plus DHA day^{-1} decreased IL-2 and IFN-γ production. Providing 1.2 g EPA plus DHA to healthy subjects aged 55–75 years resulted in decreased lymphocyte proliferation (Thies *et al.*, 2001c), but did not affect IL-2 or IFN-γ production (Thies *et al.*, 2001c). Inclusion of oily fish providing 1.2 g EPA plus DHA day^{-1} in the diet of volunteers consuming a low-fat, low-cholesterol diet decreased lymphocyte proliferation, IL-2 production and the delayed-type hypersensitivity response to seven recall antigens (Meydani *et al.*, 1993). In contrast to these observations, there are reports of no effect of 3.2 g EPA plus DHA day^{-1} on lymphocyte proliferation and IL-2 and IFN-γ production (Yaqoob *et al.*, 2000) by peripheral-blood lymphocytes and of no effect of 4.6 g EPA plus DHA day^{-1} on lymphocyte proliferation and IL-2 production (Endres *et al.*, 1993). Thus, feeding moderate amounts of long-chain n-3 PUFAs is not clearly immunosuppressive, although feeding high amounts might be.

Mechanisms of the Effect of Dietary Fatty Acids on Immune Function

While it is widely recognized that dietary fatty acids can potentially alter immune and inflammatory responses, current understanding of how they act is incomplete. Several candidate mechanisms have been proposed, including alterations in membrane structure and composition, changes in membrane-mediated functions and signals (i.e. proteins, eicosanoids), changes in gene expression and effects on the development of the immune system (Fig. 4.3).

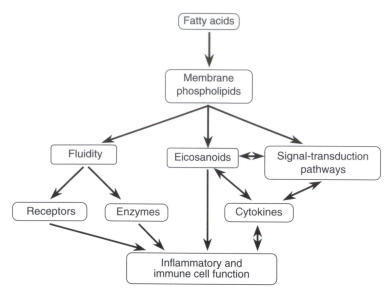

Fig. 4.3. Mechanisms whereby fatty acids might exert effects on immune cell function.

Alterations in membrane structure and composition

Immune-cell activation results in both *de novo* synthesis and an increased turnover of membrane phospholipids (e.g. Resch *et al.*, 1972; Ferber *et al.*, 1975). Therefore, essential fatty acids would be required for the synthesis of new membranes during immune-cell responses, especially those involving increased membrane synthesis and turnover (e.g. cell proliferation, phagocytosis).

The fluidity of the plasma membrane or of regions of the plasma membrane is important in the functioning of cells (see Stubbs and Smith, 1984). The fluidity of a membrane is determined by its lipid components and their fatty-acid composition (Stubbs and Smith, 1984). Membrane fluidity is an important regulator of phagocytosis (Calder *et al.*, 1990). The function of the immune system depends on interactions between different cell types and, through effects on membrane composition, dietary fatty acids have the potential to influence these interactions. For example, the interaction of cytotoxic T-cells with target cell membranes, a necessary interaction to induce effector function, is affected by the fluidity of the plasma membrane of the T-cells (Bialick *et al.*, 1984). Cell culture experiments have demonstrated that changes in fatty-acid composition of immune cells alter membrane fluidity (e.g. Calder *et al.*, 1994), but this has been less easy to demonstrate after dietary manipulations (e.g. Yaqoob *et al.*, 1995), probably because the fatty acid composition changes induced by diet are less extreme than those seen in culture and because, in the intact animal, mechanisms to counter the fluidizing effect of increasing the PUFA content of membranes (e.g. insertion of cholesterol) can be achieved more readily than in culture.

Since there has been significant focus on the effects of n-6 and n-3 PUFAs in inflammation and immunity, the proportions of those classes of fatty acids in immune cells are of interest. The exact proportion of arachidonic acid in human immune cells varies according to cell type and the lipid fraction examined (Gibney and Hunter, 1993; Sperling *et al.*, 1993). The phospholipids of human mononuclear cells (an approximately 70 : 20 : 10 mixture of T lymphocytes, B lymphocytes and monocytes purified from human blood) contain 6–10% linoleic acid, 1–2% dihomo-γ-linolenic acid (DGLA) and 15–25% arachidonic acid (Gibney and Hunter, 1993; Yaqoob *et al.*, 2000; see Table 4.2). In contrast, the proportions of n-3 fatty acids are low: α-linolenic acid is generally found only in trace amounts and EPA and DHA comprise only 0.1–0.8% and 2–4%, respectively (Gibney and Hunter, 1993; Yaqoob *et al.*, 2000; see Table 4.2).

Animal studies show that decreasing the availability of linoleic acid in the diet, especially by replacing it with n-3 fatty acids (either α-linolenic acid or long-chain n-3 fatty acids), results in decreased proportions of all n-6 fatty acids, including arachidonic acid, in immune-cell phospholipids (Marshall and Johnston, 1985; Lokesh *et al.*, 1986; Brouard and Pascaud, 1990; Yaqoob *et al.*, 1995; Jeffery *et al.*, 1996; Peterson *et al.*, 1998; Robinson and Field, 1998; Wallace *et al.*, 2000, 2001; Robinson *et al.*, 2001). When α-linolenic acid is added to the human diet in significant quantities, it appears in immune cells and there is also an increase in the proportion of EPA, although the proportion of DHA may not be elevated (Caughey *et al.*, 1996). More moderate increases in the amount of α-linolenic acid in the human diet appear to have a limited impact on immune-cell fatty-acid composition (Healy *et al.*, 2000; Thies *et al.*, 2001c). When fish oil is provided in the human diet, the proportions of EPA and DHA in immune cells are significantly elevated and the n-6/n-3 PUFA ratio is decreased (Lee *et al.*, 1985; Endres *et al.*, 1989; Fisher *et al.*, 1990; Molvig *et al.*, 1991; Gibney and Hunter, 1993; Sperling *et al.*, 1993; Caughey *et al.*,

Table 4.2. Fatty-acid composition of human mononuclear cells before and after supplementation of the diet with evening primrose oil or fish oil. Healthy volunteers supplemented their diet with 9 g evening primrose oil (providing 1 g γ-linolenic acid) day^{-1} or with 9 g fish oil (providing 3.2 g EPA plus DHA) day^{-1} for 8 weeks. Mononuclear cells were isolated by standard techniques and the fatty-acid composition determined. (Data are mean ± standard error of mean (SEM) for six subjects per group and are taken from Yaqoob *et al.*, 2000.)

	Fatty acid (g 100 g^{-1} of total fatty acids)			
	Evening primrose oil		Fish oil	
Fatty acid	Before	After	Before	After
Dihomo-γ-linolenic acid	1.2 ± 0.4	2.2 ± 0.4[a]	1.3 ± 0.5	1.9 ± 0.5
Arachidonic acid	20.6 ± 2.1	21.2 ± 0.5	22.3 ± 0.8	18.8 ± 1.3[a]
EPA	1.0 ± 0.3	1.1 ± 0.4	0.8 ± 0.4	2.8 ± 0.2[a]
DHA	2.7 ± 0.4	2.6 ± 0.4	1.9 ± 0.5	3.3 ± 0.3

[a]Indicates significantly different from before supplementation.

1996; Healy *et al.*, 2000; Yaqoob *et al.*, 2000; Thies *et al.*, 2001c; see Table 4.2) in a dose-dependent manner. Similar effects occur in neutrophils, monocytes and T and B lymphocytes (Gibney and Hunter, 1993). In many studies, the degree of enrichment of EPA is greater than that of DHA (e.g. 300% vs. 95%: Yaqoob *et al.*, 2000), although this probably depends upon the relative amounts of EPA and DHA in the fish oil preparation. The incorporation of the long-chain n-3 fatty acids is at least partly at the expense of arachidonic acid (see Table 4.2) and is considered to be near maximal 4 weeks after a dietary change (e.g. Healy *et al.*, 2000; Yaqoob *et al.*, 2000; Thies *et al.*, 2001c). Since n-3 PUFAs oxidize more readily than n-6 PUFAs, they may increase susceptibility of cellular membranes to lipid peroxidation. Increased free radical production has been demonstrated in animals fed diets rich in n-3 PUFAs. The risk of oxidation associated with increased intake of n-3 PUFA has been shown to be minimized by intake of extra antioxidants, such as vitamin E.

Alterations in membrane-mediated functions and signals

Alterations in the function of membrane proteins

Changes in plasma membrane structural characteristics can change the activity of proteins that serve as ion channels, adhesion molecules, transporters, receptors, signal transducers or enzymes (Stubbs and Smith, 1984; Clandinin *et al.*, 1991). Many membrane-associated proteins in immune cells have been shown to be modulated by membrane lipid changes. For example, feeding 5% w/w long-chain n-3 PUFAs to rats resulted in a higher proportion of T- and B-cells and macrophages expressing the transferrin receptor (CD71) after stimulation with mitogen (Robinson and Field, 1998), although feeding a higher amount of fish oil did not induce this effect (Yaqoob *et al.*, 1994b). The binding of cytokines to their receptor has been reported to be altered with changes in membrane composition (Grimble and Tappia, 1995). Additionally, the expression of several cell surface molecules was reported to be altered after fish oil feeding (Sanderson *et al.*, 1995; Hughes *et al.*, 1996; Robinson and Field, 1998; Sanderson and Calder, 1998a; Field *et al.*, 2000; Hughes and Pinder, 2000; Robinson *et al.*, 2001). Many of these molecules are involved in the co-stimulation processes necessary for lymphocyte activation, and some of the effects are suggestive of improved cell-mediated immune function.

Changes in membrane-mediated signals (signal transduction)

Lipids, derived from either endogenous or exogenous sources, affect many cell signalling pathways via a variety of mechanisms. Many of the established cell signalling molecules are generated directly from membrane phospholipids (e.g. inositol-1,4,5-trisphosphate, diacylglycerol, phosphatidic acid, choline, ceramide, platelet-activating factor, arachidonic acid). These have important roles in regulating the activity of proteins involved in immune-cell responses.

The concentration and/or composition of lipid-derived signalling molecules have been shown to be sensitive to n-3 PUFA availability either in cell culture (Jenski *et al.*, 1995) or through the diet (Huang *et al.*, 1992; Fowler *et al.*, 1993; Sperling *et al.*, 1993; Marignani and Sebaldt, 1995; Jolly *et al.*, 1997; Sanderson and Calder, 1998b). This may be due to either altered activity of the enzymes that generate the signals or to altered composition of the substrate molecules. There is evidence to support each of these possibilities (see Miles and Calder, 1998). For example, lymphocyte phospholipase Cγ activity is reduced after feeding a diet rich in fish oil, which might account for the decreased generation of signalling molecules observed (Sanderson and Calder, 1998b). There is also evidence that arachidonic acid released from the plasma membrane has a direct role in regulating some immune-cell functions, such as natural killer cell granule release and cell-mediated toxicity (Cifone *et al.*, 1993). In addition, arachidonic acid is an intracellular activator of the nicotinamide adenine dinucleotide phosphate (NADPH) oxidase enzyme in neutrophils (Sakata *et al.*, 1987), and enrichment of arachidonic acid in neutrophil membranes is reported to increase the oxidative burst of neutrophils (Badwey *et al.*, 1981, 1984; Hardy *et al.*, 1991). Dietary lipids have been demonstrated to influence the pattern of fatty acids released from lymphocytes (Sanderson *et al.*, 2000).

Changes in eicosanoid synthesis

A key link between fatty acids, inflammation and immune function is a group of bioactive mediators termed eicosanoids (prostaglandins, leucotrienes, thromboxanes), which are synthesized from 20-carbon PUFAs (Fig. 4.4). The two

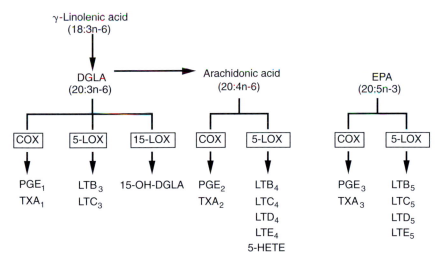

Fig. 4.4. Outline of synthesis of eicosanoids from 20-carbon n-6 and n-3 polyunsaturated fatty acids. COX, cyclo-oxygenase; DGLA, dihomo-γ-linolenic acid; EPA, eicosapentaenoic acid; HETE, hydroxyeicosatetraenoic acid; LOX, lipoxygenase; LT, leucotriene; PG, prostaglandin; TX, thromboxane.

major pathways for eicosanoid synthesis are via the enzymes cyclo-oxygenase (COX) and lipoxygenase (LOX). These enzymes initiate pathways that result in the production of prostaglandins/thromboxanes and leucotrienes/hydroxy-eicosatrienoic acids/lipoxins, respectively. Membrane arachidonic acid is the main precursor of these mediators, giving rise to dienoic prostaglandins (e.g. PGE_2) and thromboxanes (TXA_2) and tetraenoic leucotrienes (e.g. LTB_4). Arachidonic acid in cell membranes is mobilized by various phospholipase enzymes, most notably phospholipase A_2, and the released arachidonic acid is the substrate for COX or one of the three LOX enzymes (Fig. 4.5). There are at least 16 different 2-series PG and these are formed in a cell-specific manner. For example, monocytes and macrophages produce large amounts of PGE_2 and PGF_2, neutrophils produce moderate amounts of PGE_2 and mast cells produce PGD_2. The LOX enzymes have different tissue distributions, with 5-LOX being found mainly in mast cells, monocytes, macrophages and granulocytes and 12- and 15-LOX being found primarily in epithelial cells. Metabolism of arachidonic acid by the 5-LOX pathway gives rise to hydroxy and hydroperoxy derivatives (5-hydroxyeicosatetraenoic acid) (5-HETE) and 5-hydroperoxy-eicosatetraenoic acid (5-HPETE), respectively) and the 4-series LT (Fig. 4.5).

Eicosanoids (particularly PGE_2 and 4-series LT) are involved in modulating the intensity and duration of inflammatory and immune responses (for reviews, see Kinsella *et al.*, 1990; Lewis *et al.*, 1990; Tilley *et al.*, 2001). The pro-inflammatory effects of PGE_2 include inducing fever, increasing vascular permeability

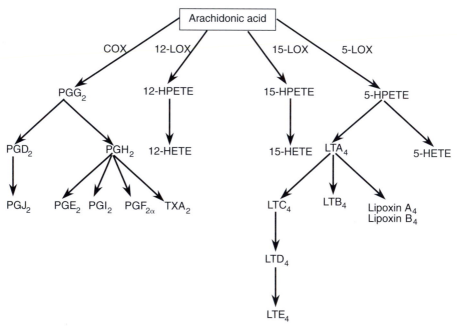

Fig. 4.5. Synthesis of eicosanoids from arachidonic acid. COX, cyclo-oxygenase; HETE, hydroxyeicosatetraenoic acid; HPETE, hydroperoxyeicosatetraenoic acid; LOX, lipoxygenase; LT, leucotriene; PG, prostaglandin; TX, thromboxane.

and vasodilatation and enhancing pain and oedema caused by other agents, such as histamine. Additionally, PGE$_2$ suppresses lymphocyte proliferation and natural killer cell activity and inhibits production of TNF-α, IL-1, IL-6, IL-2 and IFN-γ (Fig. 4.6); thus, in these respects, PGE$_2$ is immunosuppressive and anti-inflammatory. PGE$_2$ does not affect the production of the T-helper 2 (Th2)-type cytokines IL-4 and IL-10, but promotes immunoglobulin E (IgE) production by B lymphocytes (Fig. 4.6). LTB$_4$ increases vascular permeability, enhances local blood flow, is a potent chemotactic agent for leucocytes, induces release of lysosomal enzymes, enhances generation of reactive oxygen species, inhibits lymphocyte proliferation and promotes natural killer cell activity (Fig. 4.7). In addition, 4-series LT regulate the production of pro-inflammatory cytokines; for example, LTB$_4$ enhances production of TNF-α, IL-1, IL-6, IL-2 and IFN-γ (Fig. 4.7). Whereas 15-HETE inhibits lymphocyte proliferation, 5-HETE enhances it. Thus, arachidonic acid gives rise to a range of mediators that have opposing effects to one another, so the overall physiological effect will be the result of the balance of these mediators, the timing of their production and the sensitivities of target cells to their effects.

Dietary fatty acids can influence eicosanoid synthesis by affecting the supply of substrates. Feeding animals or humans increased amounts of fish oil results in a decrease in the amount of arachidonic acid in the membranes of most cells in the body, including those involved in inflammation and immunity,

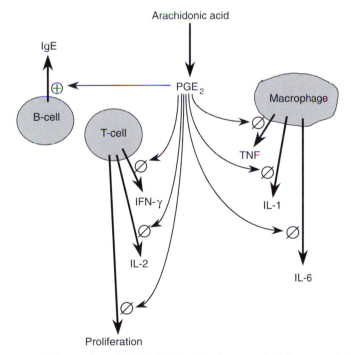

Fig. 4.6. Immunoregulatory roles of PGE$_2$. IFN-γ, interferon-γ; IgE, immunoglobulin E; IL, interleukin; PG, prostaglandin; TNF, tumour necrosis factor.

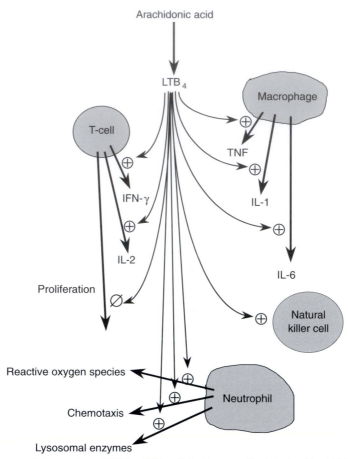

Fig. 4.7. Immunoregulatory roles of LTB$_4$. IFN-γ, interferon-γ; IL, interleukin; LT, leucotriene; TNF, tumour necrosis factor.

such as monocytes, macrophages, neutrophils and lymphocytes (*see* earlier section). This means that there is less arachidonic acid available for the synthesis of eicosanoids. Consequently, dietary fish oil decreases the production of arachidonic acid-derived eicosanoids from animal (Lokesh *et al.*, 1986; Brouard and Pascaud, 1990; Yaqoob and Calder, 1995; Peterson *et al.*, 1998; Fig. 4.8) and human (Lee *et al.*, 1985; Endres *et al.*, 1989; Meydani *et al.*, 1991; Sperling *et al.*, 1993; Caughey *et al.*, 1996) immune cells. EPA is also a substrate for the COX and LOX enzymes, resulting in the synthesis of the trienoic prostanoids (*e.g.* PGE$_3$) and pentaenoic leucotrienes (*e.g.* LTB$_5$) (Fig. 4.4). The eicosanoids produced from EPA are often less biologically potent than the analogues synthesized from arachidonic acid. For example, LTB$_5$ is only about 10% as potent as LTB$_4$ as a chemotactic agent and in promoting lysosomal enzyme release (*see* Kinsella *et al.*, 1990). Since dietary fish oil leads to decreased PGE$_2$ production, it is often stated that feeding n-3 lipids should result in a reversal of the effects of PGE$_2$. Thus, fish oil is expected to

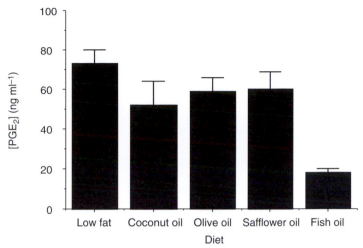

Fig. 4.8. Effect of dietary fish oil on the production of prostaglandin E_2 (PGE_2) by macrophages. Mice were fed for 8 weeks on a low-fat (25 g kg^{-1} maize oil) diet or on diets containing 200 g kg^{-1} of either hyrogenated coconut oil, olive oil, safflower oil or fish oil. Thioglycollate-elicited peritoneal macrophages were prepared and cultured with bacterial lipopolysaccharide (10 μg ml^{-1}) for 8 h. The medium was collected and PGE_2 concentrations were measured by ELISA. (Data are from Yaqoob and Calder, 1995.)

result in less inflammation, enhanced cytokine production by monocytes/ macrophages and Th1 lymphocytes and enhanced lymphocyte proliferation (Fig. 4.9). The reduction in the generation of arachidonic acid-derived mediators that accompanies fish oil consumption has led to the idea that fish oil is anti-inflammatory and might enhance immune function (Fig. 4.9). However, the *in vivo* situation is likely to be more complex than this, because PGE_2 is not the sole mediator produced from arachidonic acid and the range of mediators produced have varying, sometimes opposite, actions (see above). Furthermore, EPA will give rise to mediators with varying actions, some of which may actually be the same as those of the analogues produced from arachidonic acid. Thus, the overall effect of fish oil feeding cannot be predicted solely on the basis of an abrogation of PGE_2-mediated effects. Furthermore, a number of the effects of n-3 PUFA have been shown to occur independent of changes in eicosanoid production (Santoli *et al.*, 1990; Calder *et al.*, 1992; Soyland *et al.*, 1993).

Changes in gene expression

Fatty acids, especially PUFAs, are known to modulate the expression of a variety of genes coding for key regulatory proteins in numerous metabolic pathways in hepatocytes and adipocytes (Clarke and Jump, 1994). These effects are mediated by both indirect mechanisms (e.g. by eicosanoids, hor-

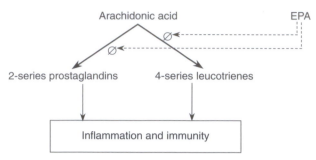

Fig. 4.9. Theoretical basis for the immunoregulatory effects of eicosapentaenoic acid (EPA).

mones) and direct effects on gene expression. There is now emerging evidence that PUFAs regulate the expression of genes for cytokines, adhesion molecules, COX, inducible nitric oxide synthase and other inflammatory proteins (Renier *et al.*, 1993; de Caterina and Libby, 1996; Khair-el-Din *et al.*, 1996; Robinson *et al.*, 1996; Curtis *et al.*, 2000; Miles *et al.*, 2000; Wallace *et al.*, 2001). Since the expression of many of these genes is regulated by the transcription factor nuclear factor kappa B (NFκB), these observations suggest that PUFAs might somehow affect the activity of this transcription factor. This might be through effects on cell signalling leading to NFκB activation. There is recent evidence that dietary fish oil affects NFκB activity (Lo *et al.*, 1999; Xi *et al.*, 2001), in a manner that is consistent with its ability to downregulate the production of inflammatory mediators.

A second group of transcription factors currently undergoing scrutiny for their role in inflammation are the peroxisome proliferator-activated receptors (PPARs). The main members of this family are PPARα and PPARγ. PPARα and γ play important roles in liver and adipose tissue, respectively (Schoonjans *et al.*, 1996). However, they are also found in inflammatory cells (Chinetti *et al.*, 1998; Ricote *et al.*, 1998). PPARs can bind, and appear to be regulated by, PUFAs and eicosanoids (Kleiwer *et al.*, 1995; Devchand *et al.*, 1996). PPARα-deficient mice have a prolonged response to inflammatory stimuli (Devchand *et al.*, 1996), suggesting that PPARα activation might be anti-inflammatory. More recently, activators of both PPARα and PPARγ have been shown to inhibit the activation of a number of inflammatory genes (Jiang *et al.*, 1998; Poynter and Daynes, 1998; Ricote *et al.*, 1998; Jackson *et al.*, 1999; Marx *et al.*, 1999; Takano *et al.*, 2000; Wang *et al.*, 2001; Xu *et al.*, 2001). Two mechanisms for the anti-inflammatory actions of PPARs have been proposed (for reviews, see Chinetti *et al.*, 2000; Delerive *et al.*, 2001). The first is that PPARs might stimulate the breakdown of inflammatory eicosanoids through the induction of peroxisomal β-oxidation. The second is that PPARs might interfere with/antagonize the activation of other transcription factors, including NFκB. Although the effect of fish oil on PPAR expression in inflammatory cells has not been reported, studies in other tissues (e.g. Berthou *et al.*, 1995) suggest that n-3 PUFAs might act by increasing the level of these anti-inflammatory transcription factors in such cells.

Effects on the development of the immune system

Despite the amount of work done in healthy adults, human diseases and animal models of disease, little work has been done on the effect of dietary PUFAs on T-cell development in the infant or young animal. However, a recent study examined the effect of altered long-chain PUFA availability on the functional indices of immune development during the first 42 days of human life (Field *et al.*, 2000). A group of clinically stable preterm infants were fed human milk, standard preterm infant formula or a preterm infant formula containing DHA (0.4%) and arachidonic acid (0.6%) for the first 42 days of life. Using blood samples obtained at 14 and 42 days of age, the effect of diet on some parameters of immune development was studied. Compared with standard formula, feeding long-chain PUFAs significantly increased the proportion of antigen mature (CD45RO+) CD4+ cells (by approximately 25%), compared with non-supplemented formula-fed infants and lowered the proportion of immature (CD45RA+) CD4+ cells to levels not different from human milk-fed infants. These changes in the sialylation of the CD45 region (RA vs. RO) are believed to reflect the maturation of the immune system (Bofill *et al.*, 1994). These data suggest that adding DHA and arachidonic acid to preterm formula may have assisted in the maturation of peripheral CD4+ cells. Between 14 and 42 days of age, the ability of peripheral mononuclear cells from unsupplemented formula-fed infants to produce IL-10 was lower than that of human milk-fed infants (Field *et al.*, 2000). IL-10 production by cells from infants fed the formula containing DHA plus arachidonic acid did not differ from that of the human milk-fed infants. Feeding the formula containing DHA plus arachidonic acid resulted in a significant decrease in the amount of secretory IL-2 receptor (SIL-2R) produced by stimulated peripheral mononuclear cells at 42 days of age, as compared with 14 days (Field *et al.*, 2000). This work supports an effect of dietary lipids, particularly long-chain PUFAs, on immune development.

Fatty Acids and Diseases Involving the Immune System

Chronic inflammatory (autoimmune) diseases

Chronic inflammatory or autoimmune diseases are often characterized by a dysregulated Th1-type response and by an inappropriate production of pro-inflammatory cytokines (e.g. TNF-α) and arachidonic acid-derived eicosanoids (e.g. PGE_2 and LTB_4). The effects of fish oil outlined above suggest that n-3 PUFAs might have a role in the prevention and therapy of chronic inflammatory diseases. In support of this idea, dietary fish oil has been shown to have beneficial clinical, immunological and biochemical effects in various animal models of human diseases. These effects include: increased survival and decreased proteinuria and anti-DNA antibodies in mice with autoimmune glomerulonephritis (Prickett *et al.*, 1983; Kelley *et al.*, 1985; Robinson *et al.*, 1985, 1986), decreased incidence and severity of joint inflammation in mice with collagen-induced arthritis (Leslie *et al.*, 1985) or rats with streptococcal cell wall-induced arthritis (Volker *et al.*, 2000) and reduced inflammation in rats with inflammatory bowel disease (Vilaseca *et al.*, 1990). These improvements are associated with abolition of pro-inflammatory cytokine production and induction of anti-inflammatory cytokines in some models (Chandrasekar and Fernandes, 1994; Fernandes *et al.*, 1994; Kleemann *et al.*, 1998; Venkatraman and Chu, 1999).

There have been a number of clinical trials assessing dietary supplementation with fish oils in several chronic inflammatory diseases in humans. N-3 PUFAs in the diet could affect the course of these diseases by altering the immune or inflammatory responses, thus modifying clinical symptoms. In some of the human trials of fish oil in inflammatory disease, anti-inflammatory effects of fish oil, including decreased production of circulating concentrations of pro-inflammatory mediators (LTB_4, TNF-α, IL-1 and C-reactive protein), were observed. Many of the short-term placebo-controlled, double-blind trials of fish oil in chronic inflammatory diseases (cyclosporin-induced nephrotoxicity and hypertension, lupus, nephritis, IgA nephropathy, Crohn's disease, ulcerative colitis) reveal significant benefit, including decreased disease activity and a lowered use of anti-inflammatory drugs (Table 4.3). However, the evidence for a beneficial effect of fish oil is strongest in rheumatoid arthritis (see Table 4.3). Further research is needed to identify which components of fish oil might be most effective, which doses should be used, what qualitative alterations of dietary fatty acids and background diet might be important, what the optimal duration of therapy should be, which disease or subsets of patients might respond and what interaction between other anti-inflammatory therapy and n-3 PUFAs might occur.

Asthma and related diseases

Eicosanoids synthesized from arachidonic acid have a role in allergic diseases: PGD_2, LTC_4, LTD_4 and LTE_4 are produced by the cells that mediate pulmonary inflammation in asthma, such as mast cells, and are believed to be the major mediators of asthmatic bronchoconstriction (Fig. 4.10). Although its action as a precursor to leucotrienes has highlighted the significance of arachidonic acid in the aetiology of allergic disease, a second link with this fatty acid has been made. This is because PGE_2 regulates the activities of lymphocytes. Of particular relevance in the context of allergic disease is the ability of PGE_2 to inhibit the production of the Th1-type cytokines IL-2 and IFN-γ without affecting the production of the Th2-type cytokines IL-4 and IL-5, and to stimulate B-cells to produce IgE (Fig. 4.10). These observations suggest that PGE_2 promotes the development of allergic disease. Since n-3 fatty acids potentially antagonize the effects of arachidonic acid, there may be a role for fish oil in treating, or in protecting against the development of, allergic diseases, including asthma. Hence, a number of trials of fish oil in asthma have been performed. Although some of these trials show fish oil-induced changes in production of some inflammatory mediators (e.g. LTB_4), a number report no effects on clinical outcomes (e.g. Arm *et al.*, 1988, 1989; see Calder and Miles, 2000). In con-

Table 4.3. Summary of clinical trials of n-3 polyunsaturated fatty acids in human chronic inflammatory diseases.

Disease	Number of double-blind, placebo-controlled studies	Doses of EPA + DHA used (g day^{-1})	Duration (weeks)	Key findings	Reviews
Rheumatoid arthritis	13	1–6.4	12–52	All studies reported improvements, including reduced duration of morning stiffness, reduced number of tender or swollen joints, reduced joint pain, reduced time to fatigue and increased grip strength. Twelve studies reported improvement in at least two clinical measures, and four studies reported improvement in at least four clinical measures. Ten studies reported decreased joint tenderness. Three studies reported significant decrease in the use of non-steroidal anti-inflammatory drugs	Volker and Garg (1996); James and Cleland (1997); Geusens (1998); Calder (2001d); Calder and Zurier (2001)
Crohn's disease	3	2.7–5.1	12–52	Two studies reported no benefit. One study reported a significant decrease in relapses. One other study, which used oily fish (100–250 g day^{-1} for 2 years), reported a significant decrease in relapses	Belluzzi and Miglio (1998)
Ulcerative colitis	4	1.8–5.4	12–52	One study reported no benefit (this study used the lowest dose of EPA plus DHA). One study reported a non-significant decrease in disease activity and a significant decrease in use of corticosteroids. Two studies reported benefit, including improved histological appearance of the colon, decreased disease activity, weight gain and decreased use of prednisolone. Two other 'open' studies reported improved symptoms, improved histological appearance of the rectal mucosa and decreased use of prednisolone	Rodgers (1998)
Psoriasis	2	1.8	8–12	One study reported significant improvement in itching, scaling and erythema. One study reported no benefit. Three open studies (providing 10–18 g EPA + DHA day^{-1} for 6–8 weeks) reported mild to moderate (two studies) or moderate to excellent (one study) improvements in scaling, itching, lesion thickness and erythema in the majority of patients. One open study that combined fish oil with a low-fat diet reported improvements	Ziboh (1998)

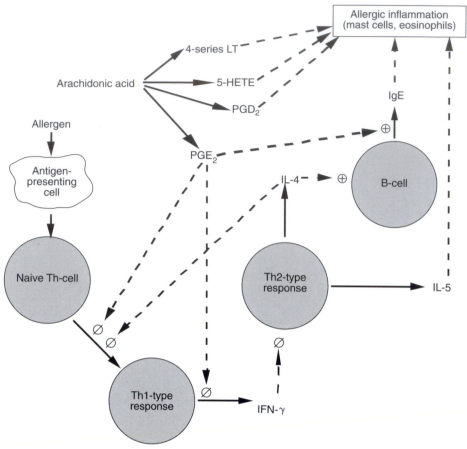

Fig. 4.10. Putative role of arachidonic acid in atopic disease. PGE_2 inhibits production of the Th1-type cytokine, IFN-γ, so allowing the production of Th2-type cytokines (e.g. IL-4) to proceed without inhibition. IL-4 promotes Ig class switching in B-cells to produce IgE; PGE_2 also directly promotes IgE production by B-cells. Thus, PGE_2 acts to promote the Th2-type response and IgE production. The 4-series LT (and some 2-series PG, such as PGD_2) are the direct mediators of allergic inflammation. HETE, hydroxyeicosatetraenoic acid; IFN, interferon; Ig, immunoglobulin; IL, interleukin; LT, leucotriene; PG, prostaglandin; Th, T-helper.

trast, some studies have shown significant clinical improvements in patients (e.g. Dry and Vincent, 1991) and there are suggestions that this type of approach may be useful in conjunction with other drug- and diet-based therapies (see Calder and Miles, 2000). Broughton *et al.* (1997) compared the effects of low-dose and high-dose fish oil in adult atopic asthmatics; the actual amount of fish oil each patient consumed was calculated according to their regular n-6 PUFA intake, such that the ratio of n-6 to n-3 fatty acid in the diet was 10:1 (low fish oil) or 2:1 (high fish oil). At baseline and after each treatment period (i.e. with low and then high fish oil), lung function was measured in response to increasing doses of methacholine. With low n-3 fatty acid ingestion, methacholine-induced respiratory distress increased. In contrast, high n-3 fatty acid ingestion resulted in improved lung function in more than 40% of subjects; all measures of respiratory function were improved in this group of patients, who also showed a markedly elevated appearance of the EPA-derived 5-series LT in their urine. However, some patients did not respond to the high n-3 polyunsaturated fatty acid intake, which in some cases worsened respiratory function. This study suggests that there may be asthmatic subjects who respond positively to fish oil intervention but others whose response may be worsened by such a dietary intervention. Thus, this therapy should be approached cautiously until more is known about the factors that determine sensitivity to n-3 PUFAs.

Endotoxaemia, sepsis and trauma

The importance of a hyperinflammatory response, characterized by overproduction of TNF-α, IL-1β, IL-6 and IL-8, in the progression of trauma patients towards sepsis is now recognized. Enhanced production of arachidonic acid-derived eicosanoids, such as PGE$_2$, is also associated with trauma and burns. The inflammatory effects of infection can be mimicked by administration of endotoxin (bacterial lipopolysaccharide). Essential fatty acid deficiency in rats increased mortality after endotoxin challenge (Cook *et al.*, 1981). Arachidonic acid administration increased mortality following endotoxin (Cook *et al.*, 1981), while feeding a high linoleic acid diet increased mortality in guinea pigs recovering from burns injury (Alexander *et al.*, 1986). Fish oil feeding or infusions enhanced the survival of guinea pigs following endotoxin challenge (Mascioli *et al.*, 1988, 1989) and decreased the accompanying metabolic perturbations in guinea pigs and rats (for references, see Calder, 1997). Mice fed fish oil and then injected with endotoxin had lower plasma TNF-α, IL-β and IL-6 concentrations than mice fed safflower oil (Sadeghi *et al.*, 1999), while fish oil-containing parenteral nutrition decreased serum TNF-α, IL-6 and IL-8 concentrations in burned rats (Hayashi *et al.*, 1998; Tashiro *et al.*, 1998). Total parenteral nutrition using fish oil as the lipid source was found to prevent the endotoxin-induced reduction in blood flow to the gut and to reduce the number of viable bacteria in mesenteric lymph nodes and liver following exposure to live bacteria (Pscheidl *et al.*, 2000). Fish oil did not, however, decrease bacterial translocation across the gut and the authors concluded that fish oil must have improved bacterial killing. Fish oil administration prior to exposure to live pathogens decreased the mortality of rats compared with vegetable oil (Barton *et al.*, 1991; Rayon *et al.*, 1997). These studies did not measure inflammatory cytokine levels, but they showed that PGE$_2$ levels were decreased by fish oil (Barton *et al.*, 1991; Rayon *et al.*, 1997). More recently, fish oil infusion after induction of sepsis by caecal ligation and puncture in rats was shown to decrease mortality (and PGE$_2$ production) compared with vegetable oil (Lanza-Jacoby *et al.*, 2001).

An understanding of the inflammatory changes occurring during sepsis and of the anti-inflammatory effects of fish oil, combined with the outcome of these animal experiments, has prompted clinical studies investigating the influence of fish oil administered either parenterally or enterally. Patients receiving parenteral fish oil following major abdominal surgery had lower serum concentrations of TNF-α and IL-6 than those receiving a control mix (Wachtler *et al.*, 1997). This study did not report clinical outcome. A large number of clinical trials (at least 20) have been performed in intensive care or surgical patients using enteral formulae containing n-3 PUFAs. The majority of these trials have used the commercially available product IMPACT®, which contains arginine, yeast RNA and n-3 PUFAs. Many of these trials report beneficial outcomes, including decreased numbers of infections and infectious or wound complications, decreased severity of infection, decreased need for mechanical ventilation, decreased progression to systemic inflammatory response syndrome and decreased length of intensive-care unit and/or total hospital stay. A comprehensive meta-analysis of 15 randomized, controlled studies using IMPACT® or Immun-Aid® (also rich in arginine, RNA and n-3 PUFAs) has been performed (Beale *et al.*, 1999). This analysis confirmed significant reductions in infection rate, number of ventilator days and length of hospital stay, but not in overall mortality. Few of the studies reviewed measured immune outcomes. However, some other studies of IMPACT®, not included in the meta-analysis, did so, focusing especially on inflammatory cytokines. Several of these studies show decreased circulating TNF-α and/or IL-6 concentrations in patients given IMPACT® or similar formulae before (Braga *et al.*, 1999; Gianotti *et al.*, 1999; Tepaske *et al.*, 2001) or after (Braga *et al.*, 1996; Wu *et al.*, 2001) major surgery. Although these observations fit with the predicted effects of n-3 PUFAs and could be used as evidence of their efficacy in the trauma and post-surgery settings, the complex nature of the formulae prevents such a clear interpretation. The effects could be due to any one of the specified nutrients (i.e. arginine, RNA, n-3 PUFAs) or to a combination of these nutrients. Indeed, the positive outcomes from the use of IMPACT® and similar formulae have often been used as evidence for the benefit of arginine in these settings (see Duff and Daly, Chapter 5, this volume).

Cancer

The immune system obviously plays an important role in anti-cancer defence. There is a progressive decrease in many immune surveillance defences in animal models of cancer (Shewchuk *et al.*, 1996) and in humans with cancer (Keissling *et al.*, 1999). A major focus of current research in immunology and oncology is the development of methods to augment host antitumour immune defences. Feeding fish oil to experimental animals protects against the development of carcinogen-induced mammary tumours, reduces the growth of mammary tumours and prevents the development of cachexia and metastatic diseases (see Cave, 1991). Although dietary fat can modulate anti-cancer defences, such as natural killer cell cytotoxicity and humoral and T-cell responses, the application of studies in healthy humans and animals to the cancer state may not be as straightforward. The influence of dietary n-3 PUFAs on the immune response may be different between healthy animals and those with suppressed immune systems (Robinson *et al.*, 2001, 2002). Tumour-bearing rats fed long-chain n-3 PUFAs as part of a low-PUFA diet had significantly increased natural killer cell cytotoxicity, a higher proportion of CD8+ and CD28+ cells that were activated (i.e. expressing CD25) and increased nitric oxide and IL-2 production after mitogen stimulation, whereas these immune enhancements were not found when n-3 PUFAs were supplemented in a high-PUFA diet.

Conclusions

Several fatty acids can potentially exert effects on inflammation and immunity. Arachidonic acid gives rise to inflammatory mediators (eicosanoids) and through these regulates the activities of inflammatory cells, the Th1 versus Th2 balance and B-cell function. It is generally considered that n-3 PUFAs act as arachidonic acid antagonists. As such, among the fatty acids, it is the n-3 PUFAs that are believed to possess the most potent immunomodulatory activities, and, among the n-3 fatty acids, those from fish oil (EPA and DHA) are more biologically potent than α-linolenic acid. Components of both natural and acquired immunity, including the production of key inflammatory mediators, can be affected by n-3 PUFAs. Although some of the effects of n-3 fatty acids may be brought about by modulation of the amount and types of eicosanoids made, it is possible that these fatty acids might exert some of their effects by eicosanoid-independent mechanisms, including actions upon intracellular signalling pathways and transcription-factor activity. There is some evidence that n-3 fatty-acid-induced effects may be of use as a therapy for acute and chronic inflammation and for disorders that involve an inappropriately activated immune response. However, more needs to be understood about the effects of individual fatty acids against different backgrounds (e.g. levels and types of fat in the diet), about the dose-response effects of n-3 PUFAs, about interactions between PUFAs and other dietary components, especially antioxidant vitamins, and about the differences in immune effects of fatty acids between health and disease.

References

Alexander, J.W. (1998) Immunonutrition: the role of ω-3 fatty acids. *Nutrition* 14, 627–633.

Alexander, J.W., Saito, H., Trocki, O. and Ogle, C.K. (1986) The importance of lipid type in the diet after burn injury. *Annals of Surgery* 204, 1–8.

Arm, J.P., Horton, C.E., Mencia-Huerta, J.M., House, F., Eiser, N.M., Clarke, T.S.H., Spur, B.W. and Lee, T.H. (1988) Effect of dietary supplementation with fish oil lipids on mild asthma. *Thorax* 43, 84–92.

Arm, J.P., Horton, C.E., Spur, B.W., Mencia-Huerta, J.M. and Lee, T.H. (1989) The effects of dietary supplementation with fish oil lipids on the airways response to inhaled allergen in bronchial asthma. *American Review of Respiratory Disease* 139, 1395–1400.

Badwey, J.A., Curnutte, J.T. and Karnovsky, M.L. (1981) Cis-polyunsaturated fatty acids induce high levels of superoxide production by human neutrophils. *Journal of Biological Chemistry* 256, 12640–12643.

Badwey, J.A., Curnutte, J.T., Robinson, J.M., Berde, C.B., Karnovsky, M.J. and Karnovsky, M.L. (1984) Effects of free fatty acids on release of superoxide and on change of shape by human neutrophils. *Journal of Biological Chemistry* 259, 7870–7877.

Barone, J., Hebert, J.R. and Reddy, M.M. (1989) Dietary fat and natural killer cell activity. *American Journal of Clinical Nutrition* 50, 861–867.

Barton, R.G., Wells, C.L., Carlson, A., Singh, R., Sullivan, J.J. and Cerra, F.B. (1991) Dietary omega-3 fatty acids decrease mortality and Kupffer cell prostaglandin E_2 production in a rat model of chronic sepsis. *Journal of Trauma* 31, 768–774.

Beale, R.J., Bryg, D.J. and Bihari, D.J. (1999) Immunonutrition in the critically ill: a systematic review of clinical outcome. *Critical Care Medicine* 27, 2799–2805.

Belluzzi, A. and Miglio, F. (1998) *n-3* Fatty acids in the treatment of Crohn's disease. In: Kremer, J. (ed.) *Medicinal Fatty Acids in Inflammation.* Birkhauser Verlag, Basle, pp. 91–101.

Berthou, L., Saladin, R., Yaqoob, P., Branellec, D., Calder, P., Fruchart, J.-C., Denefle, P., Auwerx, J. and Staels, B. (1995) Regulation of rat liver apolipoprotein A-I, apoliporotein A-II and acyl CoA oxidase gene expression by fibrates and dietary fatty acids. *European Journal of Biochemistry* 232, 179–187.

Bialick, R., Gill, R., Berke, G. and Clark, W.R. (1984) Modulation of cell-mediated cytotoxicity function after alteration of fatty acid composition *in vitro. Journal of Immunology* 132, 81–87.

Billiar, T., Bankey, P., Svingen, B., Curran, R.D., West, M.A., Holman, R.T., Simmons, R.L. and Cerra, F.B. (1988) Fatty acid uptake and Kupffer cell function: fish oil alters eicosanoid and monokine production to endotoxin stimulation. *Surgery* 104, 343–349.

Blok, W.L., Katan, M.B. and van der Meer, J.W.M. (1996) Modulation of inflammation and cytokine production by dietary (*n-3*) fatty acids. *Journal of Nutrition* 126, 1515–1533.

Blok, W.L., Deslypere, J.-P., Demacker, P.N.M., van der Ven-Jongekrijg, J., Hectors, M.P.C., van der Meer, J.M.W. and Katan, M.B. (1997) Pro- and anti-inflammatory cytokines in healthy volunteers fed various doses of fish oil for 1 year. *European Journal of Clinical Investigation* 27, 1003–1008.

Bofill, M., Akbar, A.N., Salmon, M., Robinson, M., Burford, G. and Janossy, G. (1994) Immature CD45RA[low]RO[low] T cells in the human cord blood. 1. Antecedents of CD45RA[+] unprimed T cells. *Journal of Immunology* 152, 5613–5623.

Braga, M., Vignali, A., Gianotti, L., Cestari, A., Profili, M. and Di Carlo, V. (1996) Immune and nutritional effects of early enteral nutrition after major abdominal operations. *European Journal of Surgery* 162, 105–112.

Braga, M., Gianotti, L., Radaelli, G., Vignali, A., Mari, G., Gentilini, O. and Di Carlo, V. (1999) Perioperative immunonutrition in patients undergoing cancer surgery. *Archives of Surgery* 134, 428–433.

British Nutrition Foundation (1999) *Briefing Paper* on n-3 *Fatty Acids and Health.* British Nutrition Foundation, London.

Brouard, C. and Pascaud, M. (1990) Effects of moderate dietary supplementations with n-3 fatty acids on macrophage and lymphocyte phospholipids and macrophage eicosanoid synthesis in the rat. *Biochimica et Biophysica Acta* 1047, 19–28.

Brouard, C. and Pascaud, M. (1993) Modulation of rat and human lymphocyte function by n-6 and n-3 polyunsaturated fatty acids and acetylsalicylic acid. *Annals of Nutrition and Metabolism* 37, 146–159.

Broughton, K.S., Johnson, C.S., Pace, B.K., Liebman, M. and Kleppinger, K.M. (1997) Reduced asthma symptoms with *n-3* fatty acid ingestion are related to 5-series leucotriene production. *American Journal of Clinical Nutrition* 65, 1011–1017.

Byleveld, P.M., Pang, G.T., Clancy, R.L. and Roberts, D.C.K. (1999) Fish oil feeding delays influenza virus clearance and impairs production of interferon-γ and virus-specific immunoglobulin A in lungs of mice. *Journal of Nutrition* 129, 328–335.

Calder, P.C. (1996) Immunomodulatory and anti-inflammatory effects of *n-3* polyunsaturated fatty acids. *Proceedings of the Nutrition Society* 55, 737–774.

Calder, P.C. (1997) *N-3* polyunsaturated fatty acids and cytokine production in health and disease. *Annals of Nutrition and Metabolism* 41, 203–234.

Calder, P.C. (1998a) Dietary fatty acids and the immune system. *Nutrition Reviews* 56, S70–S83.

Calder, P.C. (1998b) Dietary fatty acids and lymphocyte functions. *Proceedings of the Nutrition Society* 57, 487–502.

Calder, P.C. (1998c) *N-3* fatty acids and mononuclear phagocyte function. In: Kremer, J.M. (ed) *Medicinal Fatty Acids in Inflammation*. Birkhauser Verlag, Basle, pp. 1–27.

Calder, P.C. (2001a) Polyunsaturated fatty acids, inflammation and immunity. *Lipids* 36, 1007–1024.

Calder, P.C. (2001b) The effect of dietary fatty acids on the immune response and susceptibility to infection. In: Suskind, R.M. and Tontisirin, K. (eds) *Nutrition, Immunity, and Infection in Infants and Children*. Lippincott Williams and Wilkins, Philadelphia, pp. 137–172.

Calder, P.C. (2001c) N-3 polyunsaturated fatty acids, inflammation and immunity: pouring oil on troubled waters or another fishy tale? *Nutrition Research* 21, 309–341.

Calder, P.C. (2001d) *N-3* Fatty acids and rheumatoid arthritis. In: Ransley, J.K., Donnelly, J.K. and Read, N.W. (eds) *Food and Nutritional Supplements in Health and Disease*. Springer Verlag, London, pp. 175–197.

Calder, P.C. and Miles, E.A. (2000) Fatty acids and atopic disease. *Pediatric Allergy and Immunology* 11 (Suppl.), 29–36.

Calder, P.C. and Zurier, R.B. (2001) Polyunsaturated fatty acids and rheumatoid arthritis. *Current Opinion in Clinical Nutrition and Metabolic Care* 4, 115–121.

Calder, P.C., Bond, J.A., Harvey, D.J., Gordon, S. and Newsholme, E.A. (1990) Uptake of saturated and unsaturated fatty acids into macrophage lipids and their effect upon macrophage adhesion and phagocytosis. *Biochemical Journal* 269, 807–814.

Calder, P.C., Bevan, S.J. and Newsholme, E.A. (1992) The inhibition of T-lymphocyte proliferation by fatty acids is via an eicosanoid-independent mechanism. *Immunology* 75, 108–115.

Calder, P.C., Yaqoob, P., Harvey, D.J., Watts, A. and Newsholme, E.A. (1994) The incorporation of fatty acids by lymphocytes and the effect on fatty acid composition and membrane fluidity. *Biochemical Journal* 300, 509–518.

Calder, P.C., Yaqoob, P., Thies, F., Wallace, F.A. and Miles, E.A. (2002) Fatty acids and lymphocyte functions. *British Journal of Nutrition*, 87, S31–S48.

Caughey, G.E., Mantzioris, E., Gibson, R.A., Cleland, L.G. and James, M.J. (1996) The effect on human tumor necrosis factor α and interleukin 1β production of diets enriched in *n-3* fatty acids from vegetable oil or fish oil. *American Journal of Clinical Nutrition* 63, 116–122.

Cavadini, C., Siega-Riz, A.M. and Popkin, B.M. (2000) US adolescent food intake trends from 1965 to 1996. *Archives of Diseases in Childhood* 83, 18–24.

Cave, W.T. Jr (1991) Dietary n-3 (w-3) polyunsaturated fatty acid effects on animal tumorigenesis. *FASEB Journal* 5, 2160–2165.

Chandrasekar, B. and Fernandes, G. (1994) Decreased pro-inflammatory cytokines and increased antioxidant enzyme gene expression by ω-3 lipids in murine lupus nephritis. *Biochemical and Biophysical Research Communications* 200, 893–898.

Chinetti, G., Griglio, S., Antonucci, M., Torra, I.P., Delerive, P., Majd, Z., Fruchart, J.C., Chapman, J., Najib, J. and Staels, B. (1998) Activation of peroxisome-activated receptors alpha and gamma induces apoptosis of human monocyte-derived macrophages. *Journal of Biological Chemistry* 273, 25573–25580.

Chinetti, G., Fruchart, J.C. and Staels, B. (2000) Peroxisome proliferator-activated receptors (PPARs): nuclear receptors at the crossroads between lipid metabolism and inflammation. *Inflammation Research* 49, 497–505.

Cifone, M.G., Botti, D., Festuccia, C., Napolitano, T., del Grosso, E., Cavallo, G., Chessa, M.A. and Santoni, A. (1993) Involvement of phospholipase A2 activation and arachidonic acid metabolism in the cytotoxic functions of rat NK cells. *Cellular Immunology* 148, 247–258.

Clandinin, M.T., Cheema, S., Field, C.J., Garg, M.L., Venkatraman, J. and Clandinin, T.R. (1991) Dietary fat: exogenous determination of membrane structure and cell function. *FASEB Journal* 5, 2761–2769.

Clarke, S.D. and Jump, D.B. (1994) Dietary polyunsaturated fatty acid regulation of gene transcription. *Annual Review in Nutrition* 14, 83–98.

Cook, J.A., Wise, W.C., Knapp, D.R. and Haslishka, P.V. (1981) Essential fatty acid deficient rats: a new model for evaluating arachidonate metabolism in shock. *Advances in Shock Research* 6, 93–105.

Cooper, A.L., Gibbons, L., Horan, M.A., Little, R.A. and Rothwell, N.J. (1993) Effect of dietary fish oil supplementation on fever and cytokine production in human volunteers. *Clinical Nutrition* 12, 321–328.

Curtis, C.L., Hughes, C.E., Flannery, C.R., Little, C.B., Harwood, J.L. and Caterson, B. (2000) n-3 Fatty acids specifically modulate catabolic factors involved in articular cartilage degradation. *Journal of Biological Chemistry* 275, 721–724.

de Caterina, R. and Libby, P. (1996) Control of endothelial leucocyte adhesion molecules by fatty acids. *Lipids* 31, S57–S63.

Delerive, P., Fruchart, J.C. and Staels, B. (2001) Peroxisome proliferator-activated receptors in inflammation control. *Journal of Endocrinology* 169, 453–459.

de Pablo, M.A. and Alvarezde Cienfuegos, G. (2000) Modulatory effects of dietary lipids on immune system functions. *Immunology and Cell Biology* 78, 31–39.

Department of Health (1994) *Nutritional Aspects of Cardiovascular Disease. Report of the Cardiovascular Review Group Committee on Medical Aspects of Food Policy.* HMSO, London.

Devchand, P.R., Keller, H., Peters, J.M., Vazquez, M., Gonzalez, F.J. and Wahli, W. (1996) The PPARα–leucotriene B4 pathway to inflammation control. *Nature* 384, 39–43.

Dry, J. and Vincent, D. (1991) Effect of fish oil diet on asthma – results of a 1-year double-blind study. *International Archives of Allergy and Applied Immunology* 95, 156–157.

Endres, S., Ghorbani, R., Kelley, V.E., Georgilis, K., Lonnemann, G., van der Meer, J.M.W., Cannon, J.G., Rogers, T.S., Klempner, M.S., Weber, P.C., Schaeffer, E.J., Wolff, S.M. and Dinarello, C.A. (1989) The effect of dietary supplementation with *n-3* polyunsaturated fatty acids on the synthesis of interleukin-1 and tumor necrosis factor by mononuclear cells. *New England Journal of Medicine* 320, 265–271.

Endres, S., Meydani, S.N., Ghorbani, R., Schindler, R. and Dinarello, C.A. (1993) Dietary supplementation with *n-3* fatty acids suppresses interleukin-2 production and mononuclear cell proliferation. *Journal of Leukocyte Biology* 54, 599–603.

Ferber, E., De Pasquale, G.G. and Resch, K. (1975) Phospholipid metabolism of stimu-
    lated lymphocytes – composition of phospholipid fatty acids. *Biochimica et
    Biophysica Acta* 398, 364–376.
Fernandes, G., Chandrasekar, B., Venkatraman, J., Tomar, V. and Zhao, W. (1994)
    Increased transforming growth factor beta and decreased oncogene expression by
    omega-3 fatty acids in the spleen delays the onset of autoimmune disease in BB/W
    mice. *Journal of Immunology* 152, 5979-5987.
Fernandes, G., Troyer, D.A. and Jolly, C.A. (1998) The effects of dietary lipids on gene
    expression and apoptosis. *Proceedings of the Nutrition Society* 57, 543–550.
Field, C.J., Thomson, C.A., Van Aerde, J.E., Parrot, A., Euler, A.R. and Clandinin, M.T.
    (2000) The lower proportion of CD45RO+ cells and deficient IL-10 production by
    formula-fed infants, as compared to human-fed infants, is corrected with supplmen-
    tation of long chain-polyunsaturated fatty acids. *Journal of Pediatric
    Gastroenterology and Nutrition* 31, 291–299.
Field, C.J., Clandinin, M.T. and van Aerde, J.E. (2001) Polyunsaturated fatty acids and
    T-cell function: implications for the neonate. *Lipids* 36, 1025–1032.
Fisher, M., Levine, P.H., Weiner, B.H., Johnson, M.H., Doyle, E.M., Ellis, P.A. and
    Hoogasian, J.J. (1990) Dietary n-3 fatty acid supplementation reduces superoxide
    production and chemiluminescence in a monocyte-enriched preparation of leuco-
    cytes. *American Journal of Clinical Nutrition* 51, 804–808.
Fowler, K.H., McMurray, D.N., Fan, Y.Y., Aukema, H.M. and Chapkin, R.S. (1993)
    Purified dietary n-3 polyunsaturated fatty acids alter diacylglycerol mass and molec-
    ular species composition in concanavalin A-stimulated murine splenocytes.
    Biochimica et Biophysica Acta 1210, 89–96.
Fujikawa, M., Yamashita, N., Yamazaki, K., Sugiyama, E., Suzuki, H. and Hamazaki, T.
    (1992) Eicosapentaenoic acid inhibits antigen-presenting cell function of murine
    splenocytes. *Immunology* 75, 330–335.
Gallai, V., Sarchielli, P., Trequattrini, A., Franceschini, M., Floridi, A., Firenze, C., Alberti,
    A., Di Benedetto, D. and Stragliotto, E. (1993) Cytokine secretion and eicosanoid
    production in the peripheral blood mononuclear cells of MS patients undergoing
    dietary supplementation with *n-3* polyunsaturated fatty acids. *Journal of
    Neuroimmunology* 56, 143–153.
Geusens, P.P. (1998) *n-3* Fatty acids in the treatment of rheumatoid arthritis. In: Kremer,
    J.M. (ed.) *Medicinal Fatty Acids in Inflammation*. Birkhauser Verlag, Basle,
    pp. 111–123.
Gianotti, L., Braga, M., Fortis, C., Soldini, L., Vignali, A., Colombo, S., Radaelli, G. and
    Di Carlo, V. (1999) A prospective, randomised clinical trial on perioperative feeding
    with an arginine-, omega-3 fatty acid-, and RNA-enriched enteral diet: effect on
    host response and nutritional status. *Journal of Parenteral and Enteral Nutrition* 23,
    314–320.
Gibney, M.J. and Hunter, B. (1993) The effects of short- and long-term supplementa-
    tion with fish oil on the incorporation of *n-3* polyunsaturated fatty acids into cells of
    the immune system in healthy volunteers. *European Journal of Clinical Nutrition*
    47, 255–259.
Grimble, R.F. (1998) Dietary lipids and the inflammatory response. *Proceedings of the
    Nutrition Society* 57, 535–542.
Grimble, R.F. and Tappia, P.S. (1995) The modulatory influence of unsaturated fatty
    acid in the biology of tumour necrosis factor. *Biochemical Society Transactions* 287,
    282–286.
Harbige, L.S. (1998) Dietary *n-6* and *n-3* fatty acids in immunity and autoimmune dis-
    ease. *Proceedings of the Nutrition Society* 57, 555–562.

Hardy, S.J., Robinson, B.S., Poulos, A., Harvey, D.P., Ferrante, A. and Murray, A.W. (1991) The neutrophil respiratory burst: response to fatty acids, N-formylmethionylleucyl phenylalanine and phorbol ester suggest divergent signalling mechanisms. *European Journal of Biochemistry* 198, 801–806.

Hayashi, N., Tashiro, T., Yamamori, H., Takagi, K., Morishima, Y., Otsubo, Y., Sugiura, T., Furukawa, K., Nitta, H., Nakajima, N., Suzuki, N. and Ito, I. (1998) Effects of intravenous omega-3 and omega-6 fat emulsion on cytokine production and delayed type hypersensitivity in burned rats receiving total parenteral nutrition. *Journal of Parenteral and Enteral Nutrition* 22, 363–367.

Healy, D., Wallace, F.A., Miles, E.A., Calder, P.C. and Newsholme, P. (2000) The effect of low to moderate amounts of dietary fish oil on neutrophil lipid composition and function. *Lipids* 35, 763–768.

Hebert, J.R., Barone, J., Reddy, M.M. and Backlund, J.Y. (1990) Natural killer cell activity in a longitudinal dietary fat intervention trial. *Clinical Immunology and Immunopathology* 54, 103–116.

Huang, S.-C., Misfeldt, M.L. and Fritsche, K.L. (1992) Dietary fat influences Ia antigen expression and immune cell populations in the murine peritoneum and spleen. *Journal of Nutrition* 122, 1219–1231.

Hubbard, N.E., Somers, S.D. and Erickson, K.L. (1991) Effect of dietary fish oil on development and selected functions of murine inflammatory macrophages. *Journal of Leukocyte Biology* 49, 592–598.

Hughes, D.A. (1998) *In vitro* and *in vivo* effects of n-3 polyunsaturated fatty acids on human monocyte function. *Proceedings of the Nutrition Society* 57, 521–525.

Hughes, D.A. and Pinder, A.C. (2000) n-3 polyunsaturated fatty acids inhibit the antigen-presenting function of human monocytes. *American Journal of Clinical Nutrition* 71, 357S–360S.

Hughes, D.A., Pinder, A.C., Piper, Z., Johnson, I.T. and Lund, E.K. (1996) Fish oil supplementation inhibits the expression of major histocompatibility complex class II molecules and adhesion molecules on human monocytes. *American Journal of Clinical Nutrition* 63, 267–272.

Jackson, S.M., Parhami, F., Xi, X.-P., Berliner, J.A., Hsueh, W.A., Law, R.E. and Demer, L.L. (1999) Peroxisome proliferator-activated receptor activators target human endothelial cells to inhibit leucocyte-endothelial cell interaction. *Arteriosclerosis, Thrombosis and Vascular Biology* 19, 2094–2104.

James, M.J. and Cleland, L.G. (1997) Dietary n-3 fatty acids and therapy for rheumatoid arthritis. *Seminars in Arthritis and Rheumatism* 27, 85–97.

James, M.J., Gibson, R.A. and Cleland, L.G. (2000) Dietary polyunsaturated fatty acids and inflammatory mediator production. *American Journal of Clinical Nutrition* 71, 343S–348S.

Jeffery, N.M., Sanderson, P., Sherrington, E.J., Newsholme, E.A. and Calder, P.C. (1996) The ratio of n-6 to n-3 polyunsaturated fatty acids in the rat diet alters serum lipid levels and lymphocyte functions. *Lipids* 31, 737–745.

Jeffery, N.M., Newsholme, E.A. and Calder, P.C. (1997) The level of polyunsaturated fatty acids and the n-6 to n-3 polyunsaturated fatty acid ratio in the rat diet both affect serum lipid levels and lymphocyte functions. *Prostaglandins, Leukotrienes and Essential Fatty Acids* 57, 149–160.

Jenski, L.J., Bowker, G.M., Johnson, M.A., Ehringer, W.D., Fetterhoff, T. and Stillwell, W. (1995) Docosahexaenoic acid-induced alteration of Thy-1 and CD8 expression on murine splenocytes. *Biochimica et Biophysica Acta* 1236, 39–50.

Jiang, C.Y., Ting, A.T. and Seed, B. (1998) PPAR-gamma agonists inhibit production of monocyte inflammatory cytokines. *Nature* 391, 82–86.

Jolly, C.A., Jiang, Y.-H., Chapkin, R.S. and McMurray, D.N. (1997) Dietary (n-3) polyunsaturated fatty acids suppress murine lymphoproliferation, interleukin-2 secretion and the formation of diacylglycerol and ceramide. *Journal of Nutrition* 127, 37–43.

Jonnalagadda, S.S., Egan, S.K., Heimbach, J.T., Harris, S.S. and Kris-Etherton, P.M. (1995) Fatty acid consumption pattern of Americans: 1987–1988 USDA Nationwide Food Consumption Survey. *Nutrition Research* 15, 1767–1781.

Keissling, R., Wasserman, K., Horiguchi, S., Kono, K., Sjoberg, J., Pisa, P. and Petersson, M. (1999) Tumor-induced immune dysfunction. *Cancer Immunology and Immunotherapy* 48, 353-362.

Kelley, D.S. and Daudu, P.A. (1993) Fat intake and immune response. *Progress in Food and Nutrition Science* 17, 41–63.

Kelley, D.S., Branch, L.B. and Iacono, J.M. (1989) Nutritional modulation of human immune status. *Nutrition Research* 9, 965–975.

Kelley, D.S., Branch, L.B., Love, J.E., Taylor, P.C., Rivera, Y.M. and Iacono, J.M. (1991) Dietary alpha-linolenic acid and immunocompetence in humans. *American Journal of Clinical Nutrition* 53, 40–46.

Kelley, D.S., Dougherty, R.M., Branch, L.B., Taylor, P.C. and Iacono, J.M. (1992) Concentration of dietary n-6 polyunsaturated fatty acids and human immune status. *Clinical Immunology and Immunopathology* 62, 240–244.

Kelley, V.E., Ferretti, A., Izui, S. and Strom, T.B. (1985) A fish oil diet rich in eicosapentaenoic acid reduces cyclooxygenase metabolites and suppresses lupus in MRL-lpr mice. *Journal of Immunology* 134, 1914–1919.

Kennedy, E.T., Bowman, S.A. and Powell, R. (1999) Dietary-fat intake in the US population. *Journal of the American College of Nutrition* 18, 207–212.

Khair-el-Din, T., Sicher, S.C., Vazquez, M.A., Chung, G.W., Stallwort, K.A., Kitamura, K., Miller, R.T. and Lu, C.Y. (1996) Transcription of the murine iNOS gene is inhibited by docosahexaenoic acid, a major constituent of fetal and neonatal sera as well as fish oils. *Journal of Experimental Medicine* 183, 1241–1246.

Kinsella, J.E., Lokesh, B., Broughton, S. and Whelan, J. (1990) Dietary polyunsaturated fatty acids and eicosanoids: potential effects on the modulation of inflammatory and immune cells: an overview. *Nutrition* 6, 24–44.

Kleemann, R., Scott, F.W., Worz-Pagenstert, U., Ratnayake, W.M.N. and Kolb, H. (1998) Impact of dietary fat on the Th1/Th2 cytokine gene expression in the pancreas and gut of diabetes-prone BB rats. *Journal of Autoimmunity* 11, 97–103.

Kleiwer, S.A., Lenhard, J.M., Willson, T.M., Patel, I., Morris, D.C. and Lehman, J.M. (1995) A prostaglandin J2 metabolite binds peroxisome proliferator-activated receptor γ and promotes adipocyte differentiation. *Cell* 83, 813–819.

Lanza-Jacoby, S., Flynn, J.T. and Miller, S. (2001) Parenteral supplementation with a fish oil emulsion prolongs survival and improves lymphocyte function during sepsis. *Nutrition* 17, 112–116.

Lee, T.H., Hoover, R.L., Williams, J.D., Sperling, R.I., Ravalese, J., Spur, B.W., Robinson, D.R., Corey, E.J., Lewis, R.A. and Austen, K.F. (1985) Effects of dietary enrichment with eicosapentaenoic acid and docosahexaenoic acid on *in vitro* neutrophil and monocyte leucotriene generation and neutrophil function. *New England Journal of Medicine* 312, 1217–1224.

Leslie, C.A., Gonnerman, W.A., Ullman, M.D., Hayes, K.C., Franzblau, C. and Cathcart, E.S. (1985) Dietary fish oil modulates macrophage fatty acids and decreases arthritis susceptibility in mice. *Journal of Experimental Medicine* 162, 1336–1349.

Lewis, R.A., Austen, K.F. and Soberman, R.J. (1990) Leukotrienes and other products of the 5-lipoxygenase pathway: biochemistry and relation to pathobiology in human diseases. *New England Journal of Medicine* 323, 645–655

Lo, C.J., Chiu, K.C., Fu, M., Lo, R. and Helton, S. (1999) Fish oil decreases macrophage tumor necrosis factor gene transcription by altering the NFkappaB activity. *Journal of Surgical Research* 82, 216–221.

Lokesh, B.R., Hseih, H.L. and Kinsella, J.E. (1986) Peritoneal macrophages from mice fed dietary (n-3) polyunsaturated fatty acids secrete low levels of prostaglandins. *Journal of Nutrition* 116, 2547–2552.

Luostarinen, R., Siegbahn, A. and Saldeen, T. (1992) Effect of dietary fish oil supplemented with different doses of vitamin E on neutrophil chemotaxis in healthy volunteers. *Nutrition Research* 12, 1419–1430.

Mann, N.J., Johnson, L.G., Warrick, G.E. and Sinclair, A.J. (1995) The arachidonic acid content of the Australian diet is lower than previously estimated. *Journal of Nutrition* 125, 2528–2535.

Marignani, P.A. and Sebaldt, R.J. (1995) Formation of second messenger diradylglycerol in murine peritoneal macrophages is altered after in vivo (n-3) polyunsaturated fatty acid supplementation. *Journal of Nutrition* 125, 3030–3040.

Marshall, L.A. and Johnston, P.V. (1985) The influence of dietary essential fatty acids on rat immunocompetent cell prostaglandin synthesis and mitogen-induced blastogenesis. *Journal of Nutrition* 115, 1572–1580.

Marx, N., Sukhova, G.K., Collins, T., Libby, P. and Plutzky, J. (1999) PPARα activators inhibit cytokine-induced vascular cell adhesion molecule-1 expression in human endothelial cells. *Circulation* 99, 3125–3131.

Mascioli, E.A., Leader, L., Flores, E., Trimbo, S., Bistrian, B. and Blackburn, G. (1988) Enhanced survival to endotoxin in guinea pigs fed iv fish oil emulsion. *Lipids* 23, 623–625.

Mascioli, E.A., Iwasa, Y., Trimbo, S., Leader, L., Bistrian, B.R. and Blackburn, G.L. (1989) Endotoxin challenge after menhaden oil diet: effects on survival of guinea pigs. *American Journal of Clinical Nutrition* 49, 277–282.

Meydani, S.N., Yogeeswaran, G., Liu, S., Baskar, S. and Meydani, M. (1988) Fish oil and tocopherol-induced changes in natural killer cell-mediated cytotoxicity and PGE$_2$ synthesis in young and old mice. *Journal of Nutrition* 118, 1245–1252.

Meydani, S.N., Endres, S., Woods, M.M., Goldin, B.R., Soo, C., Morrill-Labrode, A., Dinarello, C. and Gorbach, S.L. (1991) Oral (*n-3*) fatty acid supplementation suppresses cytokine production and lymphocyte proliferation: comparison between young and older women. *Journal of Nutrition* 121, 547–555.

Meydani, S.N., Lichtenstein, A.H., Cornwall, S., Meydani, M., Goldin, B.R., Rasmussen, H., Dinarello, C.A. and Schaefer, E.J. (1993) Immunologic effects of national cholesterol education panel step-2 diets with and without fish-derived *n-3* fatty acid enrichment. *Journal of Clinical Investigation* 92, 105–113.

Miles, E.A. and Calder, P.C. (1998) Modulation of immune function by dietary fatty acids. *Proceedings of the Nutrition Society* 57, 277–292.

Miles, E.A., Wallace, F.A. and Calder, P.C. (2000) Dietary fish oil reduces intercellular adhesion molecule 1 and scavenger receptor expression on murine macrophages. *Atherosclerosis* 152, 43–50.

Molvig, J., Pociot, F., Worsaae, H., Wogensen, L.D., Baek, L., Christensen, P., Mandrup-Poulsen, T., Andersen, K., Madsen, P., Dyerberg, J. and Nerup, J. (1991) Dietary supplementation with ω-3 polyunsaturated fatty acids decreases mononuclear cell proliferation and interleukin-1β content but not monokine secretion in healthy and insulin-dependent diabetic individuals. *Scandinavian Journal of Immunology* 34, 399–410.

Peterson, L.D., Jeffery, N.M., Thies, F., Sanderson, P., Newsholme, E.A. and Calder, P.C. (1998) Eicosapentaenoic and docosahexaenoic acids alter rat spleen leucocyte fatty acid composition and prostaglandin E_2 production but have different effects on lymphocyte functions and cell-mediated immunity. *Lipids* 33, 171–180.

Poynter, M.E. and Daynes, R.A. (1998) Peroxisome proliferator-activated receptor alpha activation modulates cellular redox status, represses nuclear factor kappa B signalling, and reduces inflammatory cytokine production in ageing. *Journal of Biological Chemistry* 273, 32833–32841.

Prickett, J.D., Robinson, D.R. and Steinberg, A.D. (1983) Effects of dietary enrichment with eicosapentaenoic acid upon autoimmune nephritis in female NZB × NZW/F1 mice. *Arthritis and Rheumatism* 26, 133–139.

Pscheidl, E., Schywalsky, M., Tschaikowsky, K. and Boke-Prols, T. (2000) Fish oil-supplemented parenteral diets normalize splanchnic blood flow and improve killing of translocated bacteria in a low-dose endotoxin rat model. *Critical Care Medicine* 28, 1489–1496.

Rayon, J.I., Carver, J.D., Wyble, L.E., Wiener, D., Dickey, S.S., Benford, V.J., Chen, L.T. and Lim, D.V. (1997) The fatty acid composition of maternal diet affects lung prostaglandin E_2 levels and survival from group B streptococcal sepsis in neonatal rat pups. *Journal of Nutrition* 127, 1989–1992.

Renier, G., Skamene, E., de Sanctis, J. and Radzioch, D. (1993) Dietary n-3 polyunsaturated fatty acids prevent the development of atherosclerotic lesions in mice: modulation of macrophage secretory activities. *Arteriosclerosis and Thombosis* 13, 1515–1524.

Resch, K., Gelfrand, E.W., Hansen, K. and Ferber, E. (1972) Lymphocyte activation: rapid changes in the phospholipid metabolism of plasma membranes during stimulation. *European Journal of Immunology* 2, 598–601.

Ricote, M., Li, A.C., Willson, T.M., Kelly, C.J. and Glass, C.K. (1998) The peroxisome proliferator-activated receptor-gamma is a negative regulator of macrophage activation. *Nature* 391, 79–82.

Robinson, D.R., Prickett, J.D., Polisson, R., Steinberg, A.D. and Levine, L. (1985) The protective effect of dietary fish oil on murine lupus. *Prostaglandins* 30, 51–75.

Robinson, D.R., Prickett, J.D., Makoul, G.T., Steinberg, A.D. and Colvin, R.B. (1986) Dietary fish oil reduces progression of established renal disease in (NZB × NZW)F1 mice and delays renal disease in BXSB and MRL/1 strains. *Arthritis and Rheumatism* 29, 539–546.

Robinson, D.R., Urakaze, M., Huang, R., Taki, H., Sugiyama, E., Knoell, C.T., Xu, L., Yeh, E.T.H. and Auron, P.E. (1996) Dietary marine lipids suppress continuous expression on interleukin-1β gene expression. *Lipids* 31, S23–S31.

Robinson, L.E. and Field, C.J. (1998) Dietary long chain (n-3) fatty acids facilitate immune cell activation in sedentary, but not exercise-trained rats. *Journal of Nutrition* 128, 498–504.

Robinson, L.E., Clandinin, M.T. and Field, C.J. (2001) R3230AC rat mammary tumor and dietary long-chain (n-3) fatty acids change immune cell composition and function during mitogen activation. *Journal of Nutrition* 131, 2021–2027.

Robinson, L.E., Clandinin, M.T. and Field, C.J. (2002) The role of dietary long chain n-3 fatty acids in membrane-mediated immune defence and R3230AC mammary tumor growth in rats: influence of dietary fat composition. *Breast Cancer Research and Treatment* 73, 145–160.

Rodgers, J.B. (1998) *n-3* Fatty acids in the treatment of ulcerative colitis. In: Kremer, J.M. (ed.) *Medicinal Fatty Acids in Inflammation*. Birkhauser Verlag, Basle, pp. 103–109.

Sadeghi, S., Wallace, F.A. and Calder, P.C. (1999) Dietary lipids modify the cytokine response to bacterial lipopolysaccharide in mice. *Immunology* 96, 404–410.

Sakata, A., Ida, E., Tominaga, M. and Onoue, K. (1987) Arachidonic acid acts as an intracellular activator of the NADPH oxidase in Fcgamma receptor mediated super-oxide generation in macrophages. *Journal of Immunology* 138, 4353–4359.

Sanderson, P. and Calder, P.C. (1998a) Dietary fish oil diminishes lymphocyte adhesion to macrophage and endothelial cell monolayers. *Immunology* 94, 79–87.

Sanderson, P. and Calder, P.C. (1998b) Dietary fish oil appears to inhibit the activation of phospholipase C-γ in lymphocytes. *Biochimica et Biophysica Acta* 1392, 300–308.

Sanderson, P., Yaqoob, P. and Calder, P.C. (1995) Effects of dietary lipid manipulation upon graft vs. host and host vs. graft responses in the rat. *Cellular Immunology* 164, 240–247.

Sanderson, P., MacPherson, G.G., Jenkins, C.H. and Calder, P.C. (1997) Dietary fish oil diminishes antigen presentation activity by rat dendritic cells. *Journal of Leukocyte Biology* 62, 771–777.

Sanderson, P., Thies, F. and Calder, P.C. (2000) Extracellular release of free fatty acids by rat T lymphocytes is stimulus-dependent and is affected by dietary lipid manipulation. *Cell Biochemistry and Function* 18, 47–58.

Santoli, D., Phillips, P.D., Colt, T.L. and Zurier, R.B. (1990) Suppression of interleukin-2-dependent human T-cell growth *in vitro* by prostaglandin E (PGE) and their precursor fatty acids. *Journal of Clinical Investigation* 85, 424–432.

Schmidt, E.B., Pedesen, J.O., Ekelund, S., Grunnet, N., Jersild, C. and Dyerberg, J. (1989) Cod liver oil inhibits neutrophil and monocyte chemotaxis in healthy males. *Atherosclerosis* 77, 53–57.

Schmidt, E.B., Varming, K., Pederson, J.O., Lervang, H.H., Grunnet, N., Jersild, C. and Dyerberg, J. (1992) Long term supplementation with *n-3* fatty acids. II. Effect on neutrophil and monocyte chemotaxis. *Scandinavian Journal of Clinical and Laboratory Investigations* 52, 229–236.

Schmidt, E.B., Varming, K., Moller, J.M., Bulow Pederson, I., Madsen, P. and Dyerberg, J. (1996) No effect of a very low dose of *n-3* fatty acids on monocyte function in healthy humans. *Scandinavian Journal of Clinical Investigation* 56, 87–92

Schoonjans, K., Staels, B. and Auwerx, J. (1996) The peroxisome proliferator activated receptors (PPARs) and their effects on lipid metabolism and adipocyte differentiation. *Biochimica et Biophysica Acta* 1302, 93–109.

Shewchuk, L.D., Baracos, V.E. and Field, C.J. (1996) Reduced splenocyte metabolism and immune function in rats implanted with the Morris-hepatoma 7777. *Metabolism* 45, 848–855.

Sinclair, A.J. and O'Dea, K. (1993) The significance of arachidonic acid in hunter-gatherer diets: implications for the contemporary Western diet. *Journal of Food Lipids* 1, 143–157.

Somers, S.D., Chapkin, R.S. and Erickson, K.L. (1989) Alteration of *in vitro* murine peritoneal macrophage function by dietary enrichment with eicosapentaenoic and docosahexaenoic acids in menhaden fish oil. *Cellular Immunology* 123, 201–211.

Soyland, E., Nenseter, M.S., Braathen, L. and Drevon, C.A. (1993) Very long chain n-3 and n-6 polyunsaturated fatty acids inhibit proliferation of human T lymphocytes *in vitro*. *European Journal of Clinical Investigation* 23, 112–121.

Sperling, R.I. (1998) The effects of *n-3* polyunsaturated fatty acids on neutrophils. *Proceedings of the Nutrition Society* 57, 527–534.

Sperling, R.I., Benincaso, A.I., Knoell, C.T., Larkin, J.K., Austen, K.F. and Robinson, D.R. (1993) Dietary ω-3 polyunsaturated fatty acids inhibit phosphoinositide formation and chemotaxis in neutrophils. *Journal of Clinical Investigation* 91, 651–660.

Stubbs, C.D. and Smith, A.D. (1984) The modification of mammalian membrane polyunsaturated fatty acid composition to membrane fluidity and function. *Biochimica et. Biophysica Acta* 779, 89–137.

Takano, H., Nagai, T., Asakawa, M., Toyozaki, T., Oka, T., Komuro, I., Saito, T. and Masuda, Y. (2000) Peroxisome proliferator-receptor activators inhibit lipopolysaccharide-induced tumor necrosis factor-alpha expression in neonatal rat cardiac myocytes. *Circulation Research* 87, 596–602.

Tashiro, T., Yamamori, H., Takagi, K., Hayashi, N., Furukawa, K. and Nakajima, N. (1998) N-3 versus n-6 polyunsaturated fatty acids in critical illness. *Nutrition* 14, 551–553.

Tepaske, R., te Velthuis, H., Oudemans-van Straaten, M., Heisterkamp, S.H., van Deventer, S.J.H., Ince, C., Eysman, L. and Keseciogu, J. (2001) Effect of preoperative oral immune-enhancing nutritional supplement on patients at risk of infection after cardiac surgery: a randomised placebo-controlled trial. *Lancet* 358, 696–701.

Thies, F., Nebe-von-Caron, G., Powell, J.R., Yaqoob, P., Newsholme, E.A. and Calder, P.C. (2001a) Dietary supplementation with eicosapentaenoic acid, but not with other long chain *n-3* or *n-6* polyunsaturated fatty acids, decreases natural killer cell activity in healthy subjects aged > 55 y. *American Journal of Clinical Nutrition* 73, 539–548.

Thies, F., Miles, E.A., Nebe-von-Caron, G., Powell, J.R., Hurst, T.L., Newsholme, E.A. and Calder, P.C. (2001b) Influence of dietary supplementation with long chain n-3 or n-6 polyunsaturated fatty acids on blood inflammatory cell populations and functions and on plasma soluble adhesion molecules in healthy adults. *Lipids* 36, 1183–1193.

Thies, F., Nebe-von-Caron, G., Powell, J.R., Yaqoob, P., Newsholme, E.A. and Calder, P.C. (2001c) Dietary supplementation with γ-linolenic acid or with fish oil decreases T lymphocyte proliferation in healthy older humans. *Journal of Nutrition* 131, 1918–1927.

Tilley, S.L., Coffman, T.M. and Koller, B.H. (2001) Mixed messages: modulation of inflammation and immune responses by prostaglandins and thromboxanes. *Journal of Clinical Investigation* 108, 15–23.

Venkatraman, J.T. and Chu, W.C. (1999) Effects of dietary omega-3 and omega-6 lipids and vitamin E on serum cytokines, lipid mediators and anti-DNA antibodies in a mouse model for rheumatoid arthritis. *Journal of the American College of Nutrition* 18, 602–613.

Vilaseca, J., Salas, A., Guarner, F., Rodriguez, R., Martinez, M. and Malagelada, J.-R. (1990) Dietary fish oil reduces progresssion of chronic inflammatory lesions in a rat model of granulomatous colitis. *Gut* 31, 539–544.

Volker, D. and Garg, M. (1996) Dietary *n-3* fatty acid supplementation in rheumatoid arthritis – mechanisms, clinical outcomes, controversies, and future directions. *Journal of Clinical Biochemistry and Nutrition* 20, 83–87.

Volker, D.H., FitzGerald, P.E.B. and Garg, M.L. (2000) The eicosapentaenoic to docosahexaenoic acid ratio of diets affects the pathogenesis of arthritis in Lew/SSN rats. *Journal of Nutrition* 130, 559–565.

Wachtler, P., Konig, W., Senkal, M., Kemen, M. and Koller, M. (1997) Influence of a total parenteral nutrition enriched with ω-3 fatty acids on leucotriene synthesis of peripheral leucocytes and systemic cytokine levels in patients with major surgery. *Journal of Trauma* 42, 191–198.

Wallace, F.A., Neely, S.J., Miles, E.A. and Calder, P.C. (2000) Dietary fats affect macrophage-mediated cytotoxicity towards tumour cells. *Immunology and Cell Biology* 78, 40–48.

Wallace, F.A., Miles, E.A., Evans, C., Stock, T.E., Yaqoob, P. and Calder, P.C. (2001) Dietary fatty acids influence the production of Th1- but not Th2-type cytokines. *Journal of Leukocyte Biology* 69, 449–457.

Wang, P., Anderson, P.O., Chen, S.W., Paulsson, K.M., Sjogren, H.O. and Li, S.L. (2001) Inhibition of the transcription factors AP-1 and NF-kappa B in CD4 T-cells by peroxisome proliferator-activated receptor gamma ligands. *International Immunopharmacology* 1, 803–812.

Wu, D. and Meydani, S.N. (1998) *n-3* Polyunsaturated fatty acids and immune function. *Proceedings of the Nutrition Society* 57, 503–509.

Wu, G.H., Zhang, Y.W. and Wu, Z.H. (2001) Modulation of postoperative immune and inflammatory response by immune-enhancing enteral diet in gastrointestinal cancer patients. *World Review of Gastroenterology* 7, 357–362.

Xi, S., Cohen, D., Barve, S. and Chen, L.H. (2001) Fish oil suppressed cytokines and nuclear factor kappaB induced by murine AIDS virus infection. *Nutrition Research* 21, 865–878.

Xu, X., Otsuki, M., Saito, H., Sumitani, S., Yamamoto, H., Asanuma, N., Kouhara, H. and Kasayama, S. (2001) PPAR alpha and GR differentially down-regulate the expression of nuclear factor-kappa B-responsive genes in vascular endothelial cells. *Endocrinology* 142, 3332–3339.

Yaqoob, P. (1998a) Lipids and the immune response. *Current Opinion in Clinical Nutrition and Metabolic Care* 1, 153–161.

Yaqoob, P. (1998b) Monounsaturated fats and immune function. *Proceedings of the Nutrition Society* 57, 511–520.

Yaqoob, P. and Calder, P.C. (1995) Effects of dietary lipid manipulation upon inflammatory mediator production by murine macrophages. *Cellular Immunology* 163, 120–128.

Yaqoob, P., Newsholme, E.A. and Calder, P.C. (1994a) Inhibition of natural killer cell activity by dietary lipids. *Immunology Letters* 41, 241–247.

Yaqoob, P., Newsholme, E.A. and Calder, P.C. (1994b) The effect of dietary lipid manipulation on rat lymphocyte subsets and proliferation. *Immunology* 82, 603–610.

Yaqoob, P., Newsholme, E.A. and Calder, P.C. (1995) Influence of cell culture conditions on diet-induced changes in lymphocyte fatty acid composition. *Biochimica et Biophysica Acta* 1255, 333–340.

Yaqoob, P., Pala, H.S., Cortina-Borja, M., Newsholme, E.A. and Calder, P.C. (2000) Encapsulated fish oil enriched in α-tocopherol alters plasma phospholipid and mononuclear cell fatty acid compositions but not mononuclear cell functions. *European Journal of Clinical Investigation* 30, 260–274.

Ziboh, V.A. (1998) The role of *n-3* fatty acids in psoriasis. In: Kremer, J.M. (ed.) *Medicinal Fatty Acids in Inflammation*. Birkhauser Verlag, Basle, pp. 45–53.

5 Arginine and Immune Function

MICHAEL D. DUFF AND JOHN M. DALY

Department of Surgery, New York Presbyterian Hospital, Weill Medical College of Cornell University and 525 East 68th Street, New York, NY 10021, USA

Introduction

Arginine is a semi-essential amino acid in mammals. While dietary arginine is not an absolute requirement under normal conditions, it can become essential at times of growth and metabolic stress, such as following trauma, sepsis or burn injuries. This dibasic amino acid is found in all mammalian cells and is an intermediate in many metabolic pathways from protein synthesis to energy storage to the clearance of nitrogenous waste. The importance of arginine for the normal functioning of the immune system has become progressively apparent over the last 15 years and has led to the development of arginine-supplemented enteral feeding regimes and the concept of immunonutrition (for a review, see Evoy *et al.*, 1998).

The Biochemistry of Arginine

The structure of the arginine molecule is shown in Fig. 5.1. It is the most basic of the amino acids, with a pK_a of 12.5, and, as such, contributes to the positive charge of proteins of which it is a component. The metabolic pathways involving arginine are complex and are outlined in Fig. 5.2. Adding to the complexity of these pathways is the varied location of the enzymes involved, both at the intracellular level (mitochondrial versus cytosolic enzymes) and between tissues. With the exception of enterocytes in neonates, no single cell type contains all the necessary enzymes for arginine synthesis (Wu and Morris, 1998).

Uptake and synthesis of arginine

Arginine is actively absorbed from the gut via a sodium-dependent transport mechanism. High arginase activity within enterocytes converts 40% of dietary

© CAB *International* 2002. *Nutrition and Immune Function*
(eds P.C. Calder, C.J. Field and H.S. Gill)

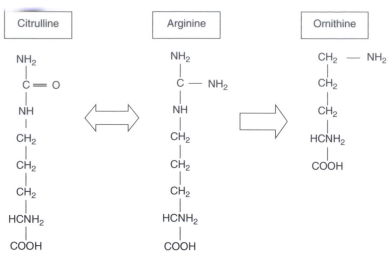

Fig. 5.1. The structures of citrulline, arginine and ornithine.

arginine to citrulline, which is released into the circulation (Castillo *et al.*, 1993). Of the arginine reaching the portal venous blood, 15% is cleared by the liver; the remainder enters the systemic circulation (O'Sullivan *et al.*, 1998). Dietary glutamine and glutamate can also be used by enterocytes to generate citrulline.

Arginine is synthesized from citrulline, primarily in the kidney, and is then released into the circulation to be taken up and used by other tissues. While arginine is also generated in large quantities by the liver, this arginine is recycled by the urea cycle within the hepatocyte, with little net production (Rabier *et al.*, 1991).

Nitric oxide pathway of arginine metabolism

No one molecule has attracted more attention in the last decade than nitric oxide (NO). This small molecule plays a pivotal role in a diverse range of functions, including vasodilatation, memory, peristalsis, penile erection, cytotoxicity and the control of various endocrine and exocrine secretions in the cardiovascular, reproductive, central nervous and immune systems (Nathan and Xie, 1994; MacMicking *et al.*, 1997). NO is synthesized from arginine by nitric oxide synthase (NOS), with the formation of citrulline. There are three known forms of this enzyme: neuronal (nNOS) and endothelial cell (ecNOS) NO synthases, which are both constitutively expressed and calcium-activated, and an inducible form (iNOS), which is controlled at the transcriptional level and is of most interest in the setting of the immune system.

iNOS expression, and hence NO production, is induced in macrophages in response to a variety of stimuli, particularly the T-helper-1 cytokines interferon (IFN)-γ and tumour necrosis factor (TNF)-α and the Gram-negative bacterial wall component endotoxin (lipopolysaccharide (LPS)). Inhibition of

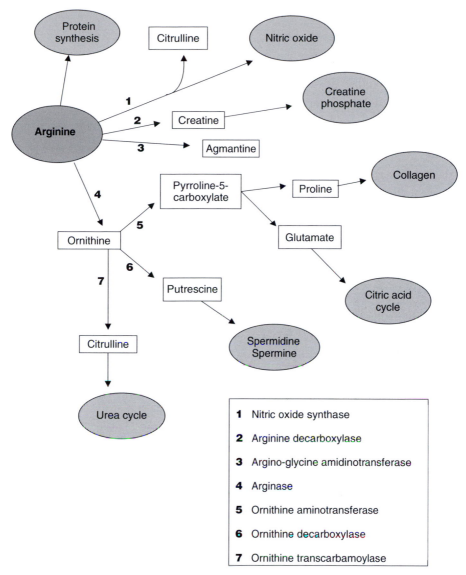

Fig. 5.2. A simplified outline of arginine metabolism, showing the major enzymes, intermediate molecules and end-points.

NO production increases the host susceptibility to viral, bacterial, fungal, protozoal and helminthic infections (MacMicking *et al.*, 1997). In addition, the anti-tumour activity of stimulated mouse macrophages is absent in iNOS knockout mice (Stuehr and Nathan, 1989). The mechanisms of NO cytotoxicity are complex, involving inhibition of DNA synthesis, mitochondrial inactivation, cell membrane lysis, cell cycle arrest, DNA strand break formation and induction of apoptosis (Burney *et al.*, 1997). In addition, NO can react with superoxide to form peroxynitrite, a powerful oxidizing agent capable of inducing cell injury and death (Samar *et al.*, 1997). Apart from its cytotoxic effects, NO is involved in regulating the expression of major histocompatibility complex (MHC) II expression in antigen-presenting cells, in modulating T-cell mitogenic responses and in the induction and suppression of many cytokines (Niedbala *et al.*, 1999; Akaike and Maeda, 2000). However, the full extent of NO involvement in the functioning of the immune system has yet to be established.

Arginase/ornithine pathways of arginine metabolism

Two forms of the arginase enzyme exist. While both forms catalyse the conversion of arginine to ornithine, they are encoded by separate gene sequences, are located in different subcellular compartments and are expressed to varying degrees in separate tissues. Type I arginase or hepatic arginase is constitutively expressed in hepatocytes. It is a cytosolic enzyme and is a central component of the urea cycle. While not constitutively present, its expression can be induced in macrophages by stimulation with T-helper-2 cytokines (especially by interleukins (IL)-4, -10 and -13) (Munder *et al.*, 1999; Chang *et al.*, 2000). Arginase II, on the other hand, is localized to the mitochondria and is found in high concentrations in kidney, brain and small intestine. Arginase II can also be induced in macrophages but by different stimuli, namely, LPS and dexamethasone (Corraliza *et al.*, 1995). The expression of both forms of arginase in macrophages is reduced by T-helper-1 cytokines, such as IFN-γ (Munder *et al.*, 1999).

Following conversion to ornithine, a number of pathways may be followed for further metabolism. What directs a cell to choose one pathway over another is not yet understood.

Urea cycle

The reactions involved in the urea cycle are shown in Fig. 5.3 and occur primarily in the liver. The function of the urea cycle is to clear nitrogenous waste, by converting ammonia to urea for excretion by the kidneys. Nitrogen can enter the cycle either through conversion to carbamoyl phosphate and subsequent passage of the carbamoyl molecule to ornithine, forming citrulline, or via glutamate to aspartate, which enters the cycle by reacting with citrulline to form arginosuccinate. Arginosuccinate lysase converts arginosuccinate to arginine, and fumarate, and arginase catalyses the degradation of arginine to ornithine with the loss of one molecule of urea. The reactions involving carbamoyl phosphate and glutamate occur in the mitochondrion, whereas the remaining reactions take place in the cytosol.

Proline

Ornithine aminotransferase catalyses the transfer of one amine residue from α-keto-glutarate to ornithine, with the formation of pyrroline-5-carboxylate,

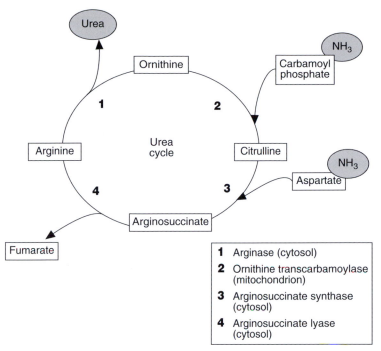

Fig. 5.3. The urea cycle.

which can then be reduced to proline or pass, via glutamate semialdehyde, to glutamate. Proline and its derivative hydroxyproline (formed *in situ* by the action of ascorbic acid) constitute 25% of the collagen molecule and therefore play a vital role in wound healing and tissue repair. Glutamate can be used by the cell for energy production, by complete oxidation to CO_2 through the citric acid cycle, or can be used for protein or amino acid synthesis.

Polyamines

The polyamines – putrescine, spermidine, spermine – are ubiquitous molecules found in all eukaryotic cells. They are synthesized from arginine via ornithine and ornithine decarboxylase, as shown in Fig. 5.2. The precise physiological role of polyamines has yet to be fully elucidated. It is known that they are required at low concentrations for cell viability and that levels increase during cell growth, differentiation and proliferation. They have been demonstrated to act through altering the three dimensional structure of tRNA thereby stimulating protein synthesis, through the phosphorylation of protein kinases, thereby accelerating intracellular signalling pathways, through modulation of transcription and mRNA turnover and through DNA editing. Inhibition of polyamine synthesis, using DL-alpha-difluoromethylornithine (DMFO) (a competitive inhibitor of ornithine decarboxylase), leads to a reduction in cell viability, cell-cycle arrest in S-phase and inhibition of cell differentiation.

Other pathways of arginine metabolism

Apart from incorporation into proteins or degradation by arginase or NOS, as described above, arginine can follow other pathways catalysed by the enzymes arginine decarboxylase and arginoglycine amidinotransferase. The latter leads to the formation of a recently discovered molecule, agmantine, which is thought to be involved in intracellular signalling. The former leads to the synthesis of phosphocreatine, an important molecule for energy storage in skeletal muscle.

Endocrine effects of arginine

Elevated plasma levels of arginine have been found to correlate with increased secretion of various hormones, including prolactin and growth hormone from the pituitary, insulin, glucagon, insulin-like growth factor 1 (IGF-1) and adrenal catecholamines (see Barbul, 1996). These hormones, in turn, can affect the functioning of the immune system. While the powerful secretagogue action of arginine is largely unexplained, a direct cholinergic effect, membrane depolarization by this highly cationic molecule and subsequent calcium influx, and the use of NO as an intermediary in cell signalling have all been demonstrated.

Prolactin

Prolactin can play a role in various stages of dendritic-cell maturation and T-helper-1 development. Prolactin induces maturation of dendritic cells from monocytes, by increasing their expression of the antigen-presenting MHC class II molecules and co-stimulatory molecules. The expression of CD40 is also up-regulated by prolactin, the final effect being increased T-cell activation. Prolactin can also stimulate the release of T-helper-1 cytokines by T-cells in the absence of dendritic cells (Matera et al., 2000).

Growth hormone

The growth hormone receptor is a member of the haematopoietin/cytokine receptor family and induces tyrosine phosphorylation through the janus kinase/signal transducer and activator of transcription (JAK/STAT) pathways. While growth hormone is not an absolute requirement for normal lymphoid and myeloid development, under situations of stress it can potentiate the cytokine responses of human T-cells, improve the antigen-presenting capability of dendritic cells, increase the numbers of haematopoietic progenitor cells in the bone marrow and induce thymic hyperplasia (Murphy and Longo, 2000).

IGF-1

IGF-1 plays an important role in the maturation of lymphocytes in the bone marrow and in their function in the periphery. In rodents, IGF-1 can restore age-related thymic involution and increase lymphocyte number and activity (Clark et al., 1993; Hinton et al., 1995). In addition, the thymotropic effects of growth hormone appear to be mediated through IGF-1.

Arginine and Immune Function – Animal Studies

Stress to the body, such as trauma with fracture or haemorrhage, burn injury or major elective surgical procedures, leads to alterations in immune functions and an attenuated immune response (Faist *et al.*, 1986). This predisposes to the development of infectious complications in the days or weeks following injury. It is estimated that, among patients who die more than 24 h after hospitalization following trauma, 75% die as a result of complications of infection and the inflammatory response (Miller *et al.*, 1982). It is in limiting this immune dysfunction that supplemental dietary arginine appears to hold most promise (see Evoy *et al.*, 1998).

Barbul and co-workers demonstrated that supplemental dietary arginine reduced trauma-induced thymic involution, lessened weight loss, improved wound healing and prolonged survival in injured rats (see Barbul, 1977). The same group also demonstrated that a dietary supplement of 1% arginine by weight increased thymic weight and the number of thymic lymphocytes in normal healthy mice and rats (see Barbul, 1986, 1996). In a burn model in guinea pigs, Saito *et al.* (1987) showed an increase in delayed hypersensitivity and in survival in arginine-supplemented animals. Madden *et al.* (1988) demonstrated a similar survival advantage in animals subjected to lethal bacterial peritonitis. This finding was replicated by Gianotti *et al.* (1993), who, in addition to improved survival, found a reduction in bacterial translocation and increased bactericidal activity in the arginine-supplemented animals.

The anti-tumour activity of arginine has been studied in a number of models, with variable results. In the setting of protein–calorie malnutrition and tumour inoculation, supplemental arginine (1% by weight) reduced the growth rate of the immunogenic neuroblastoma C1300 and improved host survival compared with glycine-supplemented controls (Fig. 5.4), while a similar effect was not seen in mice bearing a poorly immunogenic neuroblastoma TBJ (Reynolds *et al.*, 1990). Similar differences have been seen in different models of breast and colon cancer. The impression is of a dual effect of arginine: improving host resistance while simultaneously improving tumour-cell survival, the end result depending on the balance between these two opposing actions. The potential benefit of arginine supplementation in cancer therapy was further highlighted in a study by Lieberman *et al.* (1992), in which mice bearing the C1300 neuroblastoma were treated with a combination of arginine and IL-2: combined therapy led to a reduction in tumour growth and prolonged host survival, compared with the control group or either treatment alone.

Mechanism(s) of Arginine Action on Immune Function

Arginine is required for the normal growth and proliferation of lymphocytes *in vitro*. While the diminished mitogenic response seen in arginine-free conditions was initially attributed to the reduction in protein and polyamine synthesis, the demonstration that normal function and DNA synthesis can be returned by the addition of NO donors (sodium nitroprusside, *S*-nitrosoacetyl penicillamine) has forced a reconsideration of this premise (Efron *et al.*, 1991).

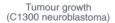

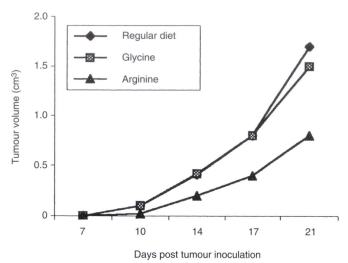

Days post tumour inoculation

Fig. 5.4. The effect of supplemental arginine on the growth of a C1300 neuroblastoma in mice with protein–calorie malnutrition (adapted from Reynolds *et al.*, 1988b).

Early mechanistic studies of the *in vivo* effect of supplemental arginine focused on T-cell activity. Increased delayed-type hypersensitivity responses, measured by foot-pad or ear-lobe thickness following inoculation of foreign material in previously sensitized hosts has been demonstrated in normal mice given supplemental arginine and in the settings of tumour, burn and sepsis (Saito *et al.*, 1987; Reynolds *et al.*, 1988b, 1990; Lewis and Langkamp-Henken, 2000). This has been found to correlate with increased T-cell mitogenesis in response to stimulation by concanavalin A, phytohaemagglutinin or tumour antigens, in addition to increases in specific T-cell cytotoxicity (Reynolds *et al.*, 1988b, 1990). Improvements in mononuclear-cell response to stimulation with concanavalin A have also been demonstrated, using cells from human subjects given arginine (Daly *et al.*, 1988). The mechanisms behind these effects remain unclear. While early reports suggested the involvement of a thymic hormone, similar effects have been produced in athymic nude mice (see Barbul, 1986). Up-regulation of IL-2 receptor expression and, in tumour-bearing mice, IL-2 production have been demonstrated and suggested as a mechanism behind increased T-cell activity (Reynolds *et al.*, 1988b). Gianotti *et al.* (1993) found that the survival advantage conferred on mice by arginine in the setting of abdominal sepsis was eliminated by the concomitant administration of the NOS inhibitor *N*-omega-nitro-L-arginine (NNA) and proposed the arginine–NO pathway as the key factor. Meanwhile, the importance of the hypothalamic–pituitary axis in arginine-mediated immune modulation was demonstrated by Barbul *et al.* (1983), who found that the thymotropic effects of supplemental arginine following injury were not reproduced in hypophysectomized rats.

In addition to the above alterations seen in T-cell functions, supplemental arginine also benefits the innate immune response, with increases in macrophage and natural killer cell cytotoxicity (Reynolds *et al.*, 1988a). The link between arginine metabolism and the tumoricidal activity of macrophages was highlighted by Mills *et al.* (1992) in a study looking at macrophage function following intraperitoneal implantation of P815 mastocytoma in naive and pre-immunized mice. Tumour rejection was associated with elevated levels of NO production and iNOS expression in peritoneal macrophages and with a reduction in arginase activity. In contrast, during times of exponential tumour growth, arginase activity was increased, with a corresponding elevation in urea and ornithine production, while NO and citrulline production were reduced. The balance between iNOS and arginase activity in macrophages has been demonstrated in many different models and is considered to be central to the shift in phenotype from wound to cytotoxic macrophage.

Both human and animal models have demonstrated the beneficial effect of arginine in wound healing. Arginine supplementation of the diet of injured rats resulted in accelerated wound healing, increased wound tensile strength and increased collagen deposition (see Barbul *et al.*, 1983). Wound healing was assessed by fresh wound strip breaking strength, fixed breaking strength and the amount of reparative collagen deposition indexed by the hydroxyproline content of implanted sponges. These findings can be explained, in part, by the increased requirement for arginine to synthesize reparative connective tissue. However, as with T-cell mitogenesis, the improvement in wound healing was not reproducible in hypophysectomized animals, suggesting a more complex mechanism.

In human studies, Kirk *et al.* (1993) examined the effect of arginine supplementation (17 g day^{-1}) on wound healing in an otherwise healthy elderly population. While epithelialization of a partial-thickness wound was not improved, collagen synthesis (as determined by hydroxyproline and protein deposition in subcutaneous polytetrafluroethylene implants) was significantly increased in those subjects given arginine.

Clinical Studies with Arginine in Patients at Risk of Sepsis and Septic Complications

The first clinical study to demonstrate a benefit from supplemental dietary arginine in surgical patients was performed in 30 patients undergoing major operations for gastrointestinal malignancy (Daly *et al.*, 1988). Patients were commenced on enteral feeding post-operatively and were randomized to receive either arginine (25 g day^{-1}) or isonitrogenous glycine (43 g day^{-1}) for 7 days. Arginine supplementation resulted in elevated plasma arginine and ornithine levels and was associated with an enhanced response of peripheral-blood lymphocytes to mitogens by day 7 and with an increased number of circulating CD4+ cells. Only the arginine-supplemented group achieved a positive nitrogen balance, which was attained by day 6 (Fig. 5.5). However, there was no difference in clinical outcome between the two groups.

CD4 (T-helper cell) expression

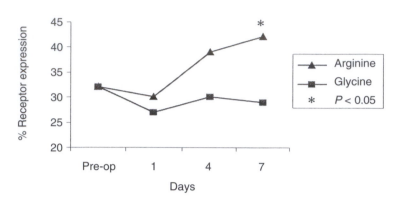

T lymphocyte activation (Con A)

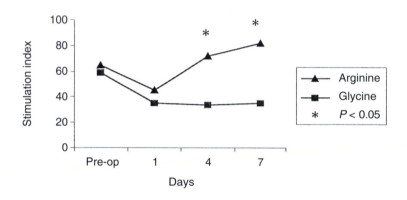

Nitrogen balance

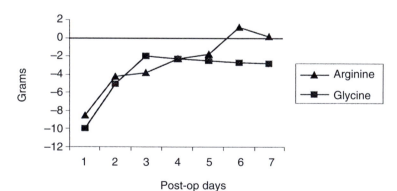

Fig. 5.5. Some immunological and metabolic effects of supplemental arginine in patients undergoing surgery for upper gastrointestinal malignancy (adapted from Reynolds *et al.*, 1990). Con A, concanavalin A.

At this time, two other dietary factors were emerging as playing an important role in modulating host defence – namely nucleotides and n-3 fatty acids. In mice fed nucleotide-free diets, supplemental RNA or uracil is required to restore cellular immunity, anti-fungal resistance, anti-bacterial resistance and, the bactericidal activity of macrophages (Van Buren *et al.*, 1994). n-3 fatty acid supplementation, in clinical and laboratory studies, has been associated with improved survival after burn injury, reduced post-injury infectious complications and diminished immunosuppression secondary to transfusion (Daly *et al.*, 1992). The proposed mechanisms of omega-3 fatty acid-induced improvements in immune function are related to an alteration of prostaglandin synthesis pathways from 2-series to 3-series prostaglandins (see Calder and Field, Chapter 4, this volume).

A study was therefore performed to examine the effect of enteral nutrition with supplemental arginine, RNA and n-3 fatty acids on immunological, metabolic and clinical outcome in patients after surgery (Daly *et al.*, 1992). Eighty-five patients requiring operations for upper gastrointestinal malignancies were randomized to receive a supplemental diet (IMPACT®, Sandoz Nutrition, Minneapolis, Minnesota, USA) or a standard enteral diet. Patients receiving the supplemental diet had a significantly greater nitrogen balance over the course of the study. Lymphocyte mitogenesis was reduced in both groups in the immediate post-operative period but returned to normal levels only in the supplemented group, by post-operative day 7. Infectious and wound complications occurred less commonly in the supplemented than in the control group (11% vs. 37%; $P = 0.02$) and mean length of hospital stay was significantly shorter in the supplemented group. A subsequent study (Daly *et al.*, 1995) used the same feeding protocol in 60 patients requiring surgery with or without adjuvant radiation/chemotherapy for upper gastrointestinal malignancy. Patients receiving the supplemental diet had fewer wound and infectious complications (10% vs. 43%; $P < 0.05$), and shorter length of hospital stay (16 vs. 22 days; $P < 0.05$) than patients receiving the standard enteral diet.

Since then, an increasing number of studies have been performed comparing immunonutrition (using one of the two formulas outlined in Table 5.1) to standard enteral feeding regimes in critically ill patients. In one of the largest such studies, a multicentre, prospective randomized trial compared early enteral nutrition by IMPACT® with standard enteral nutrition in 296 patients in intensive care units (Bower *et al.*, 1995). While mortality rates and infectious complications were the same in the treatment groups, subgroup analysis showed two interesting results. First, the mean length of hospital stay of septic patients was significantly reduced ($P < 0.05$). Second, in the 100 patients who were able to complete the total planned intake of the enteral diet within the first 7 days, there was a significant reduction in infectious complications (0.54 ± 0.78 vs. 0.94 ± 0.87) between the supplemented and control groups.

Comparing the same feeding formula with standard enteral nutrition, Braga *et al.* (1998) looked at 60 patients undergoing surgery for malignancy. While there was no demonstrable difference in the incidence of infectious complications between the two groups, the infectious complications occurring in the patients receiving the supplemental diet were assessed as being significantly less severe.

Kudsk *et al.* (1996) prospectively randomized 35 severely injured trauma patients to an enteral diet containing glutamine, arginine, n-3 fatty acids and

Table 5.1. Compositions of two enteral feeding formulae.

Component	Content 1000 kcal^{-1}	
	IMPACT®	Immun-Aid®
Protein (g)	56	37
Free arginine (g)	12.5	14
Free glutamine (g)	0	9
Other free amino acids (g)	0	20
Nucleic acids (g)	1.2	1
Total fat (g)	27.8	22
n-3 fatty acids (g)	2.8	1
Vitamins and minerals	Selectively enriched above 100% US RDA	

RDA, recommended daily allowance.

nucleotides (Immun-Aid®, McGaw, Irvine, California, USA) or to an isonitrogenous, isocaloric diet to investigate the effect on septic outcome. Significantly fewer major infectious complications developed in patients who received the supplemental diet than in the control group (6% vs. 41%; $P = 0.02$). Hospital stay was also significantly shorter.

One study to date has shown improvement in the mortality rate in patients receiving immunonutrition (Galban *et al.*, 2000). This was a prospective, randomized, multicentre study of 176 septic patients in intensive care units: 89 patients received IMPACT®, while 87 patients received a standard high-protein enteral feed. The mortality rate was reduced in the treatment group compared with the control group (17 of 89 vs. 28 of 87; $P < 0.05$), and this was most marked in moderately ill patients with APACHE (Acute Physiological and Chronic Health Evaluation) II scores between 10 and 15 (1 of 26 vs. 8 of 29; $P = 0.02$). There was also a significant difference in the incidence of bacteraemia between the two groups (7 of 89 vs. 19 of 87; $P = 0.01$) and in the number of patients developing more than one nosocomial infection (5 of 89 vs. 17 of 87; $P = 0.02$).

In a prospective, randomized, double-blind trial Senkal *et al.* (1999) examined the effects of IMPACT® enteral nutrition compared with the standard enteral diet, when commenced 5 days pre-operatively in patients with upper gastrointestinal-tract malignancy. These authors used as end-points the incidence of postoperative infectious complications, the cost of treating these complications, and the overall cost-effectiveness of immunonutrition. One hundred and fifty-four patients were eligible for analysis. The number of patients developing infectious complications after day 3 was significantly reduced in the immunonutrition group (7 of 78 vs. 16 of 76; $P = 0.04$), as was the total number of complication events (14 vs. 27; $P = 0.05$). While the total number of patients developing complications (10 of 78 vs. 18 of 76) and the mean length of stay (22.2 ± 4.1 days vs. 25.8 ± 3.8 days) in the treated group were decreased, these values did not reach statistical significance ($P = 0.08$ and $P = 0.09$, respectively). Despite higher product costs, the savings accrued by a substantially lower complication rate led to better cost-effectiveness in the group receiving immunonutrition.

Atkinson *et al.* (1998) performed a prospective, randomized, double-blind, controlled clinical trial in a heterogeneous group of critically ill patients in an intensive care unit. Infectious complications were not reported in this study, but, in the subgroup of patients ($n = 101$) who successfully achieved early enteral nutrition (> 2.5 l in the first 72 h), there was a significant reduction in the requirement for mechanical ventilation and in the length of hospital stay in the immunonutrition group.

In a meta-analysis of 12 studies containing 1482 critically ill patients, Beale *et al.* (1999) sought to address the clinical benefits derived from immunonutrition (IMPACT® or Immun-Aid®) over standard enteral feeds. This detailed analysis found that there was no overall effect on mortality. However, there were significant reductions in infection rate ($P = 0.006$), ventilator days ($P = 0.04$) and length of hospital stay ($P = 0.0002$) in the immunonutrition group. These benefits were found to be most impressive among surgical patients.

Conclusion

The favourable modulatory effects of arginine in the immune system have been well documented in animal models and some have been reproduced in humans. The most prominent effect of supplemental arginine is in abrogating trauma-induced immunosuppression – in particular, the reductions seen in T-cell mitogenesis, delayed-type hypersensitivity response, macrophage and natural killer cell cytotoxicity and the improvement of wound healing. In the clinical setting, immunonutrition, comprising supplemental arginine, nucleic acids and n-3 fatty acids, has been demonstrated to reduce infectious complications (e.g. see Table 5.2) and length of hospital stay in critically ill patients.

Table 5.2. The incidence of septic complications in prospective randomized trials comparing arginine-supplemented patients with non-supplemented controls.

				Infectious complications	
Patient cohort	Author	N	Experimental diet	Experimental	Control
Cancer surgery	Daly *et al.* (1992)	85	IMPACT®	11[a]	37
Cancer surgery	Daly *et al.* (1995)	60	IMPACT®	10[a]	43
Cancer surgery	Braga *et al.* (1998)	60	IMPACT®	10	15
Cancer surgery	Senkal *et al.* (1999)	164	IMPACT®	18[a]	35
Trauma	Brown *et al.* (1994)	37	IMPACT®	16[a]	56
Trauma	Kudsk *et al.* (1996)	33	Immun-Aid®	6[a]	41
Trauma	Moore *et al.* (1994)	98	Immun-Aid®	0[a]	11
Mixed ICU	Bower *et al.* (1995)	296	IMPACT®	6[b]	13
Mixed ICU	Galban *et al.* (2000)	181	IMPACT®	8[a,b]	22

[a]$P < 0.05$ vs. control group.
[b]Bacteraemia.
ICU, intensive care unit.

References

Akaike, T. and Maeda, H. (2000) Nitric oxide and virus infection. *Immunology* 101, 300–308.

Atkinson, S., Sieffert, E. and Bihari, D. (1998) A prospective randomized double-blind clinical trial of enteral immunonutrition in the critically ill. *Critical Care Medicine* 26, 1164–1172.

Barbul, A. (1977) Arginine: a thymotropic and wound healing promoting agent. *Surgical Forum* 28, 101.

Barbul, A. (1986) Arginine: biochemistry, physiology and therapeutic implications. *Journal of Parenteral and Enteral Nutrition* 10, 227–238.

Barbul, A. (1996) Arginine. In: Fisher, J.E. (ed.) *Nutrition and Metabolism in the Surgical Patient*. Little, Brown, New York, pp. 411–421.

Barbul, A., Rettura, G., Levenson, S.M. and Seifter, E. (1983) Wound healing and thymotropic effects of arginine: a pituitary mechanism of action. *American Journal of Clinical Nutrition* 37, 786–794.

Beale, R., Bryg, D. and Bihari, D. (1999) Immunonutrition in the critically ill: a systematic review of clinical outcome. *Critical Care Medicine* 27, 2799–2805.

Bower, R.H., Cerra, F.B., Bershadsky, B., Licari, J.J., Hoyt, D.B., Jensen, G.L., Van Buren, C.T., Rothkopf, M.M., Daly, J.M. and Adelsberg, B.R. (1995) Early enteral administration of a formula (IMPACT) supplemented with arginine, nucleotides, and fish oil in intensive care unit patients: results of a multicenter prospective randomised clinical trial. *Critical Care Medicine* 23, 436–449.

Braga, M., Gianotti, L., Vignali, A., Cestari, A., Bisagni, P. and Di Carlo, V. (1998) Artificial nutrition after major abdominal surgery: impact of route of administration and composition of the diet. *Critical Care Medicine* 26, 24–30.

Brown, R.O., Hunt, H., Mowatt-Larssen, C.A., Wojtysiak, S.L., Henningfield, M.F. and Kudsk, K.A. (1994) Comparison of specialised and standard enteral formulas in trauma patients. *Pharmacotherapy* 14, 314–320.

Burney, S., Tamir, S., Gal, A. and Tannenbaum, S.R. (1997) A mechanistic analysis of nitric oxide-induced cellular toxicity. *Nitric Oxide* 1, 130–144.

Castillo, L., Chapman, T.E., Yu, Y.M., Ajami, A., Burke, J.F. and Young, V.R. (1993) Dietary arginine uptake by the splanchnic region in adult humans. *American Journal of Physiology* 265, E532–E539.

Chang, C.I., Zoghi, B., Liao, J.C. and Kuo, L. (2000) The involvement of tyrosine kinases, cyclic AMP/protein kinase A, and p38 mitogen-activated protein kinase in IL-13-mediated arginase I induction in macrophages: its implications in IL-13-inhibited nitric oxide production. *Journal of Immunology* 165, 2134–2141.

Clark, R., Strasser, J., McCabe, S., Robbins, K. and Jardieu, P. (1993) Insulin-like growth factor-1 stimulation of lymphopoiesis. *Journal of Clinical Investigation* 92, 540–548.

Corraliza, I.M., Soler, G., Eichmann, K. and Modolell, M. (1995) Arginase induction by suppressors of nitric oxide synthesis (IL-4, IL-10 and PGE2) in murine bone-marrow-derived macrophages. *Biochemical and Biophysical Research Communications* 206, 667–673.

Daly, J.M., Reynolds, J., Thom, A., Kinsley, L., Dietrick-Gallagher, M., Shou, J. and Ruggieri, B. (1988) Immune and metabolic effects of arginine in the surgical patient. *Annals of Surgery* 208, 512–521.

Daly, J.M., Lieberman, M.D., Goldfine, J., Shou, J., Weintraub, F., Rosato, E.F. and Lavin, P. (1992) Enteral nutrition with supplemental arginine, RNA, and omega-3

fatty acids in patients after operation: Immunologic, metabolic and clinical outcome. *Surgery* 112, 56–67.

Daly, J.M., Weintraub, F.N., Shou, J., Rosato, E.F. and Lucia, M. (1995) Enteral nutrition during multimodality therapy in upper gastrointestinal cancer patients. *Annals
of Surgery* 221, 327–338.

Efron, D.T., Kirk, S.J., Regan, M.C., Wasserkrug, H.L. and Barbul, A. (1991) Nitric
oxide generation from L-arginine is required for optimal peripheral blood DNA synthesis. *Surgery* 110, 327–334.

Evoy, D., Lieberman, M.D., Fahey, T.J. and Daly, J.M. (1998) Immunonutrition: the role
of arginine. *Nutrition* 14, 611–617.

Faist, E., Kupper, T.S., Baker, C.C., Chaudry, I.H., Dwyer, J. and Baue, A.E. (1986)
Depression of cellular immunity after major injury: its association with posttrau-
matic complications and its reversal with immunomodulation. *Archives of Surgery*
121, 1000–1005.

Galban, C., Montejo, J.C., Mesejo, A., Marco, P., Celaya, S., Sanchez-Segura, J.M.,
Farre, M. and Bryg, D.J. (2000) An immune-enhancing enteral diet reduces mortal-
ity and episodes of bacteremia in septic intensive care unit patients. *Critical Care
Medicine* 28, 643–648.

Gianotti, L., Alexander, J.W., Pyles, T. and Fukushima, R. (1993) Arginine-supplemented diets improve survival in gut-derived sepsis and peritonitis by modulating
bacterial clearance: the role of nitric oxide. *Annals of Surgery* 217, 644–653.

Hinton, P.S., Peterson, C.A., Lo, H.C., Yang, H., McCarthy, D. and Ney, D.M. (1995)
Insulin-like growth factor-I enhances immune response in dexamethasone-treated
or surgically stressed rats maintained with total parenteral nutrition. *Journal of
Parenteral and Enteral Nutrition* 19, 444–452.

Kirk, S.J., Hurson, M., Regan, M.C., Holt, D.R., Wasserkrug, H.L. and Barbul, A. (1993)
Arginine stimulates wound healing and immune function in elderly human beings.
Surgery 114, 155–160.

Kudsk, K.A., Minard, G., Croce, M.A., Brown, R.O., Lowrey, T.S., Pritchard, F.E.,
Dickerson, R.N. and Fabian, T.C. (1996) A randomised trial of isonitrogenous
enteral diets after severe trauma: an immune enhancing diet reduces septic complications. *Annals of Surgery* 224, 531–540.

Lewis, B. and Langkamp-Henken, B. (2000) Arginine enhances *in vivo* immune
responses in young, adult and aged mice. *Journal of Nutrition* 130, 1827–1830.

Lieberman, M.D., Nishioka, K., Redmond, P. and Daly, J.M. (1992) Enhancement of
interleukin-2 immunotherapy with L-arginine. *Annals of Surgery* 215, 157–165.

MacMicking, J., Xie, Q. and Nathan, C. (1997) Nitric oxide and macrophage function.
Annual Review of Immunology 15, 323–350.

Madden, H.P., Breslin, R.J., Wasserkrug, H.L., Efron, G. and Barbul, A. (1988)
Stimulation of T-cell immunity by arginine enhances survival in peritonitis. *Journal
of Surgical Research* 44, 658–663.

Matera, L., Mori, M., Geuna, M., Buttiglieri, S. and Palestro, G. (2000) Prolactin in
autoimmunity and antitumor defence. *Journal of Neuroimmunology* 109, 47–55.

Miller, S.E., Miller, C.L. and Trunkey, D.D. (1982) The immune consequences of injury.
Surgical Clinics of North America 62, 167–181.

Mills, C.D., Shearer, J., Evans, R. and Caldwell, M.D. (1992) Macrophage arginine
metabolism and the inhibition or stimulation of cancer. *Journal of Immunology*
149, 2709–2714.

Moore, F.A., Moore, E.E., Kudsk, K.A., Brown, R.O., Bower, R.H., Koruda, M.J., Baker,
C.C. and Barbul, A. (1994) Clinical benefits of an immune-enhancing diet for early
post-injury enteral feeding. *Journal of Trauma* 37, 607–615.

Munder, M., Eichmann, K., Moran, J.M., Centeno, F., Soler, G. and Modolell, M. (1999) Th1/Th2-regulated expression of arginase isoforms in murine macrophages and dendritic cells. *Journal of Immunology* 163, 3771–3777.

Murphy, W.J. and Longo, D.L. (2000) Growth hormone as an immunomodulating therapeutic agent. *Immunology Today* 21, 211–213.

Nathan, C. and Xie, Q.W. (1994) Nitric oxide synthases: roles, tolls, and controls. *Cell* 78, 915–918.

Niedbala, W., Wei, X.Q., Piedrafita, D., Xu, D. and Liew, F.Y. (1999) Effects of nitric oxide on the induction and differentiation of Th1 cells. *European Journal of Immunology* 29, 2498–2505.

O'Sullivan, D., Brosnan, J.T. and Brosnan, M.E. (1998) Hepatic zonation of the catabolism of arginine and ornithine in the perfused rat liver. *Biochemical Journal* 330, 627–632.

Rabier, D., Narcy, C., Bardet, J., Parvy, P., Saudubray, J.M. and Kamoun, P. (1991) Arginine remains an essential amino acid after liver transplantation in urea cycle enzyme deficiencies. *Journal of Inherited Metabolic Disease* 14, 277–280.

Reynolds, J.V., Daly, J.M., Zhang, S., Evantash, E., Shou, J., Sigal, R. and Ziegler, M. (1988a) Immunomodulatory effects of arginine. *Surgery* 104, 142–151.

Reynolds, J.V., Thom, A.K., Zhang, S.M., Ziegler, M.M., Naji, A. and Daly, J.M. (1988b) Arginine, protein malnutrition and cancer. *Journal of Surgical Research* 45, 513–522.

Reynolds, J.V., Daly, J.M., Shou, J., Sigal, R., Ziegler, M.M. and Naji, A. (1990) Immunological effects of arginine in tumor-bearing and non-tumor-bearing hosts. *Annals of Surgery* 211, 202–210.

Saito, H., Trocki, O., Wang, S.L., Gonce, S.J., Joffe, S.N. and Alexander, J.W. (1987) Metabolic and immune effects of dietary arginine supplementation after burn. *Archives of Surgery* 122, 784–789.

Samar, B., Tamir, S., Gal, A. and Tannenboum, S.R. (1997) A mechanistic analysis of nitric oxide-induced cellular toxicity. *Nitric Oxide: Biology and Chemistry* 1, 130–144.

Senkal, M., Zumtobel, V., Bauer, K.H., Marpe, B., Wolfram, G., Frei, A., Eickhoff, U. and Kemen, M. (1999) Outcome and cost-effectiveness of perioperative enteral immunonutrition in patients undergoing elective upper gastrointestinal surgery. *Archives of Surgery* 134, 1309–1316.

Stuehr, D.J. and Nathan, C.F. (1989) Nitric oxide: a macrophage product responsible for cytostasis and respiratory inhibition in tumor target cells. *Journal of Experimental Medicine* 169, 1543–1555.

Van Buren, C.T., Kulkarni, A.D. and Rudolph, F.B. (1994) The role of nucleotides in adult nutrition. *Journal of Nutrition* 124, 160S–164S.

Wu, G. and Morris, S.M. (1998) Arginine metabolism: nitric oxide and beyond. *Biochemical Journal* 336, 1–17.

6 Glutamine and the Immune System

PHILIP C. CALDER[1] AND PHILIP NEWSHOLME[2]

[1]Institute of Human Nutrition, School of Medicine, University of Southampton, Bassett Crescent East, Southampton SO16 7PX, UK; [2]Department of Biochemistry, Conway Institute of Biomolecular and Biomedical Research, University College Dublin, Belfield, Dublin 4, Republic of Ireland

Glutamine Synthesis and Interorgan Transport

Glutamine (Fig. 6.1) is the most abundant free amino acid in the bloodstream and in the body. It contributes about 50% of the free α-amino acid pool within the human body and is quantitatively the most important amino acid involved in inter-organ nitrogen transport (Lund and Williamson, 1985). Classically, glutamine is a non-essential amino acid. Indeed, it can be synthesized in many cells and tissues of the body. The immediate precursor of glutamine is glutamate and the enzyme responsible for glutamine synthesis is glutamine synthetase (Fig. 6.2). In turn, glutamate can be formed from 2-oxoglutarate by transamination. Thus, the transamination reaction serves to transfer amino groups from amino acids to glutamine via glutamate (Fig. 6.2). Although any amino acid can potentially participate in the transamination reaction with 2-oxoglutarate, it is considered that the branched-chain amino acids play an important role in amino-group donation. The ammonia for the glutamine synthetase reaction could be generated from any deamination reaction; however, it is likely that in muscle the glutamate dehydrogenase and AMP deaminase reactions play important roles here.

Although many tissues can synthesize glutamine, only certain tissues are able to release significant amounts of it into the bloodstream. These include the lung, brain, skeletal muscle and perhaps adipose tissue. Because of its large mass, skeletal muscle is considered to be the most important glutamine producer in the body (see Elia and Lunn, 1997). In skeletal muscle, glutamine contributes approximately 60% of the total free amino acid pool and it has a concentration of approximately 20 mM (Bergstrom et al., 1974; Lund, 1981). It is estimated that skeletal muscle releases up to 9 g of glutamine day^{-1} (Elia and Lunn, 1997). This is a greater amount of glutamine than that typically provided by the diet (approximately 5 g day^{-1}). It is estimated that about 60% of glutamine released by human skeletal muscle in healthy individuals comes from de novo synthesis, with the remaining 40% coming from protein breakdown (Hankard et al., 1995).

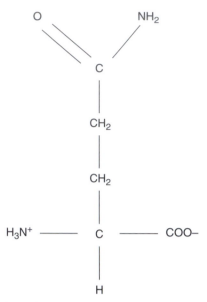

Fig. 6.1. The structure of glutamine.

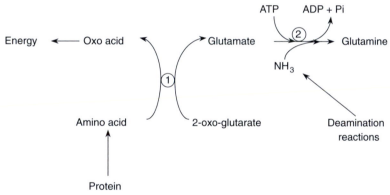

Fig. 6.2. The pathway of glutamine biosynthesis. Enzymes are indicated as: 1, transaminase; 2, glutamine synthetase.

Once released from skeletal muscle, glutamine acts as an interorgan nitrogen transporter (Lund and Williamson, 1985; Newsholme *et al.*, 1989; see Fig. 6.3). The plasma glutamine concentration in healthy adult humans is typically in the range 0.5–0.8 mM, with a mean concentration of approximately 0.65 mM. Important users of glutamine include the kidney (see Tizianello *et al.*, 1982), liver (see Haussinger, 1989), small intestine (see Windmueller and Spaeth, 1974; Souba, 1991) and cells of the immune system (for reviews, see Calder, 1994, 1995a; Wilmore and Shabert, 1998; Calder and Yaqoob, 1999; Newsholme *et al.*, 1999; Newsholme, 2001). Glutamine has a number of metabolic roles in these user organs (Table 6.1).

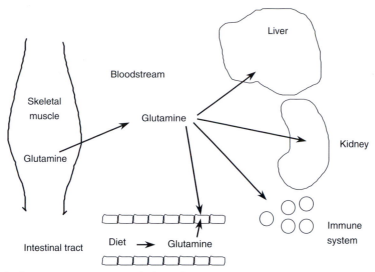

Fig. 6.3. Inter-organ transport of glutamine.

Table 6.1. Metabolic roles of glutamine.

Organ	Metabolic role of glutamine
Liver	Glucose synthesis (C skeleton)
	Amino acid synthesis
	Urea synthesis
	Glutathione synthesis (via glutamate)
Kidney	Glucose synthesis (C skeleton)
	Energy (C skeleton)
	Acid–base balance
Small intestine	Energy (C skeleton)
Immune system	Energy (C skeleton)
All tissues	Protein synthesis
	Purine synthesis (RNA, DNA)
	Pyrimidine synthesis (RNA, DNA)

In the liver, the carbon skeleton of glutamine is an important precursor for glucose synthesis, while glutamine itself can be used for the synthesis of other amino acids and proteins, with excess nitrogen disposed of via ureagenesis. Glutamine can also be used as the precursor for the glutamate portion of glutathione, which is synthesized primarily in the liver. In the kidney, glutamine participates in acid–base balance, donating its amido and amino nitrogens to join with protons to form ammonium ions, which are excreted in the urine. The remaining carbon skeleton can be used to generate energy or as a precursor for glucose synthesis (gluconeogenesis). Glutamine is the major energy source in the small intestine and is an important energy source for immune cells. Glutamine is a nitrogen donor for the synthesis of purines and pyrimidines.

Since these are the building blocks of RNA and DNA, this role of glutamine is likely to be a particularly important one in cells that have high rates of division and/or of protein secretion. These include cells of the immune system and cells of the small intestine, such as enterocytes.

The importance of glutamine to cell survival and proliferation *in vitro* was first reported by Ehrensvand *et al.* (1949) but was more fully described by Eagle *et al.* (1956). Glutamine needed to be present at ten- to 100-fold in excess of any other amino acid in cell culture and could not be replaced by glutamate or glucose. This work led to the development of the first tissue-culture medium, which contained essential growth factors, glucose, 19 essential and non-essential amino acids at approximately physiological concentrations and a high concentration of glutamine (2 mM).

Glutamine Metabolism by Cells of the Immune System

The possible fates of glutamine carbon are shown in Fig. 6.4. One possible rate-determining step in the pathway of glutamine utilization is that catalysed by the enzyme phosphate-dependent glutaminase (hereafter referred to as glutaminase), which is found within mitochondria. The activity of glutaminase is high in all lymphoid organs examined, including lymph nodes, spleen, thymus, Peyer's patches and bone marrow (Ardawi and Newsholme, 1985), and in lymphocytes (Ardawi, 1988a; Keast and Newsholme, 1990), macrophages (Newsholme *et al.*, 1986), and

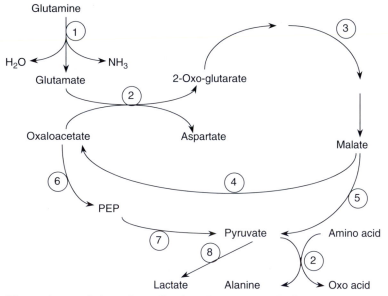

Fig. 6.4. The pathway of glutamine utilization. Enzymes are indicated as: 1, glutaminase; 2, transaminase, 3; enzymes of part of the citric acid cycle; 4, malate dehydrogenase; 5, malic enzyme; 6, phosphoenolpyruvate carboxykinase; 7, pyruvate kinase; 8, lactate dehydrogenase. PEP phosphoenolpyruvate.

neutrophils (Curi *et al.*, 1997). Glutaminase activity increases in the popliteal lymph node in response to an immunological challenge (Ardawi and Newsholme, 1982). Consistent with the high activity of glutaminase, glutamine is utilized at a high rate by cultured lymphocytes (Ardawi and Newsholme, 1983; Brand, 1985; Ardawi, 1988a; Brand *et al.*, 1989; O'Rourke and Rider, 1989), macrophages (Newsholme *et al.*, 1987; Newsholme and Newsholme, 1989; Spolarics *et al.*, 1991) and neutrophils (Curi *et al.*, 1997; see Table 6.2). Mitogenic stimulation of lymphocytes increases both glutaminase activity (Brand, 1985) and the rate of glutamine utilization (Ardawi and Newsholme, 1983; Brand, 1985; Ardawi, 1988a; Brand *et al.*, 1989; O'Rourke and Rider, 1989). Glutamine utilization by macrophages was increased by bacillus Calmette–Guérin (BCG) activation *in vivo* or by bacterial lipopolysaccharide (LPS) stimulation *in vitro* (Murphy and Newsholme, 1998). The major products of glutamine utilization by cultured lymphocytes and macrophages are glutamate, aspartate, lactate and ammonia, although alanine and pyruvate are also produced and some glutamine (approx. 25%) is completely oxidized (Ardawi and Newsholme, 1983; Brand, 1985; Newsholme *et al.*, 1987; Ardawi, 1988a; Brand *et al.*, 1989; Newsholme and Newsholme, 1989; O'Rourke and Rider, 1989). Macrophages are known to have a large oxidative capacity and their rate of O_2 consumption (515 nmol h^{-1} mg^{-1} protein) is similar to those of sheep heart (696 nmol h^{-1} mg^{-1} protein) and rat liver (520 nmol h^{-1} mg^{-1} protein) *in vitro* (Newsholme, 1987). Newsholme (1987) calculated ATP generation rates for isolated, incubated macrophages, taking into account oxygen utilized by the NADPH oxidase of these cells. The ATP generation rate in the presence of both glucose and glutamine was 930 nmol h^{-1} mg^{-1} protein, based on known pathways of metabolism. Glucose contributed 62% and glutamine 38% of the energy requirement of the cell. Since the ATP concentration of the macrophage is approximately 7 nmol mg^{-1} protein (Newsholme *et al.*, 1987), the total ATP concentration of the cell must have been turned over at least twice per minute. It has been calculated that glutamine can contribute up to 35% of the energy requirement of other immune cells in culture (Spolarics *et al.*, 1991).

Table 6.2. Rates of utilization of glucose or glutamine and of production of various metabolites by isolated mouse macrophages, rat lymphocytes or rat neutrophils. Rates of formation of $^{14}CO_2$ are from ^{14}C-labelled glucose or glutamine. (Data are from Ardawi and Newsholme, 1983; Newsholme *et al.*, 1987; Curi *et al.*, 1997.)

Cell type	Addition	Rate of utilization (nmol h^{-1} mg^{-1} cell protein)		Rate of production (nmol h^{-1} mg^{-1} cell protein)			
		Glucose	Glutamine	Lactate	Glutamate	Aspartate	$^{14}CO_2$
Macrophage	Glucose	355	–	632	–	–	11
	Glutamine	-	186	33	137	25	9
Lymphocyte	Glucose	42	–	91	–	–	1.5
	Glutamine	-	223	9	132	59	6.1
Neutrophil	Glucose	460	–	550	–	–	2.4
	Glutamine	-	770	320	250	68	6.5

Glutamine and Immune-cell Functions

Introduction

The high rate of glutamine utilization by neutrophils, macrophages and lymphocytes and its increase when these cells are challenged suggests that provision of glutamine might be important to the function of these cells and so to the ability to mount an efficient immune response. Over 30 years ago, it was reported that the addition of asparaginase or glutaminase to cultures of lymphocytes prevented the cells from proliferating (Hirsch, 1970; Simberkoff and Thomas, 1970). Furthermore, asparaginase treatment of animals leads to immunosuppression (Brambilla *et al.*, 1970; Chakrabaty and Friedman, 1970; Ashworth and MacLennan, 1974; Kafkewitz and Bendich, 1983). The immunosuppressive effect of asparaginase was shown to be due to its ability to hydrolyse glutamine and so decrease its availability to the immune system (Ashworth and MacLennan, 1974; Durden and Distasio, 1981; Kafkewitz and Bendich, 1983). These observations suggest that a supply of glutamine is required for the immune system to function optimally. A number of specific immunomodulatory actions of glutamine have now been reported.

Influence of glutamine on T lymphocyte proliferation *in vitro*

The proliferative response of rat (Ardawi and Newsholme, 1983; Szondy and Newsholme, 1989), mouse (Griffiths and Keast, 1990; Yaqoob and Calder, 1997) and human (Chuang *et al.*, 1990; Parry-Billings *et al.*, 1990a; Chang *et al.*, 1999a, b) lymphocytes to T-cell mitogens is dependent upon the availability of glutamine: in the absence of glutamine, these cells do not proliferate, but, as the glutamine concentration in the culture medium increases, lymphocyte proliferation increases (Fig. 6.5). Lymphocyte proliferation increases greatly over the glutamine concentration range between 0.01 and 1 mM and appears to be maximal at normal physiological concentrations. Other amino acids, including glutamate, aspartate and arginine, cannot substitute for glutamine to support lymphocyte proliferation (Ardawi and Newsholme, 1983; Calder, 1995b). However, hydrolysable dipeptides that contain glutamine (e.g. alanyl-glutamine or glycyl-glutamine) can act as a replacement for glutamine to support *in vitro* T lymphocyte proliferation (Brand *et al.*, 1989; Kweon *et al.*, 1991; Kohler *et al.*, 2000).

Influence of glutamine on B lymphocyte differentiation *in vitro*

The differentiation of B lymphocytes into antibody-synthesizing cells *in vitro* is glutamine-dependent and increases greatly over the physiological range of glutamine concentrations (Crawford and Cohen, 1985). This effect of glutamine cannot be mimicked by glutamate or asparagine.

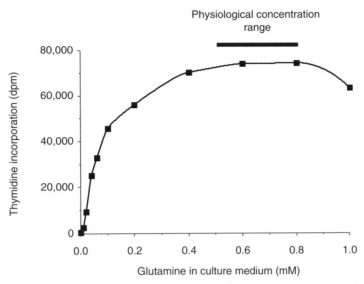

Fig. 6.5. Effect of glutamine on human blood lymphocyte proliferation *in vitro*. dpm, disintegrations per minute. P.C. Calder data are previously unpublished.

Influence of glutamine on macrophage functions *in vitro*

In contrast to lymphocytes, which are rapidly dividing cells, macrophages are terminally differentiated cells that have lost their ability to divide. However, they remain very active cells, characterized by high rates of phagocytosis, protein secretion and membrane recycling. The level of cell surface expression of various molecules involved in phagocytosis and in antigen presentation (major histocompatibility complex (MHC) II) on human blood monocytes is influenced by the concentration of glutamine in which the cells are cultured (Spittler *et al.*, 1995, 1997). This is associated with increased function (i.e. increased phagocytosis of immunoglobulin (Ig) G or complement opsonized particles and increased antigen presentation) with increasing glutamine availability (Spittler *et al.*, 1995, 1997). Glutamine availability influenced the phagocytic uptake of unopsonized yeast-cell walls (Parry-Billings *et al.*, 1990a) and of opsonized sheep red blood cells (Wallace and Keast, 1992) by incubated murine macrophages. The dipeptide alanyl-glutamine can replace glutamine to support *in vitro* phagocytosis by rat macrophages (Kweon *et al.*, 1991).

Influence of glutamine on neutrophil functions *in vitro*

Addition of glutamine to cultures of blood neutrophils taken from patients with burns or post-surgery improved the defective anti-microbial activities (e.g. decreased reactive oxygen species production, phagocytosis and bactericidal activity) of those cells (Ogle *et al.*, 1994; Furukawa *et al.*, 1997, 2000a, b). A study by Garcia *et al.* (1999) suggests a mechanism by which glutamine may promote increased antimicrobial activity by neutrophils in stress states: 2 mM extracellular glutamine was able to attenuate the adrenaline-induced inhibition of superoxide production in these cells, suggesting that glutamine may protect cells from the suppressive effects of stress hormones.

Influence of glutamine on cytokine production *in vitro*

Increased availability of glutamine enhanced interleukin (IL)-2 production by concanavalin A (Con A)-stimulated rat (Calder and Newsholme, 1992), mouse (Yaqoob and Calder, 1997) and human (Rohde *et al.*, 1996a; Yaqoob and Calder, 1998; Chang *et al.*, 1999b) lymphocytes and also increased expression of the IL-2 receptor on stimulated rat lymphocytes (Yaqoob and Calder, 1997). The latter study also reported that the proportion of CD4+ lymphocytes increased with increasing concentration of glutamine in the culture medium (Yaqoob and Calder, 1997). Interferon (IFN)-γ production by human blood lymphocytes was enhanced with increasing availability of glutamine (Heberer *et al.*, 1996; Rohde *et al.*, 1996a; Yaqoob and Calder, 1998; Chang *et al.*, 1999b), with maximum production occurring at a concentration below 0.5 mM.

Wallace and Keast (1992) demonstrated that murine macrophages stimulated with bacterial LPS secreted increasing amounts of IL-1 as the supply of glutamine increased, while more recently Murphy and Newsholme (1999) reported similar enhancement of tumour necrosis factor (TNF)-α release by rat macrophages with increasing glutamine availability. Glutamine addition to cultured rat macrophages stimulated with LPS increased IL-1β and IL-6 mRNA and secreted protein levels (Yassad *et al.*, 2000). In contrast to the observations with rodent macrophages, production of TNF-α, IL-1β and IL-6 by human blood monocytes (Rohde *et al.*, 1996a; Yaqoob and Calder, 1998) and lymphocytes (Heberer *et al.*, 1996) appears to be little affected by glutamine availability, although one study suggests otherwise for IL-6 production (Peltonen *et al.*, 1997). IL-8 production by LPS-stimulated human blood monocytes was markedly increased with increasing glutamine concentration (Murphy and Newsholme, 1999).

Glutamine feeding studies in healthy animals

A recent study compared the effects of feeding mice for 2 weeks on a diet that included 200 g casein kg^{-1}, providing 19.6 g glutamine kg^{-1}, or a glutamine-enriched diet, which provided 54.8 g glutamine kg^{-1}, partly at the expense of casein. Spleen lymphocytes from mice fed on the glutamine-enriched diet proliferated better in response to Con A than those from mice fed on the control diet (Kew *et al.*, 1999). The glutamine-enriched diet also increased the proportion of CD4+ lymphocytes in the spleen and increased the proportion of stimulated lymphocytes bearing the IL-2 receptor. IL-2, but not IFN-γ, production was significantly greater for Con A-stimulated spleen lymphocytes from mice fed the glutamine-enriched diet (Kew *et al.*, 1999), while the production of all three cytokines investigated (TNF-α, IL-1β and IL-6) was greater for LPS-stimulated macrophages from mice fed the glutamine-enriched diet (Wells *et al.*, 1999). These observations suggest that increasing the amount of glutamine in the murine diet enhances the ability of both macrophages and T lymphocytes to respond to stimulation, at least in terms of cytokine production. Feeding rats a glutamine-free diet for 7 days resulted in decreased mucosal wet weight and a decreased number of intraepithelial lymphocytes (Horvath *et al.*, 1996). This study suggests that glutamine is required for maintenance of the gut-associated immune system.

Plasma and Muscle Glutamine Levels in Catabolic Stress

One of the early responses to stress that occurs in skeletal muscle is the increased rate of export of glutamine from the intracellular free amino acid pool. This lowers the intracellular glutamine concentration, leading to protein breakdown and *de novo* synthesis of glutamine from other amino acids. Glutamine synthetase in skeletal muscle is up-regulated by glucocorticoids (Max *et al.*, 1988) and by TNF-α (Chakrabarti, 1998), and glucocorticoids increase glutamine efflux from skeletal muscle (Muhlbacher *et al.*, 1984; Parry-Billings *et al.*, 1990b). Thus, there appears to be an attempt in stress states to increase the supply of glutamine from muscle to the rest of the body. Nevertheless, glucocorticoid treatment decreases skeletal muscle and plasma glutamine concentrations (Muhlbacher *et al.*, 1984; Parry-Billings *et al.*, 1990b), suggesting that the demand for glutamine exceeds the supply.

Animal studies indicate that intramuscular and plasma glutamine concentrations are decreased in catabolic-stress situations, such as in sepsis and cancer cachexia and following burn injury and surgery (Table 6.3). In humans, plasma glutamine levels are lowered (by up to 50%) by sepsis, major injury and burns and following surgery (see Table 6.4). A recent study reported that low plasma glutamine concentration (< 0.42 mM) at admission to intensive care was associated with higher severity of illness and higher mortality (Oudemans-van Straaten *et al.*, 2001). In humans, the skeletal-muscle glutamine concentration is lowered by more than 50% in catabolic stress (see Table 6.4). These observations indicate that a significant depletion of the skeletal-muscle glutamine pool is characteristic of catabolic stress. The lowered plasma glutamine concentrations that occur are most probably the result of demand for glutamine (by the liver, kidney, gut and immune system) exceeding the supply, and it is proposed that glutamine be considered a conditionally essential amino acid during catabolic stress (Lacey and Wilmore, 1990; Wilmore and Shabert, 1998). It has been suggested that the lowered plasma glutamine availability contributes, at least in part, to the immunosuppression that accompanies such situations (Newsholme and Calder, 1997). Because of the apparent immunostimulatory actions of glutamine described above, it seems sensible to provide glutamine for patients following surgery, radiation treatment or bone-marrow transplantation or suffering from injury, sepsis or burns.

Table 6.3. Effect of catabolic stress on plasma and muscle glutamine concentrations in animals. Values separated by → indicate the concentrations observed in control and stressed animals, respectively.

Model	Plasma glutamine (mM)	Skeletal-muscle glutamine (mM)	Reference
Rat injury	ND	9.9 → 5.9	Albina *et al.* (1987)
Rat sepsis	1.1 → 0.8	3.8 → 1.5	Parry-Billings *et al.* (1989)
Rat cancer cachexia	1.0 → 0.8	5.1 → 2.3	Parry-Billings *et al.* (1991)
Rat burn injury	0.7 → 0.5	4.1 → 2.7	Ardawi (1988b)
Dog burn injury	0.7 → 0.5	7.6 → 6.0	Stinnett *et al.* (1982)
Pig post-surgery	0.3 → 0.2	ND	Deutz *et al.* (1992)

ND, not determined.

Table 6.4. Effect of stress on plasma and muscle glutamine concentrations in humans. Values separated by → indicate the concentrations observed in healthy controls and in patients with the indicated catabolic stress, respectively.

Catabolic stress	Plasma glutamine (mM)	Skeletal-muscle glutamine (mM)	Reference
Trauma/burns	0.60 → 0.70	20.0 → 10.0	Furst *et al.* (1979)
Injury	0.78 → 0.51	20.5 → 9.1	Askanazi *et al.* (1980)
Sepsis	0.53 → 0.37	19.3 → 6.7	Roth *et al.* (1982)
Sepsis	0.78 → 0.62	20.5 → 9.5	Askanazi *et al.* (1980)
Sepsis	0.38 → 0.30	22.0 → 4.0	Milewski *et al.* (1982)
Burns	0.62 → 0.30	ND	Parry-Billings *et al.* (1990a)
Burns	0.83 → 0.50	ND	Stinnett *et al.* (1982)
Surgery	0.65 → 0.48	ND	Parry-Billings *et al.* (1992a)
Surgery	0.46 → 0.36	ND	Lund *et al.* (1986)
Surgery	0.69 → 0.59	18.8 → 9.5	Askanazi *et al.* (1978)
Surgery	0.60 → 0.70	20.0 → 10.0	Askanazi *et al.* (1980)
Surgery	0.62 → 0.48	ND	Powell *et al.* (1994)

ND, not determined.

There are also reports of decreased plasma glutamine concentrations after endurance exercise (Parry-Billings *et al.*, 1992b; Rohde *et al.*, 1996b; Castell *et al.*, 1997) and athletic training (Keast *et al.*, 1995; Hack *et al.*, 1997) and in the overtrained athlete (Parry-Billings *et al.*, 1992b).

Effect of Exogenous Glutamine on Immune Function and Survival in Animal Models of Infection and Trauma

A number of animal studies have been performed to investigate the effect of glutamine on the ability to withstand challenges with various pathogens or tumour bearing. Glutamine-supplemented parenteral nutrition improved survival (75% vs. 45% in the control group receiving standard parenteral nutrition) in rats following caecal ligation and puncture (Ardawi, 1991). Likewise, intravenous glutamine improved survival (92% vs. 55% in the control group) following an intraperitoneal injection of live *Escherichia coli* into rats (Inoue *et al.*, 1993). Parenteral administration of alanyl-glutamine into rats improved survival (86% vs. 44% in the control group) in response to intraperitoneally infused *E. coli* (Naka *et al.*, 1996). Suzuki *et al.* (1993) fed mice for 10 days on diets containing casein or casein supplemented with 20 g or 40 g glutamine kg^{-1} and then inoculated them intravenously with live *Staphylococcus aureus*. Over the following 20 days, during which the mice were maintained on the same diets they had been fed prior to infection, 80% of the control animals died, while mortality was 60% in the 20 g glutamine kg^{-1} group and 30% in the 40 g glutamine kg^{-1} group. Another study showed that inclusion of glutamine in parenteral nutrition decreased mortality to intratracheally inoculated *Pseudomonas* (23% and 30% mortality at 24 and 48 h in the glutamine group vs. 55% and 75% mortality at 24 and 48 h in the control group) (DeWitt *et al.*, 1999). In addition to enhanced survival, these studies showed that glutamine improved nitrogen balance diminished the sepsis-induced decrease in muscle glutamine concentration and decreased muscle protein breakdown (Ardawi, 1991), increased plasma glutamine concentration (Inoue *et al.*, 1993), increased intestinal function and/or integrity (Inoue *et al.*, 1993; Naka *et al.*, 1996), and enhanced muscle protein synthesis (Ardawi, 1991; Naka *et al.*, 1996). These studies did not measure indices of immune function. However, Yoo *et al.* (1997) reported that proliferation of blood lymphocytes from *E. coli*-infected piglets was significantly higher if the piglets consumed a diet containing 40 g glutamine kg^{-1} compared with a diet that did not contain glutamine. Shewchuk *et al.* (1997) reported that Con A-stimulated proliferation of spleen lymphocytes taken from tumour-bearing rats fed a diet containing an increased amount of glutamine was greater than that of those taken from rats fed a standard casein-containing diet. Furthermore, infusion of alanyl-glutamine into tumour-bearing rats increased the *in vitro* phagocytic capacity of alveolar macrophages (Kweon *et al.*, 1991), while infusion into septic rats increased *in vitro* proliferation of mitogen-stimulated blood lymphocytes (Yoshida *et al.*, 1992). These studies indicate that provision of glutamine either parenterally or enterally increases the function of various immune cells and that this might account for the enhanced resistance to infection observed in other studies.

A series of studies has examined the influence of glutamine on the gut-associated and respiratory lymphoid systems in mice undergoing various challenges. Parenteral glutamine or alanyl-glutamine maintained the lymphocyte yield from Peyer's patches and intestinal integrity in mice given an intranasal inoculation of influenza virus (Li *et al.*, 1997, 1998). More recently, enteral glutamine was found to increase total cellularity of Peyer's patches (and spleen) in LPS-treated mice (Manhart *et al.*, 2000); this effect was mainly due to an increase in T-cell number. In another recent study, inclusion of glutamine in parenteral nutrition improved the concentration of secretory immunoglobulin A in the intestinal lumen and improved intestine IL-4 and IL-10 concentrations (Kudsk *et al.*, 2000).

In an animal model of haemorrhagic shock, standard parenteral nutrition decreased the *ex vivo* release of TNF-α and IL-6 by LPS-stimulated gut mononuclear cells and spleen macrophages and was associated with injury to the gut mucosa and bacterial translocation into the mesenteric lymph nodes (Schroder *et al.*, 1998). Inclusion of alanyl-glutamine and glycyl-glutamine in the parenteral regimen improved mucosal structure and prevented the fall in *ex vivo* IL-6, but not TNF-α, release (Schroder *et al.*, 1998).

Provision of Glutamine in Catabolic-stress States in Humans

The provision of glutamine or glutamine 'precursors' (glutamine-containing dipeptides, *N*-acetylglutamine, 2-oxoglutarate, branched-chain amino acids), usually by the parenteral route, has been used in various catabolic situations in humans. In most cases, the intention was not to support the immune system but rather to maintain nitrogen balance, muscle mass and/or gut integrity (for a review, see Furst *et al.*, 1997). Nevertheless, the maintenance of plasma glutamine concentrations in such a group of patients very much at risk of immunosuppression might have the added benefit of maintaining immune function.

The provision of glutamine intravenously for patients following bone-marrow transplantation resulted in a lower level of infection (12% of patients with clinical infections vs. 42% in the control group) and a shorter stay in hospital (29 ± 1 days vs. 36 ± 2 days) than for patients receiving glutamine-free parenteral nutrition (Ziegler *et al.*, 1992). A later report by this group (Ziegler *et al.*, 1998) showed that glutamine treatment resulted in greater numbers of total lymphocytes, T lymphocytes and CD4+ lymphocytes (but not B lymphocytes or natural killer cells) in the bloodstream after the patients were discharged. The authors suggested that glutamine specifically enhances T lymphocyte number and that this might be responsible for the diminished infection rate observed.

Very low-birth-weight babies who received a glutamine-enriched premature feeding formula (providing 0.3 g glutamine kg^{-1} body weight day^{-1}) had a much lower rate of sepsis (11% vs. 31%) than babies who received a standard formula (Neu *et al.*, 1997). In a study of patients in intensive care, glutamine provision decreased mortality compared with standard parenteral nutrition (43% vs. 67%) and changed the pattern of mortality (Griffiths *et al.*, 1997). Neither of these studies reported immunological outcomes of the treatments. However, another study of patients in intensive care reported that enteral glutamine increased the blood CD4:CD8 ratio (Jensen *et al.*, 1996). In a more recent study, in which patients received enteral glutamine vs. standard enteral feed from within 48 h of the trauma, there was a significant reduction in the 15-day incidence of pneumonia (17% vs. 45% in the control group), bacteraemia (7% vs. 42%) and severe sepsis (4% vs. 26%) in the glutamine group, although this was not associated with reduced mortality (Houdijk *et al.*, 1998). Parenteral administration of glutamine into patients postcolorectal surgery increased mitogen-stimulated proliferation of blood lymphocytes (O'Riordain *et al.*, 1994), suggesting that glutamine does improve T lymphocyte function in patients at risk of sepsis; glutamine did not affect *ex vivo* TNF or IL-6 production. In another study, post-operative patients who received alanyl-glutamine parenterally had increased blood lymphocyte numbers, increased *ex vivo* production of cysteinyl leucotrienes by blood neutrophils and a shorter stay in hospital (Morlion *et al.*, 1998). Most recently, infusion of a parenteral mixture containing glycyl-glutamine for 48 h after major abdominal surgery resulted in better maintenance of the human leucocyte antigen (HLA)-DR expression on circulating monocytes than in control patients who received a standard parenteral mixture (Spittler *et al.*, 2001). There was no effect of the glutamine dipeptide on production of TNF-α or IL-6 by LPS-stimulated whole blood (Spittler *et al.*, 2001). Patients with oesophageal cancer being treated with radiochemotherapy had higher blood lymphocyte counts and better lymphocyte proliferative responses if they consumed glutamine (30 g day^{-1}) for 28 days (Yoshida *et al.*, 1998). These studies indicate that glutamine is able to maintain lymphocyte numbers and (some) immune-cell responses in patients normally at risk of immunosuppression and infection.

In addition to a direct immunological effect, glutamine, even provided parenterally, improves the gut barrier function in patients at risk of infection (van der Hulst *et al.*, 1993). This would have the benefit of decreasing the translocation of bacteria from the gut and so eliminating a key source of infection. Animal studies indicate that providing glutamine does decrease bacterial translocation (Burke *et al.*, 1989).

Role of Glutamine in the Pathogenesis of Type 1 Diabetes

Since glutamine appears to act to promote lymphocyte activity, it has been proposed that increased availability of glutamine could play a role in the pathogenesis of some autoimmune conditions, such as type 1 diabetes (Wu *et al.*, 1991). Indeed, the administration of the anti-glutamine-utilization drug acivicin delayed or stopped the progression of the disease in diabetes-prone rats (Misra *et al.*, 1996). Addition of the glutaminase inhibitor 6-diazo-5-oxo-norleucine to macrophages before exposure to rat pancreatic β cells *in vitro* virtually abolished the lytic capacity of the macrophage towards the target β cells (Murphy and Newsholme, 1999). The glutamine concentration in the plasma of moderately ketoacidotic diabetics at diagnosis is significantly elevated compared with that of age- and sex-matched normal control individuals (P. Newsholme, unpublished observations), adding further weight to the argument that this amino acid is important to the pathogenic process.

Mechanism of Glutamine Action

There has been much speculation about the mechanism by which glutamine acts to preserve, or even improve, immune function. Similar metabolic characteristics apply to various cells of the immune system, despite the fact that their cell biology is different. Hence any hypothesis must explain high rates of glutamine utilization in cells with widely different cell-biological characteristics. As

indicated earlier, glutamine makes a significant contribution to energy generation in cells of the immune system. However, oxidation of glutamine is only
partial and immune cells can, and do, generate energy from other substrates
(see Calder, 1995a). These observations suggest that the importance of glutamine to immune function is not simply through its action as an energy-yielding
substrate. Another suggestion is that glutamine metabolism can generate intermediates for the synthesis of purines and pyrimidines and so provides the
building blocks for mRNA and DNA. However, the rate of synthesis of
nucleotides in lymphocytes is reported to be much less than the rate of glutamine utilization (Szondy and Newsholme, 1989). On the basis of 'metabolic
control logic', it was suggested that the importance of a high rate of glutamine
utilization in immune cells relates to maintenance of a high flux through the
pathway of glutaminolysis (i.e. the pathway of partial glutamine oxidation (Fig.
6.4)), which would allow high sensitivity to regulatory molecules controlling
biosynthetic pathways (Newsholme et al., 1989). This hypothesis has proved
difficult to test. While the capacity for rapid cell division is retained by isolated
lymphocytes, this does not apply to isolated neutrophils or macrophages, which
are terminally differentiated cells with little capacity for cell division. However,
neutrophils and macrophages have a large phagocytic capacity (requiring a
high rate of lipid turnover and synthesis) and a high secretory activity. The
mechanism by which glutamine can act to allow high rates of secretory-product
formation and release and sustain cell proliferation must account for the diverse
nature of these secretory products and the requirements for cell division and
should include at least one common metabolic product.

NADPH is required by the enzymes responsible for the formation of the
reactive species nitric oxide and superoxide, inducible nitric oxide synthase
(iNOS) and NADPH oxidase, respectively. NADPH is also required for the formation of reduced glutathione (see below) and for de novo synthesis of DNA,
RNA and fatty acids. Glutamine, via metabolism involving NADP+-dependent
malate dehydrogenase (malic enzyme (enzyme 5 in Fig. 6.4)), can generate considerable NADPH for cell requirements. The NADP+-dependent malate dehydrogenase step will result in the formation of pyruvate, which can either be
converted to lactate (ending the pathway of glutaminolysis) or be converted to
acetyl-coenzyme A (CoA) and on to CO_2. Thus, depending upon the energy
demands placed on the cell, glutamine may be partially oxidized in the pathway
of glutaminolysis or may be fully oxidized, but the outcome of metabolism in
either case is NADPH production. Glucose may also, via metabolism through
the pentose-phosphate pathway, generate NADPH. However, during periods of
active pinocytosis and phagocytosis, glucose carbon may be diverted towards
lipid synthesis and therefore the pentose-phosphate pathway may be compromised (Newsholme et al., 1996). Additionally, glutamine carbon may be used
for new amino acid synthesis in periods of active synthesis and secretion. It is
possible that NADPH is the 'common factor' that links the diverse effects that
glutamine has in cells of the immune system (Newsholme, 2001). Evidence in
support of this hypothesis is provided by the enhancing effect of glutamine on
superoxide generation in neutrophils and monocytes (Garcia et al., 1999; Saito
et al., 1999; Furukawa et al., 2000a, b) and recent in vitro data that cell prolifer-

ation in response to growth factors is positively related to the level of superoxide produced intracellularly (Suh *et al.*, 1999). Superoxide generation in cells requires the electron-donating ability of NADPH if generated via the enzyme NADPH oxidase, which directly reduces molecular oxygen. The latter enzyme is quantitatively the most significant source of superoxide in immune cells.

It is also possible that the importance of glutamine relates to its many roles as a biosynthetic precursor. Of particular importance may be its role as the precursor of glutamate for the synthesis of glutathione. Glutathione is a tripeptide antioxidant composed of glutamate, cysteine and glycine (see also Grimble, Chapter 7, this volume). Glutathione concentrations in the liver, lung, small intestine and immune cells fall in response to infection, inflammatory stimuli and trauma. The fall in hepatic glutathione concentration and in the export of glutathione from the liver can be prevented by provision of oral glutamine for rats (Hong *et al.*, 1992; Welbourne *et al.*, 1993). Glutamine-enriched parenteral nutrition elevated plasma glutathione concentration in rats (Denno *et al.*, 1996; Cao *et al.*, 1998) and promoted the release of glutathione from the rat gut into the bloodstream (Cao *et al.*, 1998).

Culture of human lymphocytes in the presence of glutathione enhances cytotoxic T-cell activity (Droge *et al.*, 1994) and depletion of intracellular glutathione diminishes lymphocyte proliferation (Chang *et al.*, 1999a) and the generation of cytotoxic T lymphocytes (Droge *et al.*, 1994). Depletion of glutathione through an exercise regimen decreased the number of CD4+ cells by 30% in a subset of individuals (Kinscherf *et al.*, 1994). Treatment with N-acetyl-cysteine (400 mg day^{-1} for 4 weeks) prevented the exercise-induced fall in intracellular glutathione concentrations and increased the number of CD4+ cells by 25%. Glutathione depletion is associated with diminished IFN-γ, but not IL-2 or IL-4, production by antigen-stimulated murine lymph-node cells (Peterson *et al.*, 1998); this effect was mediated by antigen-presenting cells and the authors suggest that glutathione acts via inducing IL-12 production by these cells to alter the T-helper (Th)1/Th2 balance in favour of a Th1 response. Thus, glutathione appears to promote a range of cell-mediated immune responses. Although glutamine is able to preserve glutathione concentrations in the liver, gut, kidney and bloodstream (see above and also Welbourne and Dass, 1982; Harward *et al.*, 1994), it is not clear whether it also preserves glutathione concentrations within immune cells. However, it was recently reported that incubation of human blood mononuclear cells with increasing concentrations of glutamine resulted in higher intracellular glutathione concentrations in both CD4+ and CD8+ cells (Chang *et al.*, 1999a). Thus, one means by which glutamine might exert its immunological effects is through maintenance of glutathione status. However, this hypothesis requires further investigation.

Conclusion

Glutamine depletion *in vivo* results in immunosuppression, and catabolic-stress situations in humans are associated with lowered plasma (and muscle) glutamine levels. Glutamine is used at a high rate by cells of the immune system and there is much evidence that key functions of these cells, tested *in vitro*, are dependent upon the provision of glutamine. Evidence is now emerging that glutamine supplied orally or intravenously improves immune function *in vivo* and in cells cultured *ex vivo*, while additionally protecting against infectious challenges. Thus, administration of glutamine or its precursors should prove beneficial as a therapy for individuals whose immune system is compromised by catabolic stress. Nevertheless, more information is required about the mechanism by which glutamine provides beneficial effects for cells of the immune system *in vivo* and *in vitro*, whether this mechanism is altered in disease states and the importance of the route of glutamine administration.

References

Albina, J.E., Henry, W., King, P.A., Shearer, J., Mastrofrancesco, B., Goldstein, L. and Caldwell, M.D. (1987) Glutamine metabolism in rat skeletal muscle wounded with α-carrageenan. *American Journal of Physiology* 252, E49–E56.

Ardawi, M.S.M. (1988a) Glutamine and glucose metabolism in human peripheral lymphocytes. *Metabolism* 37, 99–103.

Ardawi, M.S.M. (1988b) Skeletal muscle glutamine metabolism in thermally-injured rats. *Clinical Science* 74, 165–172.

Ardawi, M.S.M. (1991) Effect of glutamine-enriched total parenteral nutrition on septic rats. *Clinical Science* 81, 215–222.

Ardawi, M.S.M. and Newsholme, E.A. (1982) Maxiumum activities of some enzymes of glycolysis, the tricarboxylic acid cycle and ketone body and glutamine utilisation pathways in lymphocytes of the rat. *Biochemical Journal* 208, 743–748.

Ardawi, M.S.M. and Newsholme, E.A. (1983) Glutamine metabolism in lymphocytes of the rat. *Biochemical Journal* 212, 835–842.

Ardawi, M.S.M. and Newsholme, E.A. (1985) Metabolism in lymphocytes and its importance in the immune response. *Essays in Biochemistry* 21, 1–44.

Ashworth, L.A.E. and MacLennan, A.P. (1974) Comparison of L-asparaginases from *Escherichia coli* and *Erwinia carotovora* as immunosuppressants. *Cancer Research* 34, 1353–1359.

Askanazi, J., Elwyn, D.H., Kinney, J.M., Gump, F.E., Michelsen, C.B., Stinchfield, F.E., Furst, P., Vinnars, E. and Bergstrom, J. (1978) Muscle and plasma amino acids after injury: the role of inactivity. *Annals of Surgery* 188, 797–803.

Askanazi, J., Carpentier, Y.A., Michelsen, C.B., Elwyn, D.H., Furst, P., Kantrowitz, L.R., Gump, F.E. and Kinney, J.M. (1980) Muscle and plasma amino acids following injury: influence of intercurrent infection. *Annals of Surgery* 192, 78–85.

Bergstrom, J., Furst, P., Noree, L.-O. and Vinnars, E. (1974) Intracellular free amino acid concentrations in human skeletal muscle tissue. *Journal of Applied Physiology* 36, 693–697.

Brambilla, G., Pardodi, S., Cavanna, M., Caraceni, C.E. and Baldini, L. (1970) The immunodepressive activity of *E. coli* L-asparaginase in some transplant systems. *Cancer Research* 30, 2665–2670.

Brand, K. (1985) Glutamine and glucose metabolism during thymocyte proliferation. *Biochemical Journal* 228, 353–361.

Brand, K., Fekl, W., von Hintzenstern, J., Langer, K., Luppa, P. and Schoerner, C. (1989) Metabolism of glutamine in lymphocytes. *Metabolism* 38, 29–33.

Burke, D.J., Alverdy, J.C., Aoys, E. and Moss, G.S. (1989) Glutamine-supplemented total parenteral nutrition improves gut immune function. *Archives of Surgery* 124, 1396–1399.

Calder, P.C. (1994) Glutamine and the immune system. *Clinical Nutrition* 13, 2–8.

Calder, P.C. (1995a) Fuel utilisation by cells of the immune system. *Proceedings of the Nutrition Society* 54, 65–82.

Calder, P.C. (1995b) Requirement of both glutamine and arginine by proliferating lymphocytes. *Proceedings of the Nutrition Society* 54, 123A.

Calder, P.C. and Newsholme, E.A. (1992) Glutamine promotes interleukin-2 production by concanavalin A-stimulated lymphocytes. *Proceedings of the Nutrition Society* 51, 105A.

Calder, P.C. and Yaqoob, P. (1999) Glutamine and the immune system. *Amino Acids* 17, 227–241.

Cao, Y., Feng, Z., Hoos, A. and Klimberg, V.S. (1998) Glutamine enhances gut glutathione production. *Journal of Parenteral and Enteral Nutrition* 22, 224–227.

Castell, L.M., Poortmans, J.R., Leclercq, R., Brasseur, M., Duchateau, J. and Newsholme, E.A. (1997) Some aspects of the acute phase response after a marathon race, and the effects of glutamine supplementation. *European Journal of Applied Physiology* 75, 47–53.

Chakrabarti, R. (1998) Transcriptional regulation of the rat glutamine synthetase gene by tumor necrosis factor-alpha. *European Journal of Biochemistry* 254, 70–74.

Chakrabaty, A.K. and Friedman, H. (1970) L-asparaginase-induced immunosuppression: effects on antibody-forming cells and antibody titres. *Science* 167, 869–870.

Chang, W.K., Yang, K.D. and Shaio, M.F. (1999a) Lymphocyte proliferation modulated by glutamine; involved in the redox reaction. *Clinical and Experimental Immunology* 117, 482–488.

Chang, W.K., Yang, K.D. and Shaio, M.F. (1999b) Effect of glutamine on Th1 and Th2 cytokine responses of human peripheral blood mononuclear cells. *Clinical Immunology* 93, 294–301.

Chuang, J.C., Yu, C.L. and Wang, S.R. (1990) Modulation of human lymphocyte proliferation by amino acids. *Clinical and Experimental Immunology* 81, 173–176.

Crawford, J. and Cohen, H.J. (1985) The essential role of glutamine in lymphocyte differentiation *in vitro*. *Journal of Cell Physiology* 124, 275–282.

Curi, T.C.P., Demelo, M.P., Deazevedo, R.B., Zorn, T.M.T. and Curi, R. (1997) Glutamine utilization by rat neutrophils: presence of phosphate-dependent glutaminase. *American Journal of Physiology* 42, C1124–C1129.

Denno, R., Rounds, J.D., Faris, R., Holejko, L.B. and Wilmore, D.W. (1996) Glutamine-enriched total parenteral nutrition enhances plasma glutathione in the resting state. *Journal of Surgical Research* 61, 35–38.

Deutz, N.E.P., Reijven, P.L.M., Athanasas, G. and Soeters, P.B. (1992) Post-operative changes in hepatic, intestinal, splenic and muscle fluxes of amino acids and ammonia in pigs. *Clinical Science* 83, 607–614.

DeWitt, R.C., Wu, Y., Renegar, K.B. and Kudsk, K.A. (1999) Glutamine-enriched total parenteral nutrition preserves respiratory immunity and improves survival to *Pseudomonas* pneumonia. *Journal of Surgical Research* 84, 13–18.

Droge, W., Schulzeosthoff, K., Mihm, S., Galter, D., Schenk, H., Eck, H.P., Roth, S. and Gmunder, H. (1994) Functions of glutathione and glutathione disulfide immunology and immunopathology. *FASEB Journal* 8, 1131–1138.

Durden, D.L. and Distasio, J.A. (1981) Characterisation of the effects of asparaginase from *Escherichia coli* and a glutaminase-free asparaginase from *Vibrio succinogenes* on specific cell-mediated cytotoxicity. *International Journal of Cancer* 27, 59–65.

Eagle, H., Oyama, V.I., Levy, M., Horton, C.L. and Fleischman, R. (1956) The growth response of mammalian cells in tissue culture to L-glutamine and L-glutamic acid. *Journal of Biological Chemistry* 218, 607.

Ehrensvard, G., Fischer, A. and Stjernholm, R. (1949) Protein metabolism of tissue cells *in vitro*: the chemical nature of some obligate factors of tissue cell nutrition. *Acta Physiologica Scandanavica* 18, 218.

Elia, M. and Lunn, P.G. (1997) The use of glutamine in the treatment of gastrointestinal disorders in man. *Nutrition* 13, 743–747.

Furst, P., Bergstrom, J., Chao, L., Larsson, J., Liljedahl, S.-O., Neuhauser, M., Schildt, B. and Vinnars, E. (1979) Influence of amino acid supply on nitrogen and amino acid metabolism in severe trauma. *Acta Chirurgica Scandinavica* 494 (Suppl.), 136–138.

Furst, P., Pogan, K. and Stehle, P. (1997) Glutamine dipeptides in clinical nutrition. *Nutrition* 13, 731–737.

Furukawa, S., Saito, H., Fukatsu, K., Hashiguchi, Y., Inaba, T., Lin, M., Inoue, T., Han, I., Matsuda, T. and Muto, T. (1997) Glutamine-enhanced bacterial killing by neutrophils from post-operative patients. *Nutrition* 13, 863–869.

Furukawa, S., Saito, H., Matsuda, T., Inoue, T., Fukatsu, K., Han, I., Ikeda, S., Hidemura, A. and Muto, T. (2000a) Relative effects of glucose and glutamine on reactive oxygen intermediate production by neutrophils. *Shock* 13, 274–278.

Furukawa, S., Saito, H., Inoue, T., Matsuda, T., Fukatsu, K., Han, I., Ikeda, S. and Hidemura, A. (2000b) Supplemental glutamine augments phagocytosis and reactive oxygen intermediate production by neutrophils and monocytes from postoperative patients *in vitro*. *Nutrition* 16, 323–329.

Garcia, C., Pithon Curi, T.C., De Lourdes Firmano, M., De Melo, M.P., Newsholme, P. and Curi, R. (1999) Effect of adrenaline on glucose and glutamine metabolism and superoxide production by rat neutrophils. *Clinical Science* 96, 549–555.

Griffiths, M. and Keast, D. (1990) The effect of glutamine on murine splenic leucocyte responses to T and B-cell mitogens. *Immunology and Cell Biology* 68, 405–408.

Griffiths, R.D., Jones, C. and Palmer, T.E.A. (1997) Six-month outcome of critically ill patients given glutamine-supplemented parenteral nutrition. *Nutrition* 13, 295–302.

Hack, V., Weiss, C., Friedmann, B., Suttner, S., Schykowski, M., Erbe, N., Benner, A., Bartsch, P. and Droge, W. (1997) Decreased plasma glutamine level and CD4+ T-cell number in response to 8 wk of anaerobic training. *American Journal of Physiology* 272, E788–E795.

Hankard, R.G., Darmaun, D., Sager, B.K., Damore, D., Parsons, W.R. and Haymond, M. (1995) Response of glutamine metabolism to exogenous glutamine in humans. *American Journal of Physiology* 32, E663–E670.

Harward, T.R., Coe, D., Souba, W.W., Klingman, N. and Seeger, J.M. (1994) Glutamine preserves gut glutathione levels during intestinal ischemia/reperfusion. *Journal of Surgical Research* 56, 351–355.

Haussinger, D. (1989) Glutamine metabolism in the liver: overview and current concepts. *Metabolism* 38 (Suppl. 1), 14–17.

Heberer, M., Babst, R., Juretic, A., Gross, T., Horig, H., Harder, F. and Spagnoli, G. (1996) Role of glutamine in the immune response in critical illness. *Nutrition* 12, S71-S72.

Hirsch, E.M. (1970) L-Glutaminase: suppression of lymphocyte blastogenic responses *in vitro*. *Science* 172, 736–738.

Hong, R.W., Rounds, J.D., Helton, W.S., Robinson, M.K. and Wilmore, D.W. (1992) Glutamine preserves liver glutathione after lethal hepatic injury. *Annals of Surgery* 215, 114–119.

Horvath, K., Jami, M., Hill, I.D., Papadimitriou, J.C., Magder, L.S. and Chanasongcram, S. (1996) Isocaloric glutamine-free diet and the morphology and function of rat small intestine. *Journal of Parenteral and Enteral Nutrition* 20, 128–134.

Houdijk, A.P.J., Rijnsburger, E.R., Jansen, J., Wesdorp, R.I.C., Weis, J.K., McCamish, M.A., Teerlink, T., Meuwissen, S.G.M., Haarman, H.J.T.M., Thijs, L.G. and van Leeuwen, P.A.M. (1998) Randomised trial of glutamine-enriched parenteral nutrition on infectious morbidity in patients with multiple trauma. *Lancet* 352, 772–776.

Inoue, Y., Grant, J.P. and Snyder, P.J. (1993) Effect of glutamine-supplemented intravenous nutrition on survival after *Escherichia coli*-induced peritonitis. *Journal of Parenteral and Enteral Nutrition* 17, 41–46.

Jensen, G.L., Miller, R.H., Talabiska, D.G., Fish, J. and Gianferante, L. (1996) A double blind, prospective, randomized study of glutamine-enriched compared with standard peptide-based feeding in critically ill patients. *American Journal of Clinical Nutrition* 64, 615–621.

Kafkewitz, D. and Bendich, A. (1983) Enzyme-induced asparagine and glutamine depletion and immune system dysfunction. *American Journal of Clinical Nutrition* 37, 1025–1030.

Keast, D. and Newsholme, E.A. (1990) Effect of mitogens on the maximum activities of hexokinase, lactate dehydrogenase, citrate synthase and glutaminase in rat mesenteric lymph node lymphocytes and splenocytes during the early period of culture. *International Journal of Biochemistry* 22, 133–136.

Keast, D., Arstein, D.L., Harper, W., Fry, R.W. and Morton, A.R. (1995) Depression of plasma glutamine concentration after exercise stress and its possible influence on the immune system. *Medical Journal of Australia* 162, 15–18.

Kew, S., Wells, S.M., Yaqoob, P., Wallace, F.A., Miles, E.A. and Calder, P.C. (1999) Dietary glutamine enhances murine T-lymphocyte responsiveness. *Journal of Nutrition* 129, 1524–1531.

Kinscherf, R., Fischbach, T., Mihm, S., Roth, S., Hohenhaus-Sievert, E., Weiss, C., Edler, L., Bartsch, P. and Droge, W. (1994) Effect of glutathione depletion and oral N-acetyl-cysteine treatment on CD4+ and CD8+ cells. *FASEB Journal* 8, 448–451.

Kohler, H., Hartig-Knecht, H., Ruggeberg, J., Adam, R. and Schroten, H. (2000) Lymphocyte proliferation is possible with low concentrations of glycyl-glutamine. *European Journal of Nutrition* 39, 103–105.

Kudsk, K.A., Wu, Y., Fukatsu, K., Zarzaur, B.L., Johnson, C.D., Wang, R. and Hanna, M.K. (2000) Glutamine-enriched total parenteral nutrition maintains intestinal interleukin-4 and mucosal immunoglobulin A levels. *Journal of Parenteral and Enteral Nutrition* 24, 270–274.

Kweon, M.N., Moriguchi, S., Mukai, K. and Kishino, Y. (1991) Effect of alanylglutamine-enriched infusion on tumour growth and cellular immune function in rats. *Amino Acids* 1, 7–16.

Lacey, J.M. and Wilmore, D.W. (1990) Is glutamine a conditionally essential amino acid? *Nutrition Reviews* 48, 297–309.

Li, J., Kudsk, K.A., Janu, P. and Renegar, K.B. (1997) Effect of glutamine-enriched TPN on small intestine gut-associated lymphoid tissue (GALT) and upper respiratory tract immunity. *Surgery* 121, 542–549.

Li, J., King, B.K., Janu, P.G., Renegar, K.B. and Kudsk, K.A. (1998) Glycyl-L-glutamine-enriched total parenteral nutrition maintains small intestine gut-associated lymphoid tissue and upper respiratory tract immunity. *Journal of Parenteral and Enteral Nutrition* 22, 31–36.

Lund, J., Stjernstrom, H., Bergholm, U., Jorfeldt, L., Vinnars, E. and Wiklund, L. (1986) The exchange of blood-borne amino acids in the leg during abdominal surgical trauma: effects of glucose infusion. *Clinical Science* 71, 487–496.

Lund, P. (1981) Metabolism of glutamine, glutamate and aspartate. In: Waterlow, J.C. and Stephen, J.M.L. (eds) *Nitrogen Metabolism in Man*. Applied Sciences, London, pp. 155–167.

Lund, P. and Williamson, D.H. (1985) Inter-tissue nitrogen fluxes. *British Medical Bulletin* 41, 251–256.

Manhart, N., Vierlinger, K., Akomeah, R., Bergmeister, H., Spittler, A. and Roth, E. (2000) Influence of enteral diets supplemented with key nutrients on lymphocyte subpopulations in Peyer's patches of endotoxin-boostered mice. *Clinical Nutrition* 19, 265–269.

Max, S.R., Hill, J., Mearow, K., Konagaya, H., Konagaya, Y., Thomas, J.W., Banner, C. and Vitkavic, L. (1988) Dexamethasone regulates glutamine synthetase expression in rat skeletal muscles. *American Journal of Physiology* 255, E397–E403.

Milewski, P.J., Threlfall, C.J., Heath, D.F., Holbrook, J.B., Wilford, K. and Irving, M.H. (1982) Intracellular free amino acids in undernourished patients with and without sepsis. *Clinical Science* 62, 83–91.

Misra, M., Duguid, W.P. and Marliss, E.B. (1996) Prevention of diabetes in the spontaneously diabetic BB rat by the glutamine antimetabolite acivicin. *Canadian Journal of Physiology and Pharmacology* 74, 163–172.

Morlion, B.J., Stehle, P., Wachter, P., Siedhoff, H.P., Koller, M., Konig, W., Furst, P. and Puchstein, C. (1998) Total parenteral nutrition with glutamine dipeptide after major abdominal surgery – a randomized, double-blind, controlled study. *Annals of Surgery* 227, 302–308.

Muhlbacher, F., Kapadia, C.R., Colpoys, M.F., Smith, R.J. and Wilmore, D.W. (1984) Effects of glucocorticoids on glutamine metabolism in skeletal muscle. *American Journal of Physiology* 247, E75–E83.

Murphy, C.J. and Newsholme, P. (1998) The importance of glutamine metabolism in murine macrophages and human monocytes to L-arginine biosynthesis and rates of nitrite or urea production. *Clinical Science* 95, 397–407.

Murphy, C. and Newsholme, P. (1999) Macrophage-mediated lysis of a β-cell line, tumour necrosis factor-α release from bacillus Calmette–Guérin (BCG)-activated murine macrophages and interleukin-8 release from human monocytes are dependent on extracellular glutamine concentration and glutamine metabolism. *Clinical Science* 96, 89–97.

Naka, S., Saito, H., Hashiguchi, Y., Lin, M.T., Furukawa, S., Inoba, T., Fukushima, R., Wada, N. and Muto, T. (1996) Alanyl-glutamine-supplemented total parenteral nutrition improves survival and protein metabolism in rat protracted bacterial peritonitis model. *Journal of Parenteral and Enteral Nutrition* 20, 417–423.

Neu, J., Roig, J.C., Meetze, W.H., Veerman, M., Carter, C., Millsaps, M., Bowling, D., Dallas, M.J., Sleasman, J., Knight, T. and Anestad, N. (1997) Enteral glutamine supplementation for very low birthweight infants decreases morbidity. *Journal of Pediatrics* 131, 691–699.

Newsholme, E.A. and Calder, P.C. (1997) The proposed role of glutamine in some cells of the immune system and speculative consequences for the whole animal. *Nutrition* 13, 728–730.

Newsholme, E.A., Newsholme, P., Curi, R., Crabtree, B. and Ardawi, M.S.M. (1989) Glutamine metabolism in different tissues: its physiological and pathological importance. In: Kinney, J.M. and Borum, P.R. (eds) *Perspectives in Clinical Nutrition*. Urban and Schwarzenberg, Baltimore, pp. 71–98.

Newsholme, P. (1987) Studies on metabolism in macrophages. D Phil thesis, University of Oxford.

Newsholme, P. (2001) Why is L-glutamine metabolism important to cells of the immune system in health, post-injury, surgery or infection? *Journal of Nutrition* 131, 2515S–2522S.

Newsholme, P. and Newsholme, E.A. (1989) Rates of utilisation of glucose, glutamine and oleate and formation of end products by mouse peritoneal macrophages in culture. *Biochemical Journal* 261, 211–218.

Newsholme, P., Curi, R., Gordon, S. and Newsholme, E.A. (1986) Metabolism of glucose, glutamine, long-chain fatty acids and ketone bodies by murine macrophages. *Biochemical Journal* 239, 121–125.

Newsholme, P., Gordon, S. and Newsholme, E.A. (1987) Rates of utilisation and fates of glucose, glutamine, pyruvate, fatty acids and ketone bodies by mouse macrophages. *Biochemical Journal* 242, 631–636.

Newsholme, P., Costa Rosa, L.F.B.P., Newsholme, E.A. and Curi, R. (1996). The importance of macrophage fuel metabolism to its function. *Cell Biochemistry and Function* 14, 1–10.

Newsholme, P., Curi, R., Curi, T.C.P., Murphy, C.J., Garcia, C. and de Melo, M.P. (1999) Glutamine metabolism by lymphocytes, macrophages and neutrophils: its importance in health and disease. *Journal of Nutritional Biochemistry* 10, 316–324.

Ogle, C.K., Ogle, J.D., Mao, J.X., Simon, J., Noel, J.G., Li, B.G. and Alexander, J.W. (1994) Effect of glutamine on phagocytosis and bacterial killing by normal and pediatric burn patient neutrophils. *Journal of Parenteral and Enteral Nutrition* 18, 128–133.

O'Riordain, M., Fearon, K.C., Ross, J.A., Rogers, P., Falconer, J.S., Bartolo, D.C.C., Garden, O.J. and Carter, D.C. (1994) Glutamine supplemented parenteral nutrition enhances T-lymphocyte response in surgical patients undergoing colorectal resection. *Annals of Surgery* 220, 212–221.

O'Rourke, A.M. and Rider, L.C. (1989) Glucose, glutamine and ketone body utilisation by resting and concanavalin A activated rat splenic lymphocytes. *Biochimica et Biophysica Acta* 1010, 342–345.

Oudemans-van Straaten, H.M., Bosman, R.J., Treskes, M., van der Spoel, H.J.I. and Zandstra, D.F. (2001) Plasma glutamine depletion and patient outcome in acute ICU admissions. *Intensive Care Medicine* 27, 84–90.

Parry-Billings, M., Leighton, B., Dimitriadis, G.D., de Vasconcelos, P.R.L. and Newsholme, E.A. (1989) Skeletal muscle glutamine metabolism during sepsis. *International Journal of Biochemistry* 21, 419–423.

Parry-Billings, M., Evans, J., Calder, P.C. and Newsholme, E.A. (1990a) Does glutamine contribute to immunosuppression after major burns? *Lancet* 336, 523–525.

Parry-Billings, M., Leighton, B., Dimitriadis, G.D., Bond, J. and Newsholme, E.A. (1990b) Effects of physiological and pathological levels of glucocorticoids on skeletal muscle glutamine metabolism in the rat. *Biochemical Pharmacology* 40, 1145–1148.

Parry-Billings, M., Leighton, B., Dimitriadis, G., Curi, R., Bond, J., Bevan, S., Colquhoun, A. and Newsholme, E.A. (1991) The effect of tumour bearing on skleletal muscle glutamine metabolism. *International Journal of Biochemistry* 23, 933–937.

Parry-Billings, M., Baigrie, R.J., Lamont, P.M., Morris, P.J. and Newsholme, E.A. (1992a) Effects of major and minor surgery on plasma glutamine and cytokine levels. *Archives of Surgery* 127, 1237–1240.

Parry-Billings, M., Budgett, R., Koutedakis, Y., Blomstrand, E., Williams, C., Calder, P.C., Pilling, S., Baigrie, R. and Newsholme, E.A. (1992b) Plasma amino acid concentrations in the overtraining syndrome: possible effects on the immune system. *Medicine and Science in Sports and Exercise* 24, 1353–1358.

Peltonen, E., Pulkki, K. and Kirvela, O. (1997) Stimulatory effect of glutamine on human monocyte activation as measured by interleukin-6 and soluble interleukin-6 receptor release. *Clinical Nutrition* 16, 125–128.

Peterson, J.D., Herzenberg, L.A., Vasquez, K. and Waltenbaugh, C. (1998) Glutathione levels in antigen-presenting cells modulate Th1 versus Th2 response patterns. *Proceedings of the National Academy of Sciences of the USA* 95, 3071–3076.

Powell, H., Castell, L.M., Parry-Billings, M., Desborough, J.P., Hall, G.M. and Newsholme, E.A. (1994) Growth hormone suppression and glutamine flux associated with cardiac surgery. *Clinical Physiology* 14, 569–580.

Rohde, T., Maclean, D.A. and Pedersen, B.K. (1996a) Glutamine, lymphocyte proliferation and cytokine production. *Scandinavian Journal of Immunology* 44, 648–650.

Rohde, T., Maclean, D.A., Hartkopp, A. and Pedersen, B.K. (1996b) The immune system and serum glutamine during a triathlon. *European Journal of Applied Physiology* 74, 428–434.

Roth, E., Funovics, J., Muhlbacher, F., Schemper, M., Mauritz, W., Sporn, P. and Fritsch, A. (1982) Metabolic disorders in severe abdominal sepsis: glutamine deficiency in skeletal muscle. *Clinical Nutrition* 1, 25–41.

Saito, H., Furukawa, S. and Matsuda, T. (1999) Glutamine as an immunoenhancing nutrient. *Journal of Parenteral and Enteral Nutrition* 23 (Suppl.), S59.

Schroder, J., Lahlke, V., Fandrich, F., Gebhardt, H., Erichsen, H., Zabel, P. and Schroeder, P. (1998) Glutamine dipeptides-supplemented parenteral nutrition reverses gut muscosal structure and interleukin-6 release of rat intestinal mononuclear cells after hemorrhagic shock. *Shock* 10, 26–31.

Shewchuk, L.D., Baracos, V.E. and Field, C.J. (1997) Dietary L-glutamine supplementation reduces growth of the Morris Hepatoma 7777 in exercise-trained and sedentary rats. *Journal of Nutrition* 127, 158–166.

Simberkoff, M.S. and Thomas, L. (1970) Reversal by L-glutamine of the inhibition of lymphocyte mitosis caused by *E. coli* asparaginase. *Proceedings of the Society of Experimental Biology* 133, 642–643.

Souba, W.W. (1991) Glutamine: a key substrate for the splanchnic bed. *Annual Review in Nutrition* 11, 285–308.

Spittler, A., Winkler, S., Gotzinger, P., Oehler, R., Willheim, M., Tempfer, C., Weigel, G., Fugger, R., Boltz-Nitulescu, G. and Roth, E. (1995) Influence of glutamine on the phenotype and function of human monocytes. *Blood* 86, 1564–1569.

Spittler, A., Holzer, S., Oehler, R., Boltz-Nitulescu, G. and Roth, E. (1997) A glutamine deficiency impairs the function of cultured human monocytes. *Clinical Nutrition* 16, 97–99.

Spittler, A., Sautner, T., Gornikiewicz, A., Manhart, N., Oehler, R., Bergmann, M., Fugger, R. and Roth, E. (2001) Postoperative glycyl-glutamine infusion reduces immunosuppression: partial prevention of the surgery induced decrease in HLA-DR expression on monocytes. *Clinical Nutrition* 20, 37–42.

Spolarics, Z., Lang, C.H., Bagby, G.J. and Spitzer, J.J. (1991) Glutamine and fatty acid oxidation are the main sources of energy in Kupffer and endothelial cells. *American Journal of Physiology* 261, G185–G190.

Stinnett, J.D., Alexander, J.W., Watanabe, C., Elwyn, D.H., Furst, P., Kantrowitz, L.R., Gump, F.E. and Kinney, J.M. (1982) Plasma and skeletal muscle amino acids following severe burn injury in patients and experimental animals. *Annals of Surgery* 195, 75–89.

Suh, Y.A., Arnold, R.S., Lassegue, B., Shi, J., Xu, X., Sorescu, D., Chung, A.B., Griendling, K.K. and Lambeth, D. (1999) Cell transformation by the superoxide-generating oxidase Mox 1. *Nature* 401, 79–82.

Suzuki, I., Matsumoto, Y., Adjei, A.A., Osato, L., Shinjo, S. and Yamamoto, S. (1993) Effect of a glutamine-supplemented diet in response to methicillin-resistant *Staphylococcus aureus* infection in mice. *Journal of Nutritional Science and Vitaminology* 39, 405–410.

Szondy, Z. and Newsholme, E.A. (1989) The effect of glutamine concentration on the activity of carbamoyl-phosphate synthase II and on the incorporation of [^{3}H]thymidine into DNA in rat mesenteric lymphocytes stimulated by phytohaemagglutinin. *Biochemical Journal* 261, 979–983.

Tizianello, A., Deferrari, G., Garibotto, G., Robabaudo, C., Asquarone, N. and Ghiggeri, G.N. (1982) Renal ammoniagenesis in an early stage of metabolic acidosis in man. *Journal of Clinical Investigation* 69, 240–250.

van der Hulst, R.R.W., van Kreel, B.K., von Meyenfeldt, M.F., Brummer, R.-J.M., Arends, J.-W., Deutz, N.E.P. and Soeters, P.B. (1993) Glutamine and the preservation of gut integrity. *Lancet* 341, 1363–1365.

Wallace, C. and Keast, D. (1992) Glutamine and macrophage function. *Metabolism* 41, 1016–1020.

Welbourne, T.C. and Dass, P.D. (1982) Function of renal γ-glutamyl-transferase: significance of glutathione and glutamine. *Life Sciences* 30, 793–801.

Welbourne, T.C., King, A.B. and Horton, K. (1993) Enteral glutamine supports hepatic glutathione efflux during inflammation. *Journal of Nutritional Biochemistry* 4, 236–242.

Wells, S.M., Kew, S., Yaqoob, P., Wallace, F.A. and Calder, P.C. (1999) Dietary glutamine enhances cytokine production by murine macrophages. *Nutrition* 15, 881–884.

Wilmore, D. and Shabert, J.K. (1998) Role of glutamine in immunologic responses. *Nutrition* 14, 618–626.

Windmueller, H.G. and Spaeth, A.E. (1974) Uptake and metabolism of plasma glutamine by the small intestine. *Journal of Biological Chemistry* 249, 5070–5079.

Wu, G., Field, C.J. and Marliss, E.B. (1991) Elevated glutamine metabolism in splenocytes from spontaneously diabetic BB rats. *Biochemical Journal* 274, 49–54

Yaqoob, P. and Calder, P.C. (1997) Glutamine requirement of proliferating T lymphocytes. *Nutrition* 13, 646–651.

Yaqoob, P. and Calder, P.C. (1998) Cytokine production by human peripheral blood mononuclear cells: differential sensitivity to glutamine availability. *Cytokine* 10, 790–794.

Yassad, A., Husson, A., Bion, A. and Lavoinne, A. (2000) Synthesis of interleukin 1 beta and interleukin 6 by stimulated rat peritoneal macrophages: modulation by glutamine. *Cytokine* 12, 1288–1291.

Yoo, S.S., Field, C.J. and McBurney, M.I. (1997) Glutamine supplementation maintains intramuscular glutamine concentrations and normalizes lymphocyte function in infected early weaned pigs. *Journal of Nutrition* 127, 2253–2259.

Yoshida, S., Hikida, S., Tanaka, Y., Yanase, A., Mizote, H. and Kaegawa, T. (1992) Effect of glutamine supplementation on lymphocyte function in septic rats. *Journal of Parenteral and Enteral Nutrition* 16, 30S.

Yoshida, S., Matsui, M., Shirouzu, Y., Fujita, H., Yamana, H. and Shirouzu, K. (1998) Effects of glutamine supplements and radiochemotherapy on systemic immune and gut barrier function in patients with advanced esophageal cancer. *Annals of Surgery* 227, 485–491.

Ziegler, T.R., Young, L.S., Benfell, K., Scheltinga, M., Hortog, K., Bye, R., Morrow, F.D., Jacobs, D.O., Smith, R.J., Antin, J.H. and Wilmore, D.W. (1992) Clinical and metabolic efficacy of glutamine-supplemented parenteral nutrition following bone marrow transplantation: a double-blinded, randomized, controlled trial. *Annals of Internal Medicine* 116, 821–828.

Ziegler, T.R., Bye, R.L., Persinger, R.L., Young, L.S., Antin, J.H. and Wilmore, D.W. (1998) Effects of glutamine supplementation on circulating lymphocytes after bone marrow transplantation: a pilot study. *American Journal of Medical Science* 315, 4–10.

7

Sulphur Amino Acids, Glutathione and Immune Function

Robert F. Grimble

Institute of Human Nutrition, School of Medicine, University of Southampton, Bassett Crescent East, Southampton SO16 7PX, UK

The Biochemistry of Sulphur Amino Acids

Sulphur amino acid metabolism

The sulphur amino acids are methionine and cysteine. Their metabolism is inter-linked. As a result of this metabolism, the sulphur moiety is incorporated into a number of end-products, three of which, glutathione, taurine and proteins, have important roles in immune function. Methionine is a nutritionally essential amino acid, due to the inability of mammals to synthesize its carbon skeleton. Cysteine is considered to be semi-essential, in that it is synthesized from methionine provided that the dietary supply of the latter is sufficient. The methyl group of methionine can be removed from and reattached to the carbon skeleton of the amino acid by a cyclical process referred to as the transmethylation pathway (Fig. 7.1). The formation of homocysteine, part way along the transmethylation pathway, is an important branch point in the metabolism of methionine. Homocysteine can be remethylated to form methionine or can be metabolized by the transulphuration pathway to form cysteine (Fig. 7.1). Both the remethylation of homocysteine and the formation of cysteine utilize serine. This latter amino acid forms the carbon skeleton of cysteine and acts as a methyl-group donor to tetrahydrofolic acid, once the methyl version of the latter compound has donated its methyl group to homocysteine during the formation of methionine.

Methionine is intimately involved in the synthesis of the polyamines spermine and spermidine, in which the carbon chain of methionine is donated to a third polyamine, putrescine, which is derived from ornithine (Fig. 7.2). The polyamines are present in high concentrations in rapidly dividing cells, such as those of an activated immune system. Their role is poorly defined but appears to be important. Polyamines have been likened to 'molecular grease', in that they are permissive metabolites, ensuring the fidelity of DNA transcription and RNA translation (Grimble and Grimble, 1998). In *in vitro* studies, cells depleted

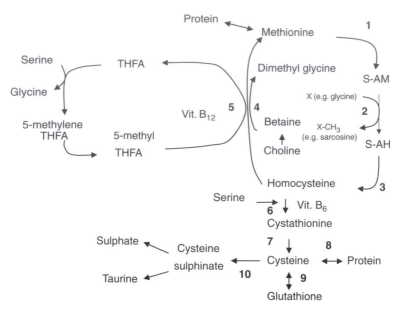

Fig. 7.1. Outline of sulphur amino acid metabolism. Enzymes: 1, methionine adenosyl transferase; 2, methyl transferase; 3, adenosyl homocysteinase; 4, betaine methyltransferase; 5, S-methyltetrahydrofolate methyl transferase; 6, cystathionine β-synthase; 7, cystathionine γ-lyase; 8, L-cysteinyl-tRNA synthetase; 9, γ-glutamyl cysteine synthase; 10, cysteine dioxygenase. S-AH, S-adenosyl homocysteine; S-AM, S-adenosyl methionine; THFA, tetrahydrofolic acid.

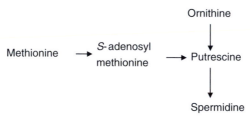

Fig. 7.2. Polyamine biosynthesis.

of polyamines exhibit increased error rates in both processes. The first enzyme in the step from ornithine to putrescine is highly induced in rapidly dividing cells.

Methionine also acts as a methyl donor in the synthesis of creatine (Fig. 7.3), which is essential for muscle energy generation through its phosphorylation to creatine phosphate. Creatine phosphate can transfer its phosphate to ADP to restore cellular ATP supplies during periods of high metabolic activity.

In addition to incorporation into proteins, cysteine can be incorporared into the key antioxidant glutathione (GSH), or converted to taurine and inorganic sulphate. The possession of an SH group by cysteine and GSH allows the formation of an S–S bridge between two molecules of cysteine or of GSH to form cystine and oxidized glutathione (GSSG), respectively. Taurine has many roles, including formation of the bile salt taurocholic acid, and is a puta-

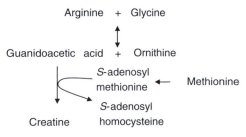

Fig. 7.3. Creatine biosynthesis.

tive antioxidant and cell membrane stabilizer. Taurine is the predominant nitrogenous compound in immune cells.

The synthesis of glutathione from its three constituent amino acids is mainly limited to the liver. Two consecutive steps are required to synthesize glutathione, each step consuming one ATP molecule (Fig. 7.4). The rate-limiting enzyme in the pathway is γ-glutamyl cysteine synthetase (step 1 of Fig. 7.4). Under normal physiological conditions, there is feedback on the activity of this enzyme by GSH. Thus, conversion of cysteine to GSH is strongly influenced by the rate of utilization/transport of GSH within and between the cells of the body. In other words, synthesis is a 'demand-led' process, provided that cysteine is available.

Glutathione is transferred to the blood and transported around the body in both plasma and cells mainly in its reduced form (GSH).

Thus, apart from protein synthesis, sulphur amino acids are involved as direct and indirect participants in pathways involved in cell replication and stabilization, antioxidant defence, assimilation of lipids and energy metabolism. As the immune response involves major changes in cell replication, oxidant stress and lipid and energy metabolism, it is not surprising that the availability of sulphur amino acids has a major impact on immune function.

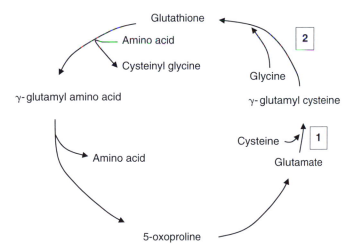

Fig. 7.4. Formation of glutathione and its role in the γ-glutamyl cycle. Enzymes: 1, γ-glutamyl cysteine synthase; 2, glutathione synthase.

Control of sulphur amino acid metabolism

The K_m values for the homocysteine transferase enzymes (steps 4 and 5 of Fig. 7.1) (which lead to the recycling of methionine) are two orders of magnitude lower than those for cystathionine synthase (step 6 of Fig. 7.1) and cystathionine γ-lyase (step 7 of Fig. 7.1) (which process methionine towards catabolism via the transulphuration pathway). Thus, at low intracellular concentrations of methionine, remethylation will be favoured over transulphuration and methionine will be conserved. When these two pathways were examined *in vivo* in rats fed diets containing 3, 15 and 30 g L-methionine kg^{-1} of diet, the percentage of methionine metabolized by the two competing pathways changed (Finkelstein and Martin, 1984, 1986). With increasing dietary methionine intake, substrate flux through the transmethylation pathway fell and flux through the transulphuration pathway increased.

Examination of the K_m values for rate-limiting enzymes processing the major cysteine metabolites provides a further insight into how sulphur amino acid metabolism is influenced by alteration in the supply of cysteine. The K_m for L-cysteinyl-tRNA synthetase (step 8 of Fig. 7.1) (essential for incorporation of cysteine into protein) is less than one-tenth of that for γ-glutamyl cysteine synthetase (step 9 of Fig. 7.1) (the rate-limiting enzyme for GSH synthesis) or cysteine dioxygenase (step 10 of Fig. 7.1) (forming cysteine sulphinate, the precursor for sulphate and taurine). Thus, under conditions of low cysteine availability, protein synthesis will be maintained and sythesis of sulphate, taurine and GSH curtailed.

From the kinetics of the key enzymes in sulphur amino acid metabolism reported above, it can be seen that, when the diet is low in sulphur amino acids, cellular methionine is highly conserved. Flux down the transulphuration pathway, which ultimately leads to methionine catabolism, increases only as dietary methionine intake increases. It can also be seen that, at low flux rates of substrate down the transulphuration pathway, conversion of cysteine into its main metabolites will be affected, so that protein synthesis will be relatively maintained while sulphate and GSH synthesis rates will fall. Synthesis of GSH and sulphate will increase in concert as increasing levels of substrate flow through the pathway. In a study in rats, seven molecules of cysteine were incorporated into GSH for every ten incorporated into protein in liver at adequate sulphur amino acid intake (Grimble and Grimble, 1998). At inadequate sulphur amino acid intake, the ratio fell to $< 3:10$. This response to a low intake of sulphur amino acids will not necessarily be advantageous since GSH is an important component of antioxidant defence. Thus, at low sulphur amino acid intakes, antioxidant defences will become weakened. The immune response makes large demands on these defences and sulphur amino acid metabolism in particular.

Sulphur Amino Acid and Glutathione Metabolism Following Infection and Injury

The immune system has a great capacity for immobilizing invading microbes, creating a hostile environment for them and bringing about their destruction (Fig. 7.5). The immune system can also become activated, in a similar way to

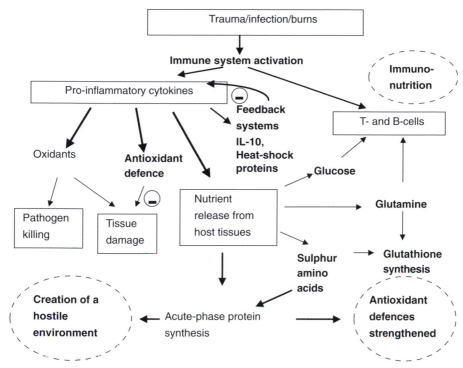

Fig. 7.5. The response of the immune system to infection and injury and the effects upon metabolism.

the response to microbial invasion, by a wide range of stimuli and conditions; these include burns, penetrating and blunt injury, the presence of tumour cells, environmental pollutants, radiation, exposure to allergens and the presence of chronic inflammatory diseases. The strength of the response to this disparate range of stimuli will vary, but it will contain many of the hallmarks of the response to invading pathogens. The immune response has a high metabolic cost, and inappropriate prolongation of the response will exert a deleterious effect upon the nutritional status of the host.

The pro-inflammatory cytokines interleukin (IL)-1, IL-6 and tumour necrosis factor (TNF)-α have widespread metabolic effects upon the body and stimulate the process of inflammation. Many of the signs and symptoms experienced after infection and injury, such as fever, loss of appetite, weight loss, negative nitrogen, sulphur and mineral balance and lethargy are caused directly or indirectly by pro-inflammatory cytokines (Fig. 7.5). The indirect effects of cytokines are mediated by actions upon the adrenal glands and endocrine pancreas, resulting in increased secretion of the catabolic hormones adrenalin, noradrenalin, glucocorticoids and glucagon. Insulin insensitivity occurs, in addition to this 'catabolic state'. The biochemistry of an infected individual is thus fundamentally changed in a way that will ensure that the immune system receives nutrients from within the body. Muscle protein is catabolized to provide amino acids for synthesizing new cells, GSH and proteins for the immune response.

Furthermore, amino acids are converted to glucose (a preferred fuel, together with glutamine, for the immune system). An increase in urinary nitrogen and sulphur excretion occurs as a result of this catabolic process. The extent of this process is highlighted by the significant increase in urinary nitrogen excretion, from 9 g day^{-1} in mild infection to 20–30 g day^{-1} following major burn or severe traumatic injury (Wilmore, 1983). The loss of nitrogen from the body of an adult during a bacterial infection may be equivalent to 60 g of tissue protein and, in a period of persistent malarial infection, equivalent to over 500 g of protein. However, during the response to infection and injury, the urinary excretion of sulphur increases to a lesser extent than that of nitrogen (Cuthbertson, 1931), suggesting that sulphur amino acids are preferentially retained and so 'spared' from catabolism. Infection with human immunodeficiency virus (HIV) has been shown to cause substantial excretion of sulphate in the urine during the asymptomatic phase of the disease (Breitkreutz *et al.*, 2000). The losses reported were equivalent to 10 g of cysteine day^{-1}, in contrast to losses of approximately 3 g day^{-1} for healthy individuals on a 'Westernized diet'. As cysteine is the precursor for both sulphate and GSH this finding may be linked with the decline in tissue glutathione pools that has been observed in HIV infection (De Rosa *et al.*, 2000). Clearly, such a depletion of antioxidant defences will not be sustainable over a long period.

Large decreases in plasma glycine, serine and taurine concentrations occur following infection and injury. These changes may be due to enhanced utilization of a closely related group of amino acids, namely, glycine, serine, methionine and cysteine. Many substances produced in enhanced amounts in response to pro-inflammatory cytokines are particularly rich in these amino acids. These substances include GSH, which comprises glycine, glutamic acid and cysteine, metallothionein (the major zinc-transport protein), which contains glycine, serine, cysteine and methionine to a composite percentage of 56%, and a range of acute-phase proteins, which contain up to 25% of these amino acids in their structure. If an increased demand for sulphur and related amino acids is created by the inflammatory response, then provision of additional supplies of these amino acids may assist the response.

Many of the components of antioxidant defence interact to maintain antioxidant status (see also Hughes, Chapter 9, Prasad, Chapter 10, and McKenzie *et al.*, Chapter 12, this volume). Glutathione and the enzymes that maintain it in its reduced form are central to effective antioxidant status. For example, when oxidants interact with cell membranes, the oxidized form of vitamin E that results is restored to its reduced form by ascorbic acid. The dehydroascorbic acid formed in this process is reconverted to ascorbic acid by interaction with the reduced form of glutathione. Subsequently, oxidized glutathione formed in the reaction is reconverted to the reduced form of glutathione by glutathione reductase (Fig. 7.6). Vitamins E and C and glutathione are thus intimately linked in antioxidant defence. The interdependence of the various nutritional components of antioxidant defence is illustrated in a study in which healthy subjects were given 500 mg ascorbic acid day^{-1} for 6 weeks (Johnston *et al.*, 1993). A 47% increase in the glutathione content of red blood cells occurred. Vitamin B$_6$ and riboflavin, which have no antioxidant properties

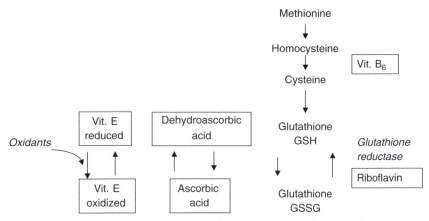

Fig. 7.6. The interaction between antioxidants in maintaining antioxidant defence.

per se, also contribute to antioxidant defences indirectly. Vitamin B_6 is the cofactor in the metabolic pathway for the biosynthesis of cysteine (Fig. 7.1). Cellular cysteine concentration is rate limiting for glutathione synthesis. Riboflavin is a cofactor for glutathione reductase, which maintains the major part of cellular glutathione in the reduced form (Fig. 7.6).

Antioxidant Defences Following Infection and Injury

Although pro-inflammatory cytokines are essential for the normal operation of the immune system, they play a major damaging role in many inflammatory diseases, such as rheumatoid arthritis, inflammatory bowel disease, asthma, psoriasis and multiple sclerosis, and in cancer (Tracey and Cerami, 1993; Grimble, 1996). They are also thought to be important in the development of atheromatous plaques in cardiovascular disease (Ross, 1993). In conditions such as cerebral malaria, meningitis and sepsis, they are produced in excessive amounts and are an important factor in increased mortality (Tracey and Cerami, 1993). Clearly, in these diseases, the cytokines are being produced in the wrong biological context. In malaria, tuberculosis, sepsis, cancer, HIV infection and rheumatoid arthritis, inflammatory cytokines bring about a loss of lean tissue, which is associated with depleted tissue GSH content and an increased output of nitrogenous and sulphur-containing excretion products in the urine (see above).

Although the body strives to maintain them, observations in experimental animals and patients indicate that antioxidant defences become depleted during infection and after injury. For example, in mice infected with influenza virus, there were 27%, 42% and 45% decreases in the vitamin C, vitamin E and glutathione contents of blood, respectively (Hennett *et al.*, 1992). In asymptomatic HIV infection, substantial decreases in glutathione concentrations in blood and lung epithelial-lining fluid have been noted (Staal *et al.*, 1992). In patients undergoing elective abdominal operations, the glutathione content of blood and skeletal muscle fell by over 10% and 42%, respectively, within 24 h of the operation (Luo *et al.*,

1996). While values in blood slowly returned to pre-operative values, concentrations in muscle were still depressed 48 h post-operatively. Furthermore, reduced tissue glutathione concentration has been noted in hepatitis C, ulcerative colitis and cirrhosis. In patients with malignant melanoma, metastatic hypernephroma and metastatic colon cancer, plasma ascorbic acid concentrations fell from normal to almost undetectable levels within 5 days of commencement of treatment with IL-2 (Grimble, 1999). In patients with inflammatory bowel disease, substantial reductions in ascorbic acid concentrations occurred in inflamed gut mucosa (Buffinton and Doe, 1995). As a general consequence of the weakening of antioxidant defences during disease that is attested to by these observations, oxidative damage is apparent in a wide range of clinical conditions in which cytokines are produced. Lipid peroxides and increased thiobarbituric acid reactive substances are present in the blood of patients with septic shock, asymptomatic HIV infection, chronic hepatitis C, breast cancer, cystic fibrosis, diabetes mellitus and alcoholic liver disease. Peroxides also increase following cancer chemotherapy, open heart surgery, bone marrow transplantation and haemodialysis. When glutathione status was reduced in rats by injection of diethyl maleate, which binds irreversibly to GSH, rendering it inactive, a sublethal dose of TNF became lethal (Zimmerman et al., 1989), thus illustrating the importance of GSH in protection from the adverse effects of pro-inflammatory cytokines. The onset of sepsis in patients leads to a transient decrease in the total antioxidant capacity of blood plasma (a functional measure of the total antioxidant content) (Cowley et al., 1996). The capacity returns to normal values over the following 5 days. However, this was not the case for patients who subsequently died, in whom values remained well below the normal range.

As well as increasing the risk of direct oxidant damage, a reduction in the strength of antioxidant defences also indirectly increases the risk of damage to the host via transcription-factor activation, leading to up-regulation of pro-inflammatory cytokine production (see below).

Glutathione and the Immune System

Direct effects of glutathione

One of the first indications that glutathione influences aspects of immune function that are related to T lymphocytes came from a study in which the GSH content of lymphocytes was measured in a group of healthy volunteers (Kinscherf et al., 1994). The numbers of helper (CD4+) and cytotoxic (CD8+) T-cells increased in parallel with intracellular glutathione concentrations up to 30 nmol mg^{-1} protein. However, the relationship between cellular glutathione concentrations and cell numbers was complex, with numbers of both subsets declining at intracellular glutathione concentrations between 30 and 50 nmol mg^{-1} protein. The study also revealed that cell numbers were responsive to long-term changes in GSH content. When the subjects engaged in a programme of intensive physical exercise daily for 4 weeks, a fall in glutathione concentrations occurred. Individuals with glutathione concentrations in the optimal range before exercise who experienced a fall in concentration after exercise showed a 30% fall in CD4+ T-cell numbers. The decline in T-cell number was prevented by administration of *N*-acetyl-cysteine (NAC) (this is metabolized to cysteine (see later)). This study suggests that immune cell function may be sensitive to a range of intracellular sulphydryl compounds, including glutathione and cysteine. In HIV+ individuals and patients with acquired immune deficiency syndrome (AIDS), a reduction in cellular and plasma glutathione has been noted (Staal *et al.*, 1992). It is unclear at present whether the depletion in lymphocyte population that occurs in these subjects is related to this phenomenon. However, in a large, randomized, double-blind, placebo-controlled trial, administration of 600 mg day^{-1} of NAC for 7 months resulted in both anti-inflammatory and immunoenhancing effects (Breitkreutz *et al.*, 2000). A decrease in plasma IL-6 concentration occurred, together with an increase in lymphocyte count and in the stimulation index of T lymphocytes in response to tetanus toxin. The precise mechanism underlying the complex effects of changes in cellular glutathione content are not clear, and whether they are related to GSH function as an antioxidant or to some other property is not apparent. However, a recent study suggests that glutathione promotes IL-12 production by antigen-presenting cells, so driving T-helper (Th) cells along the Th1 pathway of differentiation (Peterson *et al.*, 1998).

Effects of other nutrients that might have an impact on glutathione status

Vitamin B$_6$

Vitamin B$_6$, although having no antioxidant properties, plays an important part in antioxidant defences, because of its action in the metabolic pathway for the formation of cysteine, which, as indicated earlier, is the rate-limiting precursor in glutathione synthesis. Vitamin B$_6$ status has widespread effects upon immune function (Rall and Meydani, 1993). Vitamin B$_6$ deficiency causes thymic atrophy and lymphocyte depletion in lymph nodes and spleen. Antigen processing is unaffected. However, the ability to make antibodies to sheep red blood cells is depressed. In human studies, the ability to make antibodies to tetanus and typhoid antigens is not seriously affected. Various aspects of cell-mediated immunity are also influenced by vitamin B$_6$ deficiency. Skin grafts in rats and mice survive longer during deficiency, and guinea pigs exhibit decreased delayed-hypersensitivity reactions to bacillus Calmette–Guérin (BCG) administration. Deficiency of vitamin B$_6$ is rare in humans but can be precipitated with the anti-tuberculosis (anti-TB) drug isoniazid. However, experimental deficiency in elderly subjects has been shown to reduce total blood lymphocyte numbers and decrease the proliferative response of lymphocytes to mitogens (Meydani *et al.*, 1991). Likewise, IL-2 production is reduced by deficiency of the vitamin. Restoration of vitamin B$_6$ intake to normal by dietary supplements restores immune function. However, intakes that are higher than current recommended values are required to normalize all immune functions, suggesting that this vitamin can only restore immune function in this way. It is unclear, at present, whether a similar situation occurs in younger subjects.

One mechanism for the effect of vitamin B_6 on immune function may be due to the importance of the vitamin in cysteine synthesis, as outlined earlier. Deficiency of the vitamin may limit the availability of cysteine for glutathione synthesis. In rats, vitamin B_6 deficiency resulted in decreases of 12 and 21% in glutathione concentrations in plasma and spleen, respectively (Takeuchi et al., 1991). In healthy young women, large doses of vitamin B_6 (27 mg day^{-1} for 2 weeks) resulted in a 50% increase in plasma cysteine content (Kang-Yoon and Kirksey, 1992), presumably by increased flux through the transulphuration pathway. As cysteine is a rate-limiting substrate for glutathione synthesis, these findings may have implications for the response to pathogens, because of the importance of glutathione in lymphocyte proliferation and antioxidant defence. However, while vitamin B_6 has cellular effects on the immune system, evidence is lacking of any effect upon the inflammatory response.

Ascorbic acid

High concentrations of vitamin C are found in phagocytic cells. While the role of vitamin C as a key component of antioxidant defence is well established (Fig. 7.6), most studies have shown only minor effects upon a range of immune functions (see Hughes, Chapter 9, this volume), except in cases where the vitamin may be acting by interacting with GSH metabolism. Unlike deficiencies in vitamins B_6, and E and riboflavin, deficiency of vitamin C does not cause atrophy of lymphoid tissue. In a study of ultramarathon runners, dietary supplementation with 600 mg day^{-1} of ascorbic acid reduced the incidence of upper respiratory-tract infections after a race by 50% (Peters et al., 1993). It is interesting to note that strenuous exercise has been shown to deplete tissue glutathione content. The interrelationship between glutathione and ascorbic acid may therefore play a role in the effect of exercise on immune function.

When immunological parameters and antioxidant status were measured in adult males fed 250 mg day^{-1} of vitamin C for 4 days, followed by 5 mg day^{-1} for 32 days, plasma ascorbic acid and glutathione decreased and impairment of antioxidant status became evident from a doubling in semen 8-hydroxydeoxyguanosine concentration (a measure of oxidative damage to nucleic acids) during the second dietary period (Jacob et al., 1991). A fall in vitamin content in peripheral-blood mononuclear cells was noted and the delayed-type hypersensitivity reaction to seven recall antigens was significantly reduced in intensity.

Mechanism of the Effect of Oxidants and Antioxidants on Inflammation and Immune Function

There is a growing body of evidence that antioxidants suppress inflammatory components of the response to infection and trauma and enhance components related to cell-mediated immunity (see Hughes, Chapter 9, Prasad, Chapter 10, and McKenzie et al., Chapter 12, this volume). The reverse situation applies when antioxidant defences become depleted.

The oxidant molecules produced by the immune system to kill invading organisms may activate at least two important families of proteins that are sensitive to changes in cellular redox state. The families are nuclear transcription factor kappa B (NFκB) and activator protein 1 (AP1). These transcription factors act as 'control switches' for biological processes, not all of which are of advantage to the individual. NFκB is present in the cytosol in an inactive form, by virtue of being bound to IκB. Phosphorylation and dissociation of IκB renders the remaining NFκB dimer active. Activation of NFκB can be brought about by a wide range of stimuli, including pro-inflammatory cytokines, hydrogen peroxide, mitogens, bacteria and viruses and their related products, and UV and ionizing radiations. The dissociated IκB is degraded and the active NFκB is translocated to the nucleus, where it binds to response elements in the promoter regions of genes. A similar translocation of AP1, a transcription factor composed of the proto-oncogenes *c-fos* and *c-jun*, from cytosol to nucleus also occurs in the presence of oxidant stress. Binding of the transcription factors is implicated in the activation of a wide range of genes associated with inflammation and the immune response, including those encoding cytokines, cytokine receptors, cell-adhesion molecules, acute-phase proteins and growth factors (Schreck *et al.*, 1991).

Unfortunately, NFκB also activates transcription of the genes of some viruses, such as HIV. This sequence of events in the case of HIV accounts for the ability of minor infections to speed the progression of individuals who are infected with HIV towards AIDS, since, if antioxidant defences are poor, each encounter with general infections results in cytokine and oxidant production, NFκB activation and an increase in viral replication. It is thus unfortunate that reduced cellular concentrations of GSH are a common feature of asymptomatic HIV infection (Staal *et al.*, 1992).

Oxidant damage to cells will indirectly create a pro-inflammatory effect by the production of lipid peroxides. This situation may lead to up-regulation of NFκB activity, since the transcription factor has been shown to be activated in endothelial cells cultured with linoleic acid, the main dietary n-6 polyunsaturated fatty acid, an effect inhibited by vitamin E and NAC (Hennig *et al.*, 1996). The interaction between oxidant stress and an impaired ability to synthesize glutathione, which results in enhanced inflammation, is clearly seen in cirrhosis, a disease that results in high levels of oxidative stress and an impaired ability to synthesize GSH (Pena *et al.*, 1999). In this study, an inverse relationship between glutathione concentration and the ability of monocytes to produce IL-1, IL-8 and TNF-α was observed. Furthermore, treatment of the patients with the GSH pro-drug oxothiazalidine-4-carboxylate (procysteine) (Fig. 7.7) increased monocyte GSH content and reduced IL-1, IL-8 and TNF-α production. Thus, antioxidants might act to prevent NFκB activation by quenching oxidants. However, not all transcription factors respond to changes in cell redox state in the same way. When rats were subjected to depletion of effective tissue GSH pools by administration of diethyl maleate, there was a significant reduction in lymphocyte proliferation in spleen and mesenteric lymph nodes (Robinson *et al.*, 1993). In an *in vitro* study using HeLa cells and cells from human embryonic kidney, both TNF and hydrogen peroxide resulted in

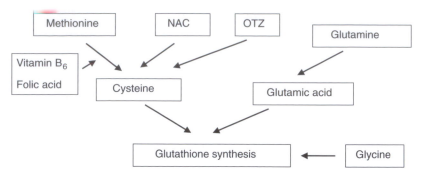

Fig. 7.7. Nutrients and drugs that are important for enhancing glutathione synthesis. NAC, *N*-acetyl cysteine; OTZ, L-2-oxothiazolidine-4-carboxylate.

activation of NFκB and AP1 (Wesselborg *et al.*, 1997). Addition of the antioxidant sorbitol to the medium suppressed NFκB activation (as expected) but (unexpectedly) activated AP1. Thus, the antioxidant environment of the cell might exert opposite effects upon transcription factors closely associated with inflammation (e.g. NFκB) and cellular proliferation (e.g. AP1). Evidence for this biphasic effect was seen when glutathione was incubated with immune cells from young adults (Wu *et al.*, 1994). A rise in cellular glutathione content was accompanied by an increase in IL-2 production and lymphocyte proliferation and a decrease in production of the inflammatory mediators prostaglandin E_2 (PGE$_2$) and leucotriene B$_4$ (LTB$_4$) Modification of the glutathione content of liver, lung, spleen and thymus in young rats, by feeding diets containing a range of casein (a protein with a low sulphur amino acid content) concentrations, changed immune cell numbers in the lung (Hunter and Grimble, 1994). It was found that, in unstressed animals, the number of lung neutrophils decreased as dietary protein intake and tissue glutathione content fell. However, in animals given an inflammatory challenge (endotoxin), liver and lung GSH concentrations increased directly in relation to dietary protein intake. Lung neutrophils, however, became related inversely with tissue glutathione content. Addition of methionine to the protein-deficient diets normalized tissue glutathione content and restored lung neutrophil numbers to those seen in unstressed animals fed a diet of adequate protein content.

Thus it can be hypothesized that antioxidants exert an immunoenhancing effect, by activating transcription factors that are strongly associated with cell proliferation (e.g. AP1), and an anti-inflammatory effect, by preventing activation of NFκB by oxidants produced during the inflammatory response.

Strategies for Modulating Tissue GSH Content and Improving Immune Function

A number of strategies have evolved to raise levels in depleted individuals. As shown in Fig. 7.7, there are three potential ways of enhancing cellular GSH content: administration of the three amino acids (cysteine, glutamic acid and glycine) that comprise the tripeptide, either singly or in various combinations; administration of cofactors for the metabolic pathways leading to GSH production, i.e. vitamin B_6, riboflavin and folic acid; and administration of synthetic compounds that become converted to precursors of GSH.

While cysteine supplies are the primary determinant of the ability to synthesize GSH, in some circumstances an insufficiency in the other two amino acids from which it is made might limit synthesis. Glutamine (a precursor of glutamate), for example, has been shown to maintain hepatic GSH in animals poisoned with acetaminophen, to enhance gut GSH synthesis in rats when given by gavage and to enhance hepatic GSH synthesis when given intravenously to rats (Cao et al., 1998). In human studies a similar effect on gut GSH concentrations was noted (O'Riordain et al., 1996). Glycine supplements have been shown to raise hepatic GSH in rats exposed to haemorrhagic shock (Spittler et al., 1999). In this condition, however, the metabolic demand for glycine is increased, since glycine is the sole nitrogen donor for haem synthesis and would therefore become rate-limiting for GSH synthesis. There are many studies that illustrate the ability of sulphur amino acid availability to influence tissue GSH concentrations (e.g. Stipanuk et al., 1992).

Studies using animal models of inflammation have shown that a low-protein diet will suppress glutathione synthesis, a situation that is reversed by the provision of cysteine or methionine (Hunter and Grimble, 1994, 1997). Beneficial effects on immune function, morbidity and mortality were observed in burned children when additional protein in the form of whey protein (the milk protein richest in sulphur amino acids) was fed (Alexander et al., 1980).

Because cysteine is unstable in its reduced form, toxic in high doses and mostly degraded in the extracellular compartment, several compounds have been used to deliver cysteine directly to cells. These include L-2-oxothiazalidine-4-carboxylate (OTZ) and NAC. OTZ is an analogue of 5-oxoproline, in which the 4-methylene moiety has been replaced with sulphur. It provides an excellent substrate for 5-oxoprolinase (an intracellular enzyme). The enzyme converts OTZ to S-carboxy-L-cysteine, which is rapidly hydrolysed to L-cysteine. NAC rapidly enters the cell and is speedily deacylated to yield L-cysteine. Recent animal and clinical trials with NAC and OTZ have demonstrated the ability of the compounds to enhance GSH status (Bernard et al., 1997; Deneke, 2000; De Rosa et al., 2000). In studies on patients with sepsis, NAC infusion was shown to increase blood GSH, decrease plasma concentrations of IL-8 and soluble TNF receptors (an index of TNF production), improve respiratory function and reduce the number of days needed in intensive care (Bernard et al., 1997; Spapen et al., 1998). While not affecting mortality rates, NAC shortened hospital length of stay by > 60%. OTZ increased whole-blood GSH in peritoneal-dialysis patients, normalized tissue GSH in rats fed a sulphur amino acid-deficient diet and decreased the extent of inflammation in a rat peritonitis model (Bernard et al., 1997). In a randomized, double-blind, controlled study on asymptomatic HIV-infected patients, oral OTZ treatment increased GSH concentrations in whole blood (Breitzkreutz et al., 2000). Other randomized studies on asymptomatic HIV+ patients in the presence and absence of anti-retroviral therapy (ART) have shown that NAC can raise blood

GSH, increase natural killer cell activity and enhance stimulation indices of T-cells incubated with mitogen or tetanus toxin (Simon *et al.*, 1994; Breitzkreutz *et al.*, 2000). Interestingly, the rise in T-cell function was accompanied by a fall in plasma IL-6 in subjects receiving ART as well as the drug. Furthermore, studies have shown that survival time was improved in HIV+ patients who maintained high concentrations of GSH in CD4+ T lymphocytes (Herzenberg *et al.*, 1997). It could therefore be surmised that improved T-cell function and reduced inflammation are modulated by improvement in antioxidant status in these patients. Alpha-lipoic acid provides a further means of enhancing tissue GSH content (Deneke, 2000). The compound is reduced to dihydrolipoic acid, which converts cystine to cysteine. This change has functional significance for glutathione status in lymphocytes, since the xc transport system, which is needed to take up cysteine into the cells, is weakly expressed and is inhibited by glutamate, while the neutral amino acid transport system, which takes up cysteine, is functional. Upon gaining entry to the immune cells, cysteine is rapidly converted to GSH. Flow-cytometric analysis of freshly prepared human peripheral-blood lymphocytes shows that lipoic acid is able to normalize a sub-population of cells with severely compromised thiol status, rather than increasing the level in all cells above normal values (Sen *et al.*, 1997). Hence lipoic acid may also prove to be a useful clinical agent for restoring cellular GSH concentration in immunocompromised subjects.

Taurine and Immune Function

Taurine, along with sulphate, can be regarded as a biochemical end-product of cysteine metabolism. However, it is apparent that taurine also plays a role in immune function. It is the most abundant free nitrogenous compound (often incorrectly classified as an amino acid) in cells. It is a membrane stabilizer and regulates calcium flux, thereby controlling cell stability. It has been shown to possess antioxidant properties and to regulate the release of pro-inflammatory cytokines in hamsters, rats and humans (Grimble, 1994; Huxtable, 1996; Kontny *et al.*, 2000).

The possibility that taurine might have immunomodulatory properties was indicated in studies in obligate carnivores, such as cats, in which taurine is an essential nutrient, due to an inability to synthesize the compound. Premature infants have similar metabolic difficulties. In cats deprived of taurine, substantial impairment of immune function occurs (Grimble, 1994). A large decline in lymphocytes, an increase in mononuclear cells and a decrease in the ability of these cells to produce a 'respiratory burst' and to phagocytose bacteria occur. There was a rise in gamma globulin concentrations in deficient animals. Spleen and lymph nodes showed regression of follicular centres and depletion of mature and immature B lymphocyte numbers. The changes were reversed by inclusion of taurine in the diets. Studies in other species have also reported effects of supplementation on immune system and function. In mice, administration of taurine prevented the decline in T-cell number that occurs with ageing and enhanced the proliferative responses of T-cells in both young and old mice

(Grimble, 1999). The effect was more marked in cells from old than from young animals. Taurine has been shown to ameliorate inflammation in trinitrobenzene sulphonic acid-induced colitis.

Taurine interacts with hypochlorous acid, produced during the 'oxidant burst' of stimulated macrophages, to produce taurine chloramine (TauCl). This compound may have important immunomodulatory properties and may be responsible for properties that have been ascribed earlier to taurine. TauCl has been shown to inhibit nitric oxide, PGE_2, TNF-α and IL-6 production from stimulated macrophages in culture and to inhibit the ability of antigen-presenting cells to process and present ovalbumin (Grimble, 1999). In *in vitro* studies with murine dendritic cells, the compound altered the balance of Th1 to Th2 cytokines, suggesting that it might play a role in maintaining the balance between the inflammatory response and the acquired immune response.

Taurolidine, which is a derivative of taurine, has been used as a bactericidal and anti-lipopolysaccharide agent. However, it may also have an immunomodulatory influence, since it is hydrolysed to taurine *in vivo*. Indeed, in a murine model of sepsis, the former compound was shown to decrease mortality (Grimble, 1999).

References

Alexander, J.W., MacMillan, B.G., Stinnett, J.D., Ogle, C.K., Bozian, R.C., Fischer, J.E., Oakes, J.B., Morris, M.J. and Krummel, R. (1980) Beneficial effects of aggressive protein feeding in severely burned children. *Annals of Surgery* 192, 505–517.

Bernard, G.R., Wheeler, A.P., Arons, M.M., Morris, P.E., La Paz, H., Russell, J.A., Wright, P.E. and the Antioxidant in ARDS Study Group (1997) A trial of antioxidants N-acetylcysteine and Procysteine in ARDS. *Chest* 112, 164–172.

Breitkreutz, R., Pittack, N., Nebe, C.T., Schuster, D., Brust, J., Beichert, M., Hack, V., Daniel, V., Edler, L. and Droge, W. (2000) Improvement of immune functions in HIV infection by sulfur supplementation: two randomized trials. *Journal of Molecular Medicine* 78, 55–62.

Buffinton, G.D. and Doe, W.F. (1995) Altered ascorbic acid status in the mucosa from inflammatory bowel patients. *Free Radical Research* 22, 131–143.

Cao, Y., Feng, Z., Hoos, A. and Klimberg, V.S. (1998) Glutamine enhances gut glutathione production. *Journal of Parenteral and Enteral Nutrition* 22, 224–227.

Cowley, H.C., Bacon, P.J., Goode, H.F., Webster, N.R., Jones, J.G. and Menon, D.K. (1996) Plasma antioxidant potential in severe sepsis: a comparison of survivors and nonsurvivors. *Critical Care Medicine* 24, 1179–1183.

Cuthbertson, D.P. (1931) The distribution of nitrogen and sulphur in the urine during conditions of increased catabolism. *Biochemical Journal* 25, 236–240.

Deneke, S.M. (2000) Thiol-based antioxidants. *Current Topics in Cell Regulation* 36, 151–180.

De Rosa, S.C., Zaretsky, M.D., Dubs, J.G., Roederer, M., Anderson, M., Green, A., Mitra, D., Watanabe, N., Nakamura, H., Tjioe, I., Deresinski, S.C., Moore, W.A., Ela, S.W., Parks, D. and Herzenberg, L.A. (2000) N-acetylcysteine replenishes glutathione in HIV infection. *European Journal of Clinical Investigation* 30, 915–929.

Finkelstein, J.D. and Martin, J.J. (1984) Methionine metabolism in mammals – distribution of homocysteine between competing pathways. *Journal of Biological Chemistry* 259, 9508–9513.

Finkelstein, J.D. and Martin, J.J. (1986) Methionine metabolism in mammals: adaptation to methionine excess. *Journal of Biological Chemistry* 261, 1582–1587.

Grimble, R.F. (1994) Sulphur amino acids and the metabolic response to cytokines. *Advances in Experimental Medicine and Biology* 359, 41–49.

Grimble, R.F. (1996) Interaction between nutrients, pro-inflammatory cytokines and inflammation. *Clinical Science* 91, 121–130.

Grimble, R.F. (1999) Theory and efficacy of antioxidant therapy. *Current Opinion in Critical Care* 2, 260–266.

Grimble, R.F. and Grimble, G.K. (1998) Immunonutrition: role of sulfur amino acids, related amino acids, and polyamines. *Nutrition* 14, 605–610.

Hennett, T., Peterhans, E. and Stocker, R. (1992) Alterations in antioxidant defences in lung and liver of mice infected with influenza A virus. *Journal of General Virology* 73, 39–46.

Hennig, B., Taborek, M., Joshi-Barve, S., Barger, S.W., Barve, S., Mattson, M.P. and McClain, C.J. (1996) Linoleic acid activates NFκB and induces NFκB dependent transcription in cultured endothelial cells. *American Journal of Clinical Nutrition* 63, 322–328.

Herzenberg, L.A., De Rosa, S.C., Dubs, J.G., Roederer, M., Anderson, M.T., Ela, S.W., Deresinski, S.C. and Herzenberg, L.A. (1997) Glutathione deficiency is associated with impaired survival in HIV disease. *Proceedings of the National Academy of Sciences of the USA* 94, 1967–1972.

Hunter, E.A.L. and Grimble, R.F. (1994) Cysteine and methionine supplementation modulate the effect of tumor necrosis factor α on protein synthesis, glutathione and zinc content of tissues in rats fed a low-protein diet. *Journal of Nutrition* 124, 2319–2328.

Hunter, E.A.L. and Grimble, R.F. (1997) Dietary sulphur amino acid adequacy influences glutathione synthesis and glutathione-dependent enzymes during the inflammatory response to endotoxin and tumour necrosis factor-α in rats. *Clinical Science* 92, 297–305.

Huxtable, R.J. (1996) Taurine past, present, and future. *Advances in Experimental Medicine and Biology* 403, 641–650.

Jacob, R.A., Kelley, D.S., Pianalto, F.S., Swendseid, M.E., Henning, S.M., Zhang, J.Z., Ames, B.N., Fraga, C.G. and Peters, J.H. (1991) Immunocompetence and oxidant defence during ascorbate depletion of healthy men. *American Journal of Clinical Nutrition* 54, 1302S–1309S.

Johnston, C.S., Meyer, C.G. and Srilakshmi, J.C. (1993) Vitamin C elevates red blood cell glutathione in healthy adults. *American Journal of Clinical Nutrition* 58, 103–105.

Kang-Yoon, S.A. and Kirksey, A. (1992) Relation of short-term pyridoxine hydrochloride supplements to plasma vitamin B_6 vitamers and amino acid concentration in young women. *American Journal of Clinical Nutrition* 55, 865–872.

Kinscherf, R., Fischbach, T., Mihm, S., Roth, S., Hohen-Sievert, E., Weiss, C., Edler, L., Bartsch, P. and Droge, W. (1994) Effect of glutathione depletion and oral N-acetyl-cysteine treatment on CD4+ and CD8+ cells. *FASEB Journal* 8, 448–451.

Kontny, E., Szczepanska, K., Kowalczewski, J., Kurowska, M., Janicka, I., Marcinkiewicz, J. and Maslinski, W. (2000) The mechanism of taurine chloramine inhibition of cytokine (interleukin-6, interleukin-8) production by rheumatoid arthritis fibroblast-like synoviocytes. *Arthritis and Rheumatism* 43, 169–177.

Luo, J.L., Hammarqvist, F., Andersson, K. and Wernerman, J. (1996) Skeletal muscle glutathione after surgical trauma. *Annals of Surgery* 223, 420–427.

Meydani, S.N., Ribaya-Mercado, J.D., Russell, R.M., Sahyoun, N., Morrow, R.D. and Gershoff, S.N. (1991) Vitamin B_6 deficiency impaires IL-2 production and lymphocyte proliferation in elderly adults. *American Journal of Clinical Nutrition* 53, 1275–1280.

O'Riordain, M.G., De Beaux, A. and Fearon, K.C. (1996) Effect of glutamine on immune function in the surgical patient. *Nutrition* 12, S82-S84.

Pena, L.R., Hill, D.B. and McClain, C.J. (1999) Treatment with glutathione precursor decreases cytokine activity. *Journal of Parenteral and Enteral Nutrition* 23, 1–6.

Peters, E.M., Goetzsche, G.M., Grobelaar, B. and Noakes, T.D. (1993) Vitamin C supplementation reduces the incidence of post-race symptoms of upper-respiratory tract infection in ultramarathon runners. *American Journal of Clinical Nutrition* 57, 170–174.

Peterson, J.D., Herzenberg, L.A., Vasquez, K. and Waltenbaugh, C. (1998) Glutathione levels in antigen-presenting cells modulate Th1 versus Th2 response patterns. *Proceedings of the National Academy of Sciences of the USA* 95, 3071–3076.

Rall, L.C. and Meydani, S.N. (1993) Vitamin B6 and immune competence. *Nutrition Reviews* 8, 217–225.

Robinson, M.K., Rodrick, M.L., Jacobs, D.O., Rounds, J.D., Collins, K.H., Saporoschetz, I.B., Mannick, J.A. and Wilmore, D.W. (1993) Glutathione depletion in rats impairs T-cell and macrophage immune function. *Archives of Surgery* 128, 29–34.

Ross, R. (1993) The pathogenesis of atherosclerosis: a perspective for the 1990s. *Nature* 362, 801–809.

Schreck, R., Rieber, P. and Baeurerle, P.A. (1991) Reactive oxygen intermediates as apparently widely used messengers in the activation of nuclear transcription factor-κB and HIV-1. *EMBO Journal* 10, 2247–2256.

Sen, C.K., Roy, S., Han, D. and Packer, L. (1997) Regulation of cellular thiols in human lymphocytes by alpha-lipoic acid: a flow cytometric analysis. *Free Radicals in Biology and Medicine* 22, 1241–1257.

Simon, G., Moog, C. and Obert, G. (1994) Effects of glutathione precursors on human immunodeficiency virus replication. *Chemical and Biological Interactions* 91, 217–224.

Spapen, H., Zhang, H., Demanet, C., Velminckx, W., Vincent, J.L. and Huyghens, L. (1998) Does N-acetyl cysteine influence the cytokine response during early human septic shock? *Chest* 113, 1616–1624.

Spittler, A., Reissner, C.M., Oehler, R., Gornikiewicz, A., Gruenberger, T., Manhart, N., Brodowicz, T., Mittlboeck, M., Boltz-Nitulescu, G. and Roth, E. (1999) Immunomodulatory effects of glycine on LPS-treated monocytes: reduced TNF-alpha production and accelerated IL-10 expression. *FASEB Journal* 13, 563–571.

Staal, F.J.T., Ela, S.W. and Roederer, M. (1992) Glutathione deficiency in human immunodeficiency virus infection. *Lancet* i, 909–912.

Stipanuk, M.H., Coloso, R.M. and Garcia, R.A.G. (1992) Cysteine concentration regulates cysteine metabolism to glutathione, sulfate and taurine in rat hepatocytes. *Journal of Nutrition* 122, 420–427.

Takeuchi, F., Izuta, S., Tsubouchi, R. and Shibata, Y. (1991) Glutathione levels and related enzyme activities in vitamin B-6 deficient rats fed a high methionine and low cysteine diet. *Journal of Nutrition* 121, 1366–1373.

Tracey, K.J. and Cerami, A. (1993) Tumor necrosis factor, other cytokines and disease. *Annual Reviews of Cell Biology* 9, 317–343.

Wesselborg, S., Bauer, M.K.A., Vogt, M., Schmitz, M.L. and Schulze-Osthoff, K. (1997) Activation of transcription factor NF-kappa B and p38 mitogen-activated protein kinase is mediated by distinct and separate stress effector pathways. *Journal of Biological Chemistry* 272, 12422–12429.

Wilmore, D.W. (1983) Alterations in protein, carbohydrate, and fat metabolism in injured and septic patients. *Journal of the American College of Nutrition* 2, 3–13.

Wu, D., Meydani, S.N., Sastre, J., Hayek, M. and Meydani, M. (1994) *In vitro* glutathione supplementation enhances interleukin-2 production and mitogenic response of peripheral blood mononuclear cells from young and old subjects. *Journal of Nutrition* 124, 655–663.

Zimmerman, R.J., Marafino, B.J. and Chan, A. (1989) The role of oxidant injury in tumor cell sensitivity to recombinant tumor necrosis factor *in vivo*. *Journal of Immunology* 142, 1405–1409.

8 Vitamin A, Infection and Immune Function

RICHARD D. SEMBA

Department of Ophthalmology, Johns Hopkins University School of Medicine, Baltimore, MD 21205, USA

Introduction

Vitamin A deficiency is a leading cause of morbidity and mortality worldwide, especially among infants, children and women in developing countries. An estimated 253 million children are at risk of immunodeficiency due to Vitamin A deficiency (World Health Organization, 1995), and millions of pregnant and lactating women are also at high risk in developing countries. Among the micronutrients, the role of vitamin A in immune function has probably been the most extensively characterized, and studies have shown a multifaceted role of vitamin A in many aspects of immunity. Vitamin A plays a role in the maintenance of mucosal surfaces, in the generation of antibody responses, in haematopoiesis and in the function of T and B lymphocytes, natural killer (NK) cells and neutrophils (for reviews, see Semba, 1994, 1998). The influence of vitamin A on different aspects of immune function is attributed to the action of vitamin A and related metabolites as modulators of gene transcription. The purpose of this chapter is to summarize the role that vitamin A plays in immune function and resistance to infectious diseases. In addition to compromising the immune system, vitamin A deficiency causes night-blindness, xerophthalmia, retardation of growth, impaired reproductive capacity and anaemia. Recently, this array of adverse health problems was described in a comprehensive manner and has been aptly termed the 'vitamin A deficiency disorders' (McLaren and Frigg, 2001).

Biochemistry and Metabolism of Vitamin A

Vitamin A is available in dietary sources as either preformed vitamin A or pro-vitamin A carotenoids. Rich dietary sources of preformed vitamin A include egg yolk, liver, butter, cheese, whole milk and cod-liver oil. In many developing countries, the consumption of foods containing preformed vitamin A is limited, and

© CAB *International* 2002. *Nutrition and Immune Function*
(eds P.C. Calder, C.J. Field and H.S. Gill)

pro-vitamin A carotenoids often comprise the major dietary source of vitamin A. The major pro-vitamin A carotenoids consist of α-carotene and β-carotene, found in such foods as dark green leafy vegetables, carrots, sweet potatoes, mangoes, and papayas and β-cryptoxanthin, found in oranges and tangerines.

Digested foods that contain preformed vitamin A are emulsified with bile salts and lipids in the small intestine. Retinol is esterified in the intestinal mucosa, packaged into chylomicrons and carried to the bloodstream via the lymphatic circulation. Pro-vitamin A carotenoids, such as β-carotene, may be converted to retinaldehyde through cleavage by carotenoid-15,15′-dioxygenase or by an asymmetrical cleavage pathway. The bioavailability of pro-vitamin A carotenoids is less than that of preformed vitamin A, due to a variety of factors, including differences in efficacy of absorption and biochemical conversion (De Pee et al., 1995; West, 2000). About 90% of the vitamin A in the body is stored in the liver as retinyl esters, and the liver has the capacity to store enough vitamin A to last for several months, with a larger storage capacity among adults than among children. Retinol is released from the liver in combination with plasma retinol-binding protein (RBP) and transthyretin (TTR). Retinol is poorly soluble in water and is carried in the blood sequestered inside the carrier proteins, RBP and TTR. Retinol seems to enter cells via specific receptors, although it is unclear whether all cells contain these receptors.

Vitamin A exerts its effects via retinoic acid and retinoid receptors, which are found in the nucleus of the cell. Retinol is converted to all-trans-retinoic acid and 9-cis-retinoic acid in the cytoplasm. Retinoic acid influences gene activation through specific receptors, which belong to the superfamily of thyroid and steroid receptors (Chambon, 1996). Retinoic acid receptors (RARs) act as transcriptional activators for many specific target genes. The RAR is expressed as several isoforms (RAR α, β and γ), and the retinoid-x receptor (RXR) is also expressed as several isoforms (RXR α, β and γ) (Kliewer et al., 1992). All-trans-retinoic acid is a ligand for RARs whereas 9-cis-retinoic acid is a ligand for both RARs and RXRs. The DNA sequences that interact with RAR and RXR are known as retinoic acid response elements. RARs and RXRs form heterodimers, which bind to DNA and control gene expression. In addition, RXRs can also form heterodimers with the thyroid hormone receptor, vitamin D_3 receptor, peroxisome proliferator activator receptors and a number of newly described 'orphan receptors'. Most retinoic acid response elements occur in the regulatory region of genes.

Vitamin A and Immune Function

Historical overview

In the years soon after its discovery, vitamin A became suspected of being a factor essential for the development of the lymphoid system and for the maintenance of mucosal surfaces of the gastrointestinal, respiratory and genitourinary tracts (Clausen, 1934; Robertson, 1934) and the high childhood morbidity and mortality in Europe and the USA in the early 20th century – comparable to those found in many developing countries today – were ascribed to the deficiency of vitamin A (Bloch, 1924). Milk, cream and butter were advocated to reduce infections in children (Bloch, 1924). Subsequently, vitamin A was evaluated in at least 30 therapeutic trials in various infections (e.g. Green and Mellanby, 1928; Ellison, 1932). It is now recognized that vitamin A modulates many different aspects of immune function, including components of both non-specific immunity (e.g. phagocytosis, maintenance of mucosal surfaces) and specific immunity (e.g. generation of antibody responses). Much of our knowledge of vitamin A and immune function is derived from experimental animal studies involving mice, rats and chickens. The effects of vitamin A deficiency on aspects of immune function are summarized in Table 8.1.

Mucosal immunity

Vitamin A deficiency impairs mucosal function through several mechanisms: (i) loss of cilia in the respiratory tract; (ii) loss of microvilli in the gastointestinal tract; (iii) loss of mucin and goblet cells in the respiratory, gastrointestinal and genitourinary tracts; (iv) squamous metaplasia with abnormal keratinization in the respiratory and genitourinary tracts; (v) alterations in antigen-specific secretory immunoglobulin A (IgA) concentrations; (vi) impairment of mucosal-associated immune-cell function; and (vii) decreased integrity of the gut. The first four were among the most striking findings described in early studies of vitamin A-deficient animals and humans (Wolbach and Howe, 1925; Blackfan and Wolbach, 1933; Sweet and K'ang, 1935). The ocular surface has also been intensively studied during vitamin A deficiency, and loss of mucin and goblet cells and squamous metaplasia of the conjunctiva and cornea are well known (McLaren, 1963; Sommer, 1982). There is a close relationship between vitamin A status and the expression of mucins (Koo *et al.*, 1999; Tei *et al.*, 2000) and keratins (Gijbels *et al.*, 1992; Darwiche *et al.*, 1993). Mucins are large glycoconjugates that are found on cell surfaces and secreted into the lumens of the gastrointestinal, respiratory and genitourinary tracts. Mucins are also secreted on the bulbar and palpebral conjunctivae of the eye. The loss of mucin that occurs in vitamin A deficiency constitutes a serious impairment of mucosal immunity.

Table 8.1. Effects of vitamin A deficiency on host defence.

Abnormal expression of keratins in the respiratory tract, genitourinary tract and ocular surface
Loss of cilia from respiratory epithelium
Loss of microvilli from small intestine
Decrease in goblet cells and mucin production in mucosal epithelia
Impaired neutrophil function
Impaired natural killer (NK) cell function and decreased number of NK cells
Impaired aspects of haematopoiesis
Shift towards T-helper type 1-like immune responses
Decrease in number and function of B lymphocytes
Impaired antibody responses to T-cell-dependent and independent antigens

---

In vitamin A-deficient chickens, the concentrations of total IgA were lower in the gut than in control animals (Rombout *et al.*, 1992). Vitamin A-deficient BALB/c mice that were challenged with influenza A virus had a lower influenza-specific IgA response than control mice (Gangopadhyay *et al.*, 1996). Vitamin A-deficient mice had significantly lower serum antibody responses against epizootic diarrhoea of infant mice (EDIM) rotavirus infection compared with control mice (Ahmed *et al.*, 1991). An impaired ability to respond with IgA antibodies to oral cholera vaccine was demonstrated in vitamin A-deficient rats (Wiedermann *et al.*, 1993a). Using the urinary lactulose/mannitol excretion test, increased gut permeability was found in vitamin A-deficient infants, and the gut integrity improved following vitamin A supplementation (Thurnham *et al.*, 2000).

NK cells

Vitamin A deficiency reduces the number of circulating NK cells and impairs NK cell cytolytic activity. NK cells play a role in anti-viral and anti-tumour immunity that is not major histocompatibility complex (MHC)-restricted, and they are involved in the regulation of immune responses. In experimental animal models, vitamin A deficiency reduced the number of NK cells in the spleen (Nauss and Newberne, 1985; Bowman *et al.*, 1990) and peripheral blood (Zhao *et al.*, 1994). The cytolytic activity of NK cells was reduced by vitamin A deficiency (Zhao *et al.*, 1994). In ageing Lewis rats, marginal vitamin A status reduced the number of NK cells in peripheral blood and the cytolytic activity of NK cells (Dawson *et al.*, 1999). There have been few studies of vitamin A status and NK cells in humans. Children with acquired immune deficiency syndrome (AIDS) who received two doses of oral vitamin A (60 mg retinol equivalents (RE)) had large increases in the number of circulating NK cells, compared with children who received placebo (Hussey *et al.*, 1996).

Neutrophils

The function of neutrophils appears to be impaired during vitamin A deficiency. Neutrophils play an important role in non-specific immunity, because they phagocytose and kill bacteria, parasites, virus-infected cells and tumour cells. Retinoic acid plays an important role in the normal maturation of neutrophils (Lawson and Berliner, 1999). Vitamin A-deficient rats had widespread defects in neutrophil function, including impaired chemotaxis, adhesion, phagocytosis and ability to generate active oxidant molecules, compared with neutrophils from controls (Twining *et al.*, 1996). In rats challenged with *Staphylococcus aureus*, impaired phagocytosis and decreased complement lysis activity were found in vitamin A-deficient rats compared with control rats (Wiedermann *et al.*, 1996). Vitamin A treatment was shown to increase superoxide production by neutrophils from Holstein calves (Higuchi and Nagahata, 2000).

Haematopoiesis

Vitamin A deficiency appears to impair haematopoiesis of some lineages, such as CD4+ lymphocytes, NK cells and erythrocytes. In humans, vitamin A deficiency has been characterized by lower total lymphocyte counts and decreased CD4+ lymphocytes in peripheral blood; furthermore, CD4+ lymphocyte counts and/or percentage increased after vitamin A supplementation of deficient individuals (Semba *et al.*, 1993a, b; Hussey *et al.*, 1996). In the vitamin A-deficient rat, lower NK-cell, B-cell and CD4+ lymphocyte counts were found in peripheral blood, and these counts responded to retinoic acid supplementation (Zhao and Ross, 1995). Retinoids have been implicated in the maturation of pluripotent stem cells to cell lineages that produce different haematopoietic cell lines, such as lymphocytes, granulocytes and megakaryocytes. Retinoids also appear to play a role in the maturation of differentiation of pluripotent stem cells into multipotent colony-forming unit granulocyte–erythroid–macrophage mixed (CFU-GEMM) cells, and differentiation and commitment of CFU-GEMM into erythroid burst-forming units (BFU-E) and then into erythroid colony-forming units (CFU-E) (Perrin *et al.*, 1997; Zermati *et al.*, 2000).

T lymphocytes

Vitamin A appears to modulate the balance between T-helper type 1- and T-helper type 2-like responses. *Trichinella spiralis* infection in mice usually stimulates strong T-helper type 2-like responses, characterized by parasite-specific IgG responses and a cytokine profile dominated by interleukin (IL)-4, IL-5 and IL-10 production. However, in vitamin A-deficient mice, infection by *T. spiralis* results in low production of parasite-specific IgG and a cytokine profile dominated by interferon (IFN)-γ and IL-12 production, more characteristic of a T-helper-1 profile (Carman *et al.*, 1992; Cantorna *et al.*, 1994, 1996). Lymphocyte responsiveness to stimulation by concanavalin A or β-lactoglobulin was higher and production of IL-2 and IFN-γ was higher in lymphocyte supernatants from vitamin A-deficient rats, compared with control rats, further supporting the idea that vitamin A deficiency modulates a shift towards T-helper type 1-like responses (Wiedermann *et al.*, 1993b). Vitamin A appears to inhibit production of IFN-γ, IL-2 and granulocyte–macrophage colony-stimulating factor (GM-CSF) by type 1 lymphocytes *in vitro* (Frankenburg *et al.*, 1998). The effect of high-level dietary vitamin A on the shift to T-helper type 2-like responses in BALB/c mice has been used to explain the apparent lack of benefit of vitamin A supplementation for acute lower respiratory infections in humans (Cui *et al.*, 2000).

Monocytes/macrophages

Retinoids appear to play a role in the differentiation and activity of cells of the monocyte/macrophage lineage. The effect of vitamin A deficiency on macrophage function is less clear, as most studies have addressed the effects of all-*trans*-retinoic acid on the function of murine macrophages (Dillehay *et al.*, 1988) or myeloid cell lines.

B lymphocytes

Vitamin A deficiency impairs the growth, activation and function of B lympho-cytes. B lymphocytes have been shown to utilize a metabolite of retinol, 14-hydroxy-4,14-*retro*-retinol, instead of retinoic acid, as a mediator for growth (Buck *et al.*, 1991). The effects of retinol and all-*trans*-retinoic acid on immunoglobulin synthesis by B lymphocytes have been examined in human cord-blood and adult peripheral-blood mononuclear cells (Israel *et al.*, 1991; Wang and Ballow 1993; Wang *et al.*, 1993; Ballow *et al.*, 1996). A T-cell-dependent antigen was used to induce differentiation of sensitized human B lymphocytes into immunoglobulin-secreting cells, and all-*trans*-retinoic acid increased the synthesis of IgM and IgG by these cells. Highly purified T lymphocytes incubated with retinoic acid enhanced IgM synthesis by cord-blood B lymphocytes, suggesting that retinoic acid modu-lates T-cell help through cytokine production (Ballow *et al.*, 1996).

Antibody responses

The hallmark of vitamin A deficiency is an impaired capacity to generate an anti-body response to T-cell-dependent antigens (Smith and Hayes, 1987; Semba *et al.*, 1992, 1994; Wiedermann *et al.*, 1993a, b) and T-cell-independent type 2 antigens, such as pneumococcal polysaccharide (Pasatiempo *et al.*, 1989). Antibody responses are involved in protective immunity to many types of infections and are the main basis for immunological protection for most types of vaccines. Depressed antibody responses to tetanus toxoid have been observed in vitamin A-deficient children (Semba *et al.*, 1992) and animals (Lavasa *et al.*, 1988; Pasatiempo *et al.*, 1990). Vitamin A deficiency appears to impair the generation of primary antibody responses to tetanus toxoid, but, if animals are replete with vitamin A prior to a sec-ond immunization, the secondary antibody responses to tetanus toxoid are compa-rable to those of control animals (Kinoshita *et al.*, 1991). These findings suggest that formation of immunological memory and class switching are intact during vitamin A deficiency, despite an impaired IgM and IgG response to primary immunization. Human peripheral-blood lymphocytes from subjects previously immunized against tetanus toxoid were used to reconstitute control and vitamin A-deficient mice with severe combined immunodeficiency (SCID). After challenge with tetanus toxoid, vitamin A-deficient SCID mice had a 2.9-fold increase in human anti-tetanus toxoid antibody, compared with a 74-fold increase in control SCID mice (Molrine *et al.*, 1995). In healthy children without vitamin A deficiency, vitamin A supplementation did not enhance antibody responses to tetanus toxoid (Kutukculer *et al.*, 2000). These findings suggest that vitamin A supplementation is unlikely to enhance anti-body responses in subjects who are not vitamin A-deficient.

Role of Vitamin A in Resistance to Infectious Disease

Vitamin A deficiency increases susceptibility to some types of infections, and there is currently an extensive literature regarding vitamin A deficiency and infection in experimental animal models (Clausen, 1934; Robertson, 1934; Scrimshaw *et al.*, 1968; Beisel, 1982; Nauss, 1986; Semba, 1994). After an extensive global survey of vitamin A deficiency, Oomen *et al.* (1964) recognized that there was a vicious circle of vitamin A deficiency and infection: 'Not only may deficiency of vitamin A itself play an important role in lowering the resistance to infection … but infectious diseases themselves predispose to and actually precipitate xerophthalmia.' There have been over 100 clinical trials of vitamin A conducted in humans, and these studies show that vitamin A supplementation can reduce morbidity and mortality due to measles and diarrhoeal disease, the morbidity of *Plasmodium falciparum* malaria and maternal morbidity and mortality related to pregnancy (see below). Vitamin A supplementation does not appear to reduce morbidity and mortality from acute lower respiratory infections or reduce mother-to-child transmission of human immunodeficiency virus (HIV) type 1 (see below).

Measles

Vitamin A supplementation reduces the morbidity and mortality from acute measles in infants and children in developing countries. Children with low circulating vitamin A concentrations had higher mortality from measles in a study from Kinshasa, Zaire (Markowitz *et al.*, 1989). An early clinical trial from London showed that vitamin A supplementation could reduce mortality in children with acute measles (Ellison, 1932). Clinical trials showed that high-dose vitamin A reduces morbidity and mortality in children with acute measles infection (Barclay *et al.*, 1987; Hussey and Klein, 1990; Coutsoudis *et al.*, 1991; Ogaro *et al.*, 1993). In acute, complicated measles, high-dose vitamin A supplementation (60 mg RE upon admission and the following day) was shown to reduce mortality by up to 80% in Cape Town, South Africa (Hussey and Klein, 1990). Vitamin A supplementation seems to reduce the infectious complications associated with measles immune suppression, such as pneumonia and diarrhoeal disease.

Vitamin A supplementation appears to modulate antibody responses to measles and increases total lymphocyte counts. Children with acute measles infection who received high-dose vitamin A supplementation (60 mg RE upon admission and the following day) had significantly higher IgG responses to measles virus and higher circulating lymphocyte counts during follow-up, compared with children who received placebo (Coutsoudis *et al.*, 1992). When vitamin A supplementation is given simultaneously with live measles vaccine, there appears to be an effect upon antibody titres to measles if maternal antibodies are present. In 6-month-old infants in Indonesia, administration of vitamin A (30 mg RE) at the time of immunization with standard-titre Schwarz measles vaccine interfered with seroconversion to measles in infants who had maternal antibody present, and significantly reduced the incidence of measles vaccine-associated rash (Semba *et al.*, 1995). A separate clinical trial also showed that vitamin A (30 mg RE) reduced antibody responses to measles virus in 9-month-old infants who had maternal antibody present, but did not interfere with overall seroconversion rates to measles (Semba *et al.*, 1997).

In Guinea-Bissau, vitamin A supplementation (30 mg RE) enhanced geometric-mean titres to measles when given simultaneously with standard-titre Schwarz measles vaccine in 9-month-old infants (Stabell Benn *et al.*, 1997). In a two-dose measles immunization schedule at ages 6 and 9 months, simultaneous vitamin A supplementation did not interfere with seroconversion to measles when measured at 18 months of age (Stabell Benn *et al.*, 1997). It was not possible to determine whether vitamin A supplementation interfered with seroconversion rates after measles vaccine in 6-month-old infants in the study in Guinea-Bissau, as with the study in Indonesia, as antibody titres were not measured until after two vaccinations. Although the results of the studies involving 6-month-old infants in Indonesia and Guinea-Bissau have been viewed as contradictory (Ross and Cutts, 1997; Stabell Benn *et al.*, 1997), the differences in the design of the measles-vaccine studies lend little validity to making direct comparisons between these two studies, and the findings may be complementary.

Diarrhoeal diseases

In developing countries, diarrhoeal diseases among children are caused by a wide variety of pathogens, including rotavirus, *Escherichia coli*, *Shigella*, *Vibrio cholerae*, *Salmonella* and *Entamoeba histolytica*. The epidemiology, clinical features, immunology and pathogenesis of diarrhoea may differ according to characteristics of the pathogen, such as production of toxins, tissue invasion, fluid and electrolyte loss and location of infection. Vitamin A supplementation or fortification has been shown to reduce the morbidity and mortality of diarrhoeal diseases among preschool children in developing countries. The reduction in diarrhoeal disease mortality appears to account for most of the reduction in overall mortality when vitamin A is given through fortification or supplementation on a community level. Clinical vitamin A deficiency is associated with diarrhoeal disease in children (Sommer *et al.*, 1984; Brilliant *et al.*, 1985; DeSole *et al.*, 1987; Gujral *et al.*, 1993; Schaumberg *et al.*, 1996). Large community-based clinical trials of vitamin A supplementation in Tamil Nadu, Nepal and Ghana show that vitamin A has a major impact upon the overall mortality of diarrhoeal disease but not on pneumonia in preschool children (Beaton *et al.*, 1993; Vitamin A and Pneumonia Working Group, 1995). The severity of diarrhoeal disease was reduced by vitamin A supplementation in a clinical trial in Brazil (Barreto *et al.*, 1994). Urinary losses of vitamin A during *Shigella* infection may be substantial in some children (Mitra *et al.*, 1998), and vitamin A supplementation (60 mg RE) has been shown to reduce morbidity in children with acute shigellosis (Hossain *et al.*, 1998). Although improvement of vitamin A status has been shown to protect against diarrhoeal diseases, it is not clear whether this is a general effect against all diarrhoeal pathogens or only against certain types of pathogens.

Acute lower respiratory infections

Acute lower respiratory infections (ALRI) are a major cause of death among children in developing countries, and major causes of ALRI include respiratory syncytial virus (RSV) infection, parainfluenza, *Haemophilus influenzae*, *Streptococcus pneumoniae* and *Bordetella pertussis*. Secondary bacterial infection with high case fatality may follow a primary viral infection in the lungs. Community-based trials failed to demonstrate any effect of vitamin A supplementation upon morbidity and mortality of ALRI (Vitamin A and Pneumonia Working Group, 1995). Hospital-based studies have also shown that high-dose vitamin A supplementation has no therapeutic effect upon the morbidity of ALRI in children (Kjolhede *et al.*, 1995; Nacul *et al.*, 1997; Fawzi *et al.*, 1998). In Chile and the USA, hospital-based trials showed that vitamin A supplementation had little impact upon RSV infection among infants and young children (Bresee *et al.*, 1996; Dowell *et al.*, 1996; Quinlan and Hayani, 1996).

High-dose vitamin A supplementation may have adverse consequences for some children who are not malnourished (Sempertegui *et al.*, 1999; Fawzi *et al.*, 2000a). In a study conducted in Dar Es Salaam, Tanzania, children hospitalized with pneumonia received high-dose vitamin A supplementation and, after discharge, they were monitored for diarrhoeal and respiratory disease. Vitamin A supplementation was associated with a higher rate of diarrhoeal disease among children who were better nourished, whereas a reduction in diarrhoeal morbidity was noted among wasted children. This apparent bidirectional effect has been termed 'the vitamin A paradox' (Griffiths, 2000). A recent controlled clinical trial conducted in Quito, Ecuador, also suggested that weekly vitamin A supplementation to children, aged 6–36 months, significantly reduced the incidence of ALRI in underweight (weight-for-age Z score < −2) children, but significantly increased the incidence of ALRI in normal-weight children (weight-for-age Z score > −1), compared with placebo (Sempertegui *et al.*, 1999).

Although vitamin A status has been shown to be related to the severity of acute respiratory infection in children (Dudley *et al.*, 1997), it is unclear why vitamin A therapy has no apparent effect in some trials upon the morbidity of acute respiratory infections among preschool children. Young age might be one contributing factor to the lack of an effect, as large community-based studies suggest that vitamin A supplementation has little effect on morbidity and mortality of infants (West *et al.*, 1995; WHO/CHD Immunisation-Linked Vitamin A Supplementation Study Group, 1998). Studies have also been conducted in populations where vitamin A deficiency is not considered a public-health problem. In the recent clinical trials involving RSV infection, the apparent lack of impact of vitamin A supplementation on RSV infection might be due to the young age of the subjects and the lack of vitamin A deficiency in the population. It would be erroneous to consider vitamin A as ineffective in increasing immunity to ALRI completely, as vitamin A supplementation has been shown to reduce the life-threatening complication of pneumonia after acute measles infection (Barclay *et al.*, 1987; Hussey and Klein, 1990).

Malaria

There is new evidence that vitamin A supplementation may help reduce the morbidity of *P. falciparum* malaria – an important observation since *P.*

falciparum causes an estimated 1–2 million deaths worldwide each year. There appears to be an association between poor vitamin A status and malaria (Stürchler *et al.*, 1987; Galan *et al.*, 1990; Friis *et al.*, 1997). A randomized, placebo-controlled clinical trial was conducted in Papua New Guinea to examine the effects of vitamin A supplementation (60 mg RE every 3 months) on malarial morbidity in preschool children aged 6–60 months (Shankar *et al.*, 1999). Weekly morbidity surveillance and clinic-based surveillance were established for monitoring acute malaria, and children were followed for 1 year. Vitamin A significantly reduced the incidence of malaria attacks by about 20–50% for all except extremely high levels of parasitaemia. Similarly, vitamin A supplementation reduced clinic-based malaria relapses, which consisted of self-solicited visits to the clinic by mothers who thought that their children should be seen because of fever. Vitamin A supplementation had little impact in children under age 12 months and the greatest effect was from 13 to 36 months of age.

HIV infection

Vitamin A supplementation may have some benefit for HIV-infected children and pregnant women in developing countries. Low plasma or serum concentrations of vitamin A or intake of vitamin A have been associated with increased disease progression and mortality and higher mother-to-child transmission of HIV (Kennedy *et al.*, 2000). Periodic high-dose vitamin A supplementation seems to reduce morbidity among children born to HIV-infected mothers (Coutsoudis *et al.*, 1995) and diarrhoeal-disease morbidity in HIV-infected children after discharge from the hospital for ALRI (Fawzi *et al.*, 1999). Vitamin A supplementation did not reduce mother-to-child transmission of HIV (Coutsoudis *et al.*, 1999; Fawzi *et al.*, 2000b). However, a trial in Durban, South Africa, showed that vitamin A supplementation reduced preterm birth (Coutsoudis *et al.*, 1999). Vitamin A supplementation does not appear to influence HIV load in the blood (Semba *et al.*, 1998). A study from Cape Town, South Africa, suggests that vitamin A supplementation modulates lymphopoiesis in children with AIDS (Hussey *et al.*, 1996).

Tuberculosis

Although malnutrition and vitamin A deficiency seem to be major risk factors for the progression of tuberculosis, clinical management usually involves chemoprophylaxis and chemotherapy alone, rather than any special concern for host nutritional status. Cod-liver oil, a rich source of vitamins A and D, was used as treatment strategy for tuberculosis for over 100 years (Williams and Williams, 1871). The role of nutrition and tuberculosis remains a major area of neglect, despite the promise that micronutrients have shown as therapy for other types of infections and the long record of the use of vitamins A and D for treatment of pulmonary and miliary tuberculosis in both Europe and the USA.

A recent clinical trial suggests that high-dose vitamin A supplementation does influence the morbidity of tuberculosis in children (Hanekom *et al.*, 1997). Studies have not been conducted to address the use of multivitamins and minerals or vitamins A plus D as adjunct therapy for tuberculosis.

Infections in pregnant and lactating women

Recent data from Nepal suggest that pregnant women with clinical vitamin A deficiency (i.e. night-blindness) are at higher risk of infectious-disease morbidity (Christian *et al.*, 1998) and mortality (Christian *et al.*, 2000b). Weekly vitamin A or β-carotene supplementation appeared to reduce the risk of infectious disease morbidity and mortality among these women, suggesting that vitamin A status may be important in pregnancy-related morbidity and mortality (West *et al.*, 1999; Christian *et al.*, 2000a). Vitamin A or β-carotene reduced all-cause mortality, and further work is needed both to replicate these findings and to determine the types of infections that might be reduced through improving vitamin A status during pregnancy. The recent trial in Nepal appears to corroborate earlier trials from England, which showed that vitamin A supplementation reduced the morbidity of puerperal sepsis (Cameron, 1931; Green *et al.*, 1931).

Conclusions and Future Directions

Vitamin A has been used as both disease-targeted and prophylactic therapy to reduce morbidity and mortality from infectious diseases for hundreds of years. Vitamin A plays an important role in haematopoiesis, the maintenance of mucosal surfaces, the function of T and B lymphocytes, NK cells and neutrophils, and the generation of antibody responses to T-cell-dependent and independent antigens. As an immune modulator, vitamin A reduces the severity but not the incidence of certain types of infections: measles, diarrhoeal diseases, malaria and, possibly, infections related to pregnancy. Vitamin A does not appear to reduce the morbidity and mortality from ALRI. As a general rule, there appears to be little value in vitamin A supplementation in populations that are already relatively well-nourished and thus clinical investigation of immune modulation by vitamin A should be focused on populations at high risk of vitamin A deficiency. Despite the tremendous advances that have been made in our understanding of the role that vitamin A plays in immune function, many gaps in knowledge remain:

- The relationship between vitamin A status in humans and the function of immune effector cells, such as neutrophils, macrophages, NK cells and cytotoxic T-cells.
- The relationship between vitamin A status in humans and the balance between T-helper type 1-like and T-helper type 2-like immune responses.
- The relationship between vitamin A status and gut integrity in humans.
- The role of vitamin A in resistance to *P. falciparum* malaria.

- The role of vitamin A in resistance to tuberculosis in humans.
- The more precise biological mechanism(s) by which vitamin A reduces measles severity.
- The more precise biological mechanism(s) by which vitamin A reduces diarrhoeal-disease severity.
- The role of vitamin A in immune senescence.
- The role of vitamin A in apoptosis.
- The relationship between vitamin A and other micronutrients (e.g. zinc) in immune modulation.
- The relationship between vitamin A status and expression of pro-inflammatory cytokines.
- The relationship between vitamin A status and specific infections during pregnancy.
- The uses of synthetic retinoids in immune modulation.

These are promising areas for future investigation, which should be addressed in order to gain further insight into the biological functions of this important vitamin.

Acknowledgements

This work was supported by the National Institute of Child Health and Human Development (HD32247, HD30042), the National Institute of Allergy and Infectious Diseases (AI41956) and the Fogarty International Center, the National Institutes of Health and the United States Agency for International Development (Cooperative Agreement HRN A-0097–00015–00).

References

Ahmed, F., Jones, D.B. and Jackson, A.A. (1991) Effect of vitamin A deficiency on the immune response to epizootic diarrhoea of infant mice (EDIM) rotavirus infection in mice. *British Journal of Nutrition* 65, 475–485.

Ballow, M., Wang, W. and Xiang, S. (1996) Modulation of B-cell immunoglobulin synthesis by retinoic acid. *Clinical Immunology and Immunopathology* 80, S73–S81.

Barclay, A.J.G., Foster, A. and Sommer, A. (1987) Vitamin A supplements and mortality related to measles: a randomised clinical trial. *British Medical Journal* 323, 160–164.

Barreto, M.L., Santos, L.M.P., Assis, A.M.O., Purificação, M., Araújo, N., Farenzena, G.G., Santos, P.A.B. and Fiaccone, R.L. (1994) Effect of vitamin A supplementation on diarrhoea and acute lower-respiratory-tract infections in young children in Brazil. *Lancet* 344, 228–231.

Beaton, G.H., Martorell, R., L'Abbe, K.A., Edmonston, B., McCabe, G., Ross, A.C. and Harvey, B. (1993) *Effectiveness of Vitamin A Supplementation in the Control of Young Child Morbidity and Mortality in Developing Countries*. ACC/SCN State-of-the-Art Nutrition Policy Discussion Paper No. 13, United Nations.

Beisel, W.R. (1982) Single nutrients and immunity. *American Journal of Clinical Nutrition* 35 (2 Suppl.), 417–468.

Blackfan, K.D. and Wolbach, S.B. (1933) Vitamin A deficiency in infants: a clinical and pathological study. *Journal of Pediatrics* 3, 679–706.

Bloch, C.E. (1924) Blindness and other diseases in children arising from deficient nutrition (lack of fat soluble A factor). *American Journal of Diseases of Childhood* 27, 139–148.

Bowman, T.A., Goonewardene, I.M., Pasatiempo, A.M.G. and Ross, A.C. (1990) Vitamin A deficiency decreases natural killer cell activity and interferon production in rats. *Journal of Nutrition* 120, 1264–1273.

Bresee, J.S., Fischer, M., Dowell, S.F., Johnston, B.D., Biggs, V.M., Levine, R.S., Lingappa, J.R., Keyserling, H.L., Petersen, K.M., Bak, J.R., Gary, H.E., Sowell, A.L., Rubens, C.E. and Anderson, L.J. (1996) Vitamin A therapy for children with respiratory syncytial virus infection: a multicenter trial in the United States. *Pediatric Infectious Diseases Journal* 15, 777–782.

Brilliant, L.B., Pokhrel, R.P., Grasset, N.C., Lepkowski, J.M., Kolstad, A., Hawks, W., Pararajasegaram, R., Brilliant, G.E., Gilbert, S., Shrestha, S.R. and Kuo, J. (1985) Epidemiology of blindness in Nepal. *Bulletin of the World Health Organization* 63, 375–386.

Buck, J., Derguini, F., Levi, E., Nakanishi, K. and Hämmerling, U. (1991) Intracellular signaling by 14-hydroxy-4,14-*retro* retinol. *Science* 254, 1654–1655.

Cameron, S.J. (1931) An aid in the prevention of puerperal sepsis. *Transactions of the Edinburgh Obstetrical Society* 52, 93–103.

Cantorna, M.T., Nashold, F.E. and Hayes, C.E. (1994) In vitamin A deficiency multiple mechanisms establish a regulatory T helper cell imbalance with excess Th1 and insufficient Th2 function. *Journal of Immunology* 152, 1515–1522.

Cantorna, M.T., Nashold, F.E., Chun, T.Y. and Hayes, C.E. (1996) Vitamin A down-regulation of IFN-γ synthesis in cloned mouse Th1 lymphocytes depends on the CD28 costimulatory pathway. *Journal of Immunology* 156, 2674–2679.

Carman, J.A., Pond, L., Nashold, F., Wassom, D.L. and Hayes, C.E. (1992) Immunity to *Trichinella spiralis* infection in vitamin A-deficient mice. *Journal of Experimental Medicine* 175, 111–120.

Chambon, P. (1996) A decade of molecular biology of retinoic acid receptors. *FASEB Journal* 10, 940–954.

Christian, P., Schulze, K., Stoltzfus, R.J. and West, K.P., Jr (1998) Hyporetinolemia, illness symptoms, and acute phase protein response in pregnant women with and without night blindness. *American Journal of Clinical Nutrition* 67, 1237–1243.

Christian, P., West, K.P., Jr, Khatry, S.K., Kimbrough-Pradhan, E., LeClerq, S.C., Katz, J., Shrestha, S.R., Dali, S.M. and Sommer, A. (2000a) Night blindness during pregnancy and subsequent mortality among women in Nepal: effects of vitamin A and beta-carotene supplementation. *American Journal of Epidemiology* 152, 542–547.

Christian, P., West, K.P., Jr, Khatry, S.K., Katz, J., LeClerq, S.C., Kimbrough-Pradhan, E., Dali, S.M. and Shrestha, S.R. (2000b) Vitamin A or beta-carotene supplementation reduces symptoms of illness in pregnant or lactating Nepali women. *Journal of Nutrition* 130, 2675–2682.

Clausen, S.W. (1934) The influence of nutrition upon resistance to infection. *Physiological Reviews* 14, 309–350.

Coutsoudis, A., Broughton, M. and Coovadia, H.M. (1991) Vitamin A supplementation reduces measles morbidity in young African children: a randomized, placebo-controlled, double-blind trial. *American Journal of Clinical Nutrition* 54, 890–895.

Coutsoudis, A., Kiepiela, P., Coovadia, H.M. and Broughton, M. (1992) Vitamin A supplementation enhances specific IgG antibody levels and total lymphocyte numbers while improving morbidity in measles. *Pediatric Infectious Diseases Journal* 11, 203–209.

Coutsoudis, A., Bobat, R.A., Coovadia, H.M., Kuhn, L., Tsai, W.Y. and Stein, Z.A. (1995) The effects of vitamin A supplementation on the morbidity of children born to HIV-infected women. *American Journal of Public Health* 85, 1076–1081.

Coutsoudis, A., Pillay, K., Spooner, E., Kuhn, L. and Coovadia, H.M. (1999) Randomized trial testing the effect of vitamin A supplementation on pregnancy outcomes and early mother-to-child transmission in Durban, South Africa. *AIDS* 13, 1517–1524.

Cui, D., Moldoveanu, Z. and Stephensen, C.B. (2000) High-level dietary vitamin A enhances T-helper type 2 cytokine production and secretory immunoglobulin A response to influenza A virus infection in BALB/c mice. *Journal of Nutrition* 130, 1322–1329.

Darwiche, N., Celli, G., Sly, L., Lancillotti, F. and DeLuca, L.M. (1993) Retinoid status controls the appearance of reserve cells and keratin expression in mouse cervical epithelium. *Cancer Research* 53(Suppl. 20), 2287–2299.

Dawson, H.D., Li, N.Q., DeCicco, K.L., Nibert, J.A. and Ross, A.C. (1999) Chronic marginal vitamin A status reduces natural killer cell number and function in ageing Lewis rats. *Journal of Nutrition* 129, 1510–1517.

De Pee, S., West, C.E., Muhilal, Karyadi, D. and Hautvast, J.G. (1995) Lack of improvement in vitamin A status with increased consumption of dark-green leafy vegetables. *Lancet* 346, 75–81.

DeSole, G., Belay, Y. and Zegeye, B. (1987) Vitamin A deficiency in southern Ethiopia. *American Journal of Clinical Nutrition* 45, 780–784.

Dillehay, D.L., Walla, A.S. and Lamon, E.W. (1988) Effects of retinoids on macrophage function and IL-1 activity. *Journal of Leukocyte Biology* 44, 353–360.

Dowell, S.F., Papic, Z., Bresee, J.S., Larrañaga, C., Mendez, M., Sowell, A.L., Gary, H.E., Anderson, L.J. and Avendaño, L.F. (1996) Treatment of respiratory syncytial virus infection with vitamin A: a randomized, placebo-controlled trial in Santiago, Chile. *Pediatric Infectious Diseases Journal* 15, 782–786.

Dudley, L., Hussey, G., Huskissen, J. and Kessow, G. (1997) Vitamin A status, other risk factors and acute respiratory infection morbidity in children. *South African Medical Journal* 87, 65–70.

Ellison, J.B. (1932) Intensive vitamin therapy in measles. *British Medical Journal* 2, 708–711.

Fawzi, W.W., Mbise, R.L., Fataki, M.R., Herrera, M.G., Kawau, F., Hertzmark, E., Spiegelman, D. and Ndossi, G. (1998) Vitamin A supplementation and severity of pneumonia in children admitted to the hospital in Dar es Salaam, Tanzania. *American Journal of Clinical Nutrition* 68, 187–192.

Fawzi, W.W., Mbise, R.L., Hertzmark, E., Fataki, M.R., Herrera, M.G., Ndossi, G. and Spiegelman, D. (1999) A randomized trial of vitamin A supplements in relation to mortality among human immunodeficiency virus-infected and uninfected children in Tanzania. *Pediatric Infectious Diseases Journal* 18, 127–133.

Fawzi, W.W., Mbise, R., Spiegelman, D., Fataki, M., Hertzmark, E. and Ndossi, G. (2000a) Vitamin A supplements and diarrheal and respiratory tract infections among children in Dar es Salaam, Tanzania. *Journal of Pediatrics* 137, 660–667.

Fawzi, W.W., Msamanga, G., Hunter, D., Urassa, E., Renjifo, B., Mwakagile, D., Hertzmark, E., Coley, J., Garland, M., Kapiga, S., Antelman, G., Essex, M. and Spiegelman, D. (2000b) Randomized trial of vitamin supplements in relation to vertical transmission of HIV-1 in Tanzania. *Journal of Acquired Immunodeficiency Syndromes* 23, 246–254.

Frankenburg, S., Wang, X. and Milner, Y. (1998) Vitamin A inhibits cytokines produced by type 1 lymphocytes *in vitro*. *Cellular Immunology* 185, 75–81.

Friis, H., Mwaniki, D., Omondi, B., Muniu, E., Magnussen, P., Geissler, W., Thiong'o, F. and Michaelsen, K.F. (1997) Serum retinol concentrations and *Schistosoma mansoni* intestinal helminths, and malarial parasitemia: a cross-sectional study in Kenyan preschool and primary school children. *American Journal of Clinical Nutrition* 66, 665–671.

Galan, P., Samba, C., Luzeau, R. and Amedee-Manesme, O. (1990) Vitamin A deficiency in pre-school age Congolese children during malaria attacks. Part 2: impact of parasitic disease on vitamin A status. *International Journal of Vitamin and Nutrition Research* 60, 224–228.

Gangopadhyay, N.N., Moldoveanu, Z. and Stephensen, C.B. (1996) Vitamin A deficiency has different effects on immunoglobulin A production and transport during influenza A infection in BALB/c mice. *Journal of Nutrition* 126, 2960–2967.

Gijbels, M.J.J., van der Harn, F., van Bennekum, A.M., Hendriks, H.F. and Roholl, P.J. (1992) Alterations in cytokeratin expression precede histological changes in epithelia of vitamin A-deficient rats. *Cell and Tissue Research* 268, 197–203.

Green, H.N. and Mellanby, E. (1928) Vitamin A as an anti-infective agent. *British Medical Journal* 2, 691–696.

Green, H.N., Pindar, D., Davis, G. and Mellanby, E. (1931) Diet as a prophylactic agent against puerperal sepsis. *British Medical Journal* 2, 595–598.

Griffiths, J.K. (2000) The vitamin A paradox. *Journal of Pediatrics* 137, 604–607.

Gujral, S., Abbi, R. and Gopaldas, T. (1993) Xerophthalmia, vitamin A supplementation and morbidity in children. *Journal of Tropical Pediatrics* 39, 89–92.

Hanekom, W.A., Potgieter, S., Hughes, E.J., Malan, H., Kessow, G. and Hussey, G.D. (1997) Vitamin A status and therapy in childhood pulmonary tuberculosis. *Journal of Pediatrics* 131, 925–927.

Higuchi, H. and Nagahata, H. (2000) Effects of vitamins A and E on superoxide production and intracellular signaling of neutrophils in Holstein calves. *Canadian Journal of Veterinary Research* 64, 69–75.

Hossain, S., Biswas, R., Kabir, I., Sarker, S., Dibley, M., Fuchs, G. and Mahalanabis, D. (1998) Single dose vitamin A treatment in acute shigellosis in Bangladeshi children: randomised double blind controlled trial. *British Medical Journal* 316, 422–426.

Hussey, G., Hughes, J., Potgieter, S., Kessow, G., Burgess, J., Beatty, D., Keraan, M. and Carlesle, E. (1996) Vitamin A status and supplementation and its effects on immunity in children with AIDS. In: *Abstracts of the XVII International Vitamin A Consultative Group Meeting, Guatemala City*. International Life Sciences Institute, Washington, DC, p. 6.

Hussey, G.D. and Klein, M. (1990) A randomized, controlled trial of vitamin A in children with severe measles. *New England Journal of Medicine* 323, 160–164.

Israel, H., Odziemiec, C. and Ballow, M. (1991) The effects of retinoic acid on immunoglobulin synthesis by human cord blood mononuclear cells. *Clinical Immunology and Immunopathology* 59, 417–425.

Kennedy, C.M., Kuhn, L. and Stein, Z. (2000) Vitamin A and HIV infection: disease progression, mortality, and transmission. *Nutrition Reviews* 58, 291–303.

Kinoshita, M., Pasatiempo, A.M.G., Taylor, C.E. and Ross, A.C. (1991) Immunological memory to tetanus toxoid is established and maintained in the vitamin A-depleted rat. *FASEB Journal* 5, 2473–2481.

Kjolhede, C.L., Chew, F.J., Gadomski, A.M. and Marroquin, D.P. (1995) Clinical trial of vitamin A as adjuvant treatment for lower respiratory tract infections. *Journal of Pediatrics* 126, 807–812.

Kliewer, S.A., Umesono, K., Mangelsdorf, D.J. and Evans, R.M. (1992) Retinoid X receptor interacts with nuclear receptors in retinoic acid, thyroid hormone and vitamin D_3 signalling. *Nature* 355, 446–449.

Koo, J.S., Jetten, A.M., Belloni, P., Yoon, Y.H., Kim, Y.D. and Nettesheim, P. (1999) Role of retinoid receptors in the regulation of mucin gene expression by retinoic acid in human tracheobronchial epithelial cells. *Biochemical Journal* 338, 351–357.

Kutukculer, N., Akil, T., Egemen, A., Kurugöl, Z., Akşit, A., Özmen, D., Turgan, N., Bayindir, O. and Çağlayan, S. (2000) Adequate immune response to tetanus toxoid and failure of vitamin A and E supplementation to enhance antibody response in healthy children. *Vaccine* 18, 2979–2984.

Lavasa, S., Kumar, L., Chakravarti, R.N. and Kumar, M. (1988) Early humoral immune response in vitamin A deficiency – an experimental study. *Indian Journal of Experimental Biology* 26, 431–435.

Lawson, N.D. and Berliner, N. (1999) Neutrophil maturation and the role of retinoic acid. *Experimental Hematology* 27, 1355–1367.

McLaren, D.S. (1963) *Malnutrition and the Eye*. Academic Press, New York.

McLaren, D.S. and Frigg, M. (2001) *Sight and Life Manual on Vitamin A Deficiency Disorders (VADD)*, 2nd edn. Task Force Sight and Life, Basle.

Markowitz, L., Nzilambi, N., Driskell, W.J., Sension, M.G., Rovira, E.Z., Nieburg, P. and Ryder, R.W. (1989) Vitamin A levels and mortality among hospitalized measles patients, Kinshasa, Zaire. *Journal of Tropical Pediatrics* 35, 109–112.

Mitra, A.K., Alvarez, J.O., Guay-Woodford, L., Fuchs, G.J., Wahed, M.A. and Stephensen, C.B. (1998) Urinary retinol excretion and kidney function in children with shigellosis. *American Journal of Clinical Nutrition* 68, 1095–1103.

Molrine, D.C., Polk, D.B., Ciamarra, A., Phillips, N. and Ambrosino, D.M. (1995) Impaired human responses to tetanus toxoid in vitamin A-deficient SCID mice reconstituted with human peripheral blood lymphocytes. *Infection and Immunity* 63, 2867–2872.

Nacul, L.C., Kirkwood, B.R., Arthur, P., Morris, S.S., Magalhães, M. and Fink, M.C.D.S. (1997) Randomised, double blind, placebo controlled clinical trial of efficacy of vitamin A treatment in non-measles childhood pneumonia. *British Medical Journal* 315, 505–510.

Nauss, K.M. (1986) Influence of vitamin A status on the immune system. In: Bauernfeind, J.C. (ed.) *Vitamin A Deficiency and Its Control*. Academic Press, Orlando, pp. 207–243.

Nauss, K.M. and Newberne, P.M. (1985) Local and regional immune function of vitamin A-deficient rats with ocular herpes simplex virus (HSV) infections. *Journal of Nutrition* 115, 1316–1324.

Ogaro, F.O., Orinda, V.A., Onyango, F.E. and Black, R.E. (1993) Effect of vitamin A on diarrhoeal and respiratory complications of measles. *Tropical and Geographical Medicine* 45, 283–286.

Oomen, H.A.P.C., McLaren, D.S. and Escapini, H. (1964) Epidemiology and public health aspects of hypovitaminosis A. *Tropical and Geographical Medicine* 4, 271–315.

Pasatiempo, A.M.G., Bowman, T.A., Taylor, C.E. and Ross, A.C. (1989) Vitamin A depletion and repletion: effects on antibody response to the capsular polysaccharide of *Streptococcus pneumoniae*, type III (SSS-III). *American Journal of Clinical Nutrition* 49, 501–510.

Pasatiempo, A.M.G., Kinoshita, M., Taylor, C.E. and Ross, A.C. (1990) Antibody production in vitamin A-depleted rats is impaired after immunization with bacterial polysaccharide or protein antigens. *FASEB Journal* 4, 2518–2527.

Perrin, M.C., Blanchet, J.P. and Mouchiroud, G. (1997) Modulation of human and mouse erythropoiesis by thyroid hormone and retinoic acid: evidence for specific effects at different steps of the erythroid pathway. *Hematology and Cell Therapy* 39, 19–26.

Quinlan, K.P. and Hayani, K.C. (1996) Vitamin A and respiratory syncytial virus infection: serum levels and supplementation trial. *Archives of Pediatric and Adolescent Medicine* 150, 25–30.

Robertson, E.C. (1934) The vitamins and resistance to infection. *Medicine* 13, 123–206.

Rombout, J.H., Sijtsma, S.R., West, C.E., Karabinis, Y., Sijtsma, O.K., van der Zijpp, A.J. and Koch, G. (1992) Effect of vitamin A deficiency and Newcastle disease virus infection on IgA and IgM secretion in chickens. *British Journal of Nutrition* 68, 753–763.

Ross, D.A. and Cutts, F.T. (1997) Vindication of policy of vitamin A with measles vaccination. *Lancet* 350, 81–82.

Schaumberg, D.A., O'Connor, J. and Semba, R.D. (1996) Risk factors for xerophthalmia in the Republic of Kiribati. *European Journal of Clinical Nutrition* 50, 761–764.

Scrimshaw, N.S., Taylor, C.E. and Gordon, J.E. (1968) *Interactions of Nutrition and Infection*. World Health Organization, Geneva.

Semba, R.D. (1994) Vitamin A, immunity, and infection. *Clinical Infectious Diseases* 19, 489–499.

Semba, R.D. (1998) Vitamin A and immunity to viral, bacterial and protozoan infections. *Proceedings of the Nutrition Society* 58, 719–727.

Semba, R.D., Muhilal, Scott, A.L., Natadisastra, G., Wirasasmita, S., Mele, L., Ridwan, E., West, K.P. Jr and Sommer, A. (1992) Depressed immune response to tetanus in children with vitamin A deficiency. *Journal of Nutrition* 122, 101–107.

Semba, R.D., Graham, N.M.H., Caiaffa, W.T., Margolick, J.B., Clement, L. and Vlahov, D. (1993a) Increased mortality associated with vitamin A deficiency during human immunodeficiency virus type 1 infection. *Archives of Internal Medicine* 153, 2149–2154.

Semba, R.D., Muhilal, Ward, B.J., Griffin, D.E., Scott, A.L., Natadisastra, G., West, K.P., Jr and Sommer, A. (1993b) Abnormal T-cell subset proportions in vitamin A-deficient children. *Lancet* 341, 5–8.

Semba, R.D., Muhilal, Scott, A.L., Natadisastra, G., West K.P., Jr and Sommer, A. (1994) Effect of vitamin A supplementation on IgG subclass responses to tetanus toxoid in children. *Clinical and Diagnostic Laboratory Immunology* 1, 172–175.

Semba, R.D., Munasir, Z., Beeler, J., Akib, A., Muhilal, Audet, S. and Sommer, A. (1995) Reduced seroconversion to measles in infants given vitamin A with measles vaccination. *Lancet* 345, 1330–1332.

Semba, R.D., Akib, A., Beeler, J., Munasir, Z., Permaesih, D., Muherdiyantiningsih, Komala, Martuti, S. and Muhilal (1997) Effect of vitamin A supplementation on measles vaccination in nine-month-old infants. *Public Health* 111, 245–247.

Semba, R.D., Lyles, C.M., Margolick, J.B., Caiaffa, W.T., Farzadegan, H., Cohn, S. and Vlahov, D. (1998) Vitamin A supplementation and human immunodeficiency virus load in injection drug users. *Journal of Infectious Diseases* 177, 611–616.

Sempertegui, F., Estrella, B., Camaniero,V., Betancourt, V., Izurieta, R., Ortiz, W., Fiallo, E., Troya, S., Rodriguez, A. and Griffiths, J.K. (1999) The beneficial effects of weekly low-dose vitamin A supplementation on acute lower respiratory infections and diarrhea in Ecuadorian children. *Pediatrics* 104, E11-E17.

Shankar, A.H., Genton, B., Semba, R.D., Baisor, M., Paino, J., Tamja, S., Adiguma, T., Wu, L., Rare, L., Tielsch, J.M., Alpers, M.P. and West, K.P., Jr (1999) Effect of vitamin A supplementation on morbidity due to *Plasmodium falciparum* in young children in Papua New Guinea: a randomised trial. *Lancet* 354, 203–209.

Smith, S.M. and Hayes, C.E. (1987) Contrasting impairments in IgM and IgG responses of vitamin A-deficient mice. *Proceedings of the National Academy of Sciences of the USA* 84, 5878–5882.

Sommer, A. (1982) *Nutritional Blindness: Xerophthalmia and Keratomalacia.* Oxford University Press, New York.

Sommer, A., Katz, J. and Tarwotjo, I. (1984) Increased risk of respiratory disease and diarrhea in children with preexisting mild vitamin A deficiency. *American Journal of Clinical Nutrition* 40, 1090–1095.

Stabell Benn, C., Aaby, P., Balé, C., Olsen, J., Michaelsen, K.F., George, E. and Whittle, H. (1997) Randomised trial of effect of vitamin A supplementation on antibody response to measles vaccine in Guinea-Bissau, West Africa. *Lancet* 350, 101–105.

Stürchler, D., Tanner, M., Hanck, A., Betschart, B., Gautschi, K., Weiss, N., Burnier, E., Del Giudice, G. and Degrémont, A. (1987) A longitudinal study on relations of retinol with parasitic infections and the immune response in children of Kikwawila village, Tanzania. *Acta Tropica* 44, 213–227.

Sweet, K.L. and K'ang, H.J. (1935) Clinical and anatomic study of avitaminosis A among the Chinese. *American Journal for Diseases of Childhood* 50, 699–734.

Tei, M., Spurr-Michaud, S.J., Tisdale, A.S. and Gipson, I.K. (2000) Vitamin A deficiency alters the expression of mucin genes by the rat ocular surface epithelium. *Investigative Ophthalmology and Visual Science* 41, 82–88.

Thurnham, D.I., Northrup-Clewes, C.A., McCullough, F.S., Das, B.S. and Lunn, P.G. (2000) Innate immunity, gut integrity, and vitamin A in Gambian and Indian infants. *Journal of Infectious Diseases* 182, S23-S28.

Twining, S.S., Schulte, D.P., Wilson, P.M., Fish, B.L. and Moulder, J.E. (1996) Vitamin A deficiency alters rat neutrophil function. *Journal of Nutrition* 127, 558–565.

Vitamin A and Pneumonia Working Group (1995) Potential interventions for the prevention of childhood pneumonia in developing countries: a meta-analysis of data from field trials to assess the impact of vitamin A supplementation on pneumonia morbidity and mortality. *Bulletin of the World Health Organization* 73, 609–619.

Wang, W. and Ballow, M. (1993) The effects of retinoic acid on *in vitro* immunoglobulin synthesis by cord blood and adult peripheral blood mononuclear cells. *Cellular Immunology* 148, 291–300.

Wang, W., Napoli, J.L. and Ballow, M. (1993) The effects of retinol on *in vitro* immunoglobulin synthesis by cord blood and adult peripheral blood mononuclear cells. *Clinical and Experimental Immunology* 92, 164–168.

West, C.E. (2000) Meeting requirements for vitamin A. *Nutrition Reviews* 58, 341–345.

West, K.P., Jr, Katz, J., Shrestha, S.R., LeClerq, S.C., Khatry, S.K., Pradhan, E.K., Adhikari, R., Wu, L.S., Pokhrel, R.P. and Sommer, A. (1995) Mortality of infants < 6 mo of age supplemented with vitamin A: a randomized, double-masked trial in Nepal. *American Journal of Clinical Nutrition* 62, 143–148.

West, K.P., Jr, Katz, J., Khatry, S.K., LeClerq, S.C., Pradhan, E.K., Shrestha, S.R., Connor, P.B., Dali, S.M., Christian, P., Pokhrel, R.P. and Sommer, A. (1999) Double blind, cluster randomised trial of low dose supplementation with vitamin A or beta carotene on mortality related to pregnancy in Nepal. *British Medical Journal* 318, 570–575.

WHO/CHD Immunisation-Linked Vitamin A Supplementation Study Group (1998) Randomised trial to assess benefits and safety of vitamin A supplementation linked to immunisation in early infancy. *Lancet* 352, 1257–1263.

World Health Organization (1995) *World Health Report: Bridging the Gaps.* World Health Organization, Geneva.

Wiedermann, U., Hanson, L.A., Holmgren, J., Kahu, H. and Dahlgren, U.I. (1993a)

Impaired mucosal antibody response to cholera toxin in vitamin A-deficient rats immunized with oral cholera vaccine. *Infection and Immunity* 61, 3957–3977.

Wiedermann, U., Hanson, L.A., Kahu, H. and Dahlgren, U.I. (1993b) Aberrant T-cell function *in vitro* and impaired T-cell dependent antibody response *in vivo* in vitamin A-deficient rats. *Immunology* 80, 581–586.

Wiedermann, U., Tarkowski, A., Bremell, T., Hanson, L.A., Kahu, H. and Dahlgren, U.I. (1996) Vitamin A deficiency predisposes to *Staphylococcus aureus* infection. *Infection and Immunity* 64, 209–214.

Williams, C.J.B. and Williams, C.T. (1871) *Pulmonary Consumption: its Nature, Varieties, and Treatment with an Analysis of One Thousand Cases to Exemplify its Duration*. Henry C. Lea, Philadelphia.

Wolbach, S.B. and Howe, P.R. (1925) Tissue changes following deprivation of fat-soluble A vitamin. *Journal of Experimental Medicine* 42, 753–778.

Zermati, Y., Fichelson, S., Valensi, F., Freyssinier, J.M., Rouyer-Fessard, P., Cramer, E., Guichard, J., Varet, B. and Hermine, O. (2000) Transforming growth factor inhibits erythropoiesis by blocking proliferation of accelerating differentiation of erythroid progenitors. *Experimental Hematology* 28, 885–894.

Zhao, Z. and Ross, A.C. (1995) Retinoic acid repletion restores the number of leucocytes and their subsets and stimulates natural cytotoxicity in vitamin A-deficient rats. *Journal of Nutrition* 125, 2064–2073.

Zhao, Z., Murasko, D.M. and Ross, A.C. (1994) The role of vitamin A in natural killer cell cytotoxicity, number and activation in the rat. *Natural Immunity* 13, 29–41.

9 Antioxidant Vitamins and Immune Function

DAVID A. HUGHES

Nutrition and Consumer Science Division, Institute of Food Research, Norwich Research Park, Norwich NR4 7UA, UK

Introduction

Oxidative stress, resulting from cumulative damage caused by reactive oxygen species (ROS), is present throughout life and is thought to be a major contributor to the ageing process. The immune system is particularly vulnerable to oxidative damage, since many immune cells produce these reactive compounds as part of the body's defence mechanisms. Higher organisms have evolved a variety of antioxidant defence systems either to prevent the generation of ROS or to intercept any that are generated. These defence systems exist in both the aqueous and membrane compartments of cells and can be enzymic or non-enzymic in nature. The enzymes contain metal ions at their active sites – these must be obtained from the diet – while the diet is the source of many non-enzymic components of the body's antioxidant defence system (e.g. antioxidant vitamins).

Reactive Oxygen Species and Antioxidant Defences

Reactive oxygen species

Free radicals are highly reactive molecules containing one or more unpaired electrons. Examples of free radicals are the superoxide anion ($O_2^-\cdot$) and the hydroxyl radical ($OH\cdot$). The term 'reactive oxygen species' is a collective one that includes not only oxygen-centred radicals but also some non-radical derivatives of oxygen, such as hydrogen peroxide (H_2O_2), singlet oxygen and hypochlorous acid (HOCl). Hydrogen peroxide can very easily break down, particularly in the presence of transition-metal ions (e.g. ferrous (Fe^{2+}) iron), to produce the hydroxyl radical, the most reactive and damaging of the oxygen free radicals:

$$H_2O_2 + Fe^{2+} \rightarrow OH\cdot + OH^- + Fe^{3+}$$

© CAB *International* 2002. *Nutrition and Immune Function*
(eds P.C. Calder, C.J. Field and H.S. Gill)

Exogenous sources of free radicals include ozone, UV radiation and cigarette smoke. Free radicals are also generated endogenously, mainly from two sources. The first is by leakage from the mitochondrial electron-transfer chain, as part of normal cellular metabolism. The second is as part of the respiratory-burst activity of leucocytes, which is involved in microbial killing.

ROS can cause damage to all of the major classes of macromolecules. They cause strand breaks in DNA (Halliwell and Aruoma, 1991), which can potentially lead to subsequent misrepair, mutation and tumour-cell formation. An example of free-radical-mediated damage to proteins is the formation of cataracts, resulting from the damage to the crystallins in the lens of the eye. However, lipids are probably most susceptible to free radical attack, particularly long chain polyunsaturated fatty acids (PUFA) that contain several double bonds. The oxidative destruction of PUFA, known as lipid peroxidation, can be extremely damaging, since it proceeds as a self-perpetuating chain reaction.

Generation of ROS in excess of the amounts that can be dealt with by the body's antioxidant protective mechanisms is thought to be a major contributor to several degenerative disorders, such as cancer and cardiovascular diseases (Table 9.1), and to the ageing process. Strong associations between diets rich in antioxidant nutrients and a reduced incidence of cancer have been observed in several epidemiological studies (Block et al., 1992; Giovannucci, 1999), and it has been suggested that a boost to the body's immune system by antioxidants might, at least in part, account for this (Bendich and Olson, 1989). Indeed, it is probably crucial to attempt to balance the production of ROS and the antioxidant defence system, ideally by dietary means rather than by taking supplements, from as early an age as possible, in order to delay the onset of, if not prevent, many age-related disorders.

The immune system appears to be particularly sensitive to oxidative stress. Immune cells rely heavily on cell–cell communication, particularly via membrane-bound receptors, to work effectively. Cell membranes are rich in PUFA, which, if peroxidized, can lead to a loss of membrane integrity, altered membrane fluidity (Baker and Meydani, 1994) and alterations in intracellular signalling and cell function. It has been shown that exposure to ROS can lead to a reduction in cell-membrane-receptor expression (Gruner et al., 1986). In addition, the production of ROS by phagocytic immune cells can damage the cells themselves if they are not sufficiently protected by antioxidants.

Table 9.1. Degenerative disorders associated with oxidative damage.

Cancer
Cardiovascular disease
Stroke
Cataract
Degeneration of the macula region of the retina
Immunosenescence
Ageing

Antioxidant defences

The enzyme superoxide dismutase decomposes superoxide radicals by converting them to hydrogen peroxide plus oxygen. Catalase and glutathione (GSH) peroxidase are enzymes that decompose peroxides, particularly hydrogen peroxide.

$$2O_2^- \cdot + 2H^+ \xrightarrow{\text{Superoxide dismutase}} H_2O_2 + O_2$$

$$2H_2O_2 \xrightarrow{\text{Catalase}} 2H_2O + O_2$$

$$2GSH + H_2O_2 \xrightarrow{\text{Glutathione peroxidase}} GSSG + 2H_2O$$
$$\text{(oxidized glutathione)}$$

There are two forms of superoxide dismutase: a mitochondrial enzyme, which contains manganese, and a cytosolic enzyme, which contains copper and zinc. Catalase contains iron, while glutathione peroxidase contains selenium. These metal ions must come from the diet. At least some of the effects that selenium, copper, zinc, iron and glutathione have on immune function relate to their roles in antioxidant defence (see Grimble, Chapter 7, Prasad, Chapter 10, Kuvibidila and Baliga, Chapter 11, and McKenzie *et al.*, Chapter 12, this volume). The diet also provides many other, non-enzymic, components of the body's antioxidant defence system. These include the antioxidants vitamins C and E and the carotenoids.

Dietary sources of antioxidant vitamins

The most important antioxidant in cell membranes is α-tocopherol, the major member of the vitamin E family. This molecule acts as a 'chain-breaking antioxidant', intercepting lipid peroxyl radicals and so terminating lipid-peroxidation chain reactions. Vitamin E is found in many dietary fats and oils, especially those containing PUFA (Table 9.2). Thus, the dietary intake of vitamin E is related to the intake of PUFA. Intakes among adults in the UK vary between 3.5 and 19.5 (median 9.3) mg α-tocopherol equivalents day^{-1} for men and

Table 9.2. Dietary sources of antioxidant vitamins.

Vitamin C	Citrus fruits, blackcurrants, kiwi fruit, strawberries Red peppers, broccoli, Brussels sprouts
Vitamin E	Whole grains, vegetable oils, wheat germ, eggs
Carotenoids	
β-carotene	Carrots, broccoli, watercress, spinach, apricots
Lycopene	Tomatoes and processed tomato products (sauce and paste)
Lutein	Peas, spinach, broccoli and dark green leafy vegetables
β-cryptoxanthin	Mandarins, satsumas, apricots, orange peppers

between 2.5 and 15.2 (median 6.7) mg day^{-1} α-tocopherol equivalents for women (Department of Health, 1991). Another group of lipid-soluble compounds that can act as antioxidants are the carotenoids, such as β-carotene, lycopene and lutein, found in highly pigmented fruits and vegetables (Mangels *et al.*, 1993). The major water-soluble free radical scavenger is ascorbic acid (vitamin C), which also plays a role in 'sparing' vitamin E, by regenerating α-tocopherol from the oxidized tocopheroxyl radical (Bendich *et al.*, 1986). The estimated average requirement for vitamin C in adults in the UK is 25 mg day^{-1} (Department of Health, 1991). More recently, attention has also focused on the antioxidant properties of plant polyphenols, found in tea and red wines (Rice-Evans, 1995), but considerably more information on the absorption, metabolism and excretion of these compounds in humans is required before their relative contribution to preventing oxidative damage can be assessed.

A balanced diet, containing at least five or six varied portions of fruits and vegetables per day, should provide an adequate supply of antioxidants for healthy individuals. Concerns regarding the taking of supplements centre around the possibilities that certain compounds might have a toxic effect if taken in doses significantly higher than can be obtained from a healthy diet and that a reliance on supplements will lead to a reduced consumption of fresh fruit and vegetables, which probably contain a multitude of compounds whose health benefits we have yet to appreciate. However, in elderly individuals, whose diet might be restricted (e.g. by loss of appetite, dental conditions) and where absorption of nutrients is impaired, there might be a case for supplementation with certain nutrients. The case is probably strongest for vitamin E, because it is impossible to obtain high intakes of this nutrient without consuming a high-fat diet. Table 9.2 identifies dietary sources of antioxidant vitamins.

Antioxidant Vitamins and Immune Function

Vitamin C and immune function

Vitamin C is found in high concentrations in white blood cells and is rapidly utilized during infection; reduced plasma concentrations are often associated with reduced immune function (see Siegel, 1993). Animal and human studies have suggested that the dietary requirements for vitamin C are increased in cancer, surgical trauma and infectious diseases (see Siegel, 1993). The belief that high intakes of vitamin C will prevent the onset of the common cold has not been substantiated scientifically, although the associated symptoms following infection appear to be reduced by a moderate intake (Coulehan *et al.*, 1974). Pauling's claims regarding the effects of vitamin C on the common cold (Pauling, 1970) inspired a great deal of research into its effect on immune function in the 1970s and early 1980s (reviewed by Thomas and Holt, 1978; Siegel, 1993). Vitamin C deficiency in the guinea pig impairs lymphocyte proliferation, the delayed-type hypersensitivity (DTH) response to tuberculin, the ability of neutrophils to kill bacteria and the activity of cytotoxic T-cells and delays the rejection of skin allografts, but has little effect on antibody responses (for references, see Siegel, 1993). Providing vitamin C to mice increased spleen lymphocyte proliferation in response to mitogens but did not affect natural killer (NK)-cell activity or the antibody response to sheep red blood cells or lipopolysaccharide (LPS) (see Siegel, 1993). Vitamin C decreased or slowed tumour development in some animal models, but not others (see Siegel, 1993). Vitamin C deficiency in humans did not impair lymphocyte proliferation or alter the number of CD4+ or CD8+ cells in the circulation (Kay *et al.*, 1982). However, Vitamin C (1–5 g daily for 3 days to several weeks) increased human T lymphocyte proliferation (Yonemoto *et al.*, 1976; Anderson *et al.*, 1980; Panush *et al.*, 1982) and neutrophil motility towards LPS-activated autologous serum (Anderson *et al.*, 1980). Some studies indicate that vitamin C increases circulating immunoglobulin (Ig) levels in humans (Prinz *et al.*, 1977; Vallance, 1977; Ziemlanski *et al.*, 1986), but other studies fail to show this (Anderson *et al.*, 1980; Panush *et al.*, 1982; Kennes *et al.*, 1983). Jacob *et al.* (1991) studied the effect of vitamin C at different levels in the diet on immune function in a group of young, healthy non-smokers. The subjects first consumed a vitamin C-deficient diet and then gradually increased their vitamin C intake (from 5 to 250 mg day^{-1}). The vitamin C-deficient diet decreased plasma and white-cell vitamin C concentrations by 50% and decreased the DTH response to seven recall antigens, but did not alter lymphocyte proliferation. Sixty or 250 mg vitamin C day^{-1} led to recovery of the DTH response, but did not affect lymphocyte proliferation. The authors suggest that the inconsistency regarding the influence of vitamin C on these two outcomes, both indicators of cell-mediated immunity, may result from the higher sensitivity of the DTH test, involvement of cells other than those isolated for *in vitro* cultures in the *in vivo* DTH response or other unknown factors. The lack of an effect on lymphocyte proliferation at an intake of 250 mg day^{-1} suggests that, at least in young individuals, only levels of vitamin C that approach pharmacological doses can produce a quantifiable effect on this parameter of immune function. It has been suggested that vitamin C intakes of 600 mg day^{-1} may be beneficial in reducing infections in individuals who undertake a large amount of physical activity: for instance, studies of marathon runners have found a significantly lower incidence of post-race upper respiratory infections in runners taking a daily supplement of 600 mg vitamin C (Peters, 1997).

One of the major problems in assessing the beneficial effects of dietary components on the immune system is the lack of a reliable marker of immune function that is known to be indicative of a long-term beneficial effect in terms of reducing the incidence of degenerative disorders in later life. Although not an immunological one, one recent study does provide an excellent example of the potential need to maintain adequate intakes of antioxidant nutrients in the middle years of life to prevent the accumulative damage caused by ROS being made manifest in later years. Jacques *et al.* (1997) examined the cross-sectional relationship between age-related lens opacities and vitamin C supplement use over a 10–12-year period in women without diagnosed cataract or diabetes. Use of vitamin C supplements for 10 years or more was associated with a 77% lower prevalence of early lens opacities and an 83% lower prevalence of moderate lens opacities, compared with women who did not use supplements. Women who consumed vitamin C supplements for less than 10 years showed no evidence of a reduced prevalence of early opacities, suggesting that long-term consumption of vitamin C supplements may substantially reduce the development of age-related lens opacities. While the use of supplements might be required to obtain sufficient intakes of vitamin C to prevent this form of oxidative damage, it is hoped that the intake required to maintain optimal immune function can be obtained from a healthy diet containing fruit and vegetables rich in antioxidants. This should be the case, since epidemiological studies of populations having a lower incidence of cancer suggest that the benefits are associated with the intake of increased amounts of these foodstuffs rather than the taking of supplements (Block *et al.*, 1992).

Vitamin C has been used to treat some clinical phagocytic cell dysfunctions. In Chediak–Higashi syndrome, which is characterized in part by defective neutrophil functions, vitamin C supplementation has been shown to increase neutrophil chemotaxis, improve bactericidal activity and reduce the length of clinical illness (Boxer *et al.*, 1976). Vitamin C also appears to be beneficial in the treatment of chronic granulomatous disease (Anderson, 1982).

Vitamin C provides important antioxidant protection for plasma lipids and lipid membranes and can also neutralize phagocyte-derived oxidants released extracelluarly, thereby preventing oxidant-mediated tissue damage, particularly at sites of inflammatory activity. Other mechanisms that have been proposed for the immunostimulatory effects of vitamin C include modulation of intracellular cyclic-nucleotide levels, modulation of prostaglandin synthesis, enhancement of cytokine production, antagonism of the immunosuppressive interaction between histamines and white blood cells and the protection of 5-lipoxygenase (Anderson *et al.*, 1990). There is a need for further research, not only into the mechanisms by which vitamin C can enhance immune-cell function, but also to define the level of intake required to maintain an optimal immune responsiveness throughout life and to reduce the incidence of degenerative disorders in later life.

Vitamin E and immune function

Since vitamin E is the most effective chain-breaking, lipid-soluble antioxidant present in cell membranes, it is considered likely that it plays a major role in maintaining cell membrane integrity by limiting lipid peroxidation by ROS.

Studies conducted in humans and animals, using either states of deficiency or supra-dietary levels, suggest strongly that vitamin E is involved in maintaining immune cell function (for a review, see Meydani and Beharka, 1998). For example, Canadian 3-year-olds with the lowest serum vitamin E levels had the lowest lymphocyte proliferative responses and serum IgM concentrations (Vobecky *et al.*, 1984). In addition, there was a positive association between plasma vitamin E levels and DTH responses and a negative association between plasma vitamin E levels and incidence of infections in healthy adults aged over 60 (see Chavance *et al.*, 1989). Administration of vitamin E to premature infants enhanced neutrophil phagocytosis (Baehner *et al.*, 1977; Chirico *et al.*, 1983) but decreased the ability of neutrophils to kill bacteria

(Baehner *et al.*, 1977); this latter effect is most probably due to a vitamin E-induced decrease in production of free radicals and related reactive species. In laboratory animals, vitamin E deficiency decreased spleen lymphocyte proliferation in response to mitogens, NK-cell activity, specific antibody production following vaccination and phagocytosis by neutrophils (for a review, see Meydani and Beharka, 1998). Vitamin E deficiency also increases susceptibility of animals to infectious pathogens (for references, see Meydani and Beharka, 1998; Han and Meydani, 1999). Vitamin E supplementation of the diet of laboratory animals enhances antibody production, lymphocyte proliferation, NK-cell activity, and macrophage phagocytosis (for references, see Meydani and Beharka, 1998). Dietary vitamin E promoted resistance to pathogens in chickens, turkeys, mice, pigs, sheep and cattle (for references, see Meydani and Beharka, 1998; Han and Meydani, 1999); some of these studies report improved immune-cell functions in the animals receiving additional vitamin E (see Han and Meydani, 1999). For example, vitamin E prevented the retrovirus-induced decrease in production of interleukin-2 (IL-2) and interferon-γ (IFN-γ) by spleen lymphocytes and in NK-cell activity in mice (Wang *et al.*, 1994).

One application of the effects of vitamin E on immune function is in the elderly. This has been investigated in both murine models and human trials. Adding vitamin E to the diet of aged mice increased lymphocyte proliferation, IL-2 production and the DTH response (Meydani *et al.*, 1986). A high level of vitamin E in the diet (500 mg kg^{-1} food) also increased NK-cell activity of spleen cells from old (but not young) mice (Meydani *et al.*, 1988). In another study, young and old mice were fed diets containing adequate (30 mg kg^{-1} diet) or high (500 mg kg^{-1} diet) levels of vitamin E for 6 weeks and infected with influenza A virus: young mice and old mice fed the high level of vitamin E had lower lung titres of virus than old mice fed the adequate vitamin E diet (Hayek *et al.*, 1997). The high level of vitamin E caused increased production of IL-2 and IFN-γ by spleen lymphocytes from influenza-infected old mice (Han *et al.*, 1998; Han and Meydani, 2000). Supplementation of the diet of elderly human subjects with 800 mg vitamin E day^{-1} for 4 weeks increased lymphocyte proliferation stimulated by concanavalin A, IL-2 production and the DTH response, but did not affect IL-1 production, the number of CD4 cells or circulating Ig concentrations (Meydani *et al.*, 1990). In a more recent study, 60, 200 and 800 mg vitamin E day^{-1} increased DTH response in elderly subjects, with 200 mg day^{-1} having the maximal effect (Meydani *et al.*, 1997). The two higher vitamin E doses improved antibody responses to hepatitis B, but only the 200 mg day^{-1} dose increased the antibody response to tetanus toxoid (Meydani *et al.*, 1997). The authors conclude that 200 mg vitamin E day^{-1} represents the optimal level for the immune response. In another study, young and elderly individuals were supplemented with 800 mg vitamin E day^{-1} for 48 days before being asked to run down an inclined treadmill for 45 min. Vitamin E supplementation was found to eliminate the age-associated difference in exercise-induced neutropenia, to prevent the exercise-induced increase in IL-1 production and to inhibit IL-6 production (Cannon *et al.*, 1991). Since these cytokines are involved in the inflammatory process and in exercise-induced muscle damage, their inhibition by vitamin E during exercise might have important implications. However, on a cautious note, studies have reported that prolonged high intakes of vitamin E (> 1000 mg day^{-1}) can lead to inhibition of neutrophil phagocytosis (Boxer, 1986). Further research is needed to assess the optimal intake of this nutrient required to provide benefit for different groups of individuals.

Cigarette smoke contains millions of free radicals per puff, and other compounds present can stimulate the formation of other highly reactive molecules (Pryor and Stone, 1993). Serum levels of vitamin E (as well as of vitamin C and β-carotene) and lung vitamin E concentrations are significantly lower in smokers compared with non-smokers and even supplementation with 2400 mg α-tocopherol equivalents day^{-1} for 3 weeks failed to restore the lung vitamin E level to that found in non-smokers (Pacht et al., 1986). Circulating phagocytes from smokers produce high levels of free radicals, which probably in part accounts for the depressed immune function observed in smokers (Johnson et al., 1990), and there is some evidence that vitamin E supplementation can reduce the overproduction of ROS by phagocytic cells from smokers (Richards et al., 1990).

Reduced vitamin E status has also been reported in human immunodeficiency virus (HIV)-infected individuals. Passi et al. (1993) found that plasma vitamin E concentrations were significantly lower in a group of 200 HIV-positive individuals compared with controls, but whether this is related to an inadequate intake of this vitamin is unclear. Dietary diaries from a group of 100 HIV-infected asymptomatic men did not indicate an inadequate intake of vitamin E, but plasma levels were low or marginally low in 74% of the men (Beach et al., 1992). In a study of patients who had developed acquired immune deficiency syndrome (AIDS), an inverse relationship was observed between serum vitamin E levels and severity of disease (Favier et al., 1994). A recent study of 49 HIV-infected subjects provided with vitamin E and vitamin C observed a significant reduction in oxidative stress and a trend towards a reduction in viral load after 3 months (Allard et al., 1998). These studies suggest that larger trials of these and other antioxidant nutrients in the treatment of HIV-infected persons should be encouraged, since there is a need to find alternative, cheaper, treatments than the combination therapies currently employed.

In terms of mechanisms of action, in addition to its role as a protective antioxidant, vitamin E, at higher intakes, is associated with a reduced production of prostaglandin E$_2$ (PGE$_2$) (e.g. Meydani et al., 1986, 1988, 1990). Since PGE$_2$ inhibits lymphocyte proliferation and NK-cell activity, it is possible that this may be one immunomodulatory mechanism of vitamin E action. It is also possible that vitamin E and, indeed, other antioxidant nutrients can influence a variety of inflammatory processes by inhibiting the activity of a transcription factor called nuclear factor kappa B (NFκB). Transcription factors are intracellular regulators of gene expression. Once activated, the transcription factor binds to the promoter region of a specific gene within the DNA in the nucleus, resulting in that gene being 'turned on'. NFκB is required for maximal transcription of many proteins that are involved in inflammatory responses, including several cytokines, such as IL-1β, IL-2 and tumour necrosis factor (TNF)-α. NFκB is a redox-sensitive transcription factor and it is thought that the generation of ROS is a vital link in mediating NFκB activation by a variety of stimuli (Lavrovsky et al., 2000).

Carotenoids and immune function

The carotenoids are a group of over 600 naturally occurring coloured pigments that are widespread in plants, of which only about 20 commonly occur in human foodstuffs. In nature, they serve two essential functions: as accessory pigments in photosynthesis, and in photoprotection. These two functions are achieved through the chemical structure of carotenoids (Fig. 9.1), which allows the molecules to absorb light and to quench singlet oxygen and free radicals.

Many epidemiological studies have shown an association between diets rich in carotenoids and a reduced incidence of many forms of cancer, and it has been suggested that the antioxidant properties of these compounds are a causative factor (Block *et al.*, 1992). Since the publication of an article by Peto *et al.* (1981), a great deal of attention has focused on the potential role of one particular carotenoid, β-carotene, in preventing cancer. Numerous publications have described epidemiological studies, *in vitro* experiments, animal studies and clinical trials that suggest that this carotenoid can protect against not only cancer, but also other oxidative damage-associated disorders, listed in Table 9.1 (reviewed by Mayne, 1996). Because the immune system plays a major role in the prevention of cancer, it has been suggested that β-carotene may enhance immune cell function (Bendich and Olson, 1989). In animals, adding carotenoids to the diet prevented stress-related thymic involution, increased the number of circulating lymphocytes, enhanced lymphocyte proliferation and cytotoxic T-cell activity and increased resistance to infective pathogens (for references, see Roe and Fuller, 1993).

Several studies have examined the effect of β-carotene on human immune function. Various doses of β-carotene have been employed in these studies, ranging from 15 mg day^{-1}, which could be achieved through the diet, up to pharmacological doses of 180 mg day^{-1}, provided over periods of 14–365 days. These studies

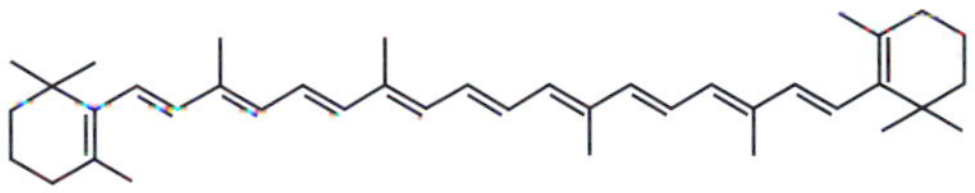

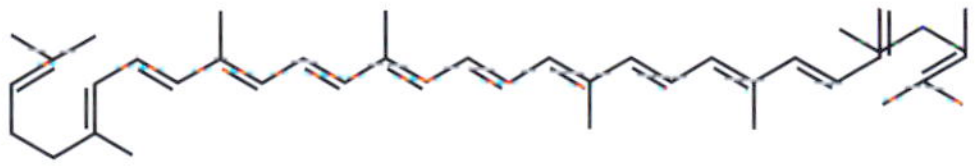

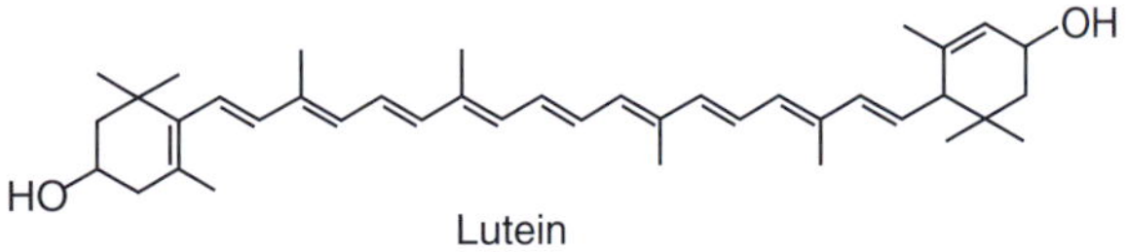

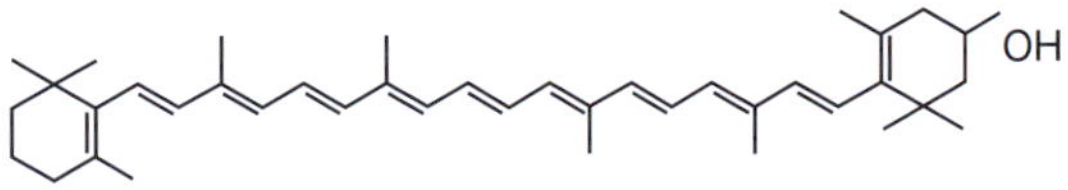

Fig. 9.1. Chemical structure of some carotenoids found in the diet.

have reported increases in the numbers of CD4+ cells or in the ratio of CD4+ to CD8+ cells in the circulation, in the percentages of lymphocytes expressing the IL-2 and transferrin receptors, and in NK-cell activity (Alexander *et al.*, 1985; Watson *et al.*, 1991; Murata *et al.*, 1994), particularly in elderly subjects. The potential for increasing the numbers of CD4+ cells led to the suggestion that β-carotene might be useful as an immunoenhancing agent in the treatment of HIV infection. Preliminary studies have shown a slight but insignificant increase in CD4+ numbers in response to β-carotene (60 mg day^{-1} for 4 weeks) in patients with AIDS (Fryburg *et al.*, 1995), but long-term effectiveness has not been reported.

Other investigators have been unable to confirm the increase in T-cell-mediated immunity in healthy individuals following β-carotene supplementation. Santos *et al.* (1996, 1997) reported the results of two studies in the elderly: a short-term, high-dose study (90 mg day^{-1} for 21 days) in women and a longer-term, lower-dose trial (50 mg alternate day^{-1} for 10–12 years) in men. Both studies concluded that there was no significant difference in T-cell function as assessed by DTH response, lymphocyte proliferation, IL-2 and PGE$_2$ production and composition of lymphocyte subsets (Santos *et al.*, 1997). However, these workers also examined the effect of β-carotene supplementation on NK-cell activity in the longer-term trial with male volunteers and observed that supplementation of the diet of older males (> 65 years) with β-carotene resulted in significantly greater NK-cell activity compared with subjects of a similar age given placebo treatment (Santos *et al.*, 1996). Since patients with Chediak–Higashi syndrome, a disorder associated with defective NK-cell function, show a higher susceptibility to tumour formation (Roder *et al.*, 1980), and homozygous mice genetically deficient in NK cell activity grow tumours and develop leukaemia more rapidly than do heterozygous littermates with normal NK-cell function (Lotzova, 1993), the enhancing effect of β-carotene on NK-cell activity has been postulated to be a link between raised intakes of this nutrient and cancer prevention. As shown in Fig. 9.2, the study by Santos *et al.* (1996) highlighted both the reduction in NK-cell activity that is observed with age and the fact that the increase in NK-cell activity observed in older males (65–86 years) following β-carotene supplementation restored it to the level seen in a group of younger males (51–64 years). The mechanism for this is unclear, but it was not due to an increase in the percentage of NK cells or to an increase in IL-2 production. The authors suggest that β-carotene may be acting directly on one or more of the lytic stages of NK-cell cytotoxicity or on NK-cell activity-enhancing cytokines other than IL-2, such as IL-12.

Individuals who are repeatedly exposed to UV light show suppression of immune function (Rivers *et al.*, 1989). Because carotenoids can provide photoprotection, several studies have assessed the ability of β-carotene to protect the immune system from UV-induced free radical damage. In one study, a group of young males were placed on a low-carotenoid diet (< 1.0 mg day^{-1} total carotenoids) and given either placebo or 30 mg β-carotene day^{-1} for 28 days prior to periodic exposure to UV light. DTH responses were significantly suppressed in the placebo group after UV treatments and the suppression was inversely proportional to plasma β-carotene concentrations in this group (Fuller *et al.*, 1992). In contrast, no significant suppression of DTH responses was seen in the β-carotene-treated group (Fuller *et al.*, 1992). The ability of β-carotene

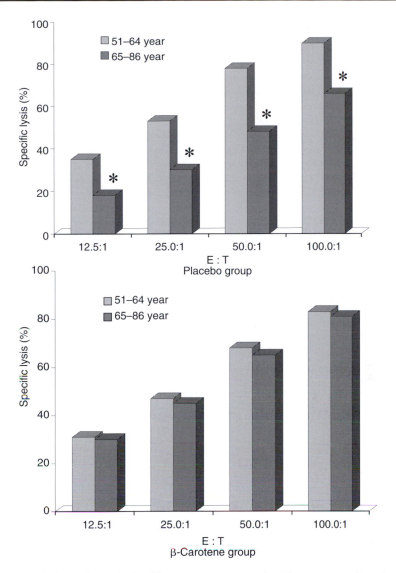

Fig. 9.2. Natural killer cell activity in different age-groups of subjects consuming placebo or β-carotene. Natural killer cell activity was determined at several effector-to-target cell ratios (E:T), using effector cells from subjects consuming placebo (*n* = 17 for 51–64 years and *n* = 13 for 65–86 years) or β-carotene (*n* = 21 for 51–64 years, and *n* =8 for 65–86 years). Data are expressed as % target-cell lysis. Reprinted from Santos *et al.* (1996) with permission by the *American Journal of Clinical Nutrition.* © American Journal of Clinical Nutrition, American Society for Clinical Nutrition.

to protect against the harmful effects of natural UV sunlight has also been demonstrated by exposing healthy female students to time- and intensity-controlled sunlight exposure: a Berlin-based study involved taking volunteers to the Red Sea and exposing areas of their skin to the sunlight by lifting discretely placed flaps in their specially designed swimsuits (Gollnick *et al.*, 1996)!

Since antigen-presenting cells initiate cell-mediated immune responses, one aspect of the immune-enhancing effect of β-carotene might be improved antigen-presenting cell function. A prerequisite for antigen presentation is the expression of major histocompatibility complex (MHC) class II molecules (human leucocyte antigen (HLA)-DR, HLA-DP and HLA-DQ) (Bach, 1985), which are present on the majority of human monocytes. The antigenic peptide is presented to the T-helper lymphocyte within a groove of the MHC class II molecule (Fig. 9.3). Since the degree of immune responsiveness of an individual has been shown to be proportional to both the percentage of MHC class II-positive monocytes and the density of these molecules on the cell surface (Janeway *et al.*, 1984), it is possible that one mechanism by which β-carotene may enhance cell-mediated immune responses is by enhancing the cell surface expression of these molecules. In addition, cell-to-cell adhesion is critical for the initiation of a primary immune response, and it has been shown that the intercellular adhesion molecule 1 (ICAM-1)–leucocyte function-associated antigen-1 (LFA-1) ligand–receptor pair is also capable of co-stimulating an immune response (Springer, 1990), enhancing T-cell proliferation and cytokine production.

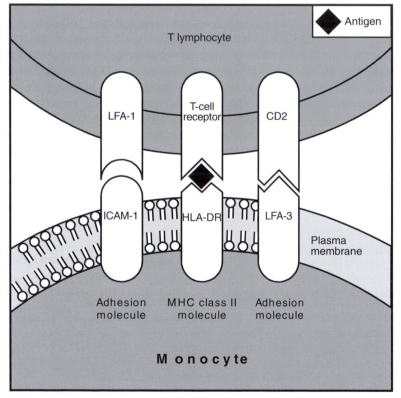

Fig. 9.3. Cell surface molecules involved in the initiation of cell-mediated immune responses. LFA, leucocyte function-associated antigen; ICAM-1, intercellular adhesion molecule 1; HLA, human leucocyte-associated antigen; MHC, major histocompatibility complex.

The effect of β-carotene supplementation (15 mg day^{-1} for 26 days; equivalent to 150 g carrots day^{-1}) on expression of MHC class II and adhesion molecules on the monocyte surface has been investigated. Following dietary supplementation, there were significant increases in plasma levels of β-carotene and in the percentages of monocytes expressing the MHC class II molecule HLA-DR and the adhesion molecules ICAM-1 and LFA-3 (Hughes *et al.*, 1997). These results suggest that moderate increases in the dietary intake of β-carotene can enhance cell-mediated immune responses within a relatively short period of time, providing a potential mechanism for the anti-carcinogenic properties attributed to this compound. The increase in surface molecule expression may also, in part, account for the ability of β-carotene to prevent the reduction in DTH response following exposure to UV radiation, since the latter can inhibit both HLA-DR and ICAM-1 expression. This finding could certainly be relevant to the preventive action of β-carotene towards skin cancer (Mathews-Roth, 1989), since immunosuppressed individuals, such as renal-transplant patients, have an increased risk of skin cancer.

As well as preventing oxidative damage, it has been suggested that β-carotene, like vitamin E, can influence immune cell function by modulating the production of PGE$_2$. This eicosanoid is the major prostaglandin (PG) synthesized by monocytes and macrophages and is known to possess a number of immunosuppressive properties (see Calder and Field, Chapter 4, this volume). It has been suggested that β-carotene might enhance immune responses by altering the activation of the arachidonic acid cascade (from which PGE$_2$ is derived), since it has been shown to be capable of suppressing the generation of arachidonic acid products *in vitro* from non-lymphoid tissues (Halevy and Sklan, 1987). This possibility requires further investigation.

There have been very few studies examining the influence of carotenoids other than β-carotene on human immune function, even though there is strong epidemiological evidence to suggest that lycopene (found in tomatoes) and lutein (found in peas, watercress and other vegetables) can protect against the development of prostate and lung cancer, respectively (Le Marchand *et al.*, 1993; Gann *et al.*, 1999). In addition, tomato intake has been found to be inversely associated with the risk of diarrhoeal and respiratory infections in young children in Sudan (Fawzi *et al.*, 2000). In terms of mechanisms of action, the effect of dietary supplementation with lycopene and lutein on the expression of monocyte surface molecules involved in antigen presentation has been investigated. It was found that these carotenoids appear to be less influential than β-carotene, when given at the same level in the diet (Hughes *et al.*, 2000). In addition, enriching the diet with lycopene (by drinking 330 ml of tomato juice daily) for 8 weeks did not modify cell-mediated immune responses in the elderly (Watzl *et al.*, 2000). In another study, performed in a group of older volunteers (over 65 years) living in Ireland, the effects of placebo, β-carotene (8.2 mg day^{-1}) and lycopene (13.3 mg day^{-1}) for 12 weeks on various parameters of cell-mediated immunity were examined. There were no significant changes in circulating T-cell subsets, mitogen-stimulated lymphocyte proliferation or surface molecule expression following any of these interventions, in spite of significant increases in the plasma levels of the carotenoids (Corridan *et al.*, 2001). The authors concluded that in well-nourished, free-living, healthy individuals, supplementation with relatively low levels of β-carotene or lycopene is not associated with either beneficial or detrimental effects on cell-mediated immunity.

Other investigators have shown an opposing effect of β-carotene and lutein upon human lymphocyte proliferation (Watzl *et al.*, 1999), emphasizing further the fact that different carotenoids might affect immune function in different ways. Therefore, in fruits and vegetables, the influence of the combination of carotenoids they contain on immune function may represent the sum total of these different effects and, indeed, the potential for synergistic effects remains to be investigated.

One possible factor to explain the different effects seen with different carotenoids might be the preferred location of these compounds within the cell and within the body. Carotenoids are lipid-soluble and thus it is thought that most will be concentrated in the lipid-rich membranes of the cell. However, their exact location may influence their effectiveness in modulating specific cellular events. Within the body, lycopene appears to be selectively taken up within the prostate, a finding that may help explain the association between higher intakes of lycopene and a reduced incidence of prostate cancer (Giovannucci, 1999). Thus, it is possible that tests on peripheral blood cells to determine immune function will not detect any localized effects, suggesting that there might be 'hidden' benefits associated with certain dietary components that we have yet to discover.

The strongest epidemiological evidence supporting a beneficial effect of carotenoids in preventing cancer is the protective effect of β-carotene intake in reducing the incidence of cancer of the lung. Carotenoid intake has been associated with a reduced lung-cancer risk in eight of eight prospective studies and in 18 of 20 retrospective studies (for a review, see Zeigler *et al.*, 1996). As a result, three major intervention trials were initiated, examining the efficacy of β-carotene in the prevention of lung cancer (Alpha-tocopherol Beta-carotene Cancer Prevention Study Group, 1994; Hennekens *et al.*, 1996; Omenn *et al.*, 1996). The failure of these trials to show a protective effect, with two of the studies showing an increase in lung cancer in smokers receiving β-carotene supplementation, has been widely publicized. The mechanism for the increased lung-cancer risk associated with the supplementation is unclear, but several suggestions have been made. Since the participants in these studies could be classified as 'high-risk' for developing lung cancer (long-term smokers or previously exposed to asbestos), it is possible that many of them had undetected tumours prior to the commencement of supplementation. The stage (or stages) of carcinogenesis that β-carotene might be effective against is unclear, but, if the effect is mediated via the immune system, it is likely to occur during the promotional stages preceding the formation of a malignant tumour. A recent analysis of the Cancer Prevention Study II (CPS-II), a prospective mortality study of more than 1 million US adults, investigated the effects of supplementation with multivitamins and/or vitamins A, C and/or E on mortality during a 7-year follow-up period. The use of a multivitamin plus vitamins A, C and/or E significantly reduced the risk of cancer in former smokers and in never-smokers, but increased the risk of lung cancer in male smokers who had used a multivitamin plus vitamins A, C and/or E, compared with men who had reported no vitamin supplement use. Interestingly, in this study, no association with smoking was seen in women (Watkins *et al.*, 2000).

One of the major unresolved dilemmas of research into β-carotene is what intake is required for optimal immune function and other health-related properties. Most studies of this compound have been undertaken at levels that are not achievable within a normal healthy diet. It is still unclear whether different intakes are associated with different outcomes or, in mechanistic studies, with different effects on various aspects of immune function. In addition, there remains the possibility that, at supra-dietary levels, β-carotene may exhibit pro-oxidant activity, particularly in the presence of high oxygen tensions, as occur in the lungs (reviewed by Palozza, 1998). Of course, the probability remains that the apparent protection of consuming a diet rich in fruits and vegetables is the result of a multifactorial effect of a number of components of these foods. In support of this, two of the prospective studies mentioned above found that higher plasma β-carotene concentrations upon entry into the trials, resulting from dietary consumption, as opposed to taking supplements, were associated with a lower risk of lung cancer (McDermott, 2000). Greater emphasis should be placed on studying the effects of enriching the diet with antioxidants via real foodstuffs rather than by supplementation.

Conclusions

Because the immune system is critically dependent on accurate cell–cell communication in order to mount a response, immune cell integrity is essential. Antioxidant nutrients help to maintain this integrity, reducing the damage caused by reactive oxygen species to cell membranes and their associated receptors, as well as modulating immune cell function by influencing the activity of redox-sensitive transcription factors and the production of cytokines and PGs. The effects of antioxidants appear to be particularly beneficial during periods of oxidative stress, whether the periods are acute, such as during infections, or chronic, such as in the elderly. However, the results of the prospective studies with β-carotene in smokers show that caution must still be taken in making recommendations regarding the taking of supplements that provide a greater intake than can be achieved by eating a diet rich in fruits and vegetables. In this regard, it is important to remember that the strongest evidence supporting a beneficial effect of antioxidant nutrients in reducing the risk of developing chronic oxidative stress-related disorders has come from epidemiological studies of populations consuming whole foods and not from supplementation studies. Further research needs to be undertaken to examine the interaction between different antioxidant nutrients and to establish the levels of intake required to optimize immune responsiveness in different sectors of the population (e.g. the elderly, cigarette smokers). In addition, greater emphasis should be placed on studying the effects of enriching the diet with antioxidants via real foodstuffs rather than by supplementation, since these foods undoubtedly contain beneficial compounds that we have still to discover.

Acknowledgement

The author would like to thank the Biotechnology and Biological Sciences Research Council for financial support.

References

Alexander, M., Newmark, H. and Miller, R.G. (1985) Oral beta carotene can increase the number of OKT4+ cells in human blood. *Immunology Letters* 9, 221–224.

Allard, J.P., Aghdassi, E., Chau, J., Tam, C., Kovacs, C.M., Salit, I.E. and Walmsley, S.L. (1998) Effects of vitamin E and C supplementation on oxidative stress and viral load in HIV-infected subjects. *AIDS* 12, 1653–1659.

Alpha-tocopherol Beta-carotene Cancer Prevention Study Group (1994) The effect of vitamin E and beta-carotene on the incidence of lung cancer and other cancers in male smokers. *New England Journal of Medicine* 330, 1029–1035.

Anderson, R. (1982) Effects of ascorbate on normal and abnormal leucocyte functions. *International Journal of Vitaminology and Nutrition Research* 23 (Suppl.), 23–34.

Anderson, R., Oosthuizen, R., Maritz, R., Theron, A. and Van Rensburg, A.J. (1980) The effect of increasing weekly doses of ascorbate on certain cellular and humoral immune functions in normal volunteers. *American Journal of Clinical Nutrition* 33, 71–76.

Anderson, R., Smit, M.J., Joone, G.K. and Van Straden, A.M. (1990) Vitamin C and cellular immune functions: protection against hypochlorous acid-mediated inactivation of glyceraldehyde-3-phosphate dehydrogenase and ATP generation in human leucocytes as a possible mechanism of ascorbate-mediated immunostimulation. *Annals of the New York Academy of Science* 587, 34–48.

Bach, F.H. (1985) Class II genes and products of the HLA-D region. *Immunology Today* 6, 89–94.

Baehner, R.L., Boxer, L.A., Allan, J.M. and Davis, J. (1977) Auto-oxidation as a basis for altered function of polymorphonuclear leucocytes. *Blood* 50, 327–335.

Baker, K.R. and Meydani, M. (1994) Beta-carotene in immunity and cancer. *Journal of Optimal Nutrition* 3, 39–50.

Beach, R.S., Mantero-Atienza, E., Shor-Posner, G., Javier, J.J., Szapocznik, J., Morgan, R., Sauberlich, H.E., Cornwell, P.E., Eisdorfer, C. and Baum, M.K. (1992) Specific nutrient abnormalities in asymptomatic HIV-1 infection. *AIDS* 6, 701–708.

Bendich, A. and Olson, J.A. (1989) Biological actions of carotenoids. *FASEB Journal* 3, 1927–1932.

Bendich, A., Machlin, L.J., Scandurra, O., Burton, G.W. and Wayner, D.D.M. (1986) The antioxidant role of vitamin C. *Free Radicals in Biology and Medicine* 2, 419–444.

Block, G., Patterson, B. and Subar, A. (1992) Fruit, vegetables, and cancer prevention: a review of the epidemiological evidence. *Nutrition and Cancer* 18, 1–29.

Boxer, L.A. (1986) Regulation of phagocyte function by alpha-tocopherol. *Proceedings of the Nutrition Society* 45, 333–334.

Boxer, L.A., Watanabe, A.M., Rister, M. and Besch, H.R. (1976) Correction of leucocyte function in Chediak–Higashi syndrome by ascorbate. *New England Journal of Medicine* 295, 1041–1045.

Cannon, J.G., Meydani, S.N., Fielding, R.A., Fiatarone, M.A., Meydani, M., Farhangmehr, M., Orencole, S.F., Blumberg, J.B. and Evans, W.J. (1991) Acute phase response in exercise. II. Associations between vitamin E, cytokines, and muscle proteolysis. *American Journal of Physiology* 260, R1235–R1240.

Chavance, M., Herbeth, B., Fournier, C., Janot, C. and Vernhes, G. (1989) Vitamin status, immunity and infections in an elderly population. *European Journal of Clinical Nutrition* 43, 827–835.

Chirico, G., Marconi, M., Colombo, A., Chiara, A., Rondini, G. and Ugazio, A. (1983) Deficiency of neutrophil phagocytosis in premature infants: influence of vitamin E supplementation. *Acta Paediatrica Scandinavica* 75, 521–524.

Corridan, B.M., O'Donoghue, M., Hughes, D.A. and Morrissey, P.A. (2001) Low-dose supplementation with lycopene or beta-carotene does not enhance cell-mediated immunity in healthy free-living elderly humans. *European Journal of Clinical Nutrition* 55, 627–635.

Coulehan, J.L., Reisinger, K.S., Rogers, K.D. and Bradley, D.W. (1974) Vitamin C prophylaxis in a boarding school. *New England Journal of Medicine* 290, 6–10.

Department of Health (1991) *Report of the Panel on Dietary Reference Values of the Committee of Medical Aspects of Food Policy: Dietary Reference Values for Food Energy and Nutrients for the United Kingdom*. HMSO, London.

Favier, A., Sappey, C., Leclerc, P., Faure, P. and Micoud, M. (1994) Antioxidant status and lipid peroxidation in patients infected with HIV. *Chemico-Biological Interactions* 91, 165–180.

Fawzi, W., Herrera, M.G. and Nestel, P. (2000) Tomato intake in relation to mortality and morbidity among Sudanese children. *Journal of Nutrition* 130, 2537–2542.

Fryburg, D.A., Mark, R.J., Griffith, B.P., Askenase, P.W. and Patterson, T.F. (1995) The effect of supplemental beta-carotene on immunological indices in patients with AIDS: a pilot study. *Yale Journal of Biology and Medicine* 68, 19–23.

Fuller, C.J., Faulkner, H., Bendich, A., Parker, R.S. and Roe, D.A. (1992) Effect of beta-carotene supplementation on photosuppression of delayed-type hypersensitivity in normal young men. *American Journal of Clinical Nutrition* 56, 684–690.

Gann, P.H., Ma, J., Giovannucci, E., Willett, W., Sacks, F.M., Hennekens, C.H. and Stampfer, M.J. (1999) Lower prostate cancer risk in men with elevated plasma lycopene levels: results of a prospective analysis. *Cancer Research* 59, 1225–1230.

Giovannucci, E. (1999) Tomatoes, tomato-based products, lycopene, and cancer: review of the epidemiologic literature. *Journal of the National Cancer Institute* 91, 317–331.

Gollnick, P.M., Hopfenmuller, W., Hemmes, C., Chun, S.C., Schmid, C., Sundermeier, K. and Biesalski, H.K. (1996) Systemic beta-carotene plus topical UV-sunscreen are an optimal protection against harmful effects of natural UV-sunlight: results of the Berlin–Eilath study. *European Journal of Dermatology* 6, 200–205.

Gruner, S., Volk, H.D., Falck, P. and Baehr, R.V. (1986) The influence of phagocytic stimuli on the expression of HLA-DR antigens; role of reactive oxygen intermediates. *European Journal of Immunology* 16, 212–215.

Halevy, O. and Sklan, D. (1987) Inhibition of arachidonic acid oxidation by beta-carotene, retinol and alpha-tocopherol. *Biochimica et Biophysica Acta* 918, 304–307.

Halliwell, B. and Aruoma, O.I. (1991) DNA damage by oxygen-derived species: its mechanisms and measurement in mammalian systems. *FEBS Letters* 281, 9–19.

Han, S.N. and Meydani, S.N. (1999) Vitamin E and infectious disease in the aged. *Proceedings of the Nutrition Society* 58, 698–705.

Han, S.N. and Meydani, S.N. (2000) Antioxidants, cytokines, and influenza infection in aged mice and elderly humans. *Journal of Infectious Diseases* 182, S74–S80.

Han, S.N., Wu, D., Ha, W.K., Smith, D.E., Beharka, A., Wang, H., Bender, B.S. and Meydani, S.N. (1998) Vitamin E supplementation increases splenocyte IL-2 and IFN-γ production of old mice infected with influenza virus. *FASEB Journal* 12, A819.

Hayek, M.G., Taylor, S.F., Bender, B.S., Han, S.N., Meydani, M., Smith, D.E., Eghtesada, S. and Meydani, S.N. (1997) Vitamin E supplementation decreases lung virus titers in mice infected with influenza. *Journal of Infectious Diseases* 176, 273–276.

Hennekens, C.H., Buring, J.E., Manson, J.E. and Stampfer, M. (1996) Lack of effect of long term supplementation with beta carotene on the incidence of malignant neoplasms and cardiovascular disease. *New England Journal of Medicine* 334, 1145–1149.

Hughes, D.A., Wright, A.J.A., Finglas, P.M., Peerless, A.C.J., Bailey, A.L., Astley, S.B., Pinder, A.C. and Southon, S. (1997) The effect of beta-carotene supplementation on the immune function of blood monocytes from healthy male non-smokers. *Journal of Laboratory and Clinical Medicine* 129, 309–317.

Hughes, D.A., Wright, A.J.A., Finglas, P.M., Polley, A.C.J., Bailey, A.L., Astley, S.B. and Southon, S. (2000) Effects of lycopene and lutein supplementation on the expression of functionally associated surface molecules on blood monocytes from healthy male non-smokers. *Journal of Infectious Diseases* 182, S11–S15.

Jacob, R.A., Kelley, D.S., Pianalto, F.S., Swendsein, M.E., Henning, S.M., Zhang, J.Z., Ames, B.N., Fraga, C.G. and Peters, J.H. (1991) Immunocompetence and oxidant defense during ascorbate depletion of healthy men. *American Journal of Clinical Nutrition* 54, 1302S–1309S.

Jacques, P.F., Taylor, A., Hankinson, S.E., Willett, W.C., Mahnken, B., Lee, Y., Vaid, K. and Lahav, M. (1997) Long-term vitamin C supplement use and prevalence of early age-related lens opacities. *American Journal of Clinical Nutrition* 66, 911–916.

Janeway, C.A., Bottomly, K., Babich, J., Conrad, P., Conzen, S., Jones, B., Kaye, J., Katz, M., McVay, L., Murphy, D.B. and Tite, J. (1984) Quantitative variation in Ia antigen expression plays a central role in immune regulation. *Immunology Today* 5, 99–104.

Johnson, J.D., Houchens, D.P., Kluwe, W.M., Craig, D.K. and Fisher, G.L. (1990) Effects of mainstream and environmental tobacco smoke on the immune system in animals and humans: a review. *CRC Critical Reviews in Toxicology* 134, 356–361.

Kay, N.E., Holloway, D.E., Hutton, S.W., Bona, N.D. and Duane, W.C. (1982) Human T-cell function in experimental ascorbic acid deficiency and spontaneous scurvy. *American Journal of Clinical Nutrition* 36, 127–130.

Kennes, B., Dumont, I., Brokee, D., Hubert, C. and Neve, P. (1983) Effect of vitamin C supplements on cell-mediated immunity in old people. *Gerontology* 29, 305–310.

Lavrovsky, Y., Chatterjee, B., Clark, R.A. and Roy, A.K. (2000) Role of redox-regulated transcription factors in inflammation, ageing and age-related diseases. *Experimental Gerontology* 35, 521–532.

Le Marchand, L., Hankin, J.H., Kolonel, L.N., Beecher, G.R., Wilkens, L.R. and Zhao, L.P. (1993) Intake of specific carotenoids and lung cancer risk. *Cancer Epidemiology Biomarkers and Prevention* 2, 183–187.

Lotzova, E. (1993) Immune surveillance and natural immunity. In: Cooper, E.L. and Nisbet-Brown, E. (eds) *Developmental Immunity*. Oxford University Press, New York, pp. 401–425.

McDermott, J.H. (2000) Antioxidant nutrients: current dietary recommendations and research update. *Journal of the American Pharmaceutical Association* 40, 785–799.

Mangels, A.R., Holden, J.M., Beecher, G.R., Forman, M.R. and Lanza, E. (1993) Carotenoid content of fruits and vegetables: an evaluation of analytical data. *Journal of the American Dietetic Association* 93, 284–296.

Mathews-Roth, M.M. (1989) Beta-carotene: clinical aspects. In: Spiller, G.A. and Scala, J. (eds) *New Protective Roles for Selected Nutrients*. Alan R. Liss, New York, pp. 17–38.

Mayne, S.M. (1996) Beta-carotene, carotenoids, and disease prevention in humans. *FASEB Journal* 10, 690–701.

Meydani, S.N. and Beharka, A.A. (1998) Recent developments in vitamin E and immune response. *Nutrition Reviews* 56, S49–S58.

Meydani, S.N., Meydani, M., Verdon, C.P., Shapiro, A.A., Blumberg, J.B. and Hayes, K.C. (1986) Vitamin E supplementation suppresses prostaglandin E_2 synthesis and enhances the immune response of aged mice. *Mechanisms of Aging and Development* 34, 191–201.

Meydani, S.N., Yogeeswaran, G., Liu, S., Baskar, S. and Meydani, M. (1988) Fish oil and tocopherol-induced changes in natural killer cell-mediated cytotoxicity and PGE_2 synthesis in young and old mice. *Journal of Nutrition* 118, 1245–1252.

Meydani, S.N., Barklund, M.P., Liu S., Meydani, M., Miller, R.A., Cannon, J.G., Morrow, F.D., Rocklin, R. and Blumberg, J.B. (1990) Vitamin E supplementation enhances cell-mediated immunity in healthy elderly subjects. *American Journal of Clinical Nutrition* 52, 557–563.

Meydani, S.N., Meydani, M., Blumberg, J.B., Leka, L.S., Siber, G., Loszewski, R., Thompson, C., Pedrosa, M.C., Diamond, R.D. and Stollar, B.D. (1997) Vitamin E supplementation and *in vivo* immune response in healthy elderly subjects: a randomized controlled trial. *Journal of the American Medical Association* 277, 1380–1386.

Murata, T., Tamai, H., Morinobu, T., Manago, M., Takenaka, H., Hayashi, K. and Mino, M. (1994) Effect of long-term administration of beta-carotene on lymphocyte subsets in humans. *American Journal of Clinical Nutrition* 60, 597–602.

Omenn, G.S., Goodman, G.E. and Thornquist, M.D. (1996) Effects of a combination of beta carotene and vitamin A on lung cancer and cardiovascular disease. *New England Journal of Medicine* 334, 1150–1155.

Pacht, E.R., Kasek, H., Mohammad, J.R., Cromwell, D.G. and Davis, W.B. (1986) Deficiency of vitamin E in the alveolar fluid of cigarette smokers: influence on alveolar macrophage cytotoxicity. *Journal of Clinical Investigation* 77, 789–796.

Palozza, P. (1998) Prooxidant actions of carotenoids in biological systems. *Nutrition Reviews* 56, 257–265.

Panush, R.E.S., Delafuente, J.C., Katz, P. and Johnson, J. (1982) Modulation of certain immunologic responses by vitamin C. III Potentiation of *in vitro* and *in vivo* lymphocyte responses. *International Journal of Vitaminology and Nutrition Research* 23, 35–47.

Passi, S., Picardo, M. and Morrone, A. (1993) Study on plasma polyunsaturated phospholipids and vitamin E, and on erythrocyte glutathione peroxidase in high risk HIV infection categories and AIDS patients. *Clinical Chemistry Enzymology Communications* 5, 169–177.

Pauling, L. (1970) *Vitamin C and the Common Cold*. W.H. Freeman, San Francisco.

Peters, E.M. (1997) Exercise, immunology and upper respiratory tract infections. *International Journal of Sports Medicine* 18(Suppl. 1), S69–S77.

Peto, R., Doll, R., Buckley, J.D. and Sporn, M.B. (1981) Can dietary beta-carotene materially reduce human cancer rates? *Nature* 290, 201–208.

Prinz, W., Bortz, R., Bregin, B. and Hersch, M. (1977) The effect of ascorbic acid supplementation on some parameters of the human immunological defense system. *International Journal of Vitaminology and Nutrition Research* 47, 248–257.

Pryor, W.A. and Stone, K. (1993) Oxidants in cigarette smoke. *Annals of the New York Academy of Science* 686, 12–28.

Rice-Evans, C. (1995) Plant polyphenols: free radical scavengers or chain-breaking antioxidants? *Biochemical Society Symposia* 61, 103–116.

Richards, G.A., Theron, A.J., Van Rensburg, C.E.J., Van Rensberg, A.J., Van Der Merwe, C.A., Kuyl, J.M. and Anderson, R. (1990) Investigation of the effects of oral administration of vitamin E and beta-carotene on the chemiluminescence responses and the frequency of sister chromatid exchanges in circulating leucocytes from cigarette smokers. *American Review of Respiratory Disease* 142, 648–654.

Rivers, J.K., Norris, P.G., Murphy, G.M., Chu, A.C., Midgley, G., Morris, J., Morris, R.W., Young, A.R. and Hawk, J.L. (1989) UVA sunbeds: tanning, photoprotection, acute adverse effects and immunological changes. *British Journal of Dermatology* 120, 767–777.

Roder, J.C., Haliotis, T., Klein, M., Korec, S., Jett, J.R., Ortaldo, J., Heberman, R.B., Katz, P. and Fauci, A.S. (1980) A new immunodeficiency disorder in humans involving NK cells. *Nature* 284, 553–555.

Roe, D.A. and Fuller, C.J. (1993) Carotenoids and immune function. In: Klurfeld, D.M. (ed.) *Nutrition and Immunology*. Plenum Press, New York, pp. 229–238.

Santos, M.S., Meydani, S.N., Leka, L., Wu, D., Fotouhi, N., Meydani, M., Hennekens, C.H. and Gaziano, J.M. (1996) Natural killer cell activity in elderly men is enhanced by beta-carotene supplementation. *American Journal of Clinical Nutrition* 64, 772–777.

Santos, M.S., Leka, L.S., Ribaya-Mercado, J.D., Russell, R.M., Meydani, M., Hennekens, C.H., Gaziano, J.M. and Meydani, S.N. (1997) Short- and long-term beta-carotene supplementation do not influence T-cell-mediated immunity in healthy elderly persons. *American Journal of Clinical Nutrition* 66, 917–924.

Siegel, B.V. (1993) Vitamin C and the immune response in health and disease. In: Klurfeld, D.M. (ed.) *Nutrition and Immunology*. Plenum Press, New York, pp. 167–196.

Springer, T.A. (1990) Adhesion receptors of the immune system. *Nature* 346, 425–434.

Thomas, W.R. and Holt, P.G. (1978) Vitamin C and immunity: an assessment of the evidence. *Clinical and Experimental Immunology* 32, 370–379.

Vallance, S. (1977) Relationship between ascorbic acid and serum proteins of the immune system. *British Medical Journal* 2, 437–438.

Vobecky, J.S., Vobecky, J., Shapcott, D. and Rola-Pleszczynski, M. (1984) Nutritional influences on humoral and cell-mediated immunity in healthy infants. *Journal of the American College of Nutrition* 3, 265.

Wang, Y., Huang, D.S., Eskelson, C.D. and Watson, R.R. (1984) Long-term dietary vitamin E retards development of retrovirus-induced dysregulation in cytokine production. *Clinical Immunology and Immunopathology* 72, 70–75.

Watkins, M.L., Erickson, J.D., Thun, M.J., Mulinare, J. and Heath, C.W., Jr (2000) Multivitamin use and mortality in a large prospective study. *American Journal of Epidemiology* 152, 149–162.

Watson, R.R., Prabhala, R.H., Plezia, P.M. and Alberts, D.S. (1991) Effect of beta-carotene on lymphocyte subpopulations in elderly humans: evidence for a dose–response relationship. *American Journal of Clinical Nutrition* 53, 90–94.

Watzl, B., Bub, A. and Rechkemmer, G. (1999) Modulation of T-lymphocyte functions by the consumption of carotenoid-rich vegetables. *British Journal of Nutrition* 82, 383–389.

Watzl, B., Bub, A., Blockhaus, M., Herbert, B.M., Luhrmann, P.M., Neuhauser-Berthold, M. and Rechkemmer, G. (2000) Prolonged tomato juice consumption has no effect on cell-mediated immunity of well-nourished elderly men and women. *Journal of Nutrition* 130, 1719–1723.

Yonemoto, R.H., Chretien, P.B. and Fehniger, T.F. (1976) Enhanced lymphocyte blastogenesis by oral ascorbic acid. *American Society of Clinical Oncology* 17, 288.

Zeigler, R.G., Mayne, S.T. and Swanson, C.A. (1996) Nutrition and lung cancer. *Cancer Causes and Controls* 7, 157–177.

Ziemlanski, S., Wartanowicz, M., Kios, A., Raczka, A. and Kios, M. (1986) The effects of ascorbic acid and alpha-tocopherol supplementation on serum proteins and immunoglobulin concentrations in the elderly. *Nutrition International* 2, 1–5.

10 Zinc, Infection and Immune Function

ANANDA S. PRASAD

Division of Hematology and Oncology, Department of Internal Medicine, Wayne State University School of Medicine, 4201 St Antoine, Detroit, MI 48201, USA

Introduction

Animal studies in the 1930s first documented the essential requirement of zinc (Zn) for the growth and survival of animals (Todd *et al.*, 1934). It was not until the 1960s that the importance of Zn deficiency for human populations was appreciated (see Prasad, 1991). Later, it became clear that Zn was also crucial for patients maintained on parenteral nutrition (Kay and Tasman-Jones, 1975). A central clinical feature of Zn deficiency in humans was the increased susceptibility to infectious diseases. Studies in the Middle East revealed that most Zn-deficient dwarfs succumbed to infections before they reached 25 years of age, leading researchers to speculate that Zn must be important for host immunity. The last two decades have witnessed a rapid growth in knowledge of the underlying mechanisms whereby Zn exerts its ubiquitous effects on immune function and disease resistance. The effects of Zn deficiency and of Zn supplementation on immune cells underscore the essential role of Zn in the normal development and function of many key tissues, cells and effectors of immunity. *In vitro* studies have elucidated the role of Zn at the cellular level and recent advances in molecular and cell biology have begun to clarify the role of Zn in gene expression, mitosis and apoptosis of lymphoid cells. It is clear that even mild Zn deficiency can impair multiple mediators of host immunity, ranging from the physical barrier of the skin to acquired cellular and humoral immunity (see Frost *et al.*, 1977; Oleske *et al.*, 1979; Good, 1981; Walsh *et al.*, 1994).

Zinc Deficiency

Most studies indicate that, among healthy adults consuming Western-style diets, Zn intake is in the range 8–12 mg day^{-1}; mean Zn intakes among adults in the UK are 11.4 mg day^{-1} for men and 8.4 mg day^{-1} for women (Department of

Health, 1991). The estimated average requirement for adults in the UK is about 7 (men) and 5.5 (women) mg day^{-1} (Department of Health, 1991). In persons suffering from marginal Zn deficiency (intake less than 5 mg day^{-1}), clinical signs consist of depressed immunity, impaired taste and smell, onset of night-blindness, impairment of memory and decreased spermatogenesis in males (Prasad *et al.*, 1961; Sandstead *et al.*, 2000). Severe Zn deficiency is character-ized by severely depressed immune function, frequent infections, bullous pustu-lar dermatitis, diarrhoea, alopecia and mental disturbances (Barnes and Moynahan, 1973). Similar effects of mild and severe Zn deficiency arise in Zn-deficient laboratory animals (see Shankar and Prasad, 1998). A rare genetic disorder, known as acrodermatitis enteropathica (AE), occurs in cattle and humans, resulting in decreased Zn absorption, accompanied by characteristic hyperpigmented skin lesions, poor growth and low plasma Zn levels (Walsh *et al.*, 1994). It is estimated that nutritional Zn deficiency may affect approxi-mately 2000 million people in the developing world.

The Cell Biology of Zinc with Relevance to the Immune System

Zinc and the cell cycle

Treatment of lymphocytes with mitogens results in a fairly rapid increase in cellu-lar Zn (see Zalewski, 1996; Shankar and Prasad, 1998; Prasad, 2000a). These findings are consistent with studies indicating a requirement for Zn during the mid to late G1 phase of the cell cycle in promotion of thymidine kinase expres-sion (Chesters *et al.*, 1993) and in another less well-defined step involved in cell transition to S phase. Activated lymphocytes take up Zn via multiple mecha-nisms, including receptors for Zn-transferrin, metallothionein, albumin and α_2-macroglobulin (see Walsh *et al.*, 1994; Shankar and Prasad, 1998; Prasad, 2000a) and also by other less well-characterized mechanisms, such as anionic channels or transporters. The Zn-dependent activity of DNA polymerase may account, in part, for the influence of Zn during the S phase of the cell cycle. Zn may also play a role in transition to the G2 and M phases. A greater proportion of S- compared with G2-phase cells was observed among mitogen-stimulated lymphocytes from mildly Zn-deficient patients suffering from sickle-cell anaemia (Prasad, 2000a). The ratio returned to normal following a period of Zn supple-mentation. The M phase of the cell cycle may also be affected by Zn deficiency, since defective tubulin polymerization is seen in tissues from Zn-deficient ani-mals (see Shankar and Prasad, 1998), and Zn is known to bind the N-terminal of tubulin, thereby stabilizing microtubule formation.

Zinc and cell replication

Zn influences the activity of multiple enzymes, which act at the very basic levels of replication and transcription. These include DNA polymerase, thymidine kinase, DNA-dependent RNA polymerase, terminal deoxyribonucleotidyl transferase and aminoacyl tRNA synthetase (Walsh *et al.*, 1994; Zalewski, 1996; Shankar and Prasad, 1998), and the family of transcriptional regulators known as Zn-finger DNA-binding proteins. In addition, Zn forms the active enzymatic sites of many metalloproteases. The activity of the major enzyme regulating DNA replication, DNA polymerase, is Zn-dependent. It is inhibited by Zn deficiency and Zn chelators and is enhanced by addition of low concentrations of Zn *in vitro*. Thymidine kinase, crucial for the synthesis of phosphorylated pyrimidines, is also very sensitive to dietary Zn depletion. Zn is, in fact, required for expression of multiple genes regulating mitosis, including thymidine kinase, ornithine decarboxylase and *c-myc*. Several transcription factors, such as nuclear factor kappa B (NFκB), metallothionein transcription factor 1 (MTF-1) and really interesting new gene (RING), contain Zn-finger-like domains, which may be influenced by changes in intracellular pools of Zn. In addition, Zn deprivation affects the activity of RNA polymerase, needed for transcription.

Zinc and lymphocyte activation

Zn plays a role in multiple aspects of T lymphocyte activation and signal transduction. Zn has been implicated in the non-covalent interaction of the cytoplasmic tails of CD4 and CD8 with the tyrosine kinase p56^{lck}, an essential protein in the early steps of T-cell activation (Turner *et al.*, 1990). Through this and possibly other pathways, Zn stimulates autophosphorylation of tyrosine residues by p56^{lck} and subsequent phosphorylation of the T-cell-receptor complex involving CD45. Zn is also involved in the activity of phospholipase C to give rise to inositol trisphosphate and diacylglycerol (see Zalewski, 1996). In addition, Zn affects the phosphorylation of proteins mediated by protein kinase C. Subsequent changes through protein phosphorylation regulate activation and cell proliferation.

Zinc and apoptosis

The major mechanism of cell death in the body and in cell culture is apoptosis, a form of cell suicide characterized by a decrease in cell volume, dramatic condensation of the chromatin and cytoplasm and fragmentation of nuclear DNA. Apoptosis is a normal physiological process, enabling a variety of important processes, from epithelial turnover to T- and B-cell development. The dysregulation of such a basic process would, therefore, have important health consequences.

Zn-deficient animals exhibit enhanced spontaneous and toxin-induced apoptosis in multiple cell types (see Zalewski and Forbes, 1993; Shankar and Prasad, 1998). Thymic atrophy is a central feature of Zn deficiency (see later). It is now known that this atrophy is accompanied by apoptotic cell death of thymocytes. Several studies have demonstrated that Zn is a regulator of lymphocyte apoptosis *in vivo* and *in vitro* (see Zalewski and Forbes, 1993; Shankar and Prasad, 1998; Prasad, 2000a). Zn supplementation decreased mycotoxin-induced apoptosis of macrophages and T-cells in mice. In addition, Zn administration to mice 48 h prior to intraperitoneal injection of endotoxin (lipopolysaccharide (LPS)) greatly abrogated subsequent apoptotic DNA cleavage in thymocytes and loss in thymic weight. *In vitro*, greater numbers of lymphocytes and thymocytes undergo apoptosis when cultured with Zn-free medium or with Zn chelators. Conversely, apoptosis of T lymphocytes induced by *in vitro* exposure to toxins and other agents is prevented by the addition of high concentrations of Zn salts. Cells could also be rescued from apoptosis with physiological levels (5–25 μM) of Zn salts if uptake was facilitated by the Zn ionophore pyrithione. It has been suggested that Zn is a major intracellular regulator of apoptosis, since lymphocytes maintain intracellular Zn at levels slightly above those needed to suppress apoptosis. In addition, a dose–response relationship exists between intracellular Zn levels and the degree of susceptibility to apoptosis.

The mechanisms whereby Zn affects apoptosis are not well understood, but it is likely that Zn acts at multiple levels. There is a good correlation between inhibition of Ca^{2+}/Mg^{2+} DNA endonuclease activity and inhibition of apoptotic DNA fragmentation (see Shankar and Prasad, 1998). Although *in vivo* data are lacking, the Ca/Zn balance may regulate endonuclease activity. Nucleoside phosphorylase, another Zn-dependent enzyme, may inhibit apoptosis by preventing the accumulation of toxic nucleotides (Prasad, 1993). Likewise, poly (ADP-ribose) polymerase, the Zn-dependent nuclear enzyme, interacts with and inhibits the Ca^{2+}/Mg^{2+} DNA endonuclease. In lymphocytes undergoing apoptosis, there is a large increase in cytoplasmic Zn, possibly originating from release of Zn from nuclear proteins.

The Role of Zinc in Antioxidant Defence

Zn plays a role in antioxidant defence, protecting cells from the damaging effects of oxygen radicals, which are generated during immune activation. Zn is a component of the cytosolic superoxide dismutase enzyme. Zn also regulates the expression of metallothionein and metallothionein-like proteins in lymphocytes, which have antioxidant activity (Prasad, 1993). Membrane Zn levels are strongly influenced by dietary Zn levels, and Zn concentrations in cell membranes appear to be important in preserving their integrity through poorly defined mechanisms involving binding to thiolate groups. Zn release from thiolate bonds can prevent lipid peroxidation. In addition, nitric oxide induces Zn release from metallothionein, the primary Zn-binding and transport protein in the body, which may limit free-radical membrane damage during inflammation. Indeed, Zn supplementation could prevent pulmonary pathology due to hyperoxia in rats (Taylor and Bray, 1991).

Thymulin

Thymulin is a nine-peptide hormone (Glu–Ala–Lys–Ser–Gln–Gly–Gly–Ser–Asn) secreted by thymic epithelial cells. Zn is bound to thymulin in a 1:1 stoichiometry via the side-chain of asparagine and the hydroxyl groups of the two serines. The binding of Zn results in a conformational change, which produces the active form of thymulin. Thymulin binds to high-affinity receptors on T-cells and promotes T-cell maturation, cytotoxicity and interleukin (IL)-2 production (see Shankar and Prasad, 1998). Thymulin activity *in vitro* and *in vivo* in both animals and humans is dependent on plasma Zn levels, such that marginal changes in Zn intake or availability affect thymulin activity (Prasad *et al.*, 1988; Shankar and Prasad, 1998). Thymulin is readily detectable in the serum of Zn-deficient patients, but is not active. The overall role of thymulin in the immuno-logical lesions caused by Zn deficiency has not been well studied. The use of thymulin as an indicator of Zn deficiency has been suggested, although thymulin concentration is also modulated by Zn-independent factors. Assays regarding Zn status and thymulin Zn saturation may prove more useful, much as the index of transferrin saturation provides useful information regarding iron status.

Zinc and Immune Function

Effects of fetal zinc deficiency on immunological development

Gestational Zn deficiency in mice and non-human primates has short- and long-term deleterious effects on the offspring. Substantial reductions are seen in lymphoid organ size and circulating immunoglobulin (Ig) levels in pups born to marginally Zn-deficient mice (Beach *et al.*, 1982). Additional murine studies showed that many of the immunodeficiencies seen at birth persisted into adult-hood, despite the pups having been raised on a normal Zn diet after weaning (Beach *et al.*, 1983). Indirect evidence for such effects in humans is also avail-able. Intrauterine growth retardation, which has been linked to maternal Zn deficiency (Dutz *et al.*, 1976), results in depressed cell-mediated immunity, which can persist for years (Dutz *et al.*, 1976; Ferguson, 1978).

Effects of zinc deficiency on barrier function

Zn deficiency damages epidermal cells, resulting in the characteristic skin lesions of AE or severe Zn deficiency (see Shankar and Prasad, 1998). Damage to the linings of the gastrointestinal and pulmonary tracts is also observed dur-ing Zn deficiency (see Shankar and Prasad, 1998).

Effects of zinc on immune-cell numbers

Lymphopenia is common in Zn-deficient humans and animals and occurs in both the central and peripheral lymphoid tissues (Walsh *et al.*, 1994). B-cell development in the bone marrow is adversely affected by Zn-deficiency (see Walsh *et al.*, 1994; Shankar and Prasad, 1998). When mice were fed a margin-ally Zn deficient diet for 30 days, the number of nucleated bone-marrow cells was reduced by one-third, with a preferential reduction in small non-granular cells. The numbers of B-cells and their precursors were reduced by nearly 75%.

Losses were predominantly in pre-B and immature B-cells, which declined by about 50% and 25%, respectively. Thus, Zn deficiency blocks development of B-cells in the marrow, resulting in fewer B-cells in the spleen.

Studies of Zn deficiency in bovine, porcine, rat and murine models and in severely Zn-deficient children describe substantial reductions in the size of the thymus (see Shankar and Prasad, 1998; Prasad, 2000a). Mice maintained on a Zn-deficient diet for as little as 2 weeks showed moderate thymic involution. After 4 weeks, the thymus retained only 25% of its original size and, at 6 weeks, only a few thymocytes remained in the thymic capsule. Thymic atrophy exceeded that of other organs and overall weight loss, which declined only 20% by 6 weeks. The reduction in thymic size and cellularity was seen mostly in the thymic cortex, where immature thymocytes develop. Such changes were not observed in control animals, confirming that Zn was responsible for the effect. Following only 1 week of normal Zn intake, thymic size increased and cellular repopulation of the cortex was seen.

Adult mice maintained for 2 weeks on a Zn-deficient diet had reduced numbers of T and B lymphocytes in peripheral blood, lymph nodes and spleen; numbers of peripheral-blood lymphocytes (and macrophages) were eventually reduced by more than 50% (see Good, 1981; Shankar and Prasad, 1998). Even marginal Zn deficiency substantially suppresses the numbers of peripheral blood immune cells in mice and in humans (Moulder and Steward, 1989; Zalewski, 1996). Zn-deficient children with AE have reduced numbers of lymphocytes, particularly T-cells, in the blood and peripheral lymphoid tissues. Decreased CD4+/CD8+ cell ratios are also seen. Recent studies in an experimental human model show that the percentage of CD8+CD73+ T lymphocytes (these are precursors to cytotoxic T lymphocytes (CTL)) is decreased in Zn deficiency (see Prasad, 2000a). This and the other effects described are reversed with Zn supplementation.

Effects of zinc deficiency and repletion on immune-cell functions

Neutrophil functions

Neutrophil chemotaxis and function are impaired in Zn-deficient animals and patients with AE and other types of Zn deficiency (see Walsh et al., 1994; Shankar and Prasad, 1998). These impairments are reversible by in vitro addition of Zn to the cells. In addition, in vitro addition of Zn improved the neutrophil response against Staphylococcus. One study observed that exercise-induced potentiation of superoxide formation by neutrophils was attenuated by Zn supplementation (Singh et al., 1994); this might be due to the role of Zn in superoxide dismutase.

Monocyte/macrophage functions

Effects on monocyte/macrophage function are also seen during Zn deficiency. In humans, the chemotactic response of monocytes from AE patients is suppressed and can be restored following addition of Zn to cells in vitro (see Walsh *et al.*, 1994; Shankar and Prasad, 1998). Monocytes from Zn-deficient mice have impaired killing of intracellular parasites, which is rapidly corrected *in vitro* by addition of Zn. Reduced macrophage phagocytosis of *Candida* has also been observed in deficient animals. In other studies, however, the ability of macrophages from Zn-deficient rodents to phagocytose particles either was enhanced and accompanied by greater numbers of Fc- and C3b-bearing cells or remained unchanged. High concentrations of Zn *in vitro* inhibited macrophage activation, mobility, phagocytosis and oxygen consumption. When marasmic children were rehabilitated with a Zn-containing regimen, monocyte phagocytic and fungicidal activity was suppressed (Schlesinger *et al.*, 1993). Since elevated Zn levels can inhibit complement activation (Montgomery *et al.*, 1979), complement-mediated phagocytosis may be adversely affected by high Zn levels. Additional studies are clearly needed to understand more fully the conditions under which Zn affects monocyte/macrophage phagocytosis.

Natural killer cell function

Human and animal studies showed decreased natural killer (NK)-cell activity in Zn deficiency (see Walsh *et al.*, 1994; Shankar and Prasad, 1998; Prasad, 2000a). NK-cell function was depressed following treatment of cells with 1,10-phenanthroline, a Zn chelator, and was reversed by readdition of Zn but not Ca or Mg. Exogenous Zn also stimulated production of interferon (IFN)-γ by human peripheral-blood NK cells (Salas and Kirchner, 1987). However, exposure of NK cells to high levels of Zn *in vitro* inhibited cytotoxicity by rendering target cells more resistant to damage. This and other reports of Zn-mediated inhibition of NK activity may be partially explained by the demonstration that the NK-cell-inhibitory receptor requires Zn (Rajagopalan *et al.*, 1995).

T- and B-cell functions

T-cell responses, such as proliferation in response to mitogens, cytotoxicity and delayed-type hypersensitivity (DTH), are suppressed during Zn deficiency and reversed by Zn supplementation (Good *et al.*, 1976; Cunningham-Rundles *et al.*, 1981; Moulder and Steward, 1989; see also Shankar and Prasad, 1998; Prasad, 2000a). Suppressed DTH responses in malnourished children are also restored following Zn supplementation (e.g. Golden *et al.*, 1978). Patients receiving total parenteral nutrition devoid of Zn had reduced T-cell responses to mitogens, which returned to normal after 20 days of Zn supplementation (Allen *et al.*, 1981). Mitogen-induced lymphocyte responses were greater after feeding rats for 14 days on a diet containing 0.1% by weight Zn than after feeding 0.004% Zn (see Chvapil *et al.*, 1976; Shankar and Prasad, 1998). In an experimental human model of Zn deficiency, the production of IL-2 and IFN-γ was decreased, whereas the production of IL-4, IL-6 and IL-10 was not affected (Beck *et al.*, 1997; Prasad *et al.*, 1997, 1999; Prasad, 2000b). IL-2 production in patients with sickle-cell disease and Zn deficiency is decreased and Zn supplementation results in increased production of IL-2 (Prasad *et al.*, 1999). Thus, Zn deficiency in humans appears to be accompanied by an imbalance of T-helper-1 and T-helper-2 function.

Since NFκB binds to the promoter enhancer area of the IL-2 and interleukin 2 receptor alpha (IL-2Rα) genes, we investigated the effect of Zn deficiency on activation of NFκB and its binding to DNA in HUT-78, a Th0 malignant human lymphoblastoid cell line (Prasad *et al.*, 2001). We showed for the first time that in Zn-deficient HUT-78 cells, phosphorylation of the NFκB-inhibitory subunit (IκB) and of IκB kinase, ubiquitination of IκB and binding of NFκB to DNA were significantly decreased in comparison with Zn-sufficient cells. Zn increased the translocation of NFκB from cytosol to nucleus. We concluded that Zn plays an important role in the activation of NFκB in HUT-78 cells, which may regulate IL-2 gene expression.

B-cell proliferative and antibody responses are inhibited by Zn deficiency (see Moulder and Steward, 1989; Walsh *et al.*, 1994; Shankar and Prasad, 1998). Interestingly, T-dependent antibody responses are more affected by Zn deficiency than T-independent ones: the plaque-forming colony responses to a T-dependent antigen (sheep red blood cells) and a T-independent antigen (dextran) were reduced 90% and 50%, respectively, in Zn-deficient mice (Fraker *et al.*, 1977, 1978, 1984, 1986). Mice fed a high-Zn diet had increased numbers of splenic plaque-forming colonies in response to T-dependent antigens (Salvin *et al.*, 1987).

Effects of high-dose zinc on immune cell functions

One study reported that 11 men receiving 300 mg Zn daily (20 times the US recommended intake) for 6 weeks experienced decreased proliferative responses of lymphocytes to mitogens and reductions in chemotaxis and phagocytosis of neutrophils (Chandra, 1984). Very high Zn intakes in adults and children can result in copper deficiency and this could be the cause of the immunosuppression (Porter *et al.*, 1977; Prasad *et al.*, 1978; Fosmire, 1990). Importantly, other larger and longer-term controlled trials of high-dose Zn supplementation in adults did not document deleterious effects on cellular immunity (Bogden *et al.*, 1988, 1990). In one study, 103 apparently healthy elderly subjects age 60 to 89 years were randomly assigned to one of three treatments: placebo, 15 mg Zn day^{-1}, or 100 mg Zn day^{-1} for 3 months (Bogden *et al.*, 1988). None of the treatments significantly altered the DTH response to a panel of seven recall antigens or *in vitro* lymphocyte proliferative responses to mitogens and antigens. Bogden *et al.* (1990) administered 100 mg Zn daily to elderly subjects for 12 months and found no deleterious immunological effects. Moreover, deleterious immunological effects were not observed in trials where clinically healthy, and otherwise normal, children received daily Zn supplementation up to twice the US recommended intake (see Shankar and Prasad, 1998). Therefore, intake of Zn twofold above the recommended intake is considered well within the safety range for preschool children and adults. As for any nutritional supplement, caution must be exercised in taking excessive doses for prolonged periods of time.

Zinc and Glucocorticoids

The release of glucocorticoid hormones from the adrenal glands can cause thymic atrophy. Since Zn deficiency raises blood glucocorticoid levels, thymic atrophy may be mediated, in part, by glucocorticoids (DePasquale-Jardieu and Fraker, 1980; Concordet and Ferry, 1993). Indeed, when adrenalectomized mice were maintained up to 6 weeks on a Zn-deficient diet, changes in thymic weight were small or absent (DePasquale-Jardieu and Fraker, 1980). In addition, when adult mice were given a slow-release corticosteroid implant, thymus size was reduced more than 80%. Steroid-implanted mice also showed large reductions in pre-B and immature B-cells in the bone marrow, suggesting that the effects of Zn deficiency on early B-cell development may also involve glucocorticoids. The contribution of glucocorticoids to the effects of Zn deficiency must, however, be interpreted with caution. Zn deficiency has profound effects on human thymocytes, which are relatively resistant to glucocorticoids (DePasquale-Jardieu and Fraker, 1980). In addition, although the thymus of Zn-deficient adrenalectomized mice remained normal in size, Zn-dependent decreases in the ratio of the areas of the cortex to the medulla still occurred. Likewise, in adrenalectomized mice, Zn deficiency reduced IgM and IgG responses to sheep red blood cells, with 50% of the loss in T-cell helper function occurring before detectable increases in plasma corticosterone. Lastly, in marginally Zn-deficient mice, loss of lymphocytes in the spleen, depressed immunity and decreased IL-2 production were observed despite the absence of thymic shrinkage or increased glucocorticoid levels.

The Influence of Zinc on Conditions Involving Immunosuppression

Individuals suffering from sickle-cell disease have depressed peripheral T-cell numbers, decreased CD4+/CD8+ T-cell ratios, loss of DTH, decreased NK-cell activity, decreased production of IL-2 and suppressed activity of thymulin (for references, see Prasad, 2000a). Zn supplementation restores these immunological parameters to near-normal levels. Likewise, in patients with Down's syndrome, Zn supplements restore immediate hypersensitivity, lymphocyte functions and neutrophil chemotaxis, and increase resistance to infection (Bjorksten *et al.*, 1980). Zn supplements also restored DTH in alcoholics and stimulated cell-mediated and humoral immunity in humans and mice with hypo-gammaglobulinaemia (for references, see Shankar and Prasad, 1998).

In elderly human beings and animals, impairments in wound healing and resistance to infection were corrected by Zn supplementation (see Prasad, 2000a), suggesting that immunodeficiency in the elderly is due in part to Zn deficiency. Low plasma Zn levels in elderly patients were associated with peripheral blood lymphopenia, although not with depressed serum IgA levels or DTH responses. Zn supplementation restored normal lymphocyte and neutrophil Zn levels, increased numbers of circulating T-cells, and improved DTH and IgG antibody responses to tetanus toxoid (for references, see Prasad, 2000a). As might be expected from these effects, increased resistance to infection was also observed.

Zinc and Infectious Diseases

Numerous animal studies indicate that Zn deficiency decreases resistance to a range of bacterial, viral, fungal and parasitic pathogens (for a review, see Shankar and Prasad, 1998), probably because of the immune impairments induced by the deficiency. Thus, the enhancing effect upon the immune response of providing Zn should translate into improved host defence and increased resistance to pathogens. However, most microorganisms require Zn for basic cellular processes (e.g. replication) and, during the acute-phase response, Zn is redistributed from the plasma to the liver and to lymphocytes (see Shankar and Prasad, 1998). It has been suggested that this is an adaptive response intended to deprive invading pathogens of Zn, facilitate immune function and prevent free-radical damage to cells. However, plasma Zn levels resulting from the acute-phase response remain generally well above the levels at which the growth of most pathogens is affected. The balance between Zn availability for host immunity and for the invading pathogen is affected by multiple factors. It appears, however, that in most cases any benefit to the pathogen of Zn availability is well compensated by the concomitant improvement in host immune function.

A number of studies have demonstrated the benefits of Zn supplementation in regard to infectious diseases in human populations (for a review, see Shankar and Prasad, 1998). Controlled trials of Zn supplementation demonstrated a reduction in the incidence and duration of acute and chronic diarrhoea by 25–30%, and in the incidence of pneumonia by up to 50% (Castillo-Duran *et al.*, 1987; Sazawal *et al.*, 1995, 1996, 1998; Ninh *et al.*, 1996; Rosado *et al.*, 1997; Roy *et al.*, 1997, 1999; Ruel *et al.*, 1997). Some studies implied that Zn may reduce clinical disease caused by *Plasmodium falciparum* (Gibson *et al.*, 1991; Bates *et al.*, 1993), and it has been demonstrated in a controlled trial carried out in Papua New Guinea that Zn supplements could reduce health-centre attendance attributable to malaria by over 35% (Shankar *et al.*, 1998). Decreased *Schistosoma mansoni* egg counts were observed among children given Zn supplements versus those given a placebo (Friis *et al.*, 1997). Humans suffering from AE also suffer fewer infections when given supranormal levels of Zn, and plasma Zn levels are substantially lower in patients with diffuse lepromatous leprosy compared with those with the more limited bacillary form (for references, see Shankar and Prasad, 1998). Zn deficiency is frequently seen in patients with human immunodeficiency virus (HIV), and disease progression is accompanied by decreased serum Zn levels and depressed lymphocyte mitogenic responses (Pifer *et al.*, 1987; Falutz *et al.*, 1988; Wang *et al.*, 1994). These changes are partially reversible by Zn supplementation.

The role of Zn in preventing and treating the common cold has been discussed for many years. It appears that Zn is effective in reducing the severity of cold symptoms. For example, in a recent placebo-controlled study, 12.8 mg of Zn was administered in lozenges to a group of subjects every 2 to 3 h while awake within 24 h of developing symptoms of the common cold (Prasad *et al.*, 2000). In the Zn-treated group, the duration and severity of cold symptoms were decreased approximately 50% in comparison with the placebo group.

Conclusion

Zn has a number of key roles relating to cell signalling, cell activation, gene expression, protein synthesis and apoptosis. Zn is crucial for the normal development of immune cells. Zn plays an important role in maintaining the activity of a range of immune cells, including neutrophils, monocytes, NK cells, B-cells and T-cells, and Zn-deficient individuals have increased susceptibility to a variety of pathogens. Providing Zn for deficient individuals improves immune function and host defence. Studies in at-risk groups indicate significant decreases in the incidence and severity of infectious disease when Zn is provided.

References

Allen, J.I., Kay, N.E. and McClain, C.J. (1981) Severe zinc deficiency in humans: association with a reversible T-lymphocyte dysfunction. *Annals of Internal Medicine* 95, 154–157.

Barnes, P.M. and Moynahan, E.J. (1973) Zinc deficiency in acrodermatitis enteropathica: multiple dietary intolerance treated with synthetic diet. *Proceedings of the Royal Society of Medicine* 66, 327–329.

Bates, C.J., Evans, P.H., Dardenne, M., Prentice, A., Lunn, P.G., Northrop-Clewes, C.A., Hoare, S., Cole, T.J., Horan, S.J. and Longmen, S.C. (1993) A trial of zinc supplementation in young rural Gambian children. *British Journal of Nutrition* 69, 243–255.

Beach, R.S., Gershwin, M.E. and Hurley, L.S. (1982) Gestational zinc deprivation in mice: persistence of immuno-deficiency for three generations. *Science* 218, 469–471.

Beach, R.S., Gershwin, M.E. and Hurley, L.S. (1983) Persistent immunological consequences of gestational zinc deprivation. *American Journal of Clinical Nutrition* 38, 579–590.

Beck, F.W.J., Prasad, A.S., Kaplan, J., Fitzgerald, J.T. and Brewer, G.J. (1997) Changes in cytokine production and T-cell subpopulations in experimentally induced zinc-deficient humans. *American Journal of Physiology* 272, E1002–E1007.

Bjorksten, B., Black, O., Gustavson, K.H., Hallmans, G., Hagloff, B. and Tarvik, A. (1980) Zinc and immune function in Down's syndrome. *Acta Paediatrica Scandinavica* 69, 183–187.

Bogden, J.D., Oleske, J.M., Lavenhar, M.A., Munves E.M., Kemp, F.W., Bruening, K.S., Holding, K.J., Denny, T.N., Guaino, M.A., Krieger, L.M. and Holland, B.K. (1988) Zinc and immunocompetence in elderly people: effects of zinc supplementation for 3 months. *American Journal of Clinical Nutrition* 48, 655–663.

Bogden, J.D., Oleske, J.M., Lavenhar, M.A., Munves, E.M., Kemp, F.W., Bruening, K.S., Holding, K.J., Denny, T.N., Guarino, M.A. and Holland, B.K. (1990) Effects of one year supplementation with zinc and other micronutrients on cellular immunity in the elderly. *Journal of the American College of Nutrition* 9, 214–225.

Castillo-Duran, C., Heresi, G., Fisberg, M. and Uauy, R. (1987) Controlled trial of zinc supplementation during recovery from malnutrition – effects on growth and immune function. *American Journal of Clinical Nutrition* 45, 602–608.

Chandra, R.K. (1984) Excessive intake of zinc impairs immune response. *Journal of the American Medical Association* 252, 1443–1446.

Chesters, J.K., Petrie, L. and Lipson, H.E. (1993) Two zinc-dependent steps during G1 to S phase transition. *Journal of Cellular Physiology* 155, 445–451.

Chvapil, M., Zukoski, C.F., Hattler, B.G., Stankova, L., Montgomery, D., Carlson, E.C. and Ludwig, J.C. (1976) Zinc and cells. In: Prasad, A.S. and Oberleas, D. (eds) *Human Health and Disease: Zinc and Copper*. Academic Press, New York, pp. 269–281.

Concordet, J.P. and Ferry, A. (1993) Physiological programmed cell death in thymocytes is induced by physical stress (exercise). *American Journal of Physiology* 265, C626–C629.

Cunningham-Rundles, C., Cunningham-Rundles, S., Iwata, T., Incefy, G., Garofalo, J.A., Menendez-Botet, C., Lewis, V., Twomey, J.J. and Good, R.A. (1981) Zinc deficiency, depressed thymic hormones, and T lymphocyte dysfunction in patients with hypogammaglobulinemia. *Clinical Immunology and Immunopathology* 21, 387–396.

Department of Health (1991) *Report of the Panel on Dietary Reference Values of the Committee of Medical Aspects of Food Policy: Dietary Reference Values for Food Energy and Nutrients for the United Kingdom*. HMSO, London.

DePasquale-Jardieu, P. and Fraker, P.J. (1980) Further characterization of the role of corticosterone in the loss of humoral immunity in zinc deficient A/J mice as determined by adrenalectomy. *Journal of Immunology* 124, 2650–2655.

Dutz, W., Rossipal, E., Ghavami, H., Vessal, K., Kohout, E. and Post, C. (1976) Persistent cell mediated immune deficiency following infantile stress during the first six months of life. *European Journal of Pediatrics* 122, 117–130.

Falutz, J., Tsoukas, C. and Gold, P. (1988) Zinc as a cofactor in human immunodeficiency virus–induced immunosuppression. *Journal of the American Medical Association* 259, 2850–2851.

Ferguson, A.C. (1978) Prolonged impairment of cellular immunity in children with intrauterine growth retardation. *Journal of Pediatrics* 93, 52–56.

Fosmire, G.J. (1990) Zinc toxicity. *American Journal of Clinical Nutrition* 51, 225–227.

Fraker, P.J., Haas, S.M. and Luecke, R.W. (1977) Effect of zinc deficiency on the immune response of young adult A/J mice. *Journal of Nutrition* 107, 1889–1895.

Fraker, P.J., DePasquale-Jardieu, R., Zwickl, C.M. and Kuecke, R.W. (1978) Regeneraiton of T-cell helper function in zinc deficient adult mice. *Proceedings of the National Academy Sciences of the USA* 75, 5660–5664.

Fraker, P.J., Hilderbrandt, K. and Luecke, R.W. (1984) Alteration of antibody-mediated responses of suckling mice to T-cell dependent and independent antigens by maternal marginal zinc deficiency: restoration of responsivity by nutritional repletion. *Journal of Nutrition* 114, 170–179.

Fraker, P.J., Gershwin, M.E., Good, R.A. and Prasad, A.S. (1986) Interrelationships between zinc and immune functions. *Federation Proceedings* 45, 1474–1479.

Friis, H., Ndhlovu, P., Mduluza, T., Kaondeva, K., Sandstrom, B., Michaelson, K.F., Vennervald, B.J. and Christensen, N.O. (1997) The effect of zinc supplementation on *Schistosoma mansoni* reinfection rate and intensities: a randomized, controlled trial among rurual Zimbabwean school children. *European Journal of Clinical Nutrition* 51, 33–37.

Frost, P., Chen, J.C., Rabbani, I., Smith, J. and Prasad, A.S. (1977) The effect of Zn deficiency on the immune response. In: Brewer, G.J. and Prasad, A.S. (eds) *Zinc Metabolism: Current Aspects in Health and Disease*. Alan R. Liss, New York, pp. 143–153.

Gibson, R.S., Heywood, A., Yaman, C., Sohlstrom, A., Thompson, L.U. and Heywood, P. (1991) Growth in children from the Wosera subdistrict, Papua New Guinea, in relation to energy and protein intakes and zinc status. *American Journal of Clinical Nutrition* 53, 782–789.

Golden, M.H.N., Golden, B.E., Harland, P.S.E.G. and Jackson, A.A. (1978) Zinc and immunocompetence in protein-energy malnutrition. *Lancet* 1, 1226–1228.

Good, R.A. (1981) Nutrition and immunity. *Journal of Clinical Immunology* 1, 3–11.

Good, R.A., Fernandes, G., Yunis, E.J., Cooper, W.C., Jose, P.C., Kramer, T.R. and Hansen, M.A. (1976) Nutritional deficiency, immunologic function, and disease. *American Journal of Pathology* 84, 599–614.

Kay, R.G. and Tasman-Jones, C. (1975) Acute zinc deficiency in man during intra-venous alimentation. *Australian and New Zealand Journal of Surgery* 45, 325–330.

Montgomery, D.W., Chvapil, M. and Zukoski, C.F. (1979) Effects of zinc chloride on guinea pig complement component activity *in vitro*: concentration-dependent inhibition and enhancement. *Infection and Immunity* 23, 424–431.

Moulder, K. and Steward, M.W. (1989) Experimental zinc deficiency: effects on cellular responses and the affinity of humoral antibody. *Clinical and Experimental Immunology* 77, 269–274.

Ninh, N.X., Thissen, J.-P., Collette, L., Gerrard, G., Khoi, H.H. and Ketelslegers, J.M. (1996) Zinc supplementation increases growth and circulating insulin-like growth factor (IGF-1) in growth retarded Vietnamese children. *American Journal of Clinical Nutrition* 63, 514–519.

Oleske, J.M., Westphal, M.L., Shore, S., Gorden, D., Bogden, J.D. and Nahmias, A. (1979) Zinc therapy of depressed cellular immunity in acrodermatitis enteropathica. *Amerian Journal of Diseases of Children* 133, 915–918.

Pifer, L.L., Wang, Y.F., Chiang, T.M., Ahokas, R., Woods, D.R. and Joyner, R.E. (1987) Borderline immunodeficiency in male homosexuals: is life-style contributory? *Southern Medical Journal* 80, 687–691.

Porter, K.G., McMaster, D., Elmes, M.E. and Love, A.H. (1977) Anaemia and low serum-copper during zinc therapy. *Lancet* ii, 774.

Prasad, A.S. (1991) Discovery of human zinc deficiency and studies in an experimental human model. *American Journal of Clinical Nutrition* 53, 403–412.

Prasad, A.S. (1993) *Biochemistry of Zinc*. Plenum Press, New York.

Prasad, A.S. (2000a) Effects of zinc deficiency on immune functions. *Journal of Trace Elements in Experimental Medicine* 13, 1–20.

Prasad, A.S. (2000b) Effects of zinc deficiency on Th1 and Th2 cytokine shifts. *Journal of Infectious Disease* 182(Suppl.1), S62-S68.

Prasad, A.S., Halsted, J.A. and Nadimi, M. (1961) Syndrome of iron deficiency anemia, hepatosplenomegaly, dwarfism and geophagia. *American Journal Medicine* 31, 532–546.

Prasad, A.S., Brewer, G.J., Schoomaker, E.B. and Rabbani, P. (1978) Hypocupremia induced by zinc therapy in adults. *Journal of the American Medical Association* 240, 2166–2168.

Prasad, A.S., Meftah, S., Abdallah, J., Kaplan, J., Brewer, G.J., Bach, J.F. and Dardenne, M. (1988) Serum thymulin in human zinc deficiency. *Journal of Clinical Investigation* 82, 1202–1210.

Prasad, A.S., Beck, F.W.J., Grabowski, S.M., Kaplan, J. and Mathog, R.H. (1997) Zinc deficiency: changes in cytokine production and T-cell subpopulations in patients with head and neck cancer and in non-cancer subjects. *Proceedings of the Association of American Physicians* 109, 68–77.

Prasad, A.S., Beck, F.W.J., Kaplan, J., Chandrasekar, P.H., Ortega, J., Fitzgerald, J.T. and Swerdlow, P. (1999) Effects of zinc supplementation on incidence of infections and hospital admissions in sickle cell disease (SCD). *American Journal of Hematology* 61, 194–202.

Prasad, A.S., Fitzgerald, J.T., Bao, B., Beck, F.W.J. and Chandrasekar, P.H. (2000) Duration of symptoms and plasma cytokine levels in patients with the common cold treated with zinc acetate. *Annals of Internal Medicine* 133, 245–252.

Prasad, A.S., Bao, B., Beck, F.W.J. and Sarkar, F.H. (2001) Zinc activates NF-kB in HUT-78 cells. *Journal of Laboratory and Clinical Medicine* 138, 250–256.

Rajagopalan, S., Winter, C.C., Wagtmann, N. and Long, E.O. (1995) The Ig-related killer cell inhibitory receptor binds zinc and requires zinc for recognition of HLA-C on target cells. *Journal of Immunology* 155, 4143–4146.

Rosado, J.L., Lopez, P., Munoz, E., Martinez, H. and Allen, L.H. (1997) Zinc supplementation reduced morbidity, but neither zinc nor iron supplementation affected growth or body composition of Mexican pre-schoolers. *American Journal of Clinical Nutrition* 65, 13–19.

Roy, S.K., Tomkins, A.M., Akramuzzaman, S.M., Behrens, R.H., Haider, R., Mahalanabis, D. and Fuchs, G. (1997) Randomised controlled trial of zinc supplementation in malnourished Bangladeshi children with diarrhoea. *Archives of Disease in Childhood* 77, 196–200.

Roy, S.K., Tomkins, A.M., Haider, R., Behra, R.H., Akramuzzaman, S.M., Mahalanabis, D. and Fuchs, G.J. (1999) Impact of zinc supplementation on subsequent growth and morbidity in Bangladeshi children with acute diarrhoea. *European Journal of Clinical Nutrition* 53, 529–534.

Ruel, M.T., Ribera, J.A., Santizo, M.C., Lonnerda, B. and Brown, K.H. (1997) Impact of zinc supplementation on morbidity from diarrhea and respiratory infections among rural Guatemalan children. *Pediatrics* 99, 808–813.

Salas, M. and Kirchner, H. (1987) Induction of interferon gamma in human leucocyte cultures stimulated by Zn^{2+}. *Clinical Immunology and Immunopathology* 45, 139–142.

Salvin, S.B., Horecker, B.L., Pan, L.X. and Rabin, B.S. (1987) The effect of dietary zinc and prothymosin on cellular immune responses of RF/J mice. *Clinical Immunology and Immunopathology* 43, 281–288.

Sandstead, H.H., Penland, J.G., Xu-Cun, C., Prasad, A.S., Alcock, N.W., Egger, N.G., Carroll, R. and Dayal, H.H. (2000) Zinc and micronutrient repletion of children. *Journal of Trace and Microprobe Techniques* 18, 523–527.

Sazawal, S., Black, R., Jalla, S., Bhan, M.K., Bhandari, N. and Sinha, A. (1995) Zinc supplementation in young children with acute diarrhea in India. *New England Journal of Medicine* 333, 839–844.

Sazawal, S., Black, R.E., Bhan, M.K., Jalla, S., Bhandari, N., Sinha, A. and Majumdar, S. (1996) Zinc supplementation reduces the incidence of persistent diarrhea and dysentery among low socioeconomic children in India. *Journal of Nutrition* 126, 443–450.

Sazawal, S., Black, R., Jalla, S., Mazumdar, S., Sinha, A. and Bhan, M.K. (1998) Zinc supplementation reduces the incidence of acute lower respiratory infections in infants and preschool children – a double-blind controlled trial. *Pediatrics* 102, 1–5.

Schlesinger, L., Arevalo, M., Arredondo, S., Lonnerdal, B. and Stekel, A. (1993) Zinc supplementation impairs monocyte function. *Acta Paedictrica* 82, 734–738.

Shankar, A.H. and Prasad, A.S. (1998) Zinc and immune function: the biological basis of altered resistance to infection. *American Journal of Clinical Nutrition* 68, 447S-463S.

Shankar, A.H., Genton, B., Baisor, M., Paino, J., Tamja, S., Adiguma, T., Wu, L., Rare, L., Bannon, D., Tielsch, J.M., West, K.P., Jr and Alpers, M.P. (1998) The influence of zinc supplementation on morbidity due to plasmodium falciparum: a randomized trial in preschool children in Papua New Guinea. *American Journal of Tropical Medicine and Hygiene* 62, 663–669.

Singh, A., Failla, M.L. and Deuster, R.A. (1994) Exercise induced changes in immune function: effects of zinc supplementation. *Journal of Applied Physiology* 76, 2298–2303.

Taylor, C.G. and Bray, T.M. (1991) Effect of hyperoxia on oxygen free radical defence enzymes in the lung of zinc-deficient rats. *Journal of Nutrition* 121, 460–466.

Todd, W.R., Elvejheim, C.A. and Hart, E.B. (1934) Zinc in the nutrition of the rat. *American Journal of Physiology* 107, 146–156.

Turner, J.M., Brodsky, M.H., Irving, B.A., Levin, S.D., Perlmutter, R.M. and Littman, D.R. (1990) Interaction of the unique N-terminal region of tyrosine kinase p56[lck] with cytoplasmic domains of CD4 and CD8 is mediated by cysteine motifs. *Cell* 60, 755–765.

Walsh, C.T., Sandstead, H.H., Prasad, A.S., Newberne, P.M. and Fraker, P.J. (1994) Zinc health effects and research priorities for the 1990s. *Environmental Health Perspectives* 102, 5–46.

Wang, Y., Liang, B. and Watson, R.R. (1994) The effect of alcohol consumption on nutritional status during murine AIDS. *Alcohol* 11, 273–278.

Zalewski, P.D. (1996) Zinc and immunity: implications for growth, survival and function of lymphoid cells. *Journal of Nutritional Immunology* 4, 39–80.

Zalewski, P.D. and Forbes, I.J. (1993) Intracellular zinc and the regulation of apoptosis. In: Lavin, M. and Watters, D. (eds) *Programmed Cell Death: the Cellular and Molecular Biology of Apoptosis.* Harwood Academic Publishers, Melbourne, pp. 73–86.

11   Role of Iron in Immunity and Infection

SOLO KUVIBIDILA*[1] AND B. SURENDRA BALIGA[2]

[1]Division of Hematology/Oncology, Department of Pediatrics, Louisiana State University Health Sciences Center, Box T8-1, 1542 Tulane Avenue, New Orleans, LA 70112, USA; [2]Department of Pediatrics, College of Medicine, University of South Alabama, 2451 Fillingim Street, Mobile, AL 36617, USA

Introduction

Iron is the fourth most common element on earth and is one of the most studied nutrients in human health (see Yip and Dallman, 1996). Iron exists in two main forms: ferric (Fe^{3+}) and ferrous (Fe^{2+}). The ease of oxidation and reduction of iron makes it a unique trace element for many cellular redox reactions. Iron is required by virtually all living cells for many biochemical reactions, especially for aerobic and anaerobic energy metabolism and cell proliferation (Cazzalo et al., 1990). In spite of our knowledge on the role of iron in human health related to haematology since the 18th century, the importance of iron in immunity was first recognized only in the late 1960s and early 1970s. This field evolved from clinical observations of an association between iron deficiency and infection (see Strauss, 1978; Humbert and Moore, 1983; Kuvibidila et al., 1989). It was later shown that some immune responses were altered by iron deficiency (see Dallman, 1987; Kuvibidila et al., 1989). This chapter will summarize the current knowledge of the effects of iron deficiency and iron overload on immunity and the implications for infection.

Iron Status

Between two-thirds and three-quarters of body iron circulates in blood in the form of haemoglobin. Iron status is evaluated by three methods: clinical evaluation, haematological and biochemical laboratory tests and therapeutic iron trials. The four blood indexes that distinguish iron deficiency, normal iron status and iron overload are serum ferritin concentration, blood haemoglobin concen-

*Corresponding author.

© CAB International 2002. Nutrition and Immune Function
(eds P.C. Calder, C.J. Field and H.S. Gill)

tration, transferrin saturation and serum transferrin receptor concentration. Iron deficiency differs from normal iron status by reduced blood levels of haemoglobin, transferrin saturation below the levels defined for age and gender, serum ferritin concentration less than 12 μg l^{-1}, and soluble transferrin receptor concentration above 9 mg l^{-1}. Groups at risk of iron deficiency include infants, young children and women of childbearing age. Iron overload differs from normal iron status by increased serum ferritin concentration (> 200 μg l^{-1}) and transferrin saturation (> 50%). Groups at risk of iron overload include individuals who receive frequent blood transfusions, such as those with beta-thalassaemia or sickle-cell disease, patients with renal disease who receive medicinal iron due to impaired erythropoiesis, people with idiopathic haemochromatosis and the Bantu of southern Africa, who frequently consume traditional beer, which is very rich in iron.

Iron Absorption and Transport

Iron is predominantly absorbed in the duodenum. In its free form, iron is a potent pro-oxidant known to induce peroxidation of lipids, proteins and nucleic acids. Extracellular iron circulates in blood bound to transferrin. One transferrin molecule has two iron-binding sites. Under physiological conditions, cells take up iron from plasma by endocytosis, whereby one transferrin molecule binds to one transferrin receptor molecule, and the complex is transferred to the cytoplasm by invagination. As a result of low pH in the endosome, iron is released to the cytoplasm, where it is either used for various cellular functions or incorporated into ferritin. Upon loss of iron, the apotransferrin–transferrin-receptor complex is transported back to the cell membrane, where apotransferrin is released into the bloodstream, and the transferrin receptor is available for a new round of transferrin binding. The mechanism by which the apotransferrin–transferrin-receptor complex is transported to the cell membrane remains unclear. However, Sainte-Marie et al. (1997) suggest that changes in free cytoplasmic calcium concentrations might be involved in the recycling of transferrin receptor.

Effects of Iron Deficiency on Immunity

Iron metabolism by T-cells and the effects of iron deficiency on T-cell functions

Resting T-cells do not express the transferrin receptor on their cell surface, and therefore either do not take up iron from their environment or take up very little (Tormey et al., 1972). Upon T-cell activation, T-cells express surface transferrin receptors in the G0/G1 phase of the cell cycle before the initiation of DNA synthesis, but after induction of interleukin (IL)-2 secretion (Neckers and Cossman, 1983). The increase in transferrin receptor concentrations is believed to be to ensure sufficient iron uptake to support the activity of ribonucleotide reductase for the biosynthesis of deoxyribonucleotides.

There are many cell-mediated immune responses that have been investigated in iron-deficient subjects and laboratory animals (Table 11.1). In children and adults, iron deficiency resulting from dietary restriction reduces the proportion of T lymphocytes in blood, although the absolute number of T-cells can be either reduced or unchanged (Chandra and Saraya, 1975; Srikantia *et al.*, 1976; Bagchi *et al.*, 1980; Prema *et al.*, 1982; Swarup-Mitra and Sinha, 1984; Kemahli *et al.*, 1988; Vydyborets, 2000). However, based on the report of Santos and Falcao (1990), it appears that iron deficiency resulting from blood loss does not reduce the proportion of T-cells in blood, but it does decrease total T-cell numbers. The discrepancy between these types of iron deficiency is probably related to the long period of time required for the development of iron deficiency by dietary restriction as compared with blood loss. The absolute numbers and proportions of CD4+ and CD8+ T-cells are either decreased or normal in iron deficiency.

In mice, iron deficiency reduces the proportion of total T-cells, helper T-cells, and cytotoxic/suppressor T-cells in the spleen (Kuvibidila *et al.*, 1990;

Table 11.1. Iron and T-cell functions.

Immune function/response	Iron deficiency: before treatment	Iron deficiency: after treatment	Iron overload
Thymus weight	↓ or ↔	↑	Not determined
Spleen weight	↑	↓	Not determined
Total lymphocytes	↓ or ↔	↑	↔
Total T-cell number (CD3+)	↓ or ↔	↑	↔
Proportion of T-cells (% CD3+)	↓	↑	↓
Proportion of CD4 cells	↓ or ↔	↔	↓
Total CD4 cells	↓ or ↔	↑	↓
Proportion of CD8 cells	↓ or ↔	↔	↑ or ↔ (↓ iron chelation)
Total CD8 cells	↓ or ↔	↔	↔
CD4/CD8 ratio	↓ or ↔	↔	↓
Delayed-type hypersensitivity	↓	↑	↓
Antibody-dependent cytotoxicity	↓	↔	
Splenic T-cell cytotoxicity	↓ (mice)	Not determined	Not determined
Lymphocyte proliferation	↓ (in most studies)	↑	↓, ↑ or ↔
Interleukin-2 secretion	↓ or ↔	↓ or ↔	↓
Interleukin-4 secretion	Not determined	Not determined	↑
Interleukin-10 secretion	Not determined	Not determined	↑
Interferon-γ secretion	↓	Not determined	↓
Hydrolysis of PIP$_2$	↓	↑	Not determined
Protein kinase C activity	↓	↑	Not determined
Protein kinase C translocation	↓	↑	Not determined
Protein kinase C mRNA	↓	Not determined	Not determined

PIP$_2$, cell-membrane phosphatidylinositol-4,5-bisphosphate; ↑, increase; ↓, decrease; ↔, no significant change from normal.

Helyar and Sherman., 1992; Table 11.2). However, it does not alter the ratio of helper to cytotoxic T-cells (Table 11.2), which is also sometimes the case in humans. Iron deficiency induces thymus atrophy in mice, but does not affect the proportion of total T-cells, helper T-cells and cytotoxic/suppressor T-cells or the ratio of helper to cytotoxic T-cells in the thymus (Kuvibidila *et al.*, 1990). The mechanisms of thymus atrophy are unclear but are probably multifactorial. Recent data suggest that iron deficiency decreases thymocyte proliferation *in vivo* but does not increase apoptosis (Kuvibidila *et al.*, 2001). A defect in endocrine function of the thymus is not likely to be responsible for thymus atrophy, since plasma thymulin concentration is normal in iron-deficient mice (Kuvibidila *et al.*, 1990).

Iron deficiency in humans and laboratory animals consistently induces anergy (Joynson *et al.*, 1972; Bhaskaram and Reddy, 1975; Chandra and Saraya, 1975; MacDougall *et al.*, 1975; Kuvibidila *et al.*, 1981; Swarup-Mitra and Sinha, 1984; Kemahli *et al.*, 1988). In most though not all studies, iron deficiency has been shown to decrease secretion of IL-2 (Galan *et al.*, 1992; Kuvibidila *et al.*, 1992; Latunde-Dada and Young, 1992; Thibault *et al.*, 1993; Omara and Blakley, 1994), and interferon (IFN)-γ (Omara and Blaker, 1994), the lymphocyte proliferative responses to mitogens (Fig. 11.1) and antigens (Joynson *et al.*, 1972; Bhaskaram and Reddy, 1975; Chandra and Saraya, 1975; MacDougall *et al.*, 1975; Kuvibidila *et al.*, 1983b, 1998, 1999; Swarup-Mitra and Sinha, 1984; Omara and Blakley, 1994) and antibody-dependent cytotoxicity (Bagchi *et al.*, 1980). Most affected immune responses in humans are corrected within 1–3 months by iron therapy.

Iron metabolism by B-cells and the effects of iron deficiency on humoral immunity

In contrast to T-cells, resting B-cells express low levels of the transferrin receptor, which implies that they continuously take up small quantities of iron (Neckers *et al.*, 1984). Upon activation with a mitogen, up to 80% of B-cells express surface transferrin receptor, and hence exhibit increased iron uptake.

Table 11.2. Distribution of B- and T-cell subsets in the spleen of iron-deficient and control mice (adapted, with permission from the American Society for Clinical Nutrition, from Kuvibidila *et al.*, 1990).

	Control (%)	Iron-deficient (%)	Pair-fed (%)
B-cells	53.6 ± 4.1	28.5 ± 9.1[a]	50.8 ± 5.5
T-cells	29.3 ± 3.6	11.4 ± 6.9[a]	26.3 ± 6.2
Helper T-cells	17.4 ± 2.6	6.5 ± 4.1[a]	16.7 ± 4.0
Suppressor T-cells	11.1 ± 1.6	4.1 ± 2.7[a]	9.9 ± 2.7
Helper T-cells/suppressor T-cells	1.6 ± 0.2	1.6 ± 0.3	1.7 ± 1.2

[a]$P < 0.001$ versus control and pair-fed mice.
Values are mean ± standard error of mean. Sample sizes are 14 control, 16 iron-deficient, 16 pair-fed mice.

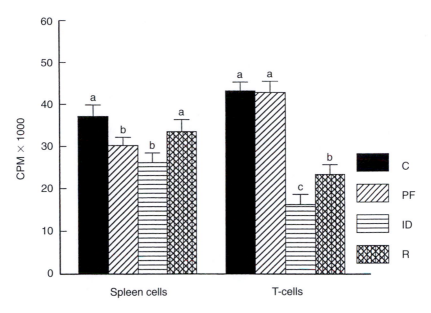

Fig. 11.1. Proliferation in response to concanavalin A of spleen cells and purified splenic T lymphocytes as a function of iron status. Values are mean ± standard error of the mean thymidine incorporation. C, control; PF, pair-fed; ID, iron-deficient; R, iron-replete; CPM, counts per minute. Bars with different letters are significantly different from each other ($P <$ 0.05). (Adapted, with permission from the American Society for Clinical Nutrition, from Kuvibidila *et al.*, 1983b.)

This suggests that iron deprivation may also affect certain B-cell functions. Indeed, murine splenic B-cell proliferation in response to bacterial lipopolysaccharide is significantly reduced by iron deficiency (Kuvibidila *et al.*, 1983a; Fig. 11.2). However, when parameters of humoral immunity are compared in iron-deficient and control individuals, it is noticed that, in general, humoral immunity is quite well preserved. The percentage and total number of B-cells and the concentration of immunoglobulins (Ig) are either unchanged or slightly increased, and antibody production in response to tetanus toxoid immunization is also normal (Table 11.3; Chandra and Saraya, 1975; Srikantia *et al.*, 1976; Bagchi *et al.*, 1980; Krantman *et al.*, 1982; Prema *et al.*, 1982). In contrast to humans, iron deficiency in laboratory animals decreases the percentage of B-cells in the spleen (Table 11.2; Kuvibidila *et al.*, 1990; Helyar and Sherman, 1992), antibody production against tetanus toxoid (Nalder *et al.*, 1972), secondary antibody response to influenza vaccine (Dhur *et al.*, 1990), the number of plaque-forming cells (Kuvibidila *et al.*, 1982) and Ig levels (Kochanowski and Sherman, 1985; Table 11.3). In addition, the number of intestinal cells containing IgM and secretory IgA (sIgA) in rats is reduced by iron deficiency, an alteration that may affect intestinal mucosal immunity (Perkkio *et al.*, 1987). The discrepancy between humans and laboratory animals could be due to species differences.

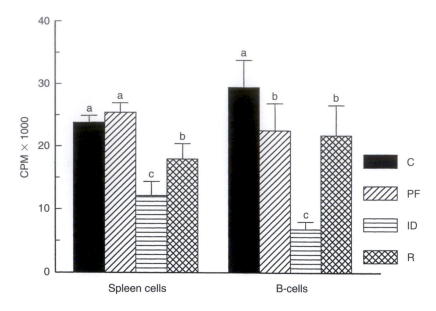

Fig. 11.2. Proliferation in response to lipopolysaccharide of spleen cells and enriched B-cell fractions as a function of iron status. Values are mean ± standard error of the mean (SEM) thymidine incorporation.C, control; PF, pair-fed; ID, iron-deficient; R, iron-replete; CPM, counts per minute. Bars with different letters are significantly different from each other (*P* < 0.05). (Adapted, with permission from the American Society for Clinical Nutrition, from Kuvibidila *et al.*, 1983b.)

Table 11.3. Iron and humoral immunity.

Immune function	Iron deficiency: before treatment	Iron deficiency: after treatment	Iron overload
% B-cells	↓, ↑ or ↔	↓	↑
Total B-cell number	↓, ↑ or ↔	↔	↑ or ↔
Immunoglobulin levels	↑ or ↔	↓	↑
SIgA, IgM, IgG	↓ (rats)	Not determined	↑[a]
Antibody production (influenza vaccine)	↓ (rats)	Not determined	Not determined
Antibody production (tetanus toxoid)	↓ in animals ↔ in humans	Not determined	↔
Plasma IgE after *Candida* infection in mice	Not determined	Not determined	↑
B-cell proliferation	↓	↑	↓ or ↔

[a]Activated cells from patients with hereditary haemochromatosis.
↓, decreased; ↑, increased; ↔, no significant change from normal.

Iron metabolism by monocytes and macrophages and the effects of iron deficiency on their functions

Although monocytes do not express transferrin receptor, macrophages do (Testa *et al.*, 1991). Macrophages differ from lymphocytes or other cell types because they up-regulate the expression of surface transferrin receptor when cultured in an iron-rich medium. This makes sense because macrophages are involved in iron storage and require iron for cytotoxic activity (Jiang and Baldwin, 1993).

Although the production of macrophage migration inhibitory factor is reduced in iron-deficient adults (Joynson *et al.*, 1972; Swarup-Mitra and Sinha, 1984), production of IL-1 is not, and macrophage cytotoxicity is only slightly reduced (Table 11.4; Bhaskaram *et al.*, 1989). *In vitro* iron chelation by desferrioxamine led to reduced secretion of tumour necrosis factor (TNF)-α by alveolar macrophages from both healthy non-smokers and smokers, which implies that iron deficiency may reduce the production of this pro-inflammatory

Table 11.4. Iron and non-specific immunity.

Immune function	Iron deficiency: before treatment	Iron deficiency: after treatment	Iron overload
Macrophage/monocyte phagocytosis	↓	Not determined	↓ or ↔
Macrophage/monocyte killing capacity	↓	Not determined	↓ or ↔
Peritoneal macrophage tumoricidal activity	↓	Not determined	Not determined
Neutrophil phagocytosis	↔	↔	↓
Neutrophil bactericidal activity	↓	↑	↓
Myeloperoxidase activity	↓	↑	Not determined
Neutrophil migration to inflammation site	↓	Not determined	Not determined
Natural killer cell activity	↓	Not determined	↓
In vivo macrophage clearance of particles	↓ (mice)	↑	Not determined
Interleukin-1 secretion	↓ in rats ↔ in humans	Not determined	↓
Interleukin-12 secretion	Not determined	Not determined	↓ for neutrophils ↔ for macrophages
Interferon-α secretion	↓	Not determined	Not determined
Tumour necrosis factor-α secretion	↓	Not determined	↔
Nitroblue reduction	↓ or ↔	Not determined	↓
Zymosan opsonization	Not determined	Not determined	↓
Nitric oxide production	Not determined	Not determined	↓ for neutrophils ↔ for macrophages
Complement C3	↓	↑	Not determined
Haemolytic activity CH50	↓ or ↔	↑	Not determined

↓, decreased; ↑, increased; ↔, no significant change from normal.

cytokine (O'Brien-Ladner *et al.*, 1998). Such an effect would be beneficial under circumstances associated with lung injury. In contrast to humans, macrophages from iron-deficient laboratory animals show reduced *in vitro* secretion of IL-1 (Helyar and Sherman, 1987) and IFN-γ (Omara and Blakley, 1994), decreased *in vivo* clearance of polyvinyl-pyrrolidone (Kuvibidila and Wade, 1987) and decreased tumoricidal activity (Kuvibidila *et al.*, 1983b).

Iron metabolism by neutrophils and the effects of iron deficiency on their functions

Iron concentrations in neutrophils are affected by the iron status of the host: they can be low in iron deficiency and elevated in iron overload. Neutrophils can take up iron from iron-saturated transferrin (Brieland and Fantone, 1991), although transferrin receptors have never been demonstrated on the neutrophil surface (Parmley *et al.*, 1983).

Several neutrophil responses have been assessed in both iron-deficient humans and laboratory animals (Table 11.4). Although neutrophil phagocytosis remains normal in iron deficiency, intracellular killing of bacteria is significantly impaired in both humans and laboratory animals (Yetgin *et al.*, 1979; Walter *et al.*, 1986; Murakawa *et al.*, 1987; Chwang *et al.*, 1988). In parallel with reduced bactericidal killing, the activity of myeloperoxidase, an iron-dependent enzyme involved in neutrophil killing of bacteria, is impaired. The impaired functions return to normal after a few weeks of iron repletion (Walter *et al.*, 1986; Murakawa *et al.*, 1987).

Iron deficiency and natural killer (NK)-cell activity

Similarly to T lymphocytes, resting NK cells do not express surface transferrin receptor, and they probably take up very little iron from the environment (Kemp, 1993). However, upon activation, they express the transferrin receptor on their surface. There is no information on the effects of iron deficiency on NK cell activity in human subjects. In rats, moderate, as well as severe, iron deficiency markedly reduces NK cytotoxicity against the YAC-1 target cell line (Spear and Sherman, 1992).

Mechanisms of impaired immunity in iron deficiency

The mechanisms by which iron deficiency impairs cell-mediated and non-specific immunity are not fully understood, but they are multifactorial (Table 11.5). They include, though are not limited to, reduced activity of iron-dependent enzymes (specifically ribonucleotide reductase), reduced cytokine secretion, a reduced number of immunocompetent T-cells and, very probably, altered signal transduction. Specific steps of signal-transduction pathways that are potentially regulated by iron remain to be identified. However, protein kinase C activity and its translo-

Table 11.5. Possible mechanisms of impaired cell-mediated immunity.

Decreased	Proportion and absolute numbers of immunocompetent T-cells
Decreased	Activity of ribonucleotide reductase
Decreased	Activity of other iron-dependent enzymes
Altered	Composition of cell-membrane phospholipids
Decreased	Hydrolysis of cell-membrane phospholipids, hence reduced production of second messengers (e.g. diacylglycerol, inositol-1,3,5-trisphosphate)
Defective	Protein kinase C activation, hence reduced phosphorylation of various factors, including membrane receptors for interleukin-2 and transferrin
Altered	Activity of other protein kinases that phosphorylate various factors that regulate cell proliferation
Altered	Concentration of free cytoplasmic calcium, factor involved in signal transduction
Altered	T-helper-1- and T-helper-2-type responses
Altered	Concentrations of receptors on T-cells and antigen-presenting cells

cation to the plasma membrane in murine spleen lymphocytes and human T-cell lines are impaired by iron deficiency (Alcantara *et al.*, 1991, 1994; Kuvibidila *et al.*, 1991, 1999; Fig. 11.3). Furthermore, iron chelation reduces production of mRNA for protein kinase C (Alcantara *et al.*, 1991, 1994). One early event in T-cell activation pathways that is also reduced by iron deprivation is the hydrolysis of cell-membrane phosphatidylinositol-4,5-bisphosphate by phospholipase C (a zinc-dependent enzyme) (Fig. 11.4) (Kuvibidila *et al.*, 1998). The end-products of this enzymatic reaction, inositol-1,3,5-trisphosphate and diacylglycerol, regulate protein kinase C activity. Both protein kinase C activation and the hydrolysis of cell-membrane phospholipids are crucial for signal transduction that leads to T-cell proliferation and many functions. The altered protein kinase C activation and hydrolysis of cell-membrane phospholipids may lead to impaired immune responses in iron-deficient humans and laboratory animals. However, a defect in the activity of other protein kinases involved in the regulation of the cell-cycle progression cannot be ruled out (Lucas *et al.*, 1995).

Effects of Iron Overload on Immunity

In contrast to the numerous studies conducted in humans and laboratory animals on the effects of iron deficiency on immune responses, less work has been conducted on the effects of iron overload on immune functions. Part of the reason for this is the fact that primary iron overload is not as common as iron deficiency. However, iron overload due to repeated blood transfusion in patients with haemoglobinopathies or renal disease is not rare.

Iron overload and T-cell functions

Patients with iron overload due to multiple transfusion (beta-thalassaemia, sickle-cell disease) generally have reduced proportions of T lymphocytes and

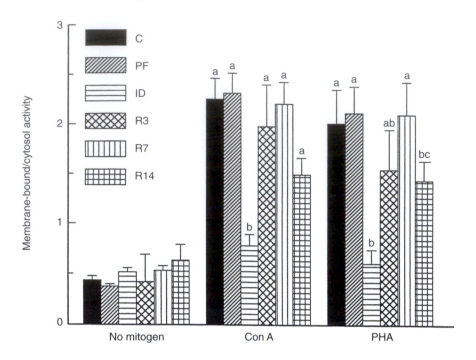

Fig. 11.3. Protein kinase C translocation from the cytosol to the cell membrane of lymphocytes as a function of iron status. Values are mean ± standard error of the mean ratio of membrane-bound protein kinase C activity to cytosolic protein kinase C activity. C, control; PF, pair-fed; ID, iron-deficient; R3, R7 and R14, iron-deficient mice that received the control diet (repletion protocol) for 3 days (R3), 7 days (R7) and 14 days (R14); Con A, concanavalin A; PHA, phytohaemagglutinin. Bars with different letters are significantly different from each other ($P < 0.05$). (Reproduced with permission from John Wiley & Sons Inc., from Kuvibidila *et al.*, 1999.)

CD4+ T-cells and a reduced ratio of CD4+/CD8+ T-cells (Gugliemo *et al.*, 1984; Kaplan *et al.*, 1984; Dwyer *et al.*, 1987; Table 11.1). Lymphocyte proliferative responses to mitogens and delayed-type hypersensitivity skin responses to antigens are also reduced in these patients (Hernandez *et al.*, 1980; Munn *et al.*, 1981; Escalona *et al.*, 1987). However, it is not always certain whether the reduction in the proportion of T-cells is due to iron overload alone or to a combination with other factors, such as alloantigen sensitization or the coexistence of other nutrient deficiencies (protein–energy malnutrition, zinc, vitamin A, vitamin E), which are also known to impair cell-mediated and non-specific immunity (Kuvibidila *et al.*, 1993). However, since iron chelation by desferrioxamine has been shown to improve lymphocyte proliferation, there is no doubt that iron overload plays some role in impaired immune responses in transfused patients. While there is no information on cytokine secretion, the percentages of CD3+, CD4+ and CD8+ T-cells are slightly increased and lymphocyte proliferative responses to mitogens are reduced in untreated patients with hereditary haemochromatosis (Bryan *et al.*, 1991). Following iron chelation, the

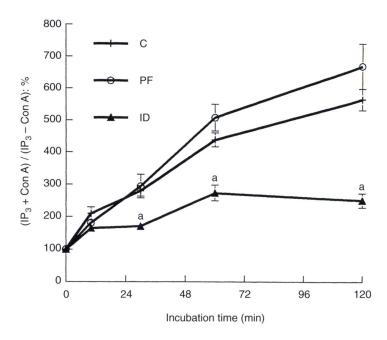

Fig. 11.4. Hydrolysis of cell-membrane phosphatidyl inositol-4,5-bisphosphate in murine lymphocytes as a function of iron status. Data are mean + standard error of the mean IP$_3$ generation in the presence of Con A/IP$_3$ generation in the absence of Con A, expressed as a percentage of that ratio at zero time. C, control; PF, pair-fed; ID, iron-deficient; Con A, concanavalin A; IP$_3$, inositol-1,3,5-trisphosphate; [a],$P < 0.01$ vs. control and pair-fed mice. (Adapted, with permission from the American Society for Nutritional Sciences, from Kuvibidila *et al.*, 1998.)

percentages of CD3+ and CD4+ T-cells returned to normal levels, while those of CD8+ decreased below normal levels.

Data on T-cell functions in laboratory animals with iron overload are inconsistent. While lymphocyte proliferation is impaired in mice (Omara and Blakley, 1994), it is increased in iron-overloaded rats (Wu *et al.*, 1990). The secretion of IL-2 (Omara and Blakley, 1994) and IFN-γ (Mencacci *et al.*, 1997) by mitogen-activated murine spleen cells is suppressed by iron overload. In contrast to this down-regulation of T-helper-1-type response, iron overload up-regulates the T-helper-2-type response: the secretion of IL-4 and IL-10 in response to *Candida albicans* is significantly increased when compared with spleen cells from mice with normal iron status (Mencacci *et al.*, 1997).

Iron overload and B-cell functions

As is the case for T-cells, very little information is available on B-cell functions in non-transfusion patients with iron overload. However, it appears that the humoral immunity is not impaired by iron overload (Table 11.3). In fact, IgG,

IgA, IgM and total Ig secretion by non-activated and pokeweed mitogen-stimulated peripheral blood mononuclear cells obtained from patients with hereditary haemochromatosis is higher than that of cells from control individuals
(Bryan et al., 1991). In patients with β-thalassaemia and those with sickle-cell
disease, B-cell numbers and Ig concentrations are elevated (Glassman et al.,
1980; Escalona et al., 1987). Serum concentrations of IgE specific for C. albicans are increased several-fold in iron-overloaded mice compared with mice
with normal iron status (Mencacci et al., 1997).

Iron overload and macrophage functions

While iron overload has no effects on the secretion of TNF-α by bacterial
lipopolysaccharide-activated alveolar macrophages, it reduces the secretion of
IL-1β (O'Brien-Ladner et al., 1998; Table 11.4). Further support for a negative
effect of iron overload on IL-1 secretion is provided by increased levels following iron chelation by desferrioxamine. Macrophage phagocytosis and the secretion of nitric oxide and IL-12 are not affected by iron overload (Mencacci et al.,
1997).

    The role of iron in microbial killing by monocytes/macrophages is complex.
Iron is required for the generation of hydroxyl radicals, which are more potent
anti-microbial agents than hydrogen peroxide and superoxide anion, which are
produced during the oxidative burst. The limited existing data suggest that
macrophage killing capacity is either normal or slightly decreased in iron overload (Brock, 1992). However, when iron is added to the culture medium,
macrophage killing capacity of certain microorganisms, such as Brucella abortus, Staphylococcus aureus and Mycobacterium tuberculosis, is increased
(Jiang and Baldwin, 1993; Byrd, 1997).

Iron overload and neutrophil functions

Iron overload also has deleterious effects on neutrophil functions. Secondary
iron overload due to multiple blood transfusions in patients with beta-thalassaemia (Cantinieaux et al., 1987) and those with renal disease (Waterlot et
al., 1985; Flament et al., 1986) is associated with reduced phagocytosis of
various microorganisms (yeast, S. aureus, Escherichia coli) (Table 11.3).
Nitroblue tetrazolium reduction, zymozan opsonization, myeloperoxidase
activity and bactericidal capacity are also impaired in patients who are iron-
overloaded due to transfusion (Waterlot et al., 1985; Cantinieaux et al.,
1987). Although there are other factors that can contribute to impaired neutrophil functions in transfused patients, the improved neutrophil phagocytosis
and bactericidal capacity following decreased body iron stores by iron chelation or increased erythropoiesis provide good evidence for the negative
effects of iron overload on neutrophil functions (Boelaert et al., 1990;
Cantinieaux et al., 1999). The secretion of nitric oxide and IL-12 by neutrophils obtained from uninfected and C. albicans-infected mice is abolished

by iron overload when compared with cells obtained from mice with normal iron status (Mencacci *et al.*, 1997).

Iron overload and NK cell function

Although NK activity is not depressed in patients with haemochromatosis (Chapman *et al.*, 1988), it is severely reduced in transfused patients with beta-thalassaemia or sickle-cell disease (Kaplan *et al.*, 1984). However, while *in vitro* incubation with desferrioxamine improved NK activity, *in vivo* administration of the same chelator to patients with beta-thalassaemia failed to correct it. This is most probably due to insufficient reduction of iron levels in NK cells or to the presence of some confounding variables that also impair NK activity. There is no information on NK activity in laboratory animals with iron overload.

Iron Status and Infection

The role of iron in cell division and cellular functions is well established. Almost all living cells, including bacteria, fungi, protozoa, mammalian cells from various tissues (including those of the immune system) require iron for DNA synthesis and many other cellular functions (Cazzalo *et al.*, 1990). In addition to its role for ribonucleotide reductase activity, iron is also a cofactor of enzymes involved in cell respiration, antioxidant defence (catalase) and neutrophil bacterial killing (myeloperoxidase). Microorganisms need iron in the concentration range of 22–220 μg l^{-1} (Payne and Finkelstein, 1978). Although an insufficient supply of iron will diminish the growth of microorganisms (Patruta and Horl, 1999), the iron in human body fluids and tissues is potentially more than sufficient to sustain optimal growth of microorganisms (Fairbank, 1988; Cook and Skikne, 1989; Cazzalo *et al.*, 1990). However, this iron is tightly bound to various proteins (haemoglobin, myoglobin, ferritin, lactoferrin, transferrin and various enzymes) and therefore is, in general, unavailable to microorganisms. On the host's side, too little iron may impair immune responses, especially those that require cell proliferation and bactericidal activity. Too much iron is toxic to cells, as it induces peroxidation of intracellular and cell-membrane macromolecules, and it may also impair immune functions. Thus, there must be a suitable amount of iron available to support immune function, while not promoting the growth of infectious agents above that with which the host defence can cope. The importance of this subtle balance probably explains the variety of observations that have been made with regard to the influence of iron status on susceptibility to infection. Some observations demonstrate that iron promotes infection, suggesting that iron deficiency is 'beneficial', as it may protect from infectious illnesses. Other observations show that iron protects from infection, which implies that iron deficiency is deleterious and may promote infection. Yet other observations indicate that iron status alone is probably insufficient to determine susceptibility to infection. Supporting data on each of these views exist in the literature and have been reviewed by other authors (Walter *et al.*, 1997; Patruta and Horl, 1999).

Evidence that iron may promote infection

Several studies have been published that suggest that iron may promote infections. For example, administration of iron, especially to neonates and school-age children, increased various types of infection (Barry and Reeve, 1977; Murray *et al.*, 1978a, b; Smith *et al.*, 1989) and, in some studies, mortality was significantly increased (see McFarlane *et al.*, 1970; Brock, 1993). In support of the idea that iron promotes infection is the observation that, during infection, the host responds by decreasing serum iron concentration and shifting it to storage in the reticuloendothelial cells; it may be that this is an attempt by the host to deprive the invading microorganisms of iron.

The situation regarding iron status and malaria is complicated by the fact that it is the red blood cell that is parasitized. The malaria parasite is totally dependent upon red blood cells of the host to complete its life cycle. This might explain the observations that malaria is more common in iron-replete than in iron-deficient individuals (Oppenheimer *et al.*, 1986) and that the levels of malaria infection and the severity of disease were increased by iron supplementation (Murray *et al.*, 1978a, b).

Evidence that iron may protect from infection and that iron deficiency may promote infection

Some studies have shown that prevention, as well as treatment, of iron deficiency by medicinal iron and food fortification reduces the rate of respiratory and non-respiratory infections (e.g. Chwang *et al.*, 1988; Hussein *et al.*, 1988).

Evidence that iron status alone may not determine susceptibility to infections

Several studies suggest that iron status does not affect susceptibility to infections (e.g. Snow *et al.*, 1991; Heresi *et al.*, 1995; Menendez *et al.*, 1997). In a study, conducted in Tanzania, of more than 800 infants, iron supplementation for 24 weeks starting at 8 weeks of age did not significantly affect the rate of malarial infection (Menendez *et al.*, 1997). Unfortunately, the rate of other types of infection was not reported. Iron fortification during the first year of life in Chilean children did not alter the rate of diarrhoeal diseases and respiratory infections (Heresi *et al.*, 1995). In fact, the rate of infection was higher in children with iron deficiency compared with children with adequate iron status, regardless of iron treatment. However, it was unclear from the paper what came first, iron deficiency or infection.

Conclusions

In spite of the numerous human and laboratory animal studies showing that many cell-mediated and non-specific immune responses are impaired in iron deficiency, the relationship between iron deficiency and infection is far less clear. Unfortunately, the issue of susceptibility to infection is very complex and depends not only on iron status, but also on many host, parasite and environmental factors (Keush, 1990). Some of these factors include exposure to microorganisms, the presence of other nutritional deficiencies, the type of population (neonates, young children, women, men, elderly), the severity and duration of iron deficiency, the type, dose and duration of iron therapy and pre-existing conditions (primary and secondary immunodeficiencies). There is no doubt that these confounding factors affect susceptibility to and severity of infection, regardless of iron status. However, based on published data, the two extremes of iron nutritional status – iron deficiency and iron overload – both have detrimental effects on cell-mediated and non-specific immunity. Iron deficiency and iron overload will therefore affect susceptibility to certain types of infections, and the severity and duration of infection will vary according to host and parasite factors (extracellular versus intracellular microorganisms). In summary, oral and intramuscular iron administration of therapeutic doses to immunocompromised (malnourished) individuals is associated with increased risk of morbidity due to malaria and other infectious diseases and should therefore be avoided. In contrast, since there is no evidence of deleterious effect of oral iron supplementation to immunocompetent individuals, prevention of iron deficiency either by iron supplementation or food fortification, should remain among the priorities of public health.

Acknowledgement

The authors' work is supported by the National Institutes of Health (NIH) Grant No. HL03144 and a Research Enhancement Grant from Louisiana State University Health Sciences Center.

References

Alcantara, O., Javors, M. and Boldt, D.H. (1991) Induction of protein kinase C mRNA in cultured lymphoblastoid T-cell by iron-transferrin but not soluble iron. *Blood* 77, 1290–1297.

Alcantara, O., Obeid, L., Hannun, Y., Ponka, P. and Boldt, D.H. (1994) Regulation of protein kinase C (PKC) by iron: effect of different iron compounds on PKC-beta and PKC-alpha expression and role of the 5′ flanking region of the PKC-beta gene in the response to ferric transferrin. *Blood* 84, 3510–3517.

Bagchi, K., Mohanram, M. and Reddy, V. (1980) Humoral immune response in children with iron deficiency. *British Medical Journal* 280, 1249–1251.

Barry, D.M.J. and Reeve, A.W. (1977) Increased incidence of gram negative neonatal sepsis with intramuscular iron administration. *Pediatrics* 60, 908–912.

Bhaskaram, C. and Reddy, V. (1975) Cell-mediated immunity in iron and vitamin-deficient children. *British Medical Journal* 3, 522.

Bhaskaram, P., Sherada, K., Sivakumar, B., Rao, K.V. and Nair, M. (1989) Effect of iron and vitamin A deficiencies on macrophage function in children. *Nutrition Research* 9, 35–45.

Boelaert, J.R., Cantinieaux, B.F., Hariga, C.F. and Fondu, P.G. (1990) Recombinant erythropoietin reverses polymorphonuclear granulocyte dysfunction in iron-overloaded dialysis patients. *Nephrology Dialysis Transplantation* 5, 504–507.

Brieland, J.K. and Fantone, J.C. (1991) Ferrous iron release from transferrin by human neutrophil-derived superoxide anion: effect of pH and iron saturation. *Archives of Biochemistry and Biophysics* 284, 78–83.

Brock, J.H. (1992) Iron and the immune system. In: Lauffer, R.B. (ed.) *Iron and Human Disease*. CRC Press, Boca Raton, Florida, pp. 161–178.

Brock, J.H. (1993) Iron and immunity. *Journal of Nutritional Immunology* 2, 47–106.

Bryan, C.F., Leech, S.H., Kumar, P., Gaumer, R., Bozelka, B. and Morgan, J. (1991) The immune system in hereditary hemochromatosis: a quantitative and functional assessment of cellular arm. *American Journal of Medical Science* 301, 55–61.

Byrd, T.F. (1997) Tumor necrosis factor alpha promotes growth of virulent mycobacterium tuberculosis in human monocytes: iron-mediated growth suppression is correlated with decreased release of TNF-alpha from iron-treated infected monocytes. *Journal of Clinical Investigation* 99, 2518–2529.

Cantinieaux, B.F., Hariga, C., Ferster, A., De-Maertaere, E., Toppet, M. and Fondu, P. (1987) Neutrophil dysfunctions in thalassemia major: the role of cell iron overload. *European Journal of Haematology* 39, 28–34.

Cantinieaux, B., Janssens, A., Boelaert J.R., Lejeune, M., Vermylen, C., Kerrels, V., Cornu, J., Winand, J. and Fondu, P. (1999) Ferritin-associated iron induces neutrophil dysfunction in hemosiderosis. *Journal of Laboratory and Clinical Medicine* 133, 353–361.

Cazzalo, M., Bergamaschi, G., Dezza, L. and Arosio, P. (1990) Manipulation of cellular iron metabolism for modulating normal and malignant cell proliferation: achievement and prospects. *Blood* 75, 1903–1919.

Chandra, R.K. and Saraya, A.K. (1975) Impaired immunocompetence associated with iron deficiency. *Journal of Pediatrics* 86, 899–902.

Chapman, D.E., Good, M.F., Powell, L.W. and Halliday, J.W. (1988) The effects of iron, iron-binding proteins and iron overload on human natural killer cell activity. *Journal of Gastroenterology and Hepatology* 3, 9–17.

Chwang, L.C., Soemantri, A.G. and Pollitt, E. (1988) Iron supplementation and physical growth of rural Indonesia children. *American Journal of Clinical Nutrition* 47, 496–501.

Cook, J.D. and Skikne, B.S. (1989) Iron deficiency and diagnosis. *Journal of Internal Medicine* 226, 349–355.

Dallman, P.R. (1987) Iron deficiency and the immune response. *American Journal of Clinical Nutrition* 46, 329–334.

Dhur, A., Galan, P., Hannoun, C., Hout, K. and Hercberg, S. (1990) Effects of iron deficiency upon the antibody response to influenza virus in rats. *Journal of Nutritional Biochemistry* 1, 629–634.

Dwyer, J., Wood, C., McNamara, J., Williams, A., Andiman, W., Rink, L., O'Connor, T. and Pearson, H. (1987) Abnormalities in the immune system of children with beta-thalassaemia major. *Experimental Immunology* 68, 621–629.

Escalona, E., Malave, I., Rodriguez, E., Araujo, Z., Inati, J., Arends, A. and Perdomo, Y. (1987) Mitogen-induced lymphoproliferative responses and lymphocyte subpopulations in patients with sickle disease. *Journal of Clinical and Laboratory Immunology* 22, 191–196.

Fairbank, V.F. (1988) Iron-deficiency anemia. In: Mazza, J.J. (ed.) *Manual of Clinical Hematology*. Little Brown, Boston, Massachusetts, pp. 1–48.

Flament, J., Goldman, M., Waterlot, Y., Dupont, E., Wybran, J. and Vanherweghem, J.L. (1986) Impairment of phagocyte oxidative metabolism in hemodialyzed patients with iron overload. *Clinical Nephrology* 25, 227–230.

Galan, P., Thibault, H., Preziosi, P. and Hercberg, S. (1992) Interleukin-2 production in iron-deficient children. *Biological Trace Element Research* 32, 421–426.

Glassman, A.B., Deas, D.V., Berlinsky, F.S. and Bennett, C.E. (1980) Lymphocytic blast transformation and peripheral lymphocyte percentages in patients with sickle cell disease. *Annals of Clinical and Laboratory Science* 10, 9–12.

Guglielmo, P., Cunsolo, F., Lombardo, T., Sortino, G., Giustolisi, R., Cacciola, E. and Cacciola, E. (1984) T-cell subset abnormalities in thalassemia intermedia: possible evidence for thymus functional deficiency. *Acta Haematologia* 72, 361–367.

Helyar, L. and Sherman, A.D. (1987) Iron deficiency and interleukin-1 production by rat leucocytes. *American Journal of Clinical Nutrition* 46, 346–352.

Helyar, L. and Sherman, R.A. (1992) Moderate and severe iron deficiency lowers numbers of spleen T lymphocyte and B lymphocyte subsets in the C57BL/6 mouse. *Nutrition Research* 12, 1113–1122.

Heresi, G., Pizarro, F., Olivares, M., Cayazzo, M., Hertampg, E., Walter, T., Murphy, R.J. and Stekel, A. (1995) Effect of supplementation with iron-fortified milk on incidence of diarrhea and respiratory infection in urban-resident infants. *Scandinavian Journal of Infectious Disease* 27, 385–389.

Hernandez, P., Cruz, C., Santos, M.N. and Ballester, J.M. (1980) Immunologic dysfunction in sickle cell anemia. *Acta Haematologica* 63, 156–161.

Humbert, J.R. and Moore, L.J. (1983) Iron deficiency and infection: a dilemma. *Journal of Pediatric Gastroenterology and Nutrition* 2, 403–406.

Hussein, M.A., Hassan, H., Abdel-Ghaffer, A.A. and Salen, S. (1988) Effects of iron supplementation on the occurrence of diarrhea among children in rural Egypt. *Food and Nutrition Bulletin* 10, 35–39.

Jiang, X. and Baldwin, C.L. (1993) Iron augments macrophage-mediated killing of *Brucella abortus* alone and in conjunction with interferon-gamma. *Cellular Immunology* 148, 397–407.

Joynson, D.H.M., Murray-Walker, D., Jacobs, A. and Dolby, A.E. (1972) Defects of cell-mediated immunity in patients with iron-deficiency anaemia. *Lancet* ii, 1058–1059.

Kaplan, J., Sanarik, S., Gitlin, J. and Lusher, J. (1984) Diminished helper to suppressor lymphocyte ratios and natural killer cell activity in recipients of repeated blood transfusions. *Blood* 64, 308–310.

Kemahli, A.S., Babacan, E. and Cavdar, A.O. (1988) Cell mediated immune responses in children with iron deficiency and combined iron and zinc deficiency. *Nutrition* 8, 129–136.

Kemp, J.D. (1993) The role of iron and iron binding proteins in lymphocyte physiology and pathology. *Journal of Clinical Immunology* 13, 81–92.

Keush, G.T. (1990) Micronutrients and susceptibility to infection. *Annals of the New York Academy of Science* 589, 181–189.

Kochanowski, B.A. and Sherman, A.R. (1985) Decreased antibody formation in iron-deficient rat pups – effect of iron repletion. *American Journal of Clinical Nutrition* 41, 278–284.

Krantman, H.J., Young, S.R., Ank, B.J., O'Donnell, C.M., Rachelefsky, G.S. and Stiehm, E.R. (1982) Immune function in pure iron deficiency. *American Journal of Diseases of Children* 136, 840–844.

Kuvibidila, S. and Wade, S. (1987) Macrophage function as studied by the clearance of ^{125}I-labeled polyvinylpyrrolidone in iron-deficient and iron-replete mice. *Journal of Nutrition* 117, 170–176.

Kuvibidila, S.R., Baliga, B.S. and Suskind, R.M. (1981) Effects of iron deficiency anemia on delayed cutaneous hypersensitivity in mice. *American Journal of Clinical Nutrition* 34, 2635–2640.

Kuvibidila, S.R., Baliga, B.S. and Suskind, R.M. (1982) Generation of plaque forming cells in iron-deficient anemic mice. *Nutrition Reports International* 26, 861–871.

Kuvibidila, S., Nauss, K.M., Baliga, B.S. and Suskind, R.M. (1983a) Impairment of blastogenic response of splenic lymphocytes from iron-deficient mice: *in vivo* repletion. *American Journal of Clinical Nutrition* 37, 15–25.

Kuvibidila, S.R., Baliga, B.S. and Suskind, R.M. (1983b) The effects of iron deficiency on cytolytic activity of mice spleen and peritoneal cells against allogenic tumor cells. *American Journal of Clinical Nutrition* 38, 238–244.

Kuvibidila, S., Baliga, S.B. and Suskind, R.M. (1989) Consequences of iron deficiency on infection and immunity. In: Lebenthal, E. (ed.) *Textbook of Gastroenterology and Nutrition in Infancy*, 2nd edn. Raven Press, New York, pp. 423–431.

Kuvibidila, S., Dardenne, M., Savino, W. and Lepault, F. (1990) Influence of iron-deficiency anemia on selected thymus functions in mice: thymulin biological activity, T-cell subsets and thymocyte proliferation. *American Journal of Clinical Nutrition* 51, 228–232.

Kuvibidila, S., Baliga, B.S. and Murthy, K.K. (1991) Impaired protein kinase C activation as one of the possible mechanisms of reduced lymphocyte proliferation in iron deficiency in mice. *American Journal of Clinical Nutrition* 54, 944–950.

Kuvibidila, S., Baliga, B.S. and Murthy, K.K. (1992) Alteration of interleukin-2 (IL-2) production in iron deficiency anemia. *Journal of Nutritional Immunology* 1, 81–88.

Kuvibidila, S., Yu, L., Ode, D. and Warrier, R.P. (1993) The immune response in protein–energy malnutrition and single nutrient deficiencies. In: Klurfeld, D.M. (ed.) *Nutrition and Immunology*. Plenum Press, New York, pp. 121–155.

Kuvibidila, S.R., Baliga, B.S., Warrier, R.P. and Suskind, R.M. (1998) Iron deficiency reduces the hydrolysis of cell membrane phosphatidyl inositol-4,5-bisphosphate during splenic lymphocyte activation in C57BL/6 mice. *Journal of Nutrition* 128, 1077–1083.

Kuvibidila, S., Kitchens, D. and Baliga, B.S. (1999) *In vivo* and *in vitro* iron deficiency reduces protein kinase C activation and translocation in murine splenic and purified T-cells. *Journal of Cellular Biochemistry* 74, 468–478.

Kuvibidila, S.R., Porretta, C., Baliga, B.S. and Leiva, L.E. (2001) Reduced thymocyte proliferation but not increased apoptosis as a possible cause of thymus atrophy in iron-deficient mice. *British Journal of Nutrition* 86, 157–162.

Latunde-Dada, G.O. and Young, A.P. (1992) Iron deficiency and immune responses. *Scandinavian Journal of Immunology* 11 (Suppl.), 207–209.

Lucas, J.J., Szepesi, A., Domenico, J., Takase, K., Tordai, A., Terada, N. and Gelfand, E.W. (1995) Effects of iron-depletion on cell-cycle progression in normal human T lymphocytes: selective inhibition of appearance of the cyclin A-associated component of the p33[cdk2] kinase. *Blood* 86, 2268–2280.

MacDougall, L.G., Anderson, R., McNab, G.M. and Katz, J. (1975) Immune response in iron-deficient children: impaired cellular defence mechanisms with altered humoral components. *Journal of Pediatrics* 86, 833–843.

McFarlane, H., Reddy, S., Adcock, K.J., Adeshina, H., Cooke, A.R. and Akene, J. (1970) Immunity, transferrin, and survival in kwashiorkor. *British Medical Journal* 4, 268–270.

Mencacci, A., Cenci, E., Boelaert, J.R., Bucci, P., Mosci, P., Fe d'Ostiani, C., Bistoni, F. and Romani, L. (1997) Iron overload alters innate and T helper cell response to *Candida albicans* in mice. *Journal of Infectious Disease* 175, 1467–1476.

Menendez, C., Kahigwa, E., Hirt, R., Vounatsou, P., Aponte, J.J., Font, F., Acosta, C.J., Schellenberg, D.M., Galindo, C.M., Kimario, J., Urassa, H., Brabin, B., Smith, T.A., Kitua, A.Y., Tanner, M. and Alanso, P.L. (1997) Randomised placebo-controlled trial of iron supplementation and malaria chemoprophylaxis for prevention of severe anaemia and malaria in Tanzanian infants. *Lancet* 350, 844–850.

Munn, C.G., Markenson, A.L., Kapadia, A. and De Sousa, M. (1981) Impaired T-cell mitogen responses in some patients with thalassemia intermedia. *Thymus* 3, 119–128.

Murakawa, H., Bland, C.E., Willis, W.T. and Dallman, P.R. (1987) Iron deficiency and neutrophil function: different rates of correction of the depressions in oxidative burst and myeloperoxidase activity after iron treatment. *Blood* 69, 1464–1468.

Murray, M.J., Murray, A.B., Murray, N.J. and Murray, M.B. (1978a) Diet and cerebral malaria: the effect of famine and re-feeding. *American Journal of Clinical Nutrition* 31, 57–61.

Murray, M.J., Murray, A.B., Murray, M.B. and Murray, C.J. (1978b) The adverse effect of iron repletion on the course of certain infections. *British Medical Journal* 2, 1113–1115.

Nalder, B.N., Mahoney, A.W., Ramakrishnan, R. and Hendricks, D.G. (1972) Sensitivity of the immunological response to nutritional status of rats. *Journal of Nutrition* 102, 535–542.

Neckers, L.M. and Cossman, J. (1983) Transferrin receptor induction in mitogen-stimulated human T lymphocytes is required for DNA synthesis and cell division and is regulated by interleukin-2. *Proceedings of the National Academy of Sciences of the USA* 80, 3494–3498.

Neckers, L.M., Yenokida, G. and James, S.P. (1984) The role of transferrin receptor in human B lymphocyte activation. *Journal of Immunology* 133, 2437–2441.

O'Brien-Ladner, A.R., Blumer, B.M. and Wesselius, L.J. (1998) Differential regulation of alveolar macrophage-derived interleukin-1 beta and tumor necrosis factor-alpha by iron. *Journal of Laboratory and Clinical Medicine* 132, 497–506.

Omara, F.O. and Blakley, B.R. (1994) The effects of iron deficiency and iron overload on cell-mediated immunity in the mouse. *British Journal of Nutrition* 72, 899–909.

Oppenheimer, S.J., Gibson, F.D., MacFarlane, S.B., Moody, J.B., Harrison, C., Spencer, A. and Bunari, O. (1986) Iron supplementation increases prevalence and effects of malaria: report on clinical studies in Papua New Guinea. *Transactions of the Royal Society of Tropical Medicine and Hygiene* 80, 603–612.

Parmley, R.T., Hajdu, I. and Denys, F.R. (1983) Ultrastructural localization of the transferrin receptor and transferrin on marrow cell surfaces. *British Journal of Haematology* 54, 633–641.

Patruta, S.L. and Horl, W. (1999) Iron and infection. *Kidney International* 55(Suppl. 69), S125–S130.

Payne, S.M. and Finkelstein, R.A. (1978) The critical role of iron in host–bacterial interaction. *Journal of Clinical Investigation* 61, 1428–1440.

Perkkio, M.V., Jansson, L.T., Dallman, P.R., Siimes, M.A. and Savilahti, E. (1987) sIgA and IgM-containing cells in intestinal mucosa of iron deficient rats. *American Journal of Clinical Nutrition* 46, 341–345.

Prema, K., Ramalakshmi, B.A., Madhavapeddi, R. and Babu, S. (1982) Immune status of anaemic pregnant women. *British Journal of Obstetrics and Gynaecology* 89, 222–225.

Sainte-Marie, J., LaFont, E.I., Pecheur E.I., Favero, J., Philippot, J.R. and Bienvenue, A. (1997) Transferrin receptor functions as a signal-transduction molecule for its own recycling via increases in the internal Ca^{2+} concentration. *European Journal of Biochemistry* 250, 689–697.

Santos, P.C. and Falcao, R.P. (1990) Decreased lymphocyte subsets and K-cell activity in iron deficiency anemia. *Acta Haematologica* 84, 118–121.

Smith, A.W., Hendrickse, R.G., Harrison, C., Hayes, R.J. and Greenwood, B.M. (1989) The effects on malaria of treatment of iron-deficiency anaemia with oral iron in Gambian children. *Annals of Tropical Paediatrics* 9, 17–23.

Snow, R.W., Byass, P., Shenton, F.C. and Greewood, B.M. (1991) The relationship between anthropometric measurements and measurements of iron status and sus-ceptibility to malaria in Gambian children. *Transactions of the Royal Society of Tropical Medicine and Hygiene* 85, 584–589.

Spear, A.T. and Sherman, A.R. (1992) Iron deficiency alters DMBA-induced tumor bur-den and natural killer cell cytotoxicity in rats. *Journal of Nutrition* 122, 46–55.

Strauss, R.G. (1978) Iron deficiency, infections, and immune function: a reassessment. *American Journal of Clinical Nutrition* 31, 660–666.

Srikantia, S.G., Prasad, J.S., Bhaskaram, C. and Krishnamachari, K.A. (1976) Anaemia and the immune response. *Lancet* i, 1307–1309.

Swarup-Mitra, S. and Sinha, A.K. (1984) Cell-mediated immunity in nutritional anaemia. *Indian Journal of Medical Research* 79, 354–362.

Testa, U., Khun, L., Petrini, M., Quaranta, M.T., Pelosi, E. and Peschle, C. (1991) Differential regulation of iron regulatory element-binding protein(s) in cell extracts of activated lymphocytes versus monocytes–macrophages. *Journal of Biological Chemistry* 266, 13925–13930.

Thibault, H., Galan, P., Selz, F., Preziosi, P., Olivier, C., Badoual, J. and Hercberg, S. (1993) The immune response in iron-deficient young children: effect of iron supple-mentation on cell-mediated immunity. *European Journal of Pediatrics* 152, 120–124.

Tormey, D.C., Imrie, R.C. and Mueller, G.C. (1972) Identification of transferrin as a lym-phocyte growth promoter in human serum. *Experimental Cell Research* 74, 163–169.

Vydyborets, S.V. (2000) An analysis of the immunity indices of patients with iron defi-ciency anemia. *Likarska Sprava* 3–4, 71–75.

Walter, T., Arredondo, S., Arevalo, M. and Stekel, A. (1986) Effect of iron therapy on phagocytosis and bactericidal activity in neutrophils of iron-deficient infants. *American Journal of Clinical Nutrition* 44, 877–882.

Walter, T., Olivares, M., Pizzaro, F. and Munoz, C. (1997) Iron, anemia, and infection. *Nutrition Reviews* 55, 111–124.

Waterlot, Y., Cantinieaux, B., Hariga-Muller, C., De-Maertelaere-Laurent, E., Vanherweghem, J.L. and Fondu, P. (1985) Impaired phagocytic activity of neu-trophils in patients receiving hemodialysis: the critical role of iron overload. *British Medical Journal* 291, 501–504.

Wu, W.H., Meydani, M., Meyani, S.N., Burklund, P.M., Blumberg, J.B. and Munro, H.N. (1990) Effects of dietary iron overload on lipid peroxidation, prostaglandin synthe-sis and lymphocyte proliferation in young and old rats. *Journal of Nutrition* 120, 280–289.

Yetgin, S., Altay, C., Ciliv, G. and Laleli, Y. (1979) Myeloperoxidase activity and bacteri-cidal function of PMN in iron deficiency. *Acta Haematologica* 61, 10–14.

Yip, R. and Dallman, P.R. (1996) Iron. In: Ziegler, E. and Filer, L.J., Jr (eds) *Present Knowledge in Nutrition*, 7th edn. International Life Sciences Institute Press, Washington, DC, pp. 276–292.

12 Selenium and the Immune System

Roddie C. McKenzie*[1], John R. Arthur[2],
Susan M. Miller[3], Teresa S. Rafferty[1] and
Geoffrey J. Beckett[3]

[1]Department of Medical and Radiological Sciences, University of
Edinburgh, Lauriston Building, Royal Infirmary of Edinburgh, Edinburgh
EH3 9YW, UK; [2]Division of Cell Integrity, Rowett Research Institute,
Bucksburn, Aberdeen AB21 9SB, UK; [3]Department of Clinical Biochemistry,
University of Edinburgh, Lauriston Building, Royal Infirmary of Edinburgh,
Edinburgh EH3 9YW, UK

Introduction

Selenium (Se) modulates immunity: Se deficiency impairs immunity, Se intakes
above those habitually consumed in many Western countries boost immunity
and high Se intakes lead to toxic effects and suppression of immunity. This
chapter will first review the metabolism of Se and its incorporation into Se-con-
taining proteins (selenoproteins), which mediate many of the immune effects of
Se. The function of individual selenoproteins will be reviewed briefly and this
will be followed by a description of the effects of Se on immunity and the protective role of Se in inflammation and viral infection.

Historical Background

Se can be highly toxic, with signs and symptoms starting to occur in humans if
the daily intake exceeds approximately 0.8–1 mg. Studies in the 1940s
suggested that Se may be a potential carcinogen, but, paradoxically, it is now
recognized that Se has powerful anti-cancer properties. Although initially it was
the toxic properties of Se that generated scientific interest, in 1957 Schwartz
and Foltz (Schwartz and Foltz, 1957) found that Se could prevent hepatic

*Corresponding author.

© CAB International 2002. Nutrition and Immune Function
(eds P.C. Calder, C.J. Field and H.S. Gill)

necrosis in vitamin E-deficient rats. This observation led to the acceptance that Se was an essential trace element. The discovery in 1973 that Se was a constitutive part of cytoplasmic glutathione peroxidase (cyGPX) provided a mechanism by which the trace element could exert its biological actions. It was thus hypothesized that Se exerted its effects through modifying the expression of this important antioxidant enzyme (Vernie, 1984). However, it soon became apparent that Se must have other means for exerting some of its biological actions, since, for example, changes in the expression of drug-metabolizing enzymes observed in Se-deficient mice could be reversed using doses of Se that had no effects on GPX expression. Labelling experiments on cells and animal tissue with ^{75}Se-selenite demonstrated that more than 35 selenoproteins, with diverse roles, are expressed by tissues. It is now widely recognized that, in addition to exerting important antioxidant activity, Se can act as a growth factor and an anti-cancer agent and is required to ensure thyroid hormone homoeostasis and optimal fertility and immune function. Although many of the biological effects of Se operate through modifying the expression of selenoenzymes, there is good evidence to suggest that some actions of Se (such as its anti-cancer properties) may operate independently of these selenoproteins (Reilly, 1993; Arthur and Beckett, 1994; Foster and Sumar, 1997; Allan *et al.*, 1999).

Selenoproteins

Synthesis

Mammalian selenoproteins contain selenocysteine residues, usually at their active sites. The importance of the selenocysteine residue lies in the fact that, at physiological pH, the residue is fully ionized, allowing it to participate effectively in redox-type reactions. In contrast, cysteine residues, which may also participate in redox reactions, are only approximately 10% ionized at physiological pH. Selenocysteine residues are incorporated at specific sites in the selenoproteins through a co-translational event directed by the UGA codon. Although the UGA codon can be recognized by the cell as a termination codon, in selenoprotein synthesis the UGA codon also signals the insertion of a selenocysteine residue. The recognition of the UGA codon to signal the insertion of a selenocysteine residue requires selenocysteine insertion sequence (SECIS) elements. In eukaryotes, the SECIS elements are located in the 3′ untranslated region of the mRNA and comprise a small number of conserved nucleotides, which form a stem–loop structure. These SECIS elements are different for each selenoprotein but form a similar-shaped stem loop and are functionally interchangeable (Berry, 1991).

The synthesis of selenocysteine and its insertion into specific selenoproteins in prokaryotes involves the products of four genes (*selA*, *selB*, *selC* and *selD*). The products are: a selenocysteine-specific tRNA species (tRNA^{Sec}) (*selC*), which carries the anticodon for UGA, the enzymes selenocysteine synthase (*selA*) and selenophosphate synthetase (*selD*), which are essential for the formation of selenocysteine-tRNA^{Sec} from seryl-tRNA^{Sec}, and the elongation factor, which specifically recognizes the selenocysteine-tRNA (*selB*) (Bermano *et al.*, 1995; Allan *et al.*, 1999).

The lack of a series of mutants has delayed the description of the mechanism of selenocysteine incorporation and selenoprotein synthesis in eukaryotes. However, two forms of the tRNA^Sec have been isolated in eukaryotes and both contain the UGA anticodon, which is functional in *Escherichia coli* (Kollmus *et al.*, 1996; Low and Berry, 1996). Like bacterial tRNA^Sec, in eukaryotes tRNA^Sec is esterified with serine and is subsequently converted to seryl-tRNA^Sec. The major steps of this co-translational event in eukaryotes are illustrated in Fig. 12.1, highlighting the role of SECIS-binding protein 2 (SBP2) and multiple selenophosphate synthetases (Mansell and Berry, 2001).

Selenoproteins that have been characterized

Although 30–40 selenoproteins have been demonstrated using isotopic labelling, only approximately 20 have been further characterized. The biological actions of some of these selenoproteins are known and are summarized in Table 12.1 (see also Holmgren, 1985, 1989; Beckett and Arthur, 1994; Burk,

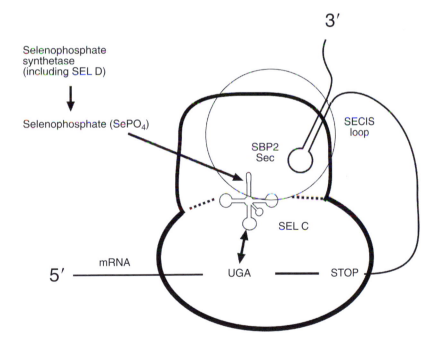

Fig. 12.1. The synthesis of specific selenoproteins. A tRNA that recognizes the stop codon UGA on mRNA forms a complex with the selenocysteine insertion sequence (SECIS) loop in the 3′ untranslated region of the mRNA. Selenophosphate converts a serine bound to the tRNA to selenocysteine; this is then incorporated into the backbone of the protein. The part of the protein complex that carries out this reaction on the ribosome is SBP2; SEL C is the tRNA and SEL D is one of the selenophosphate synthetases.

Table 12.1. Properties of selenoproteins.

Selenoprotein family	Member	Where found	Structural features	Role
Glutathione peroxidase (GPX)	Cytoplasmic GPX (cyGPX)	All cells	Tetramer: four identical subunits (molecular weight 19–25 kDa). Each subunit has a glutathione-binding site and a single selenocysteine residue at the active site	Catalyses reduction of a variety of hydroperoxides, including H_2O_2 and fatty-acid hydroperoxides
	Phospholipid hydroperoxide GPX (PHGPX)	Cytosol and membranes of many cells. High activity in testis	Monomer (molecular weight 19 kDa)	Catalyses reduction of a variety of hydroperoxides, especially fatty-acid and cholesterol hydroperoxides
	Extracellular GPX	Plasma. Synthesized mainly in proximal tubules of kidney; also by thyrocytes	Tetramer	? Accounts for all hydroperoxide-reducing activity of plasma
	Gastrointestinal GPX	Closely related to cyGPX		? Protection of gastrointestinal tract against ingested hydroperoxides
Iodothyronine deiodinase (ID)	ID I	Liver and kidney provide 80% of plasma T3		Thyroid hormone metabolism: catalyses 5- and 5'-monodeiodination of iodothronines (including thyroid hormones). 5'-Deiodination promotes conversion of T4 to its active form T3; 5-deiodination promotes conversion of T4 to the inactive reverse T3

		Structure	Distribution	Function
Iodothyronine deiodinase (ID)	ID II		Brain, CNS, Placenta, pituitary	Catalyses 5'-monodeiodination of iodothyronines (including thyroid hormones)
	ID III		Brain, CNS, Placenta, pituitary	Catalyses 5-monodeiodination of iodothyronines (including thyroid hormones)
Selenoprotein P		Up to ten selenocysteine residues, nine of which are located at the carboxyl terminus	Extracellular (accounts for 40% of plasma Se)	Function not known
Thioredoxin reductase	At least three isoforms exist	FAD-containing homodimer with a single selenocysteine residue near the carboxyl terminus of each subunit chain	All tissues	Along with thioredoxin (substrate) and NADPH (cofactor) forms a powerful dithiol-disulphide oxidoreductase system. Can catalyse the reduction of a variety of chain substrates. Thioredoxin involved as hydrogen donor for ribonucleotide reductase (key step of DNA synthesis). Involved in many cell functions (cell growth, apoptosis inhibition, maintenance of cellular redox state)
Selenoprotein W	Four forms identified (in the rat)		Intracellular. High amounts in brain, muscle, testis and spleen; low amount in liver	? Antioxidant

CNS, central nervous system; NADPH, nicotinamide adenine dinucleotide phosphate; FAD, flavin adenine dinucleotide.

1994; Sunde, 1994; Arthur *et al.*, 1997; St Germain and Galton, 1997; Burk and Hill, 1999; Arner and Holmgren, 2000).

Hierarchy of Selenium Supply in Selenium Deficiency

When Se intake is limited there is a clear hierarchy of Se supply, both to different tissues and to different selenoenzymes within a tissue. Thus, it appears that regulatory mechanisms exist, which ensure that, in Se deficiency, Se levels are maintained in certain priority organs and selenoproteins. Se is well retained by brain, endocrine and reproductive organs, indicating the relative importance of the trace element for the biological functions of these organs. In contrast, Se is lost rapidly from liver and muscle. Within a tissue, iodothyronine deiodinase I and phospholipid hydroperoxide GPX (PHGPX) take priority for expression over cyGPX in Se deficiency (Behne *et al.*, 1988; Bermano *et al.*, 1995).

The mechanisms that regulate the supply of Se to selenoproteins have probably evolved, at least in part, to cope with differing amounts of the micronutrient in the diet. The processes whereby dietary Se finds its way into selenocysteine within specific selenoproteins are complicated, allowing for regulation at many levels. The major portion of Se in the diet is probably in the form of the amino acid selenomethionine. This amino acid is the seleno analogue of methionine and can take part in many of the metabolic pathways for the sulphur-containing amino acid. Se is also found in the diet as selenocysteine and as various inorganic salts, such as selenite and selenate. There is also a large variety of selenosulphur compounds, but quantitatively these may only represent a very small portion of the dietary total Se. Once selenomethionine is absorbed into an animal, it can be metabolized in a similar fashion to methionine and can be incorporated non-specifically into proteins (Fig. 12.2).

The rate of incorporation of selenomethionine is very dependent on the adequacy of methionine levels. Thus, when methionine is limiting, larger portions of selenomethionine are incorporated, due to a mass-action effect. Conversely, when higher levels of methionine are consumed, less selenomethionine is incorporated. Similarly, it is possible that any selenocysteine absorbed into the animal is also incorporated non-specifically into protein. This non-specific incorporation of Se into protein has no known physiological role, although these amino acids may provide a source of Se for production of specific selenoproteins during Se deficiency.

Incorporation of Se into specific selenoproteins requires the complex mechanism described previously. The selenophosphate synthetases operating in this mechanism produce selenophosphate from ATP and a form of Se, which is chemically similar to selenide. Many of the inorganic Se compounds that are absorbed from the diet would be reduced by molecules such as glutathione to selenide-like compounds (Fig. 12.2). However, Se from selenomethionine has to go through a transamination pathway and then reduction. Thus, in mammalian tissue, there are non-specifically incorporated seleno amino acids and selenocysteine incorporated at the active site of the selenoproteins.

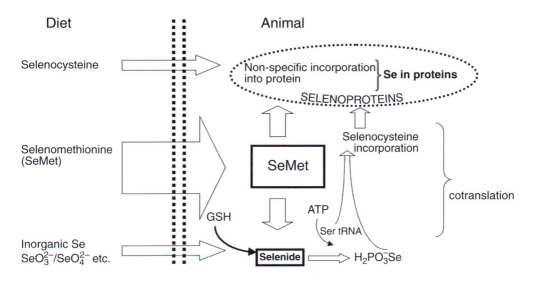

Fig. 12.2. Some pathways of selenium (Se) metabolism. The different forms of Se in the diet are absorbed and the major pool of selenomethionine passes either non-specifically into proteins instead of methionine or passes through an inorganic intermediate similar to selenide, which is then specifically incorporated into selenoproteins. Not shown are the pathways for methylation of excess Se, prior to excretion. GSH, glutathione.

Se metabolism is thus a complex process and this is perhaps not surprising, given the potential chemical reactivity of inorganic Se compounds. The Se as selenocysteine at the active site of enzymes is a very efficient biological catalyst and large amounts of non-specific incorporation of the amino acid might lead to inappropriate biochemical reactions within the body. The predominance of selenomethionine as a dietary source of the micronutrient provides a relatively inert source, which through well-regulated metabolic pathways can be specifically incorporated into the active site of the specific selenoproteins (for a review, see Daniels, 1996).

Effects of Selenium on the Immune System

Studies over the past 30 years have demonstrated that an adequate Se intake is essential for both cell-mediated and humoral (antibody-mediated) immunity (for reviews, see Spallholz *et al.*, 1990; Kiremidjian-Schumacher and Roy, 1998; McKenzie *et al.*, 1998; Kiremidjian-Schumacher *et al.*, 2000; Rayman, 2000). The immunomodulatory effects of Se occur through three principal mechanisms: (i) anti-inflammatory effects of selenoproteins or selenocompounds; (ii) selenoenzymes or Se compounds altering the redox state of the cell by acting as antioxidants; and (iii) through the generation of cytostatic and anti-cancer compounds as products of Se metabolism.

Effects of selenium on respiratory burst and microbe killing

The respiratory burst is a microbicidal reaction that takes place in neutrophils and monocyte/macrophages. Using a partial reduction of oxygen, it produces superoxide ($O_2^-\cdot$), hydrogen peroxide (H_2O_2) and other reactive oxygen species (ROS) that kill bacteria. As a defence mechanism, it is extremely effective, but the host must be able to remove the peroxides that are generated in the process; otherwise, host cell damage will result. Superoxide is converted by superoxide dismutase to H_2O_2, which can, if not removed, decompose to the extremely reactive hydroxyl radical ($OH\cdot$) (see Trenam et al., 1992).

In the 1970s, it was realized that Se deficiency led to decreased GPX activity and an inability to produce a respiratory-burst reaction that was effective at killing microbes (Spallholz et al., 1990). The reason for this is that the production of $O_2^-\cdot$ is sensitive to H_2O_2, which damages the $O_2^-\cdot$-generating enzyme. This loss of respiratory-burst reaction impairs effective killing of bacteria and results in granuloma formation (a mass of activated, but ineffective, leucocytes) and an inability of the host to eliminate microbes (references in Spallholz et al., 1990). Furthermore, nitric oxide (NO) is used by a variety of host cells to destroy bacteria and viruses. Reaction of NO with $O_2^-\cdot$ leads to the formation of peroxynitrite ($ONOO^-$), which causes oxidative damage to lipids, proteins and DNA (references in McKenzie, 2000). In Se deficiency, there is an impaired capability to detoxify organic and inorganic peroxides, generated by oxidative stress or through general metabolism. As a consequence, damage to macromolecules and cell membranes can occur.

Effects of selenium on eicosanoid metabolism

Potent lipid modulators of inflammation are synthesized from arachidonic acid cleaved from membrane phospholipids by the action of phospholipases A_2 and C, followed by the action of cyclo-oxygenase (see Fig. 12.3; see also Calder and Field, Chapter 4, this volume). This family of metabolites of arachidonic acid, known collectively as eicosanoids (Gerritsen, 1996), has both pro-inflammatory and immunosuppressive properties (see Calder and Field, Chapter 4, this volume). Furthermore, the excessive generation of hydroperoxides formed by the lipoxygenase and cyclo-oxygenase enzymes in circulating leucocytes can lead to oxidative damage to endothelial cells.

The leucotrienes (LTs), such as LTB_4, are pro-inflammatory compounds (see Calder and Field, Chapter 4, this volume). Some, like LTB_4, are important chemoattractants for neutrophils, bringing them into the inflamed tissue. The LTB_4 synthase enzyme requires reduction of 12-hydroperoxyeicosatetraenoic acid (12-HPETE) by the PHGPX or other GPX enzymes (reviewed in Parnham and Graf, 1987; Spallholz et al., 1990). Se deficiency results in decreased LTB_4 synthesis and impaired neutrophil chemotaxis. Diminished peroxidase capacity in Se deficiency also leads to a decrease in the synthesis of prostacyclins (Cao et al., 2000). These mediators prevent arterial thrombosis and platelet aggregation. Instead, Se deficiency promotes the synthesis of thromboxanes, which cause platelet aggregation. Platelet degranulation results in the release of pro-inflammatory mediators, including vasoactive amines, eicosanoids and pro-inflammatory cytokines. Thromboxane synthesis and platelet aggregation and activation are decreased by Se (Zbikowska *et al.*, 1999).

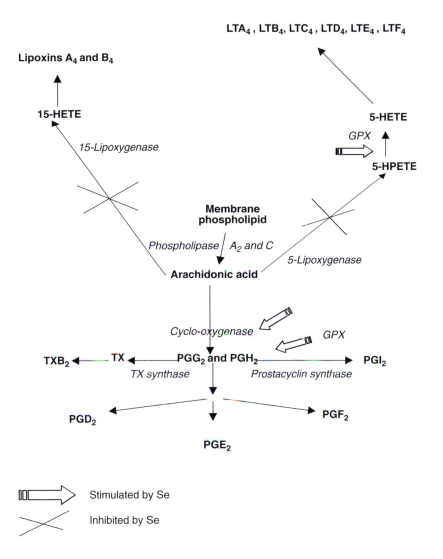

Fig. 12.3. The effects of selenium (Se) on the production of eicosanoids. The enzymes catalysing each step are indicated in italic. GPX indicates either a GPX or the phospholipid hydroperoxide GPX. Reactions stimulated or inhibited by Se are indicated. Cyclo-oxygenase is a key enzyme in eicosanoid synthesis. High levels of peroxides inactivate cyclo-oxygenase; these can be broken down by GPX – thus GPX is an activator of cyclo-oxygenase. PGG_2 and PGH_2 are unstable endoperoxides, which are converted to thromboxanes (TX), prostacyclins (PGI_2) or prostaglandins (PG). 5-HETE, 5-hydroxyeicosatetraenoic acid. LT, lakotriene.

Effects of selenium on lymphocytes and killer cells

Se supplementation stimulates several activities of lymphocytes, natural killer (NK) cells and lymphokine-activated killer cells (summarized in Figs 12.4 and 12.5). Preservation of protein structure is partly Se-dependent, because of the role of thioredoxin reductases in maintaining proteins in their correctly folded configuration. For cell-mediated immunity to function, interaction between many immunologically active proteins and their receptors needs to occur. Interleukin (IL)-2 is a vitally important paracrine growth and activation cytokine for immune cells (see Devereux, Chapter 1, this volume). A major immunostimulatory effect of Se is by Se-induced up-regulation of expression of the α and β subunits of the IL-2 receptor, which are expressed on many immune cells and notably on T and B lymphocytes. This increases the ability of these cells to respond to IL-2. Stimulation with IL-2 from activated CD4+ T-helper cells then potentiates the cytotoxicity of killer cells, increases numbers of lymphocytes, promotes antibody production by B lymphocytes and improves the responsiveness of immature bone-marrow cells to other cytokines in order to produce immune-cell precursors. The combination of IL-2 and interferon gamma binding to monocytes and macrophages boosts resistance to and killing of microbes (Kiremidjian-Schumacher et al., 1996).

Se also causes increases in the cytotoxicity of CD8+ cells, increases CD4+ cell numbers and responses to mitogens and greater survival of CD4+ cells in human immunodeficiency virus (HIV)-infected patients (for references, see Spallholz et al., 1990; Kiremidjian-Schumacher et al., 1996, 2000; Kiremidjian-Schumacher and Roy, 1998; McKenzie et al., 2002). The diminished proliferative response of lymphocytes to mitogenic stimuli in aged mice can be reversed by dietary Se supplementation, acting by up-regulation of the IL-2 receptor (Roy et al., 1995). Se supplementation also appears to reverse the age-related decline in NK-cell function in elderly humans (Ravaglia et al., 2000). The loss of NK-cell activity is one means by which cancer cells may evade immune-mediated destruction.

The thioredoxin reductases and the GPXs protect host cells from their own respiratory-burst reaction. The thioredoxin reductases also have the ability to inactivate NK lysin, a protein produced by cytotoxic cells to kill bacteria and tumour cells. In Se deficiency, it is possible that host cells are vulnerable to damage from both types of 'friendly fire'. Proof of the importance of this mechanism is that tumour cells often have elevated levels of thioredoxin reductase, which protects them from NK lysin. Thus, Se deficiency weakens the immune response at several key points.

In 1973, it was discovered that mice fed Se-enriched diets had increased titres for immunoglobulin G (IgG) and IgM antibodies and had higher levels of complement proteins. Most studies since then in various animals and in humans have confirmed that Se alone or in combination with vitamin E raises B-cell numbers and antibody production in response to vaccination. Studies showing that Se supplementation increases antibody production, complement responses and cell-mediated killing are catalogued in Spallholz et al. (1990) and McKenzie et al. (1998). Studies in farm animals have shown that Se

Se deficiency   **Se supplemented**

NEUTROPHILS

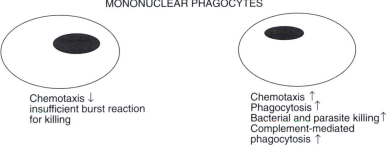

But much inflammation
and less microbe killing
Chemotaxis ↓

More microbicidal,
Chemotaxis ↑
Cell numbers ↑

MONONUCLEAR PHAGOCYTES

Chemotaxis ↓
insufficient burst reaction
for killing

Chemotaxis ↑
Phagocytosis ↑
Bacterial and parasite killing ↑
Complement-mediated
phagocytosis ↑

NATURAL AND LYMPHOKINE-ACTIVATED KILLER CELLS

↑ Tumour- or
virus-infected
target-cell killing

CYTOKINE RELEASE AND ADHESION MOLECULE EXPRESSION

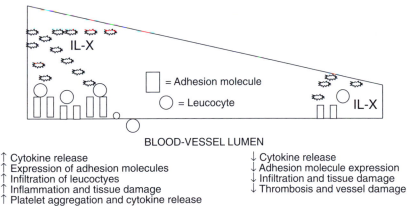

IL-X

☐ = Adhesion molecule

◯ = Leucocyte

IL-X

BLOOD-VESSEL LUMEN

↑ Cytokine release   ↓ Cytokine release
↑ Expression of adhesion molecules ↓ Adhesion molecule expression
↑ Infiltration of leucoctyes   ↓ Infiltration and tissue damage
↑ Inflammation and tissue damage   ↓ Thrombosis and vessel damage
↑ Platelet aggregation and cytokine release

Fig. 12.4. Effects of selenium (Se) deficiency (left-hand column) or Se supplementation (right-hand column) on cells and molecules mediating innate immunity. ↑ signifies an increase in activity or numbers and ↓ denotes a decline in activity or numbers. Ros, reactive oxygen species. IL-X, various interleukins.

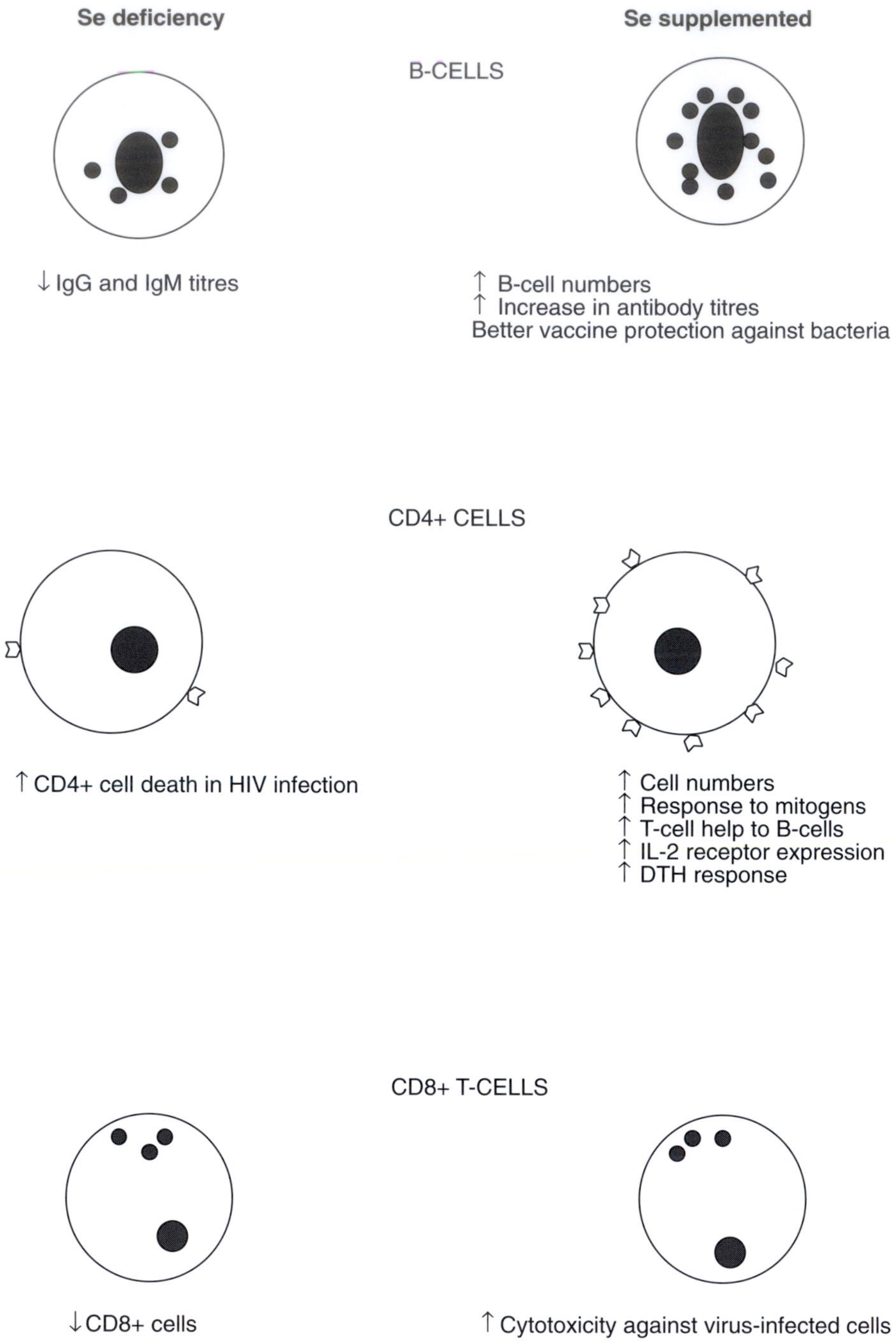

Se deficiency

Se supplemented

B-CELLS

↓ IgG and IgM titres

↑ B-cell numbers
↑ Increase in antibody titres
Better vaccine protection against bacteria

CD4+ CELLS

↑ CD4+ cell death in HIV infection

↑ Cell numbers
↑ Response to mitogens
↑ T-cell help to B-cells
↑ IL-2 receptor expression
↑ DTH response

CD8+ T-CELLS

↓ CD8+ cells

↑ Cytotoxicity against virus-infected cells

Fig. 12.5. Effects of selenium (Se) deficiency (left-hand column) or Se supplementation (right-hand column) on cells and molecules mediating acquired immunity. ↑ signifies an increase in activity or numbers and ↓ denotes a decline in activity or numbers. HIV, human immunodeficiency virus; IL-2, interleukin-2; DTH, delayed-type hypersensitivity; Ig, immunoglobulin.

deficiency increases the severity of and mortality from parasitic, viral, fungal and bacterial infections. It is now common farm practice to supplement animal feed with Se to boost growth and disease resistance. However, excessive amounts of Se (equivalent to > 400 μg day^{-1} in humans) were found to lead to toxic effects and immune suppression (Spallholz *et al.*, 1990).

Anti-inflammatory effects of selenium

Effects on cell signalling and gene transcription

Se compounds have anti-inflammatory properties, probably resulting from their ability to influence the redox state of the cell and to remove ROS (Parnham and Graf, 1987). Recently, it has been realized that ROS serve as secondary messengers within cells, conveying signals of oxidative damage from the plasma membrane through the cellular signalling cascades by influencing kinase activity and by regulating the induction of transcription factors and their DNA-binding ability in the nucleus (Lander, 1997; McKenzie *et al.*, 2002). Many protein–protein and protein–DNA interactions require thiol groups or cysteine residues on the proteins to be in a reduced state. This can be regulated by the thioredoxin reductase/thioredoxin system. The complexities of these interactions are still being unravelled. However, two key anti-inflammatory targets of Se are the transcription factors, activated protein 1 (AP-1) and nuclear factor kappa B (NFκB). These factors and the genes encoding them are activated by changes in the redox state of the cell and oxidative stress, such as may be caused by chemicals or radiation. For example, ROS activate a protease, which cleaves the inhibitory subunit from the inactive NFκB in the cytoplasm, allowing the activated NFκB to move to the nucleus, where it activates gene transcription. Many pro-inflammatory cytokine genes have binding sites for these factors in their promoter regions. Se prevents gene induction by metabolizing ROS to prevent transcription-factor activation and possibly by inhibiting binding of the transcription factor to its response element on the DNA (reviewed in McKenzie *et al.*, 2002).

Effects of selenium on cytokines and adhesion molecules

Se compounds block the constitutive expression of IL-1, IL-6, tumour necrosis factor alpha (TNF-α) and IL-8 in skin cells (see Figs 12.4 and 12.6). Induction of these pro-inflammatory cytokines leads to up-regulation of adhesion molecules on endothelial cells and binding and recruitment of leucocytes to damaged tissue (Fig. 12.4). These cytokines also activate leucocytes, increasing their release of inflammatory mediators. IL-8 acts as a potent chemoattractant for neutrophils and T-cells. Endothelial cells grown under Se-deficient conditions and stimulated with TNF-α bind more neutrophils than endothelial cells from Se-replete controls and have higher levels of E-selectin, P-selectin and intercellular adhesion molecule-1 expression (see Maddox *et al.*, 1999; McKenzie *et al.*, 2002).

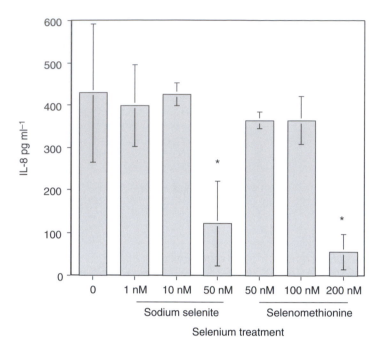

Fig. 12.6. Inhibition of cytokine release from normal human keratinocytes in culture by selenium. Primary keratinocytes were supplemented with either sodium selenite or selenomethionine for 24 h prior to the media being collected and the protein levels measured by ELISA. Control cells had no selenium added. Results are expressed as the mean ± standard error of the mean, $n = 3$. Significant difference from the control cells, * $P < 0.05$. IL-8, interleukin-8.

Conversely, Beck and Levander have shown that Se deficiency down-regulates the production of certain cytokines in the hearts of mice infected with a cardiotoxic virus. Mice fed Se-deficient diets did not differ in the production of IL-1 from the Se-replete controls, but mRNA for IL-6, a co-stimulant for IL-2 production, was decreased in Se deficiency. A decrease in the production of mRNA for TNF-α was also observed and the authors suggest that the decrease in the availability of these cytokines could radically disrupt anti-viral immunity (Beck and Levander, 1998).

Cytokines can also be induced by non-specific damage to DNA. When skin cells (keratinocytes) are irradiated with ultraviolet B radiation (UVB), thymidine dimer formation (cross-linking of adjacent pyrimidines), single-strand breaks in DNA and oxidative damage to DNA occur. Two cytokines induced by DNA damage are TNF-α and IL-10. In the skin, TNF-α causes emigration of the Langerhans cells, the principal dendritic antigen-presenting cells in the skin. Without these antigen-presenting cells, local immune suppression occurs and neoplastic cells cannot be readily detected. Release of IL-10 potentiates this situation by inhibiting the release of pro-inflammatory cytokines and by inhibiting antigen presentation and cell-mediated immune responses. Se, as selenite or selenomethionine, protects keratinocytes from oxidative DNA damage and the UVB-induced release of IL-10 and TNF-α proteins, as well as inhibiting UVB induction of the pro-inflammatory cytokines, IL-6 and IL-8. Peroxynitrite can cause DNA single-strand breaks; strand breakage is prevented by GPX and thioredoxin reductase. Overall, Se can prevent cytokine release in response to DNA damage, preventing inflammation and helping to prevent immune suppression following UVB irradiation (reviewed in McKenzie, 2000).

Cytokines can also influence the expression of selenoproteins. The immunosuppressive cytokine transforming growth factor β inhibits GPX gene transcription (Mostert *et al.*, 1999). Also, activation of a plasmid construct consisting of the selenoprotein P promoter linked to a reporter gene was suppressed by treatment of cells harbouring the construct with IL-1β, interferon-γ or TNF-α (Dreher *et al.*, 1997).

Effects of selenium on the skin immune system

The skin is the frontier of the immune system, the interface of the body with the external environment and the site of exposure of the immune system to mutagenic and oxidative damage from UV radiation (reviewed in Duthie *et al.*, 1999). Oxidizing agents are also produced by commensal microorganisms that reside on the skin. Se has been shown to have a vital role in protecting the skin from carcinogenesis and from oxidative damage (reviewed in McKenzie, 2000). In mice, dietary Se supplements or even topical application of Se significantly decrease the incidence of skin tumours, tumour size and mortality. Mice on Se-deficient diets also have significantly lower numbers of Langerhans cells in the skin, which may result from increased secretion of TNF-α, which triggers emigration of these dendritic cells. In humans, low Se intake has been correlated with increased incidence of skin cancer, but it is not clear yet whether Se supplements protect humans from skin damage and malignancy (reviewed in McKenzie, 2000).

In vitro, selenite and selenomethionine protect keratinocytes from UVB-induced cell death by necrosis and apoptosis. The mechanisms are thought to involve protection from lipid peroxidative damage to membranes, a decrease in oxidative DNA damage and inhibition of caspase-3, one of the proteases involved in triggering apoptosis (reviewed in McKenzie, 2000). For maximum protection, at least 12 h preincubation of the cells with the Se compounds is necessary, suggesting that the protection is mediated by selenoproteins. The GPX family seem to have an important role in this protection; for example, the molluscum contagiosum virus, which causes skin papules, carries an open reading frame encoding a GPX-like transcript. Transfection of this cDNA into keratinocytes protects them from UVB-induced cell death (Shisler *et al.*, 1998). Furthermore, unlike catalase, which also breaks down H_2O_2, GPX is not inactivated by UVB. Tanning of the skin protects against UVB, and thioredoxin reductase has been proposed to regulate the production of the melanin tanning pigment (reviewed in McKenzie, 2000). Thus, Se plays an important role in protecting the skin immune system from oxidative damage and carcinogenesis.

Effects of selenium on viral infections

Oxidative stress is produced during viral infections and contributes to the pathology of the disease. Nutritional deficiencies can exacerbate the problem (reviewed in Beck and Levander, 1998). The Coxsackie B3 virus, which is implicated in the pathology of Keshan disease, mutates to a more cardiotoxic form when passaged through Se-deficient mice (see Beck, 1999). This seems to be a common theme for RNA viruses and it has been proposed that the oxidizing environment of an Se-deficient host may contribute to faster mutation of the viral genome (Beck *et al.*, 1995). These viruses lack proofreading capability and this contributes to their high mutation rates. Beck and Levander (1998) have noted that the severe forms of the influenza virus, demonstrating a large degree of antigenic drift, have evolved in Se-deficient parts of China and that HIV is thought to have evolved in areas of Central Africa where Se intake is very low. The importance of selenoenzymes for anti-viral protection was demonstrated in experiments where mice were fed gold thioglucose or gold sodium thiomalate, which inhibit selenocysteine residues. In these animals, injection with normally non-lethal Semliki Forest virus or Sindbis viruses was fatal (Beck and Levander, 1998). Furthermore, injection of non-virulent Coxsackie B3 virus into GPX knockout mice led to mutation to a more virulent strain (Beck, 1999).

The long terminal repeat of HIV controls replication and is activated by binding of NFκB, which is regulated by the cell redox state and oxidative stress. TNF-α stimulates NFκB activation in T-cells. As we have described, Se compounds can inhibit TNF-α release. An inverse correlation between plasma Se concentration, red-cell GPX activity and the progression of acquired immune deficiency syndrome (AIDS) has been shown (reviewed in Chen *et al.*, 1997; McKenzie *et al.*, 2002). In culture, Se supplementation of HIV-infected monocytes and CD4+ T-cells inhibits TNF-α-induced viral replication (Hori *et al.*, 1997). Thus, it seems that Se may be useful in the treatment of AIDS (Chen *et al.*, 1997). Dietary Se supplements have been used for the treatment of hepatitis-B-induced liver cancer in China. The incidence of hepatitis-B-virus-induced liver cancer in humans decreased in a previously Se-deficient, hepatitis-B+ population given Se supplements of 200 μg day^{-1}.

Viruses illustrate the importance of the GPX system in protection from ROS. Several different viral genomes (HIV, Ebola, molluscum and hepatitis C) encode GPX-like molecules (Zhang *et al.*, 1999). This presumably protects them against the ROS produced by host phagocytes.

The Relationship between Selenium Intake and Other Diseases

Overview

The intakes of Se recommended by health authorities in different countries vary between 50 and 70 μg day^{-1}. These values are based on the observation that such intakes should produce maximal expression of extracellular GPX (eGPX) in plasma or cyGPX activity in red cells. Thus, the Se requirements are based on biochemical parameters and, as yet, there is no consensus as to other biochemical or physiological effects of Se status that may be used to determine optimal intake. The recognition that the anti-cancer effects of Se in humans can occur at intakes of 200 μg day^{-1} or more suggests that a reappraisal of optimal Se intake may be needed.

Daily Se intakes of humans can vary across the globe from less than 5 μg day^{-1} up to 3000 μg day^{-1}. However, these intakes represent extremes and, in most cases, Se intakes are between 30 and 200 μg day^{-1}. With regard to human health issues, most debate revolves around whether intakes of 30–75 μg day^{-1} are associated with an increased incidence of a range of diseases, including cardiovascular disease and cancers. Low dietary Se intake has been implicated in the development of numerous health disorders in humans. These include Kashin–Beck disease, cancer, cardiovascular disease (including Keshan disease), muscular dystrophy, malaria, alopecia areata, pregnancy hypertension syndrome, altered immune function, male infertility and even AIDS (reviewed in Rayman, 2000). Patients on long-term parenteral nutrition without Se supplementation in their formulation run the risk of Se deficiency, which is manifested in myopathy and cardiomyopathy. Low Se status (low Se and erythrocyte GPX activity) in the elderly was correlated with lower tri-iodothyrinine (T3)-to-thyroxine (T4) ratios, due to raised T4 concentrations, and was seen with advancing age (Olivieri *et al.*, 1996). Se supplementation decreased the serum T4 concentration in these patients. The age-related decline in T3 content was ascribed to the requirement for iodothyronine-5′-deiodinase, which is a selenoprotein, to catalyse the conversion of T4 to T3. A deficiency in T4-to-T3 conversion will impair general metabolism, including immunity.

Cancer

In 1965, Shamberger and Rudolph demonstrated a significant reduction of skin-cancer incidence in carcinogen-treated mice given a topical application of sodium selenite. This initiated a great number of subsequent studies, using animal models, which consistently demonstrated the anti-carcinogenic nature of Se. The anti-cancer effects seem to be of two types: one is the ability to protect against DNA damage and to bolster immune effectiveness and the second is the ability of selenocompounds to cause growth inhibition and apoptosis of tumour cells, while leaving normal cells unaffected (reviewed in Combs and Clark, 1999; Ganther, 1999). Se compounds inhibit the cellular oncogene AP-1, which is required for cell growth. Other selenocompounds, such as selenodiglutathione, do not kill normal cells, but cause apoptosis of tumour cells by inducing the tumour suppressor protein, p53, and apoptosis (Lanfear *et al.*, 1994). For p53 to bind to DNA, thiol groups on nine critical cysteine residues must be in a reduced state, this is mediated by thioredoxin. Inactivation of thioredoxin reductase prevents activation of a functional p53 (references in McKenzie *et al.*, 2002). Se compounds also prevent metastasis and angiogenesis of tumours, possibly by inhibition of release of cytokines, such as IL-8.

In humans, some, but not all, epidemiological studies have suggested an inverse correlation between Se intake and the prevalence of malignancy. The most convincing evidence for Se having an anti-cancer effect in humans comes from a recent randomized, double-blind, placebo-controlled, supplementation study (Combs and Clark, 1999). In this study, 1300 subjects from the USA received 200 μg of Se daily (given as Se-rich yeast) or a placebo for approximately 5 years. Total cancer incidence was 42% lower in the Se-supplemented group compared with the placebo group, with significant decreases in the incidence of prostate, gastric and colorectal cancers. Similarly, the total death rate from malignancy was 52% lower in the subjects who received Se supplementation when compared with the placebo group. The multicentre PRECISE trial has recently been started in the USA, Finland, Denmark, Sweden and the UK with a view to extending these observations to European populations (Rayman, 2000).

Cardiovascular disease

The risk of developing atherosclerosis and heart disease may be higher in people who have a low dietary Se intake. Endothelial dysfunction is a primary factor in the pathogenesis of atherosclerosis. Laboratory-based research has provided considerable evidence to suggest that Se may be beneficial to the endothelium and thus help to prevent atherosclerotic disease. Se supplementation of cell cultures protects the endothelium from oxidative damage and can alter platelet function, cytokine signalling and transcription of pro-atherogenic adhesion molecules (Fig. 12.4).

The contribution of Se deficiency to the pathogenesis of cardiovascular disease was originally suggested from epidemiological studies that correlated low Se content of forage crops, drinking water and blood with regional mortality rates from cardiovascular disease (Schamberger et al., 1979). Other studies have failed to confirm this link. Huttunen (1997) postulated that the conflicting data from these studies can be explained by a threshold effect of Se intake on the risk of cardiovascular disease; that is, in populations with low Se status, a correlation between serum Se and cardiovascular risk is observed, while populations with a high Se intake (serum Se levels > 45 μg l^{-1}) would show no such correlation (Korpela, 1993). There are data that support this 'threshold hypothesis' (Kardinaal et al., 1997): from the ten centres across nine European countries, only one (Germany, with the lowest measured Se concentrations) demonstrated a statistically significant inverse association between toenail Se levels and risk of myocardial infarction.

Conclusion

In conclusion, Se deficiency seriously impairs cell-mediated and humoral immunity and appears to play a part in the pathogenesis and exacerbation of some chronic inflammatory and viral diseases. Dietary Se supplements may be a useful additional therapy in the treatment of some of these conditions. However, excessive Se intakes also impair immune function.

References

Allan, C.B., Lacourciere, G.M. and Stadtman, T.C. (1999) Responsiveness of selenoproteins to dietary selenium. *Annual Review of Nutrition* 19, 1–16.

Arner, E.S.J. and Holmgren, A. (2000) Physiological functions of thioredoxin and thioredoxin reductase. *European Journal of Biochemistry* 267, 6102–6109.

Arthur, J.R. and Beckett, G.J. (1994) Newer aspects of micronutrients in at risk groups: new metabolic roles for selenium. *Proceedings of the Nutrition Society* 53, 615–624.

Arthur, J.R., Nicol, F., Mitchell, J.H. and Beckett, G.J. (1997) Selenium and iodine deficiencies and selenoprotein function. *Biomedicine and Environmental Science* 10, 1–7.

Beck, M.A. (1999) Selenium and host defence towards viruses. *Proceedings of the Nutrition Society* 58, 707–711.

Beck, M.A. and Levander, O.A. (1998) Dietary oxidative stress and the potentiation of viral infection. *Annual Review of Nutrition* 18, 93–116.

Beck, M.A., Shi, Q., Morris, V.C. and Levander, O.A. (1995) Rapid genomic evolution of nonvirulent Coxsackie virus B3 in selenium deficient mice results in selection of identical virulent isolates. *Nature Medicine* 1, 433–436.

Beckett, G.J. and Arthur, J.R. (1994) The iodothyronine deiodinases and 5'-deiodination. *Baillière's Clinical Endocrinology and Metabolism* 8, 285–304.

Behne, D., Hilmert, H., Scheid, S., Gessner, H. and Elger, W. (1988) Evidence for specific selenium target tissues and new biologically important selenoproteins. *Biochimica et Biophysica Acta* 966, 12–21.

Bermano, G., Nicol, F., Dyer, J.A., Sunde, R.A., Beckett, G.J., Arthur, J.R. and Hesketh, J.E. (1995) Tissue specific regulation of selenoenzyme gene expression during selenium deficiency in rats. *Biochemical Journal* 311, 425–430.

Berry, M.J. (1991) Recognition of UGA as a selenocysteine codon in type-1 deiodinase requires sequences in the 3' untranslated region. *Nature* 353, 273–276.

Burk, R.F. (1994) Selenoprotein P: a selenium-rich extracellular glycoprotein. *Journal of Nutrition* 124, 1891–1897.

Burk, R.F. and Hill, K.E. (1999) Orphan selenoproteins. *Bioessays* 21, 231–237.

Cao, Y.Z., Reddy, C.C. and Sordillo, L.M. (2000) Altered eicosanoid biosynthesis in selenium-deficient endothelial cells. *Free Radicals in Biology and Medicine* 28, 381–389.

Chen, C.Y., Zhou, J.Y. and Xu, H.B. (1997) Advances in the studies of relationship between selenium and human immunodeficiency virus. *Progress in Biochemistry and Biophysics* 24, 327–330.

Combs, G.F. and Clark, L.C. (1999) Selenium and cancer. In: Heber, D., Blackburn, G.L. and Go, V.L.W. (eds) *Nutritional Oncology*. Academic Press, San Diego, pp. 215–222.

Daniels, L.A. (1996) Selenium metabolism and bioavailability. *Biological Trace Element Research* 54, 185–199.

Dreher, I., Jakobs, T.C. and Kohrle, J. (1997) Cloning and characterization of the human selenoprotein P promoter: response of selenoprotein P expression to cytokines in liver cells. *Journal of Biological Chemistry* 272, 29364–29371.

Duthie, M.S., Kimber, I. and Norval, M. (1999) The effects of ultraviolet radiation on the human immune system. *British Journal of Dermatology* 140, 995–1009.

Foster, D.J. and Sumar, S. (1997) Selenium in health and disease. *Critical Reviews in Food Science and Nutrition* 37, 211–228.

Ganther, H.E. (1999) Selenium metabolism, selenoproteins and mechanisms of cancer prevention: complexities with thioredoxin reductase. *Carcinogenesis* 20, 1657–1666.

Gerritsen, M.E. (1996) Physiological and pathophysiological roles of eicosanoids in the microcirculation. *Cardiovascular Research* 32, 720–732.

Holmgren, A. (1985) Thioredoxin. *Annual Reviews of Biochemistry* 54, 237–271.

Holmgren, A. (1989) Thioredoxin and glutaredoxin systems. *Journal of Biological Chemistry* 264, 13963–13966.

Hori, K., Hatfield, D., Maldarelli, F., Lee, B.J. and Clouse, K.A. (1997) Selenium supplementation suppresses tumor necrosis factor alpha-induced human immunodeficiency virus type 1 replication *in vitro*. *AIDS Research and Human Retrovirology* 13, 1325–1332.

Huttunen, J.K. (1997) Selenium and cardiovascular diseases – an update. *Biomedical and Environmental. Science* 10, 220–226.

Kardinaal, A.F., Kok, F.J., Kohlmeier, L., Martin-Moreno, J.M., Ringstad, J., Gomez-Aracena, J., Mazaev, V.P., Thamm, M., Martin B.C., Aro, A., Kark, J.D., Delgado-Rodriguez, M., Riemersma, R.A., van 't Veer, P. and Huttunen, J.K. (1997) Association between toenail selenium and risk of acute myocardial infarction in European men: the EURAMIC Study: European Antioxidant Myocardial Infarction and Breast Cancer. *American Journal of Epidemiology* 145, 373–379.

Kiremidjian-Schumacher, L. and Roy, M. (1998) Selenium and immune function *Zeitschrift für Ehrnahrungswissenschaft* 37(Suppl. 1), 50–56.

Kiremidjian-Schumacher, L., Roy, M., Wishe, H.I., Cohen, M.W. and Stotzky, G. (1996) Supplementation with selenium augments the functions of natural killer and lymphokine-activated killer cells. *Biological Trace Element Research* 52, 227–239.

Kiremidjian-Schumacher, L., Roy, M. and Glickman, R. (2000) Selenium and immunocompetence in patients with head and neck cancer. *Biological Trace Element Research* 73, 97–111.

Kollmus, H., Flohè, L. and McCarthy, J.E.G. (1996) Analysis of eukaryotic mRNA structures directing cotranslational incorporation of selenocysteine. *Nucleic Acid Research* 24, 1195–1201.

Korpela, H. (1993) Selenium in cardiovascular disease. *Journal of Trace Elements and Electrolytes in Health and Disease* 7, 115.

Lander, H.M. (1997) An essential role for free radicals and derived species in signal transduction. *FASEB Journal* 11, 118–124.

Lanfear, J., Fleming, J., Wu, L., Webster, G. and Harrison, P.R. (1994) The selenium metabolite selenodiglutathione induces p53 and apoptosis. *Carcinogenesis* 15, 1387–1392.

Low, S.C. and Berry, M.J. (1996) Knowing when not to stop: selenocysteine incorporation in eukaryotes. *Trends in Biological Sciences* 21, 203–208.

McKenzie, R.C. (2000) Selenium, ultraviolet radiation and the skin. *Clinical and Experimental Dermatology* 25, 1–7.

McKenzie, R.C., Rafferty, T.S. and Beckett, G.J. (1998) Selenium: an essential element for immune function. *Immunology Today* 19, 342–345.

McKenzie, R.C., Arthur, J.R. and Beckett, G.J. (2002) Selenium and the regulation of cell signalling, growth and survival: molecular and mechanistic aspects. *Antioxidant and Redox Signalling* 4, 339–351.

Maddox, J.F., Aherne, K.M., Reddy, C.C. and Sordillo, L.M. (1999) Increased neutrophil adherence and adhesion molecule mRNA expression in endothelial cells during selenium deficiency. *Journal of Leukocyte Biology* 65, 658–664.

Mansell, J.B. and Berry, M.J. (2001) Towards a mechanism for selenocysteine incorporation in eukaryotes. In: Hatfield, D.L. (ed.) *Selenium, its Molecular Biology and Role in Human Health.* Kluwer Academic Publishers, Boston, pp. 69–80.

Mostert, V., Dreher, I., Kohrle, J. and Abel, J. (1999) Transforming growth factor-beta inhibits expression of selenoprotein P in cultured human liver cells. *FEBS Letters* 460, 23–26.

Olivieri, O., Girelli, D., Stanzial, A.M., Rossi, L., Bassi, A. and Corrocher, R. (1996) Selenium, zinc, and thyroid hormones in healthy subjects: low T3/T4 ratio in the elderly is related to impaired Se status. *Biological Trace Element Research* 51, 31–41.

Parnham, M.J. and Graf, E. (1987) Selenoorganic compounds and the therapy of hydroperoxide-linked pathological conditions. *Biochemical Pharmacology* 36, 3095–3102.

Ravaglia, G., Forti, P., Maioli, F., Bastagli, L., Facchini, A., Mariani, E., Savarino, L., Sassi, S., Cucinotta, D. and Lenaz, G. (2000) Effect of micronutrient status on natural killer cell immune function in healthy free-living subjects aged > 90 y. *American Journal of Clinical Nutrition* 71, 590–598.

Rayman, M.P. (2000) The importance of selenium to human health. *Lancet* 356, 233–241.

Reilly, C. (1993) Selenium in health and disease. *Australian Journal of Nutrition and Dietetics* 50, 136–144.

Roy, M., Kiremidjian-Schumacher, L., Wishe, H.I., Cohen, M.W. and Stotzky, G. (1995) Supplementation with selenium restores age-related decline in immune cell function. *Proceedings of the Society of Experimental Biology and Medicine* 209, 369–375.

St Germain, D.L. and Galton, V.A. (1997) The deiodinase family of selenoproteins. *Thyroid* 7, 655–668.

Schwartz, K. and Foltz, C.M. (1957) Selenium as an integral part of factor 3 against dietary necrotic liver degeneration. *Journal of the American Chemical Society* 79, 3292–3293.

Shamberger, R.J. and Rudolph, G. (1966) Protection against cocarcinogenesis by antioxidants. *Experientia* 22, 116–118.

Shamberger, R.J., Willis, C.C. and McCormack, L.J. (1979) Selenium and heart disease III. Blood selenium and heart mortality in 19 states. In: Hemphill, D.D. (ed.) *Trace Substances in Environmental Health XIII.* University of Missouri, Columbia, pp. 59–63.

Shisler, J.L., Senkevich, T.G., Berry, M.J. and Moss, B. (1998) Ultraviolet-induced cell death blocked by a selenoprotein from a human dermatotropic poxvirus. *Science* 279, 102–105.

Spallholz, J.E., Boylan, L.M. and Larsen, H.S. (1990) Advances in understanding selenium's role in the immune system. *Annals of the New York Academy of Sciences* 587, 123–139.

Sunde, R.A. (1994) Molecular biology of selenoproteins. *Annual Review of Nutrition* 10, 451–478.

Trenam, C.W., Blake, D.R. and Morris, C.J. (1992) Skin inflammation – reactive oxygen species and the role of iron. *Journal of Investigative Dermatology* 99, 675–682.

Vernie, L.N. (1984) Selenium in carcinogenesis. *Biochimica et Biophysica Acta* 738, 203–217

Zbikowska, H.M., Wachowicz, B. and Krajewski, T. (1999) Selenium compounds inhibit the biological activity of blood platelets. *Platelets* 10, 185–190.

Zhang, W., Ramanathan, C.S., Nadimpalli, R.G., Bhat, A.A., Cox, A.G. and Taylor, E.W. (1999) Selenium-dependent glutathione peroxidase modules encoded by RNA viruses. *Biological Trace Element Research* 70, 97–116.

13 Probiotics and Immune Function

HARSHARNJIT S. GILL AND MARTIN L. CROSS

Institute of Food, Nutrition and Human Health, Massey University, Palmerston North, New Zealand

Introduction: Microbes and the Intestinal Environment

Microorganisms represent an essential, functioning component of the mammalian intestinal lumen. While the stomach is sparsely populated by acid-tolerant microbes, post-gastric sites support an increasing microbial population density, which in humans can reach concentrations of up to 10^{11} bacteria g^{-1} of lumen contents in the large intestine (Salminen *et al.*, 1998). Indeed, the human body contains approximately tenfold as many bacterial cells as somatic cells. Colonization of the human intestinal tract by microorganisms begins perinatally, when a newborn baby first encounters maternal and environmental microbes during and immediately following delivery. As neonatal development continues, there is a succession of colonization of the infant's developing intestinal tract by major groups of bacteria, which, under normal circumstances, begins to stabilize during weaning (Mitsuoka and Hayakawa, 1973). A stable intestinal microflora is typically attained post-weaning and during early childhood, and forms an essential component of the functioning human body. Perturbations of this resident microflora (for example, by external stressors, dramatic alterations of the diet or antibiotic treatment) can lead to a deterioration of physiological function and decline in health, including poor digestion and nutrient assimilation, immune dysfunctions and susceptibility to infection by diarrhoea-causing pathogens.

The intestinal microflora constitutes a metabolically active microbial environment, dominated by a relatively low diversity of genera, which, in the gut of healthy individuals, exist as part of a stable community (Fuller, 1992). Under normal circumstances, these resident gut bacteria cause neither pathogenesis nor inflammation in the host, but instead contribute to health maintenance, by forming a barrier layer against colonization by pathogens and by aiding in nutrient digestion and assimilation (Salminen *et al.*, 1998). In addition, the resident intestinal microflora plays other important physiological roles in health maintenance: deconjugating potentially damaging oxidative metabolites and toxins in the gut; degrading potentially allergenic food proteins; regulating cholesterol and triglyceride uptake; increasing vitamin biosynthesis; and providing immunosurveillance signals to limit intestinal-tract inflammation. Thus, a stable, properly functioning and active intestinal-tract microflora is essential to the continuance of human health.

Probiotic Supplementation of the Intestinal Microflora

Among the most predominant microbes in the human intestinal tract are the Gram-positive lactic acid-producing genera *Lactobacillus* and *Bifidobacterium*. Lactobacilli and bifidobacteria are also common fermentative microbes in yoghurt, cheese and soured vegetable foods (such as sauerkraut and suguki). The majority of fermentative microorganisms present in such foodstuffs are susceptible to low stomach pH and bile-salt secretions and cannot survive gastric processing. However, following oral delivery, a few strains are able to survive gastric transit and can persist in the intestinal lumen. These strains are thus able to transiently colonize the gut by integrating into the existing microflora, and are termed 'probiotics'.

Probiotics can be defined as dietary supplements containing living microbes that are able to persist in (or transiently colonize) the human intestinal tract and impart a beneficial influence on host physiology, such that this effect is able to improve health. This process is particularly important at times when the normal indigenous microflora has been perturbed: at this point, exogenously supplied probiotics of a defined species/strain are able to temporarily colonize the intestinal tract and stabilize the microfloral composition, thus restoring the vital physiological functioning of the microbial community. Thus, the use of probiotics in health improvement relies on the principle that exogenous microbes (from food sources) augment the beneficial physiological effects of the normal (indigenous) gut microflora.

Among the many purported physiological influences of probiotic microorganisms, a large proportion of research attention over the last decade has focused on the interaction of probiotics with the immune system (Salminen *et al.*, 1998). It is evident that several probiotic strains of lactic acid bacteria (LAB) are able to influence the immune system and, in many cases, this effect has been linked to a measurable improvement in health. The immune system comprises innate and adaptive components, and these play vital interacting roles in health maintenance, in both regulating and stimulating the body's responses.

Probiotics and the Immune System: Regulation and Stimulation

With regard to the role that the immune system plays in health maintenance and improvement, the traditional viewpoint has been one of immunity as a defence system against intrinsic (neoplasms and tumours) and extrinsic disease-causing agents (pathogens). However, this definition forms only part of the picture. Through control and orchestration of immune responses, the immune system is also able to regulate inflammatory events and control or limit the development of pathologies. This occurs mainly via the production of modulatory hormones (cytokines) that are able to shape and modify the character of a developing immune or inflammatory reaction (see Devereux, Chapter 1, this volume). In this context, it should be realized that gut-dwelling microbes are far from passive inhabitants of the intestinal-tract mucosa in an inert immunological sense. Paradoxically, it is the very signals generated by gastrointestinal (GI)-tract microbial interactions with the immune system that probably constitute the beneficial impact of probiotics on health. Clinical case studies have indicated that children raised in environments rich in early-life bacterial exposure (including lactobacilli-containing foods) develop fewer immune dysfunctional diseases than those experiencing more sterile environments (Alm *et al.*, 1999). In this case, it has been suggested that early stimulation by 'appropriate' bacterial signals may regulate the development of the immune system, such that immunopathologies (e.g. atopic reactions and mucosal allergies) are limited (Matricardi *et al.*, 1999). Indeed, a recent study has shown that supplementing the diets of newborn babies with the probiotic *Lactobacillus rhamnosus* (strain GG) can effectively reduce the incidence of atopic eczema during infancy and early childhood (Kalliomaki *et al.*, 2001), suggesting that augmentation of the neonatal intestinal microflora with exogenous bacteria can provide the bacterial signals necessary to combat allergic sensitization.

There is also more direct evidence that orally delivered probiotic organisms can interact with the immune system to limit pathologies. Further studies on *L. rhamnosus* GG have indicated that this probiotic can alleviate immune-mediated atopy following oral delivery to infants or to nursing mothers (Majamaa and Isolauri, 1997; Isolauri *et al.*, 2000), can partially control immune-mediated inflammatory responses in adults (via regulation of leucocyte inflammatory receptor expression) (Pelto *et al.*, 1998) and can reduce the incidence and severity of infant diarrhoea concomitant with an increase in circulating antibody responses (Kaila *et al.*, 1992; Majamaa *et al.*, 1995; Table 13.1). Clearly, there is scope to exploit the beneficial effects of probiotics on the immune system, with a view to the development of safe, dietary adjuncts/food-borne alternatives to pharmaceutical intervention for the control of a wide range of human pathologies (Elmer *et al.*, 1996).

Immune Signalling by Orally Delivered Probiotics

The first point of contact for orally delivered probiotics with intestinal tissues occurs as the microorganisms form lectin-like attachments to epithelial cells of the intestinal tract, as they begin to colonize the mucosa (Fuller, 1992). Recent research has shown that human intestinal epithelial cells are immunocompetent and can transcribe cytokine messenger RNA in response to contact with probiotic bacteria (Delneste *et al.*, 1998). This response is heightened in cells that have been subjected to cytokine activation (e.g. during an inflammatory reaction) and is accompanied by an up-regulation of cell surface receptors.

Table 13.1. Clinical evidence of immune stimulation by probiotic microorganisms.

Microorganism	Immunological effect	Subjects	Reference
Lactobacillus acidophilus La1/*Lactobacillus johnsonii*; *Lactobacillus rhamnosus* HN001; *Bifidobacterium bifidum* Bb12; *Bifidobacterium lactis* HN019	↑ Phagocytic activity of blood mononuclear and polymorphonuclear cells	Healthy adult and elderly volunteers	Schiffrin *et al.* (1995, 1997); Donnet-Hughes *et al.* (1999); Arunachalam *et al.* (2000); Chiang *et al.* (2000); Gill and Rutherfurd (2001); Gill *et al.* (2001a, b); Sheih *et al.* (2001)
Lactobacillus casei Shirota; *Bifidobacterium lactis* HN019	↑ Tumoricidal activity of blood mononuclear cells	Healthy adult and elderly volunteers; patients with colorectal cancer	Sawamura *et al.* (1994); Chiang *et al.* (2000); Gill *et al.* (2001a,b,c); Sheih *et al.* (2001)
Lactobacillus brevis Labre; *Bifidobacterium lactis* HN019	↑ Production of interferons (cytokines) by peripheral blood mononuclear cells *in vitro* and pro-interferon enzymes in circulation	Healthy adult and elderly volunteers	de Simone *et al.* (1989, 1993); Kishi *et al.* (1996; Aattouri and Lemonnier (1997); Arunachalam *et al.* (2000)
Lactobacillus rhamnosus GG; *Bifidobacterium breve* YIT4064	↑ Anti-rotavirus antibody responses during infection	Children with rotavirus diarrhoea	Kaila *et al.* (1992); Majamaa *et al.* (1995); Yasui *et al.* (1999b)
Lactobacillus rhamnosus GG	↑ Specific antibody responses following vaccination	Volunteer adult vaccinees	Link-Amster *et al.* (1994); Isolauri *et al.* (1995); Fangac *et al.* (2000)

During the regulation of potential inflammatory events, it now seems that bacterial signalling from the gut microflora plays an important role in the communication between gut epithelial cells and associated intraepithelial lymphocytes. *In vitro* studies with the CaCo-2 human intestinal epithelial cell line have shown that fermentative (*Lactobacillus sakei*) and probiotic (*Lactobacillus johnsonii*) species can induce the expression of the anti-inflammatory mediator transforming growth factor (TGF)-β, but not pro-inflammatory cytokines, such as tumour necrosis factor (TNF)-α or interleukin (IL)-1β. Addition of leucocytes to CaCo-2 *Lactobacillus* co-cultures promotes the production of pro-inflammatory molecules by the epithelial cells, but also induces secretion of the leucocyte-derived anti-inflammatory mediator IL-10 (Haller *et al.*, 2000). Thus, the picture that emerges is that gut microflora and/or probiotic microbes play an active role in the maintenance of gut homoeostasis by inducing the release of anti-inflammatory mediators and that, under pro-inflammatory conditions, the cross-talk between epithelial cells and leucocytes augments this regulatory role via additional cytokine mediation. In this context, contact between gut-dwelling bacteria and intestinal cells may be considered part of the routine microbial signalling processes of a healthy gut microflora, forming a homoeostatic mechanism for the regulation of intestinal inflammation. Indeed, removal of these routine signals at the gut epithelial surface can lead to a breakdown in these regulatory immune mechanisms and consequently promote aggressive and uncontrolled inflammatory responses (Kuhn *et al.*, 1993; Kulkarni and Karlsson, 1993).

While it has been suggested that routine signalling between resident/probiotic microbes and gut epithelial cells plays a maintenance role for gut homoeostasis, it is arguably direct immunostimulation by an interaction of the microbes with lymphoid foci that has received most research attention. In this situation, the interactions are quite different: microbes traverse the epithelial boundary and contact leucocytes directly (e.g. in the organized capsular foci of Peyer's patches), enabling direct immunoactivation. Evidence for this direct interaction has been obtained experimentally in animal models (de Simone *et al.*, 1987; Yasui *et al.*, 1989; Herias *et al.*, 1999; Perdigon *et al.*, 1999), and has an important consequence: unlike immunoinflammatory events that take place solely in the common mucosal immune system, immunostimulation via lymphoid foci facilitates ready access of messenger cells to the systemic circulation, via drainage to the mesenteric lymph node and thoracic duct. Thus, the consequence of an interaction between probiotic bacteria and lymphoid foci in the GI tract could include effects on systemic immune responses involving circulating leucocytes (Perdigon *et al.*, 1988, 1995). Several Gram-positive bacterial cell-wall components (including lipoteichoic acid, peptidoglycan and muramyl dipeptide) have been shown to bind leucocyte pattern-recognition receptors, including the endotoxin receptor (CD14), Toll 2 and type I macrophage scavenger receptor (Dunne *et al.*, 1994; Cleveland *et al.*, 1996; Cauwels *et al.*, 1997; Dziarski *et al.*, 1998), and this could represent the mechanism by which probiotics are able to stimulate the immune system directly.

Immunoregulation and Stimulation by Probiotics: Laboratory and Clinical Studies

Although the primary site of immunological signalling is at the gut mucosal interface, there is evidence that the immunomodulatory effects of probiotics can be expressed systemically. Typically, this is manifested by changes in leucocyte or humoral function, which can be assessed by *ex vivo* assays. To date, several compartments of the immune system have been identified as affected by probiotic delivery, including lymphocyte function (proliferation, cytokine secretion and cellular cytotoxicity); innate cell defences (e.g. phagocytosis, oxidative radical production, lysosomal enzyme secretion); natural cytocidal function of macrophages and natural killer (NK) cells, and antibody responses (both in terms of total immunoglobulin (Ig) levels and antigen-specific responses) (Table 13.1). In addition, there is evidence that oral delivery of probiotics can influence cellular phenotype expression, both at the mucosal interface and systemically, to reflect a state of activation.

Probiotic effects on lymphocytes

The majority of research to characterize probiotic effects on lymphocyte function has utilized animal models for study. Oral delivery of different strains of *Lactobacillus* has been shown to confer an increased capacity for splenic lymphocytes to proliferate in response to T-cell and B-cell mitogenic stimulation (Vesely *et al.*, 1985; de Simone *et al.*, 1987; Kirjavainen *et al.*, 1999; Gill *et al.*, 2000) and, in at least one case, this general enhancement of lymphocyte function has also been demonstrated at the local level in lymphoid foci of the intestinal tract (i.e. Peyer's patches) (Perdigon *et al.*, 1991). What is not clear at the moment is whether this enhanced capacity for lymphocytes to undergo activation/mitosis is due to increases in population levels (i.e. proportionally more lymphocytes) and/or increases in responsiveness to stimuli (i.e. lymphocytes at a heightened state of preactivation). However, a study by Perdigon *et al.* (1999) has shown that T-helper (CD4+) lymphocyte numbers are increased in the gut-associated lymphoid tissue (GALT) following oral delivery of *Lactobacillus casei*, providing evidence that probiotic stimulation can increase the size of lymphocyte populations.

Oral delivery of probiotics has also been shown to increase the capacity of systemic lymphocytes to secrete T-cell cytokines in response to appropriate *in vitro* stimulation. Some strains of *Lactobacillus* and *Bifidobacterium* have been demonstrated to increase the capacity of murine splenic lymphocytes (Pereyra *et al.*, 1991; Gill, 1998; Matsuzaki and Chin, 2000) and human peripheral-blood lymphocytes (Solis-Pereyra and Lemonnier, 1991) to secrete the cytokine interferon-γ (IFN-γ), following mitogen stimulation *in vitro*. Clinical studies have confirmed that certain probiotic LAB can induce increased expression of both type I and type II interferons among peripheral blood mononuclear cells (Kishi *et al.*, 1996; Aattouri and Lemonnier 1997; Solis-Pereyra *et al.*, 1997; Arunachalam *et al.*, 2000; Table 13.2).

Table 13.2. Health benefits of probiotic microorganisms that interact with the immune system.

Microorganism	Immunological effect	Health benefit	Reference
Lactobacillus acidophilus	↑ Production of anti-allergy cytokine (IFN-γ)	↓ Eosinophil count in asthmatic subjects; ↓ IgE levels in elderly subjects with nasal allergies	Trapp *et al.* (1993); Wheeler *et al.* (1997)
Lactobacillus rhamnosus GG	↓ Expression of inflammatory receptor molecules in milk-hypersensitive subjects; ↓ expression of pro-allergy cytokine (IL-4) in milk-hypersensitive subjects	↓ Atopic responses in milk-hypersensitive infants and adults	Sutas *et al.* (1996b); Majamaa & Isolauri (1997); Pelto *et al.* (1998); Kalliomaki *et al.* (2001)
Lactobacillus rhamnosus GG	↑ Anti-pathogen antibody responses	Promotes recovery from acute rotavirus diarrhoea in children; reduces viral shedding	Kaila *et al.* (1992); Majamaa *et al.* (1995)
Lactobacillus casei Shirota	↑ Cellular immune responses	↓ Tumour recurrence in adult bladder cancer patients following resection	Sawamura *et al.* (1994); Aso *et al.* (1995)

IFN-γ, interferon-γ; IL-4, interleukin-4; IgE, immunoglobulin E.

Probiotic effects on innate cell defences

A large body of work concerned with definition of probiotic effects on the immune system has focused on innate cell responses. Early studies had shown that oral delivery of *L. casei* probiotic strains to mice could activate mononuclear phagocytes for increased phagocytic activity and lysosomal enzyme production and that this enhancement could be detected in cells derived from peritoneal exudates (Perdigon *et al.*, 1986, 1988). Subsequent studies have confirmed that certain strains of probiotic LAB can prime peritoneal macrophage populations for enhanced phagocytosis, lysosomal enzyme production and free radical oxidant production (Perdigon *et al.*, 1988; Gill, 1998; Matsuzaki and Chin, 2000). Further studies in murine models have reported that probiotic feeding can also enhance the activity of blood-derived phagocytes and that both mononuclear (monocyte) and polymorphonuclear (neutrophil) populations are stimulated by probiotics (Gill *et al.*, 2000). Human studies have confirmed this effect in circulating phagocytes of adult subjects (Schiffrin *et al.*, 1995; Donnet-Hughes *et al.*, 1999; Yoon *et al.*, 1999; Chiang *et al.*, 2000; O'Mahony *et al.*, 2000; Sheih *et al.*, 2001) including the elderly (Arunachalam *et al.*, 2000; Gill *et al.*, 2001a, b, c; Table 13.1).

In common with studies on the effects on lymphocyte proliferation, it is at present unclear whether oral probiotic delivery enhances phagocytic cell function as a reflection of increased cell numbers and/or increased cellular avidity to phagocytose. It is likely that bacterial signalling will activate a general release of phagocytically active cells into circulation (Herich *et al.*, 1999), and this is possibly achieved by microbial stimulation of phagocytic precursor cells. It is important to note that mononuclear phagocytes, in particular, are also capable of secreting immunomodulatory cytokines and that stimulation of these cells by oral probiotics has been shown to increase production of key cytokines, which modify and shape the character of the immune response (Tejada-Simon *et al.*, 1999b). Thus, it is possible that phagocyte activation is the first and key event in immune stimulation by probiotics and that enhanced phagocytic capacity is a reliable index of this activation, prior to the initiation of downstream events, such as cytokine-mediated enhancement of leucocyte cytotoxicity and lymphocyte activation.

Studies in murine models have shown that the cytocidal activity of splenic leucocytes can also be increased following delivery of certain strains of probiotics. Systemic priming of mice with viable *L. casei* (Shirota strain) can enhance *ex vivo* tumoricidal activity of splenic NK cells and macrophages (Kato *et al.*, 1983, 1984) and can also increase cytocidal activity against cytomegalovirus-infected target T-cells (Ohashi *et al.*, 1988). Oral delivery of *L. rhamnosus* HN001 or *L. casei* Shirota to mice has also been shown to increase *ex vivo* NK-cell tumoricidal activity (Gill *et al.*, 2000; Matsuzaki and Chin, 2000). In human studies, feeding of *L. rhamnosus* (strain HN001) or *Bifidobacterium lactis* (strain HN019) has been demonstrated to up-regulate peripheral blood NK-cell-mediated cytotoxicity against tumour cells (Chiang *et al.*, 2000; Gill *et al.*, 2001a, b, c; Sheih *et al.*, 2001; Table 13.1).

Probiotic effects on antibody responses

Several studies have investigated the ability of probiotics to regulate antibody production. Initial animal studies showed that probiotics were able to potentiate systemic antibody responses to parenterally delivered foreign antigens in mice (Portier *et al.*, 1993) and that serum levels of IgG and IgM isotypes were elevated (Perdigon *et al.*, 1991, 1999). Subsequent studies have indicated that probiotic strains such as *L. rhamnosus* HN001 or *B. lactis* HN019 can potentiate antibody responses to both systemically and orally administered T-dependent antigens in mice and that increases in specific antibody titre can be measured in both the serum and intestinal-tract secretions, the latter involving a rise in IgA levels (Yasui *et al.*, 1989; Yasui and Ohwaki, 1991; Herias *et al.*, 1999; Tejada-Simon *et al.*, 1999a; Gill *et al.*, 2000). Since the major GI antibody secretion is derived from plasma cells of the lamina propria, these results suggest that probiotics are able to stimulate the mucosal immune system, possibly via direct interaction with immunocompetent T-cells of the GI tract. Indeed, recent studies in mice have indicated that probiotic LAB are able to increase the mucosal density of IgM- and IgA-secreting plasma cells in both gut epithelial and broncho-alveolar lymphoid tissues (Bibas Bonet *et al.*, 1999; Perdigon *et al.*, 1999).

Under disease conditions, animal studies have also indicated that probiotic delivery can increase GI tract and systemic antibody responses to bacterial pathogens, including *Escherichia coli* (Perdigon *et al.*, 1990, 1991), *Shigella sonnei* (Nader de Marcias *et al.*, 1992) and *Salmonella typhimurium* (Paubert-Braquet *et al.*, 1995; Shu *et al.*, 2000). Clinical studies have demonstrated that the orally delivered probiotic *L. rhamnosus* GG can also increase the frequency of pathogen-specific and total antibody-secreting cells in children during convalescence from rotavirus diarrhoea (Kaila *et al.*, 1992; Majamaa *et al.*, 1995). However, in the case of non-infectious diseases, such as atopy, it appears that certain probiotic bacteria are able to exert a regulatory, rather than enhancing, effect on antibody production. Several studies have shown that IgE responses in allergen-primed mice can be attenuated by the oral or systemic delivery of probiotic LAB (Matsuzaki *et al.*, 1998; Shida *et al.*, 1998; Yasui *et al.*, 1999a; Matsuzaki and Chin, 2000), suggesting that an ability to regulate immune responses may play an important role. Indeed, *in vitro* studies by Murosaki *et al.* (1998) have shown that adding *L. casei* (Shirota strain) to cultures of allergen-reactive murine splenocytes can directly suppress IgE production.

Health Benefits of Probiotic-mediated Immunomodulation

As described previously, probiotics are capable of modulating the immune system via both immunostimulation and immunoregulation, and thus have the potential to have an impact on health status and disease conditions that have an inherent immune component. In the case of immunostimulation, probiotics may provide a boosting of the immune system in key aspects of effector mechanisms that are tailored towards combating infectious diseases or intrinsic pathologies, such as neoplasm development. In addition, the ability of probiotics to stimulate cytokine secretion may provide an important immunoregula tory function for the control of immune dysfunctional conditions, such as chronic inflammation and allergies. Research that has sought to investigate these potential outlets for probiotics in health has drawn on both animal studies and human clinical trials for supportive evidence.

Probiotics and infectious diseases

There is clear evidence that certain probiotic LAB strains are able to potentiate pathogen-specific antibody responses, both in animal models and in humans. Yasui *et al.* (1999b) have demonstrated that mice immunized with influenza vaccine and fed *Bifidobacterium breve* (strain YIT4064) as a probiotic developed enhanced virus-specific antibody responses and showed greater protection against respiratory challenge than non-probiotic-fed mice. In addition, some studies have confirmed an increase in innate and lymphoid cell-mediated events in pathogen-infected mice, which may contribute to enhanced disease resistance. Shu *et al.* (2000) have recently shown that the probiotic *B. lactis* HN019 could enhance pathogen-specific antibody responses in *S. typhimurium*-infected mice, as well as promoting increased peritoneal cell phagocytosis and splenic lympho-proliferative potential; correlation analyses indicated that elevated immune function in probiotic-fed mice corresponded with reduced pathogen translocation in these mice and promoted enhanced survival. Other strains of bifidobacteria (such as *B. breve*) have been shown to increase murine antibody titres in nursing dams and to provide increased protection to weanling mice against rotavirus (Yasui *et al.*, 1995; Fukushima *et al.*, 1999). Recent studies have confirmed this phenomenon in weanling piglets that have been fed *B. lactis* HN019, which exhibit enhanced cellular and humoral immunity and increased protection against naturally acquired weanling diarrhoea (Shu *et al.*, 2001).

In human studies, the probiotic *L. rhamnosus* GG has been shown to promote recovery from both rotavirus and non-bloody diarrhoea in children and infants (Raza *et al.*, 1995; Saxelin, 1997), by reducing virus shedding as well as the duration and intensity of diarrhoeal disease (Table 13.2). Two studies have demonstrated a concomitant rise in the frequency of antibody-secreting plasma cells in the circulation of probiotic-fed children, strongly suggesting that enhanced humoral immunity plays a role in reducing convalescence time by aiding viral elimination (Kaila *et al.*, 1992; Majamaa *et al.*, 1995). Studies using *B. breve* have shown that oral administration of this probiotic to hospitalized children can also support a reduction in both the incidence of diarrhoea and of viral shedding, concomitant with elevated titres of anti-rotavirus IgA antibody in the stools (Araki *et al.*, 1999).

Probiotics and tumour growth

Several studies in animal models have investigated the effects of probiotic administration on immune responses and tumour regression. Initial studies had indicated that systemically delivered LAB cells could potentiate *ex vivo* leuco-cyte tumoricidal and lymphoproliferative responses and could limit the growth of both primary and secondary tumours at several tissue sites *in vivo* (Kato *et al.*, 1981, 1983). More recent studies have focused on the use of orally deliv-ered probiotics and anti-tumour immunity. *L. casei* Shirota has received a great deal of research attention. Orally delivered *L. casei* Shirota was shown to reduce the establishment and growth of inoculated syngeneic sarcoma cells in BALB/c mice, concomitant with an increased lymphoproliferative response and capacity to secrete the cytokine IL-2 by splenic T-cells in these animals (Yokokura, 1994). Furthermore, growth of secondary tumours was inhibited in probiotic-fed mice following tumour resection, again linked to enhanced lym-phocyte responsiveness (Kato *et al.*, 1994). *Lactobacillus plantarum* (strain L-137) has also been shown to retard the growth of implanted P3881D tumour cells in syngeneic DBA/2 mice, and in this case the mechanism was suggested to be a systemic elevation of the pro-cellular-immunity cytokine IL-12, favour-ing anti-tumour cellular immune responses (Murosaki *et al.*, 2000).

Additional studies on *L. casei* Shirota have indicated that this strain may also have anti-carcinogenic effects related to enhanced immune activity. Takagi *et al.* (1999) have recently demonstrated that mice fed the probiotic developed fewer systemic tumours following injection of the hydrocarbon carcinogen 3-methylcholanthrene and that lymphoproliferative responses and the IL-2-secreting activity of splenic T-cells were retained, while the comparative immune responses in non-probiotic-fed mice declined markedly during tumour development. In similar studies, probiotic-containing yoghurt has been shown to limit intestinal-tract tumour development in mice injected with the carcino-gen 1,2-dimethylhydrazine (Perdigon *et al.*, 1998), and this reduction was asso-ciated with enhanced infiltrations of CD4+ T lymphocytes into the intestinal tissues in these mice. Other strains of *Lactobacillus* have also been shown to limit the incidence and mean developmental size of colonic adenocarcinomas in Sprague–Dawley rats fed 1,2-dimethylhydrazine (Balansky *et al.*, 1999; McIntosh *et al.* 1999), although associated immune responses were not investi-gated in these studies. A further anti-cancer mechanism of probiotics involves the deconjugation of potentially mutagenic enzymes in the gut lumen, although this mechanism is not thought to have an immune component.

No longitudinal clinical trials have yet been undertaken to determine the potentially protective effects of immunoactive probiotics in the reduction of tumour incidence/development. However, a few studies have investigated the ability of probiotic LAB strains to retard tumour growth in cancer patients. *L. casei* Shirota was shown to reduce the recurrence of superficial bladder cancer in adult patients following resection (Aso *et al.*, 1995) and also to delay the onset of tumour recurrence (Aso *et al.*, 1992; Table 13.2). Although associated cellular immune parameters were not reported in these studies, work in adult colon-can-cer patients has shown that oral *L. casei* Shirota delivery can enhance circulating NK-cell activity (Sawamura *et al.*, 1994), suggesting that tumour limitation may be the result of enhanced immunoactivity imparted by the probiotic. In contrast, however, a recent study has reported that *L. casei* Shirota does not enhance NK-cell tumoricidal activity in healthy adult subjects (Spanhaak *et al.*, 1998).

Probiotics and the control of immune dysfunctions

The immune system plays an essential role in the regulation of inflammatory-type diseases, and consequently a dysfunction of the immune system can lead to exacerbation of disease. Due to their potential for immune regulation, it has been suggested that probiotics offer potential for the alleviation of several immuno-inflammatory diseases. Perhaps most attention has been given to the ability of probiotics to regulate allergic/atopic responses. In animal studies, *L. casei* Shirota has been shown to reduce cutaneous anaphylaxis in allergen-sensitized mice following dermal challenge (Yasui *et al.*, 1999a). Both *L. casei* Shirota and *L. plantarum* L-137 have been shown to exhibit anti-allergy properties in mice, reportedly due to their ability to induce high-level systemic expression of IL-12 (Murosaki *et al.*, 1998; Kato *et al.*, 1999), which can down-regulate allergic responses. Indeed, some strains of lactobacilli have been shown to elevate systemic levels of IL-12 following oral delivery (Murosaki *et al.*, 1999; Tejada-Simon *et al.*, 1999a), suggesting that this is a major mechanism by which probiotics effect anti-allergy-type immunoregulation.

In human studies of allergic disease, there is longitudinal evidence that consumption of probiotic-supplemented yoghurt over a period of 1 year can lower the circulating levels of IgE and reduce nasal allergies in elderly subjects (Halpern *et al.*, 1991; Trapp *et al.*, 1993; Table 13.2). Wheeler *et al.* (1997) have shown that shorter-term consumption of probiotics (i.e. 1 month) by adult allergy sufferers can generate a trend towards reduced peripheral blood eosinophil counts and increased IFN-γ-secreting activity of lymphocytes, suggesting that probiotic-induced anti-allergy immune regulation may be effective in humans also. A report by Pelto *et al.* (1998) demonstrated an alternative mechanism for the ability of *L. rhamnosus* GG to limit hypersensitivity responses in subjects with cows'-milk allergy, namely, that the probiotic can prevent the up-regulation of pro-inflammatory receptors on leucocytes (a response that normally precedes GI tract inflammation in milk-sensitive subjects). Other potential mechanisms by which probiotics might limit food-hypersensitivity responses include their ability to stabilize the gut intestinal barrier against macromolecular sensitization (Majamaa and Isolauri, 1997) and/or the enzymatic hydrolysis of potentially allergenic macromolecules (Rokka *et al.*, 1997). In the latter case, an additional mechanism may be the generation of immunoregulatory peptides from milk substrates by the enzymatic action of probiotics, since Sutas *et al.* (1996a, b) have shown that milk or casein hydrolysed with *L. rhamnosus* GG invokes lower levels of pro-allergy immune responses in antigen-stimulated peripheral blood lymphocytes from milk-sensitive subjects than do intact macromolecules.

In addition to anti-allergy immunoregulation, several studies have suggested that probiotics could be used to combat inflammatory-type diseases. There is some evidence that dietary consumption of immunoregulating LAB might assist in combating autoimmune diseases, including juvenile chronic arthritis (Malin *et al.*, 1996), although the potential mechanism for this is uncertain. A recent report has shown that a diet rich in lactobacilli could decrease subjective symptoms of arthritis among rheumatoid patients, although whether this effect was a result of anti-inflammatory immune regulation is uncertain (Nenonen *et al.*, 1998). The potential use of probiotics to augment the routine immune signalling events of the gut microflora, as a means of restoring vital anti-inflammatory immunoregulatory control mechanisms, has recently gained a great deal of attention as a promising means of combating inflammatory bowel disease (Gionchetti *et al.*, 2000). However, definitive proof for the effectiveness of this mechanism remains to be obtained.

Overview and Conclusions

It is clear, from the foregoing discussions, that there is significant evidence, both experimental and clinical, to indicate that certain strains of probiotic organisms can modulate the immune system of the host. The two major impacts that have been demonstrated so far include immunostimulation and immunoregulation. Immunostimulation involves an elevation of immune function(s) to a heightened state of responsiveness, and may provide an important role in conditions where an elevation of immune function is not achievable by conventional means or in boosting responses among individuals with sub-optimal immunity. Experimentally, several strains of *Lactobacillus* and *Bifidobacterium* have been shown to boost humoral antibody responses to experimentally administered T-cell-dependent antigens (Portier *et al.*, 1993; Perdigon *et al.*, 1995; Gill *et al.*, 2000). In human studies, *Lactobacillus* GG has been shown to enhance the humoral immune response to orally administered rotavirus and *Salmonella typhi* vaccines (Isolauri *et al.*, 1995; Fangac *et al.*, 2000), while *B. breve* enhances IgA antibody responses to poliomyelitis vaccine (Fukushima *et al.*, 1998), thus providing evidence of the potential use of probiotics as oral adjuvants to boost immune responses at the gut mucosal surface. Future uses of probiotics may be expanded to their use as oral adjuvants to promote immune responses against vaccines that currently can only be administered parenterally – for example, to boost circulating antibody responses to orally administered influenza vaccine (Maassen *et al.*, 2000).

A further role for immune-stimulating probiotics is their use in boosting immune function in individuals with suboptimally functioning immunity. *Lactobacillus* GG has already been mentioned as an oral immunostimulator to enhance antibody responses in children combating rotavirus infection, and probiotics may prove very useful in this context of boosting immunity among malnourished children or infants with poorly developed sensitization. At the other end of the age spectrum, probiotics may prove useful in boosting immunity among elderly subjects. Studies have shown that senescence of the immune system can predispose the elderly to infectious and non-infectious diseases and that a decline in immune function with age can contribute to decreased life expectancy (Roberts-Thomson *et al.*, 1974; Goodwin, 1995). Immunosenescence is characterized by a suboptimal functioning of the cellular immune system in particular, mainly involving T-cell-mediated responses but also some NK-cell and phagocyte functions (Lesourd and Meaume, 1994; Butcher *et al.*, 2000; Solana and Mariani, 2000). In this respect, it has been demonstrated that

L. rhamnosus (strain HN001) and *B. lactis* (strain HN019) are both effective at boosting cellular immune function among healthy middle-aged and elderly subjects (Arunachalam *et al.*, 2000; Chiang *et al.*, 2000; Gill and Rutherfurd, 2001; Gill *et al.*, 2001a, b, c; Sheih *et al.*, 2001). Thus, certain probiotic strains may offer benefit to elderly consumers by stimulating the very compartments of the immune system that are adversely affected by ageing.

The immunoregulatory role of probiotics has probably received the greatest degree of attention in experimental research. A large proportion of this work has thus far focused on probiotic LAB, which induce the anti-allergy cytokines IL-12 and IFN-γ, for their potential use in preventing atopic responses and combating allergies. Yet there is still only limited clinical evidence that orally delivered probiotics are effective at combating allergic symptoms among at-risk groups (Trapp *et al.*, 1993; Wheeler *et al.*, 1997). In contrast, there is gathering clinical evidence that certain probiotic strains can be used effectively in neonatal and paediatric care to provide the necessary bacterial signals which, in early life, enable the immune system to develop appropriately and to avoid allergic sensitization (Isolauri *et al.*, 2000; Kalliomaki *et al.*, 2001).

Other potential uses of immunoregulatory probiotics (e.g. in controlling inflammatory diseases at the gut surface) have only recently begun to attract research attention (Venturi *et al.*, 1999), partly because the microbial : gut mucosal signalling mechanisms are only beginning to be understood by microbiological researchers (Haller *et al.*, 2000). A recent pilot study (Gupta *et al.*, 2000) showed promising preliminary results for the use of *L. rhamnosus* GG as a dietary supplement to reduce clinical indices of GI-tract inflammation in children with Crohn's disease. As research starts to define the interactions of the gut microflora and the immune system in the maintenance of health, so it is likely that new avenues for dietary intervention will become the focus of research efforts.

The Future for Probiotics in Immune Health

For both immunostimulatory and immunoregulatory roles, contemporary research has already identified a few promising strains of immunoactive probiotics (predominantly LAB) and these strains either are currently being commercialized or are near commercialization. An on-going need for research in this area is for continued safety monitoring, particularly among individuals with pre-existing health conditions. For example, among patients with active autoimmune conditions, probiotic strains that stimulate cellular immune function must receive particular and thorough attention to avoid the potential for disease exacerbation; moreover, the safety of probiotics in subjects with deficient immune systems (e.g. acquired immune deficiency syndrome (AIDS) patients) should be considered. That aside, the essential requirement in all of these cases is not only that the probiotic under consideration is effective at influencing immunity but that it influences the immune system in the appropriate manner and, moreover, that this action contributes in a meaningful way to health improvement. In the former case, this suggests that well-designed and appropriate clinical trials are conducted to determine the impact of any probiotic on the immune system and that this research is conducted on the target population (with regard to demographics, etc.) (Meydani and Ha, 2000). In the latter case, where an effect of probiotics on the immune system has already been demonstrated, there remains the need to correlate immunoactivity with health improvement. In many cases (e.g. boosting of anti-tumour immunity) such evidence will only come from longitudinal/cross-sectional studies of significant duration (Macfarlane and Cummings, 1999). Nevertheless, major progress in the use of defined probiotics for health improvement is likely to become apparent in the coming decade.

References

Aattouri, N. and Lemonnier, D. (1997) Production of interferon induced by *Streptococcus thermophilus*: role of CD4[+] and CD8[+] lymphocytes. *Journal of Nutritional Biochemistry* 8, 25–31.

Alm, J., Swartz, J., Lilja, G., Scheynius, A. and Pershagen, G. (1999) Atopy in children of families with an anthroposophic lifestyle. *Lancet* 353, 1485–1488.

Araki, T., Shinozaki, T., Irie, Y. and Miyazawa, Y. (1999) Trial of oral administration of *Bifidobacterium breve* for the prevention of rotavirus infection. *Journal of the Japanese Association of Infectious Diseases* 73, 305–310.

Arunachalam, K., Gill, H.S. and Chandra, R.K. (2000) Enhancement of natural immune function by dietary consumption of *Bifidobacterium lactis* (HN019). *European Journal of Clinical Nutrition* 54, 1–5.

Aso, Y., Akaza, H. and Kotake, T. (1992) Prophylactic effect of a *Lactobacillus casei* preparation on the recurrence of superficial bladder cancer. *Urology International* 49, 125–129.

Aso, Y., Akaza, H. and Kotake, T. (1995) Preventive effect of a *Lactobacillus casei* preparation on the recurrence of superficial bladder cancer in a double-blind trial. *European Urology* 27, 104–109.

Balansky, R., Gyosheva, B., Ganchev, G., Mircheva, Z., Minkova, S. and Georgiev, G. (1999) Inhibitory effects of freeze-dried milk fermented by selected *Lactobacillus bulgaricus* strains on carcinogenesis induced by 1,2-dimethylhydrazine in rats and by diethylnitrosamine in hamsters. *Cancer Letters* 147, 125.

Bibas Bonet, M.E., de Petrino, S.F., Meson, O., de Budeguer, M.V. and Perdigon, G. (1999) Optimal effect of *Lactobacillus delbruecki* subsp. *bulgaricus*, among other lactobacilli species, on the number of IgA and mast cells associated with the mucosa in immunosuppressed mice. *Food and Agricultural Immunology* 11, 259–267.

Butcher, S., Chahel, H. and Lord, J.M. (2000) Ageing and the neutrophil: no appetite for killing? *Immunology* 100, 411–416.

Cauwels, A., Wan, E., Leismann, M. and Tuomanen, E. (1997) Coexistence of CD14-dependent and independent pathways for stimulation of human monocytes by Gram-positive bacteria. *Infection and Immunity* 65, 3255–3260.

Chiang, B.L., Sheih, Y.H., Wang, L.H. and Gill, H.S. (2000) Enhancement of immunity by *Bifidobacterium lactis*: optimisation and definition of cellular responses. *European Journal of Clinical Nutrition* 54, 849–855.

Cleveland, M.G., Gorham, J.D., Murphy, T.L., Tuomanen, E. and Murphy, K.M. (1996). Lipoteichoic acid preparations of gram-positive bacteria induce interleukin-12 through a CD14-dependent pathway. *Infection and Immunity* 64, 1906–1912.

Delneste, Y., Donnet-Hughes, A. and Schiffrin, E.J. (1998) Functional foods: mechanisms of action on immunocompetent T-cells. *Nutrition Reviews* 56, S93-S98.

de Simone, C., Vesely, R., Negri, R., Bianchi Salvadori, B., Zanzoglu, S., Cilli, A. and Lucci, L. (1987) Enhancement of immune response of murine Peyer's patches by a diet supplemented with yoghurt. *Immunopharmacology and Immunotoxicology* 9, 87–100.

de Simone, C., Bianchi Salvadori, B., Jirillo, E., Baldinelli, L., Bitonti, F. and Vesely, R. (1989) Modulation of immune activities in humans and animals by dietary lactic acid bacteria. In: Chandan, R.C. (ed.) *Yogurt Nutritional and Health Properties.* John Libbey Eurotext, London, pp. 201–213.

de Simone, C., Vesely, R., Bianchi Salvadori, B. and Jirillo, E. (1993) The role of probiotics in modulation of the immune system in man and in animals. *International Journal of Immunotherapy* 9, 23–28.

Donnet-Hughes, A., Rochat, F., Serrant, P., Aeschlimann, J.M. and Schiffrin, E.J. (1999) Modulation of nonspecific mechanisms of defence by lactic acid bacteria: effective dose. *Journal of Dairy Science* 82, 863–869.

Dunne, D.W., Resnick, D., Greenberg, J., Krieger, M. and Joiner, K.A. (1994) The type I macrophage scavenger receptor binds to gram-positive bacteria and recognizes lipoteichoic acid. *Proceedings of the National Academy of Sciences of the USA* 91, 1863–1867.

Dziarski, R., Tapping, R.I. and Tobias, P.S. (1998) Binding of bacterial peptidoglycan to CD14. *Journal of Biological Chemistry* 273, 8680–8690.

Elmer, G.W., Surawicz, C.M. and McFarland, L.V. (1996) Biotherapeutic agents: a neglected modality for the prevention and treatment of selected intestinal and vaginal infections. *Journal of the American Medical Association* 272, 870–876.

Fangac, H., Elinaa, T., Heikkib, A. and Seppoa, S. (2000) Modulation of humoral immune response through probiotic intake. *FEMS Immunology and Medical Microbiology* 29, 47–52.

Fukushima, Y., Kawata, Y., Hara, H., Terada, A. and Mitsuoka, T. (1998) Effect of a probiotic formula on intestinal immunoglobulin A production in healthy children. *International Journal of Food Microbiology* 42, 39–44.

Fukushima, Y., Kawata, Y., Mizumachi, K., Kurisaki, J. and Mitsuoka, T. (1999) Effect of bifidobacteria feeding on fecal flora and production of immunoglobulins in the lactating mouse. *International Journal of Food Microbiology* 46, 193–197.

Fuller, R. (1992) *History and Development of Probiotics: Probiotics – the Scientific Basis.* Chapman & Hall, London.

Gill, H.S. (1998) Stimulation of the immune system by lactic cultures. *International Dairy Journal* 8, 535–544.

Gill, H.S. and Rutherfurd, K.J. (2001) Probiotic supplementation to enhance human natural immunity: effects of a newly characterised immunostimulatory strain (*Lactobacillus rhamnosus* HN001) on leucocyte phagocytosis. *Nutrition Research* 21, 183–189.

Gill, H.S., Rutherfurd, K.J., Prasad, J. and Gopal, P.K. (2000) Enhancement of natural and acquired immunity by *Lactobacillus rhamnosus* (HN001), *Lactobacillus acidophilus* (HN017) and *Bifidobacterium lactis* (HN019). *British Journal of Nutrition* 83, 167–176.

Gill, H.S., Cross, M.L., Rutherfurd, K.J. and Gopal, P.K. (2001a) Dietary probiotic supplementation to enhance cellular immunity in the elderly. *British Journal of Biomedical Science* 58, 94–96.

Gill, H.S., Rutherfurd, K.J., Cross, M.L. and Gopal, P.K. (2001b) Enhancement of immunity in the elderly by dietary supplementation with the probiotic *Bifidobacterium lactis* HN019. *American Journal of Clinical Nutrition* 74, 833–839.

Gill, H.S., Rutherfurd, K.J. and Cross, M.L. (2001c) Dietary probiotic supplementation enhances natural killer cell activity in the elderly: an investigation of age-related immunological changes. *Journal of Clinical Immunology* 21, 264–271.

Gionchetti, P., Rizzello, F., Venturi, A., Brigidi, P., Matteuzzi, D., Bazzocchi, G., Poggioli, G., Miglioli, M. and Campieri, M. (2000) Oral bacteriotherapy as maintenance treatment in patients with chronic pouchitis: a double-blind, placebo-controlled trial. *Gastroenterology* 119, 305–309.

Goodwin, J.S. (1995) Decreased immunity and increased morbidity in the elderly. *Nutrition Reviews* 53, S41-S45.

Gupta, P., Andrew, H., Kirschner, B.S. and Guandalini, S. (2000) Is *Lactobacillus* GG helpful in children with Crohn's disease? Results of a preliminary, open-label study. *Journal of Pediatric Gastroenterology and Nutrition* 31, 453–457.

Haller, D., Bode, C., Hammes, W.P., Pfeifer, A.M., Schiffrin, E.J. and Blum, S. (2000) Non-pathogenic bacteria elicit a differential cytokine response by intestinal epithelial cell/leucocyte co-cultures. *Gut* 47, 79–87.

Halpern, G.M., Vruwink, K.G., Van De Water, J., Keen, C.L. and Gershwin, M.E. (1991) Influence of long-term yoghurt consumption in young adults. *International Journal of Immunotherapy* 7, 205–210.

Herias, M.V., Hessle, C., Telemo, E., Midtvedt, T., Hanson, L.A. and Wold, A.E. (1999) Immunomodulatory effects of *Lactobacillus plantarum* colonizing the intestine of gnotobiotic rats. *Clinical and Experimental Immunology* 116, 283–290.

Herich, R., Bomba, A., Nemcova, R. and Gancarcikova, S. (1999) The influence of short-term and continuous administration of *Lactobacillus casei* on basic haematological and immunological parameters in gnotobiotic piglets. *Food and Agricultural Immunology* 11, 287–295.

Isolauri, E., Joensus, J., Suomalainen, H., Luomala, M. and Vesikari, T. (1995) Improved immunogenicity of oral D XRRV reabsorbant rotavirus vaccine by *Lactobacillus casei* GG. *Vaccine* 13, 310–312.

Isolauri, E., Arvola, T., Sutas, Y., Moilanen, E. and Salminen, S. (2000) Probiotics in the management of atopic eczema. *Clinical and Experimental Allergy* 30, 1604–1610.

Kaila, M., Isolauri, E., Soppi, E., Virtanen, E., Laine, S. and Arvilommi, H. (1992) Enhancement of the circulating antibody secreting cell response in human diarrhoea by a human *Lactobacillus* strain. *Pediatric Research* 32, 141–144.

Kalliomaki, M., Salminen, S., Arvillommi, H., Kero, P., Koskinen, P. and Isolauri, E. (2001) Probiotics in primary prevention of atopic disease: a randomised placebo-controlled trial. *Lancet* 357, 1076–1079.

Kato, I., Yokokawa, T. and Mutai, M. (1981) Antitumor activity of *Lactobacillus casei* in mice. *Gann* 72, 517–523.

Kato, I., Yokokura, T. and Mutai, M. (1983) Macrophage activation by *Lactobacillus casei* in mice. *Microbiology and Immunology* 27, 611–618.

Kato, I., Yokokura, T. and Mutai, M. (1984) Augmentation of mouse natural killer cell activity by *Lactobacillus casei* and its surface antigens. *Microbiology and Immunology* 28, 209–217.

Kato, I., Endo, K. and Yokokura, T. (1994) Effects of oral administration of *Lactobacillus casei* on antitumor responses induced by tumor resection in mice. *International Journal of Immunopharmacology* 16, 29–36.

Kato, I., Tanaka, K. and Yokokura, T. (1999) Lactic acid bacterium potently induces the production of interleukin-12 and interferon-γ by mouse splenocytes. *International Journal of Immunopharmacology* 21, 121–131.

Kirjavainen, P.V., El-Nezami, H.S., Salminen, S.J., Ahokas, J.T. and Wright, P.F. (1999) The effect of orally administered viable probiotic and dairy lactobacilli on mouse lymphocyte proliferation. *FEMS Immunology and Medical Microbiology* 26, 131–135.

Kishi, A., Uno, K., Matsubara, Y., Okuda, C. and Kishida, T. (1996) Effect of the oral administration of *Lactobacillus brevis* subsp. *coagulans* on interferon-α producing capacity in humans. *Journal of the American College of Nutrition* 15, 408–412.

Kuhn, R., Lohler, J., Rennick, D., Rajewsky, K. and Muller, W. (1993) Interleukin-10-deficient mice develop chronic enterocolitis. *Cell* 75, 263–274.

Kulkarni, A.B. and Karlsson, S. (1993) Transforming growth factor β-knockout mice: a mutation in one cytokine gene causes a dramatic inflammatory disease. *American Journal of Pathology* 143, 3–9.

Lesourd, B.M. and Meaume, S. (1994) Cell mediated immunity changes in ageing: relative importance of cell subpopulation switches and of nutritional factors. *Immunology Letters* 40, 235–242.

Link-Amster, H., Rochat, F., Saudan, K.Y., Mignot, O. and Aeschlimann, J.M. (1994) Modulation of a specific humoral immune response and changes in intestinal flora mediated through fermented milk intake. *FEMS Immunology and Medical Microbiology* 10, 55–64.

Maassen, C.B., van Holten-Neelen, C., Balk, F., den Bak-Glashouwer, M., Leer, R.J., Laman, J.D., Boersma, W.J. and Claassen, E. (2000) Strain-dependent induction of cytokine profiles in the gut by orally-administered *Lactobacillus* strains. *Vaccine* 18, 2613–2623.

Macfarlane, G.T. and Cummings, J.H. (1999) Probiotics and prebiotics: can regulating the activities of intestinal bacteria benefit health? *British Medical Journal* 318, 999–1003.

McIntosh, G.H., Royle, P.J. and Playne, M.J. (1999) A probiotic strain of *L. acidophilus* reduces DMH-induced large intestinal tumors in male Sprague–Dawley rats. *Nutrition and Cancer* 35, 153–159.

Majamaa, H. and Isolauri, E. (1997) Probiotics: a novel approach in the management of food allergy. *Journal of Allergy and Clinical Immunology* 99, 179–185.

Majamaa, H., Isolauri, E., Saxelin, M. and Vesikari, T. (1995) Lactic acid bacteria in the treatment of acute rotavirus gastroenteritis. *Journal of Pediatric Gastroenterology and Nutrition* 20, 333–338.

Malin, M., Verronen, P., Mykkanen, H., Salminen, S. and Isolauri, E. (1996) Increased bacterial urease activity in faeces in juvenile chronic arthritis: evidence of altered intestinal microflora? *British Journal of Rheumatology* 35, 689–694.

Matricardi, P.M., Rosmini, F., Rapicetta, M., Gasbarrini, G. and Stroffolini, T. (1999) Atopy, hygiene, and anthroposophic lifestyle. *Lancet* 354, 430.

Matsuzaki, T. and Chin, J. (2000) Modulating immune responses with probiotic bacteria. *Immunology and Cell Biology* 78, 67–73.

Matsuzaki, T., Yamazaki, R., Hashimoto, S. and Yokokura, T. (1998) The effect of oral feeding of *Lactobacillus casei* strain Shirota on immunoglobulin E production in mice. *Journal of Dairy Science* 81, 48–53.

Meydani, S.N. and Ha, W.K. (2000) Immunologic effects of yogurt. *American Journal of Clinical Nutrition* 71, 861–872.

Mitsuoka, T. and Hayakawa, K. (1973) The fecal flora in man. I. Composition of the fecal flora of various age groups. *Zentralbl Bakteriologi* 223, 333–342.

Murosaki, S., Yamomoto, Y., Ito, K., Inokuchi, T., Kusaka, H., Ikeda, H. and Yoshikai, Y. (1998) Heat-killed *Lactobacillus plantarum* L-137 suppresses naturally fed antigen-specific IgE production by stimulation of IL-12 production in mice. *Journal of Allergy and Clinical Immunology* 102, 57–64.

Murosaki, S., Muroyama, K., Yamamoto, Y., Kusaka, H., Liu, T. and Yoshikai, Y. (1999) Immunopotentiating activity of nigerooligosaccharides for the T helper 1-like immune response in mice. *Bioscience, Biotechnology and Biochemistry* 63, 373–378.

Murosaki, S., Muroyama, K., Yamamoto, Y. and Yoshikai, Y. (2000) Antitumor effect of heat-killed *Lactobacillus plantarum* L-137 through restoration of impaired inter-leukin-12 production in tumor-bearing mice. *Cancer Immunology and Immunotherapy* 49, 157–164.

Nader de Macias, M.E., Apella, M.C., Romero, N.C., Gonzalez, S.N. and Oliver, G. (1992) Inhibition of *Shigella sonnei* by *Lactobacillus casei* and *Lact. acidophilus*. *Journal of Applied Bacteriology* 73, 407–411.

Nenonen, M.T., Helve, T.A., Rauma, A.L. and Hanninen, O.O. (1998) Uncooked, lacto-bacilli-rich, vegan food and rheumatoid arthritis. *British Journal of Rheumatology* 37, 274–281.

Ohashi, T., Yoshida, A. and Minamishima, Y. (1988) Host-mediated antiviral activity of *Lactobacillus casei* against cytomegalovirus infection in mice. *Biotherapy* 1, 27–39.

O'Mahony, L., Feeney, M., Dunne, C., O'Halloran, S., Murphy, L., Kiely, B., O'Sullivan, G., Shanahan, F. and Collins, J.K. (2000) Probiotic bacteria and the human immune system. In: Buttriss, J. and Saltmarsh, M. (eds) *Functional Foods – Claims and Evidence*. Royal Society of Chemistry, London, pp. 63–69.

Paubert-Braquet, M., Gan, X.H., Gaudichon, C., Hedef, N., Serikoff, A., Bouley, C., Bonavida, B. and Braquet, P. (1995) Enhancement of host resistance against *Salmonella typhimurium* in mice fed a diet supplemented with yogurt or milks fermented with various *Lactobacillus casei* strains. *International Journal of Immunotherapy* 11, 153–161.

Pelto, L., Isolauri, E., Lilius, E.M., Nuutila, J. and Salminen, S. (1998) Probiotic bacteria down-regulate the milk-induced inflammatory response in milk-hypersensitive sub-jects but have an immunostimulatory effect in healthy subjects. *Clinical and Experimental Allergy and Immunology* 28, 1474–1479.

Perdigon, G., de Macias, M.E.N., Alvarez, S., Oliver, G. and de Ruiz Holgado, A.P. (1986) Effect of perorally administered lactobacilli on macrophage activation in mice. *Infection and Immunity* 53, 404–410.

Perdigon, G., de Macias, M.E., Alvarez, S., Oliver, G. and de Ruiz Holgado, A.P. (1988) Systemic augmentation of the immune response in mice by feeding fermented milks with *Lactobacillus casei* and *Lactobacillus acidophilus*. *Immunology* 63, 17–23.

Perdigon, G., de Macias, M.E., Alvarez, S., Oliver, G. and de Ruiz Holgado, A.P. (1990) Prevention of gastrointestinal infection using immunobiological methods with milk fermented with *Lactobacillus casei* and *Lactobacillus acido*philus. *Journal of Dairy Research* 57, 255–264.

Perdigon, G., Alvarez, S. and de Ruiz Holgado, A.P. (1991) Immunoadjuvant activity of *Lactobacillus casei*: influence of the dose on the secretory immune response and protective capacity in intestinal infections. *Journal of Dairy Research* 58, 485–496.

Perdigon, G., Alvarez, S., Rachid, M., Aguero, G. and Gobbato, N. (1995) Probiotic bacteria for humans: clinical systems for evaluation of effectiveness. *Journal of Dairy Science* 78, 1597–1606.

Perdigon, G., Valdez, J.C. and Rachid, M. (1998) Antitumour activity of yogurt: study of possible immune mechanisms. *Journal of Dairy Research* 65, 129–138.

Perdigon, G., Vintini, E., Alvarez, S., Medina, M. and Medici, M. (1999) Studies of the possible mechanisms involved in the mucosal immune system activation by lactic acid bacteria. *Journal of Dairy Science* 82, 1108–1114.

Pereyra, B.S., Falcoff, R., Falcoff, E. and Lemonnier, D. (1991) Interferon induction by *Lactobacillus bulgaricus* and *Streptococcus thermophilus* in mice. *European Cytokine Network* 2, 299–303.

Portier, A., Boyaka, N.P., Bougoudogo, F., Dubarry, M., Huneau, J.F., Tome, D., Dodin, A. and Coste, M. (1993) Fermented milks and increased antibody responses against cholera in mice. *International Journal of Immunotherapy* 9, 217–224.

Raza, S., Graham, S. and Allen, S.J. (1995) *Lactobacillus* GG promotes recovery from acute non bloody diarrhoea in Pakistan. *Pediatric Infectious Diseases Journal* 14, 107–111.

Roberts-Thomson, I.C., Whittingham, S., Youngchaiyud, U. and Mackay, I.R. (1974) Ageing, immune response, and mortality. *Lancet* 7877, 368–370.

Rokka, T., Syvaoja, E.L., Tuomine, J. and Korhonen, H. (1997) Release of bioactive peptides by enzymatic proteolysis of *Lactobacillus* GG fermented UHT milk. *Milchwissenschaft* 52, 675–678.

Salminen, S., Bonley, C., Bourron-Ruanlt, M., Cummings, J.H., Franck, A., Gibson, G.R., Isolauri, E., Moreau, M.C., Roberfroid, M. and Rowland, I. (1998) Functional food science and gastrointestinal physiology and function. *British Journal of Nutrition* 80, S147-S171.

Sawamura, A., Yamaguchi, Y., Toge, T., Nagata, N., Ikeda, H., Nakanishi, K. and Asakura, A. (1994) Enhancement of immuno-activities by oral administration of *Lactobacillus casei* in colorectal cancer patients. *Biotherapy* 8, 1567–1572.

Saxelin, M. (1997) *Lactobacillus* GG – a human probiotic strain with thorough clinical documentation. *Food Reviews International* 13, 293–313.

Schiffrin, E.J., Rochar, F., Link-Amster, H., Aeschlimann, J.M. and Donnet-Hughes, A. (1995) Immunomodulation of human blood cells following the ingestion of lactic acid bacteria. *Journal of Dairy Science* 78, 491–497.

Schiffrin, E.J., Brassart, D., Servin, A., Rochat, F. and Donnet-Hughes, A. (1997) Immune modulation of blood leucocytes in humans by lactic acid bacteria: criteria for strain selection. *American Journal of Clinical Nutrition* 66, 515S-520S.

Sheih, Y.H., Chiang, B.L., Wang, L.H., Liao, C.K. and Gill, H.S. (2001) Systemic immunity-enhancing effects in healthy subjects following dietary consumption of the lactic acid bacterium *Lactobacillus rhamnosus* HN001. *Journal of the American College of Nutrition* 20(Suppl. 2), 149–156.

Shida, K., Makino, K., Morishita, A., Takamizawa, K., Hachimura, S., Ametani, A., Sato, T., Kumagai, Y., Habu, S. and Kaminogawa, S. (1998) *Lactobacillus casei* inhibits antigen-induced IgE secretion through regulation of cytokine production in murine splenocyte cultures. *International Archives of Allergy and Immunology* 115, 278–287.

Shu, Q., Rutherfurd, K.J., Fenwick, S.G., Prasad, J., Gopal, P.K. and Gill, H.S. (2000) Dietary *Bifidobacterium lactis* (HN019) enhances resistance to oral *Salmonella typhimurium* infection in mice. *Microbiology and Immunology* 44, 213–222.

Shu, Q., Qu, F. and Gill, H.S. (2001) Probiotic treatment using *Bifidobacterium lactis* HN019 reduces weanling diarrhea associated with rotavirus and *Escherichia coli* infection in a piglet model. *Journal of Pediatric Gastroenterology and Nutrition* 33, 171–177.

Solana, R. and Mariani, E. (2000) NK and NK/T-cells in human senescence. *Vaccine* 18, 1613–1620.

Solis-Pereyra, B. and Lemonnier, D. (1991) Induction of 2–5A synthetase activity and interferon in humans by bacteria used in dairy products. *European Cytokine Network* 2, 137–140.

Solis-Pereyra, B., Aattouri, N. and Lemonnier, D. (1997) Role of food in the stimulation of cytokine production. *American Journal of Clinical Nutrition* 66, 521S-525S.

Spanhaak, S., Havenaar, R. and Schaafsma, G. (1998) The effect of consumption of milk fermented by *Lactobacillus casei* strain Shirota on the intestinal microflora and immune parameters in humans. *European Journal of Clinical Nutrition* 52, 899–907.

Sutas, Y., Soppi, E., Korhonen, H., Syvaoja, E.L., Saxelin, M., Rokka, T. and Isolauri, E. (1996a) Suppression of lymphocyte proliferation *in vitro* by bovine caseins hydrolyzed with *Lactobacillus casei* GG-derived enzymes. *Journal of Allergy and Clinical Immunology* 98, 216–224.

Sutas, Y., Hurme, M. and Isolauri, E. (1996b) Down-regulation of anti-CD3 antibody-induced IL-4 production by bovine caseins hydrolysed with *Lactobacillus* GG-derived enzymes. *Scandinavian Journal of Immunology* 43, 687–689.

Takagi, A., Matsuzaki, T., Sato, M., Nomoto, K., Morotomi, M. and Yokokura, T. (1999) Inhibitory effect of oral administration of *Lactobacillus casei* on 3-methylcholan-threne-induced carcinogenesis in mice. *Medical Microbiology and Immunology* 188, 111–116.

Tejada-Simon, M.V., Lee, J.H., Ustunol, Z. and Pestka, J.J. (1999a) Ingestion of yogurt containing *Lactobacillus acidophilus* and *Bifidobacterium* to potentiate immunoglobulin A responses to cholera toxin in mice. *Journal of Dairy Science* 82, 649–660.

Tejada-Simon, M.V., Ustunol, Z. and Pestka, J.J. (1999b) *Ex vivo* effects of lactobacilli, streptococci, and bifidobacteria ingestion on cytokine and nitric oxide production in a murine model. *Journal of Food Protection* 62, 162–169.

Trapp, C.L., Chang, C.C., Halpern, G.M., Keen, C.L. and Gershwin, M.E. (1993) The influence of chronic yogurt consumption on populations of young and elderly adults. *International Journal of Immunotherapy* 9, 53–64.

Venturi, A., Gionchetti, P., Rizzello, F., Johansson, R., Zucconi, E., Brigidi, P., Matteuzzi, D. and Campieri, M. (1999) Impact on the composition of the faecal flora by a new probiotic preparation: preliminary data on maintenance treatment of patients with ulcerative colitis. *Alimentary Pharmacology and Therapeutics* 13, 1103–1108.

Vesely, R., Negri, R., Bianchi Salvadori, B.B., Lavezzari, D. and De Simone, C. (1985) Influence of a diet additioned with yogurt on the immune system. *Journal of Immunology and Immunopharmacology* 1, 30–35.

Wheeler, J.G., Shema, S., Bogle, M.L., Shirrell, A., Burks, A.W., Pittler, A. and Helm, R.M. (1997) Immune and clinical impact of *Lactobacillus acidophilus* on asthma. *Annals of Allergy Asthma and Immunology* 79, 229–233.

Yasui, H. and Ohwaki, M. (1991) IgA production and intestinal microflora: augmentation of IgA production by *Bifidobacterium breve*. *Japanese Journal of Clinical Microbiology* 24, 426–430.

Yasui, H., Mike, A. and Ohwaki, M. (1989) Immunogenicity of *Bifidobacterium breve* and change in antibody production in Peyer's patches after oral administration. *Journal of Dairy Science* 72, 30–35.

Yasui, H., Kiyoshima, J. and Ushijima, H. (1995) Passive protection against rotavirus-induced diarrhea of mouse pups born to and nursed by dams fed *Bifidobacterium breve* YIT4064. *Journal of Infectious Disease* 172, 403–409.

Yasui, H., Shida, K., Matsuzali, T. and Yokokura, T. (1999a) Immunomodulatory function of lactic acid bacteria. *Antonie van Leeuwehhoek* 76, 383–389.

Yasui, H., Kiyoshima, J., Hori, T. and Shida, K. (1999b) Protection against influenza virus infection of mice fed *Bifidobacterium breve* YIT4064. *Clinical and Diagnostic Laboratory Immunology* 6, 186–192.

Yokokura, T. (1994) Anti-tumor and immune stimulating activities of *Lactobacillus casei*. *Japanese Journal of Dairy Food Science* 43, 141–150.

Yoon, H., Dubarry, M., Bouley, C., Meredith, C., Portier, A., Tome, D., Renevot, O., Blachon, J.L., Dugas, B., Drewitt, P. and Postaire, E. (1999) New insights in the validation of systemic biomarkers for the evaluation of the immunoregulatory properties of milk fermented with yogurt culture and *Lactobacillus casei* (Actimel (R)): a prospective trial. *International Journal of Immunotherapy* 15, 79–89.

14 Role of Local Immunity and Breast-feeding in Mucosal Homoeostasis and Defence against Infections

PER BRANDTZAEG

Laboratory for Immunohistochemistry and Immunopathology (LIIPAT), Institute of Pathology, University of Oslo, Rikshospitalet, N-0027 Oslo, Norway

Introduction

The mammalian host defence has successfully handled environmental confrontations for millions of years. To this end, numerous genes involved in innate and acquired (adaptive) immune protection have been subjected to evolutionary modifications, thus being shaped according to the microbial pressure and environmental (including dietary) impact. In humans, this modulation has been influenced by various ways of living, such as hunting, fishing, gathering, agriculture and animal husbandry.

In the process of evolution, the mucosal immune system has generated two arms of adaptive defence: (i) antigen exclusion, performed by secretory antibodies of the immunoglobulin (Ig)A and IgM classes, to modulate or inhibit surface colonization of microorganisms and dampen penetration of potentially dangerous soluble agents; and (ii) suppressive mechanisms to avoid local and peripheral overreaction (hypersensitivity) against innocuous substances bombarding the mucosal surfaces (Fig. 14.1). The latter arm is referred to as 'oral tolerance' when induced via the gut against dietary antigens (Brandtzaeg, 1996a); it probably explains why overt and persistent hypersensitivity to food proteins is relatively rare (Bischoff *et al.*, 2000). Similar down-regulatory mechanisms apparently operate against antigens from the commensal microbial flora (Duchmann *et al.*, 1997; Karlsson *et al.*, 1999; Helgeland and Brandtzaeg, 2000).

Oral tolerance generally seems to be a rather robust adaptive immune function, in view of the fact that more than a ton of food may pass through the

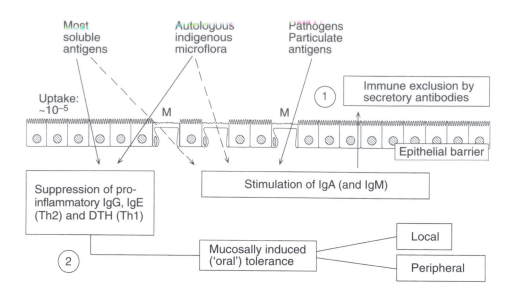

Fig. 14.1. Schematic depiction of two major adaptive immune mechanisms operating at mucosal surfaces. (1) Immune exclusion limits epithelial colonization of pathogens and inhibits penetration of harmful foreign material. This first line of defence is principally mediated by secretory antibodies of the immunoglobulin (Ig)A (and IgM) class in cooperation with various non-specific innate protective factors (not shown). Secretory immunity is preferentially stimulated by pathogens and other particulate antigens taken up through thin membrane (M) cells located in the dome epithelium covering inductive mucosa-associated lymphoid tissue (see Fig. 14.3). (2) Penetrating innocuous soluble environmental and dietary antigens (magnitude of uptake indicated), as well as the autologous indigenous microbial flora, are less stimulatory for secretory immunity (self-limiting responses, broken arrows), but induce suppression of pro-inflammatory humoral immune responses (IgG and T-helper-2 (Th2) cytokine-dependent IgE antibodies), as well as Th1 cytokine-dependent delayed-type hypersensitivity (DTH). The homoeostatic Th1/Th2 balance is regulated by a complex and poorly defined phenomenon called mucosal or 'oral' tolerance (see Fig. 14.5), which exerts down-regulatory effects both locally and in the periphery. (Modified from Brandtzaeg *et al.*, 1999a.)

gut of an adult every year, resulting in substantial uptake of intact antigens even in the healthy state. Nevertheless, the neonatal period is particularly critical in terms of mucosal defence, in regard to both infections and priming for allergic disease (Holt and Jones, 2000). This is so because the mucosal barrier function and the immunoregulatory network are poorly developed for a variable period after birth (Brandtzaeg *et al.*, 1991; Holt, 1995). Notably, the post-natal development of mucosal immune homoeostasis appears to depend on the establishment of a normal commensal microbial flora, as well as on the adequate timing and dose of dietary antigens when first introduced (Brandtzaeg, 1996b, 1998; Helgeland and Brandtzaeg, 2000).

Antibody-mediated Defence in the Neonate

Striking species differences

The enterocytes of mammals play a vital role in defence of the neonate, not only by forming a mechanical barrier but also by transferring breast-milk-derived maternal antibodies from the gut lumen, thus providing passive systemic immunity in the newborn period. This enterocytic Ig transmission differs remarkably among species. In the ungulate (horse, cattle, sheep, pig), the whole length of the intestine is involved in a non-selective protein uptake, including all Ig isotypes, in a poorly defined pinocytic process. Because colostrum of these animals is particularly rich in IgG, this antibody class will preferentially reach the circulation of the neonate via its gut epithelium during the two first postnatal days, after which so-called 'gut closure' takes place (Mackenzie, 1990). Rodents, on the other hand, express an Fc receptor specific for IgG apically on neonatal enterocytes in the proximal small intestine. This receptor (FcRn), which disappears at weaning, has been particularly well characterized on enterocytes of the neonatal rat; it is a major histocompatibility complex (MHC) class I-related molecule, associated with β_2-microglobulin (Simister and Mostov, 1989). Complexes of FcRn and IgG are internalized in clathrin-coated pits at the base of the microvilli; binding of the ligand takes place in the acidic luminal environment, and IgG release occurs at physiological pH on the basolateral face of the enterocyte, after which the receptor is recycled.

In contrast to the animal species mentioned above, the human fetus acquires maternal IgG via the placenta (Mackenzie, 1990) and perhaps, to some extent, from swallowed amniotic fluid via FcRn expressed by fetal enterocytes (Israel *et al.*, 1993). Indeed, a bidirectional transport mechanism for IgG was recently demonstrated in a human intestinal epithelial cell line (Dickinson *et al.*, 1999), but the functional significance of FcRn on enterocytes in the human newborn remains unknown. Intestinal uptake of secretory IgA (SIgA) antibodies after breast-feeding appears of little or no importance in the support of systemic immunity (Ogra *et al.*, 1977; Klemola *et al.*, 1986), except perhaps in the preterm infant (Weaver *et al.*, 1991). Although gut closure in humans normally seems to occur mainly before birth, a patent mucosal barrier function may not be established until after 2 years of age; the different variables involved in this process are poorly defined (van Elburg *et al.*, 1992). Interestingly, the post-natal colonization of commensal bacteria is important both to establish (Hooper *et al.*, 2001) and to regulate (Neish *et al.*, 2000) an appropriate epithelial barrier.

Immediately after birth, the mucosae are bombarded by a large variety of microorganisms, as well as by protein antigens from the environment, the latter particularly in formula-fed infants. The mucosal surface to be protected is enormous, probably more than 100 times that of the skin. In fact, the various mucosae are favoured as portals of entry by the majority of infectious agents, allergens and carcinogens. In most mucosal tissues, the epithelial barrier is monolayered and therefore quite vulnerable, so the defence of this large surface area is a formidable task. Nevertheless, most babies growing up under privileged conditions show remarkably good resistance to infections if their innate non-specific mucosal defence mechanisms are normally developed. This can be explained by the fact that immune protection of their mucosae is additionally provided by maternal IgG antibodies, which are distributed in interstitial tissue fluid at a concentration 50–60% of the intravascular level. In the first postnatal period, only occasional traces of SIgA and SIgM normally occur in the intestinal juice, whereas some IgG is more often present. This might be a result of external FcRn-mediated transmission or, perhaps more probably, it reflects passive epithelial 'leakage' from the highly vascularized lamina propria, which, particularly after 34 weeks of gestation, contains readily detectable maternal IgG (Brandtzaeg et al., 1991). However, an optimal mucosal barrier function in the neonatal period unquestionably depends on an adequate supply of breast milk, as highlighted in relation to mucosal infections, especially in developing countries (Anon., 1994). In the Westernized part of the world, the anti-infectious protective value of breast-feeding is clinically most apparent in preterm infants (Hylander et al., 1998).

Critical role of breast-feeding

When much of the transferred maternal IgG has been catabolized around 2 months of age, the infant becomes still more dependent on antibodies from breast milk for specific humoral immunity. At least 90% of the pathogens attacking humans use the mucosae as portals of entry; mucosal infections are in fact a major killer of children below the age of 5 years, being responsible for more than 14 million deaths of children annually in developing countries. Diarrhoeal disease alone claims a toll of 5 million children per year, or about 500 deaths every hour. These sad figures document the need for mucosal vaccines against common infectious agents, in addition to the importance of advocating breast-feeding. Convincing epidemiological documentation suggests that the risk of dying from diarrhoea is reduced 14–24 times in nursed children (Hanson et al., 1993; Anon., 1994). Indeed, exclusively breast-fed infants are better protected against a variety of infections (Pisacane et al., 1994; Wold and Hanson, 1994; Newman, 1995; Wright et al., 1998) and apparently also against allergy, asthma (Saarinen and Kajosaari, 1995; Oddy et al., 1999; Kull et al., 2001) and coeliac disease (Brandtzaeg, 1997a). Interestingly, experiments in neonatal rabbits strongly suggest that SIgA is a crucial anti-microbial component of breast milk (Dickinson et al., 1998). The role of secretory antibodies for mucosal homoeostasis is furthermore supported by the fact that knockout mice lacking SIgA and SIgM show increased mucosal leakiness (Johansen et al., 1999).

After the peak of passive immunity mediated by maternal IgG and antibodies from breast milk, the survival of the infant will, to an increasing extent, depend on its own adaptive immune responses. At mucosal surfaces, such responses are largely expressed by local antibody production (Brandtzaeg et al., 1999a). The cellular basis for this first-line humoral defence is the fact that exocrine glands and secretory mucosae contain most of the body's activated B-cells, terminally differentiated to Ig-producing blasts and plasma cells (collectively called immunocytes). These cells produce mainly dimers and some larger polymers of IgA (collectively called pIgA), which, along with pentameric IgM, can be actively transported through the serous type of secretory epithelia (Brandtzaeg, 1973, 1974a, b, 1975; Brandtzaeg *et al.*, 1968), including lactating mammary glands (Brandtzaeg, 1983), to act in a first-line mucosal defence (Fig. 14.2). As discussed later, this function depends on the epithelial polymeric Ig receptor (pIgR), which consists of a transmembrane glycoprotein, also known as membrane secretory component (SC).

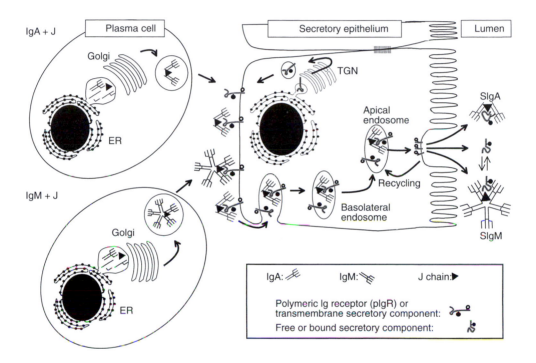

Fig. 14.2. Model for local generation of secretory immunoglobulin (Ig)A and secretory IgM. J-chain-containing dimeric IgA (IgA + J) and pentameric IgM (IgM + J) are produced by local plasma cells (left). Polymeric Ig receptor (pIgR) or membrane secretory component (SC) is synthesized by secretory epithelial cell in the rough endoplasmic reticulum (ER) and matures in the Golgi complex by terminal glycosylation (●-). In the trans-Golgi network (TGN), pIgR is sorted for delivery to the basolateral plasma membrane. The receptor becomes phosphorylated (○-) on a serine residue in its cytoplasmic tail. After endocytosis, ligand-complexed and unoccupied pIgR is delivered to basolateral endosomes and sorted for transcytosis to apical endosomes. Some recycling from basolateral endosomes to the basolateral surface may occur for unoccupied pIgR (not shown). Receptor recycling also takes place at the apical cell surface as indicated, although most pIgR is cleaved to allow extrusion of SIgA, SIgM and free SC to the lumen. During epithelial translocation, covalent stabilization of SIgA regularly occurs (disulphide bond between bound SC and one IgA subunit indicated), whereas free SC in secretions stabilizes the non-covalently bound SC in SIgM (dynamic equilibrium indicated). (Modified from Brandtzaeg *et al.*, 1999a.)

IgA-producing immunocytes are normally undetectable in human intestinal mucosa before 10 days of age but thereafter a rapid increase takes place, although IgM immunocytes usually remain predominant up to 1 month (Brandtzaeg et al., 1991; Brandtzaeg, 1996b, 1998). Adult salivary IgA levels are reached quite late in childhood, but only a small increase of IgA-producing cells has been reported to take place in the intestinal mucosa after 1 year. These observations have been made in industrialized countries; a faster development of the IgA immune system is usually seen in children from developing countries, reflecting the adaptability of mucosal immunity according to the environmental antigenic load, as discussed below. This should not detract from the fact that breast-feeding is highly desirable for both its immunological and its nutritional value (Børresen, 1995).

Immune Induction in Mucosa-associated Lymphoid Tissue (MALT)

Integration and regionalization

Lymphoid cells are located in three distinct compartments in the gut: organized gut-associated lymphoid tissue (GALT), the lamina propria and the surface epithelium. GALT comprises the Peyer's patches, the appendix and numerous solitary lymphoid follicles, especially in the large bowel (O'Leary and Sweeney, 1986). All these lymphoid structures are believed to represent inductive sites for intestinal immune responses (Brandtzaeg et al., 1999a). The lamina propria and epithelial compartment constitute effector sites but are nevertheless important in terms of cellular expansion and differentiation within the mucosal immune system. GALT and other MALT structures (see below) are covered by a characteristic follicle-associated epithelium (FAE), which contains membrane (M) cells (Figs 14.1 and 14.3). These specialized thin epithelial cells are particularly effective in the uptake of live and dead antigens from the gut lumen, especially when they are of a particulate nature (Hathaway and Kraehenbuhl, 2000). Many enteropathogenic infectious bacterial and viral agents use the M cells as portals of entry.

GALT structures resemble lymph nodes with B-cell follicles, intervening T-cell areas and a variety of antigen-presenting cell (APC) subsets, but there are no afferent lymphatics supplying antigens for immunological stimulation. Therefore, the exogenous stimuli must come directly from the gut lumen, probably in the main via the M cells. Among the T-cells, the CD4+ helper subset predominates, the ratio between CD4 and CD8 cells being similar to that of other peripheral T-cell populations (Brandtzaeg et al., 1999a). In addition, B-cells aggregate together with T-cells in the M cell pockets, which thus represent the first contact site between immune cells and luminal antigens (Brandtzaeg, 2001; Yamanaka et al., 2001). The B-cells may perform important antigen-presenting functions in this compartment, perhaps promoting antibody diversification and immunological memory or contributing to tolerance induction (Brandtzaeg et al., 1999b). Other types of professional APCs, macrophages and dendritic cells (DCs), are located below the FAE and between the follicles.

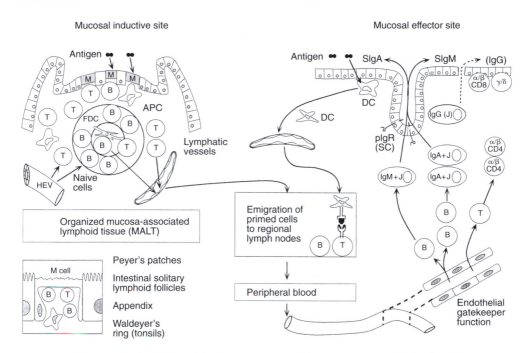

Fig. 14.3. Schematic depiction of the human mucosal immune system. Inductive sites are constituted by regional mucosa-associated lymphoid tissue (MALT) with their B-cell follicles and M cell (M)-containing follicle-associated epithelium, through which exogenous antigens are actively transported to reach professional antigen-presenting cells (APCs), including B-cells (B) and follicular dendritic cells (FDCs). In addition, mucosal dendritic cells (DCs) may capture antigens and migrate via draining lymph to regional lymph nodes, where they become active APCs, which stimulate T-cells (T) for positive or negative (down-regulatory) immune responses. Naive B- and T-cells enter MALT (and lymph nodes) via high endothelial venules (HEVs). After being primed to become memory/effector B- and T-cells, they migrate from MALT and regional lymph nodes via lymph and peripheral blood for subsequent extravasation at mucosal effector sites. This process is directed by the profile of adhesion molecules and chemokines expressed on the microvasculature, the endothelial cells thus exerting a 'gatekeeper' function for mucosal immunity. The intestinal lamina propria is illustrated with its various immune cells, including B lymphocytes, J-chain-expressing immunoglobulin (Ig)A and IgM plasma cells, IgG plasma cells with a variable J-chain level (J), and CD4+ T-cells. Additional features are the generation of secretory IgA (SIgA) and secretory IgM (SIgM) via pIgR (SC)-mediated epithelial transport, as well as paracellular leakage of smaller amounts (broken arrow) of serum-derived and locally produced IgG antibodies into the lumen. Note that IgG cannot interact with J chain to form a binding site for pIgR. The distribution of intraepithelial lymphocytes (mainly T-cell receptor α/β+CD8+ and some γ/δ+ T-cells) is schematically depicted. Insert (lower left corner) shows details of an M cell and its 'pocket' containing various cell types.

Pioneer studies performed in animals almost 30 years ago demonstrated that immune cells primed in GALT are functionally linked to mucosal effector sites by an integrated migration or 'homing' pathway (Brandtzaeg, 1996a). T-cells activated by microbial and other antigens in GALT preferentially differentiate to CD4+ helper cells, which, aided by DCs and the secretion of cytokines, such as transforming growth factor (TGF)-β and interleukin (IL)-10, induce the differentiation of antigen-specific B-cells to predominantly IgA-committed plasma blasts. These blasts proliferate and differentiate further on their route through mesenteric lymph nodes and the thoracic duct into the bloodstream (Fig. 14.3). Thereafter, they home preferentially to the gut mucosa, where they complete their terminal differentiation to IgA-producing plasma cells (see below). As reviewed elsewhere (Brandtzaeg et al., 1999a, c), this migration of lymphoid cells is facilitated by 'homing receptors' interacting with ligands on the microvascular endothelium at the effector site ('addressins'), with an additional fine-tuned navigation mechanism conducted by chemoattractant cytokines (chemokines). Under normal conditions, therefore, the local microvasculature exerts a 'gatekeeper' function to allow selective extravasation of primed lymphoid cells belonging to the mucosal immune system (Fig. 14.3).

Although GALT constitutes the major part of MALT, induction of mucosal immune responses can also take place in the palatine tonsils and other lymphoepithelial structures of Waldeyer's pharyngeal ring, including nasal-associated lymphoid tissue (NALT), such as the adenoids in humans (Brandtzaeg, 1999; Brandtzaeg et al., 1999b, c), and probably also bronchus-associated lymphoid tissue (BALT). Because BALT is lacking in normal lungs of newborns and adults (Pabst and Gehrke, 1990; Tschernig et al., 1995), Waldeyer's ring may represent a significant component of human MALT. Accumulating evidence suggests that a certain regionalization exists in the mucosal immune system, especially a dichotomy between the gut and the upper aerodigestive tract with regard to homing properties and terminal differentiation of B-cells (Brandtzaeg et al., 1999a, b, c). This disparity may be explained by microenvironmental differences in the antigenic repertoire as well as the adhesion molecules and chemokines involved in preferential local leucocyte extravasation. It appears that primed immune cells selectively home to effector sites corresponding to the inductive sites where they were initially triggered by antigens. Such regionalization within the 'common' or integrated mucosal immune system has to be taken into account in the development of local vaccines.

B-cell homing to mammary glands

Lactating mammary glands are part of the integrated mucosal immune system, and milk antibodies reflect antigenic stimulation of MALT in the gut as well as in the airways. This fact has been documented by showing that SIgA from breast milk exhibits antibody specificities for an array of common intestinal and respiratory pathogens (Goldman, 1993). The secretory antibodies are thus highly targeted against infectious agents in the mother's environment, which are those likely to be encountered by the infant during its first weeks of life. Therefore, breast-feeding represents an ingenious immunological integration of mother and child (Fig. 14.4). Although the protection provided by this humoral defence mechanism is most readily demonstrable in populations living in poor sanitary conditions (Hanson et al., 1993; Anon., 1994), a beneficial clinical effect is also apparent in the industrialized world (Wold and Hanson, 1994),

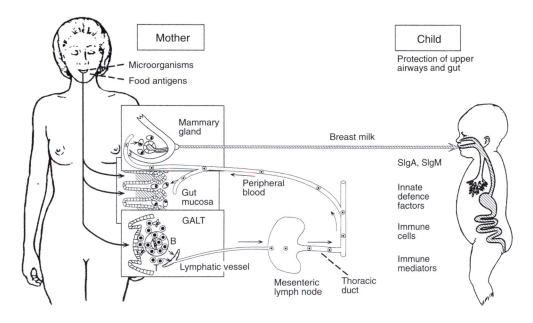

Fig. 14.4. Integration of mucosal immunity between mother and the newborn. The figure emphasizes migration (arrows) of primed B- (and probably T-) cells from gut-associated lymphoid tissue (GALT), such as Peyer's patches, via lymph and peripheral blood to lactating mammary glands. This distribution of precursors for immunoglobulin (Ig)A plasma cells beyond the gut mucosa is crucial for glandular production and subsequent occurrence in breast milk of secretory antibodies (SIgA and SIgM) specific for enteric antigens (microorganisms and food proteins). By this mechanism, the breast-fed infant will receive relevant secretory antibodies directed against the microflora initially colonizing its mucosae (reflecting the mother's microflora) and hence be better protected both in the gut and in the upper airways by SIgA and SIgM (hatched areas), in the same way as the mother's gut mucosa is protected by similar antibodies (hatched areas).

even in relation to relatively common diseases, such as otitis media and acute lower respiratory tract infections (Pisacane *et al.*, 1994; Newman, 1995; Golding *et al.*, 1997).

   Antibodies to various dietary antigens, such as cow's milk proteins (Savilahti *et al.*, 1991) and gluten (Juto and Holm, 1992), are also present in breast milk. However, little is known about the preferential site where soluble luminal antigens exert immune priming. Thus, dietary proteins may be taken up mainly through the extensive epithelial surfaces covering the diffuse immunological effector tissue of the intestinal mucosa rather than by M cells, and may therefore be largely transported to the mesenteric lymph nodes. As discussed below, their fate and possible immune-inductive or tolerogenic effects will depend on how they are handled locally and whether they reach lymph or portal blood (Brandtzaeg *et al.*, 1987; Sanderson and Walker, 1993; Brandtzaeg, 1996a).

Post-natal Development of Mucosal Immunity

Activation of the local B-cell system

Peyer's patches are the best studied MALT structures and start to develop in fetal life (Cornes, 1965; Husband and Gleeson, 1990), with discrete T- and B-cell areas being apparent as early as 19 weeks of gestation (Spencer and MacDonald, 1990). The primary lymphoid follicles seem to be generated around follicular dendritic cells (FDCs). However, lymphoid hyperplasia, with secondary follicles containing germinal centres (signifying B-cell activation), does not occur until shortly after birth (Bridges *et al.*, 1959; Spencer *et al.*, 1986a; Gebbers and Laissue, 1990); this reflects the dependency of MALT on exogenous environmental stimulation. Furthermore, animal studies have shown an absence of secondary follicles in Peyer's patches of germ-free mice (Parrott, 1976). The germinal-centre B-cells express small amounts of membrane IgA, along with less IgM or IgG (Butcher *et al.*, 1982). Such isotype skewing reflects differentiation to precursors for IgA-producing cells. The drive for isotype switching towards IgA, together with J-chain expression, in B-cells is much more evident in Peyer's patches than in other MALT structures, but the reasons for this are unclear (Brandtzaeg *et al.*, 1999a, b). The combination of IgA and J-chain production is a prerequisite for the generation of SIgA antibodies (Fig. 14.2).

The retarded post-natal immune activation of MALT parallels the functionally decreased systemic immunocompetence in the newborn period (MacDonald and Spencer, 1993; Holt, 1995; Holt and Jones, 2000). Thus, peripheral CD4+ T-cells of infants show a reduced capacity for the production of interferon (IFN)-γ (Taylor and Bryson, 1985; Holt *et al.*, 1992) and IL-4 (Lewis *et al.*, 1991), as well as for B-cell help (Splawski and Lipsky, 1991; MacDonald and Spencer, 1993). One reason might be that there are relatively few circulating memory (CD45RO+) T-cells in infancy. Interestingly, the responsiveness of neonatal naive (CD45RA+) T-cells does not differ significantly from that of virgin counterparts in adults, and more recent animal studies suggest that the chief explanation for the apparent immunological immaturity is to be found in a deficient APC function (Ridge *et al.*, 1996). Thus, in the neonate macrophages, DCs and B-cells are all unable to deliver adequate co-stimulatory signals to naive T-cells (Lu *et al.*, 1979; Taylor and Bryson, 1985; Morris *et al.*, 1992; Ridge *et al.*, 1996).

Homing of primed lymphoid cells to mucosal effector sites

After antigen-induced activation, proliferation and partial differentiation in MALT, lymphoid memory and effector cells migrate rapidly via regional lymph nodes and the peripheral blood circulation to various secretory effector sites (Fig. 14.3). The presence of SIgA antibodies to bovine β-lactoglobulin in neonatal breast milk ('witch milk') from infants fed cow's milk formula (Roberton *et al.*, 1986) documents such early postnatal homing of primed intestinal B-cells to mammary glands. However, very few B-cells with IgA-producing capacity are actually present in the blood of newborns (< 8 per million mononuclear cells), although this number is remarkably increased (~ 600 per million mononuclear cells) after 1 month, reflecting the progressive exogenous stimulation of GALT (Nahmias *et al.*, 1991). An initial early elevation of Ig-producing cells can be seen in preterm infants, especially in those with intrauterine infections, although the IgM class not unexpectedly dominates in such cases (Stoll *et al.*, 1993). Altogether, these observations support the notion that mucosal immune cells are competent even before birth, at least during the final trimester, but that APCs need to undergo an activation process initiated by exogenous 'danger signals' enabling them to provide sufficient co-stimulatory signals to naive T-helper (Th) cells (Medzhitov and Janeway, 1997). This is further supported by the finding that fetal lamina propria T-cells (mainly CD4+) can be activated by mitogens or bacterial super-antigens *in vitro* (MacDonald and Spencer, 1993).

In this context, it is also interesting to note that intraepithelial lymphocytes (IELs) are present in human intestinal epithelium as early as 11 weeks of gestation (Orlic and Lev, 1977). As in adults, fetal IELs occur mainly in the villi of the small intestine and are dominated by CD3+ CD8+ T-cells (Brandtzaeg *et al.*, 1998). Their numbers increase throughout the gestational period (Spencer *et al.*, 1986b), which suggests that the migration of IELs into the epithelium is, to some extent, antigen-independent. However, stimulation by luminal factors clearly determines the numbers of IELs, as shown by their rapid post-natal increase, up to tenfold by the age of 1–2 years (Cerf-Bensussan and Guy-Grand, 1991; Machado *et al.*, 1994); this probably reflects the development of GALT, from which the intestinal IEL precursors may largely be derived (Guy-Grand *et al.*, 1978; Dunkley and Husband, 1987; Cuff *et al.*, 1993). In a similar manner, germ-free animals have few IELs. Moreover, conventionalization of germ-free mice and rats has demonstrated a marked stimulatory effect of the commensal intestinal microflora and also its apparent impact on the T-cell receptor (TCR) repertoire of IELs (Helgeland and Brandtzaeg, 2000).

Effects of antigen exposure and nutrition on secretory immunity

The degree of antigenic and mitogenic exposure is decisive not only for the post-natal development of IELs, but also for the secretory immune system. Antigenic constituents of food clearly exert a stimulatory effect on the intestinal B-cell system, as suggested by the occurrence of fewer lamina propria IgA immunocytes both in mice fed on hydrolysed milk proteins (Sagie *et al.*, 1974) and in parenterally fed babies (Knox, 1986). Likewise, mice given total parenteral (intravenous) nutrition have reduced numbers of B- and T-cells in the gut, as well as decreased SIgA levels (Li *et al.*, 1995a, b; Janu *et al.*, 1997), and they show impaired SIgA-dependent influenza-specific immunity (Renegar *et al.*, 2001). The effect of food in the gut lumen could be direct immune stimulation or mediated via release of gastrointestinal neuropeptides. The indigenous microbial flora is also extremely important for secretory immunity, as shown by the fact that the intestinal IgA system of germ free or specific pathogen-free mice is normalized after about 4 weeks of conventionalization (Crabbé et al., 1970; Horsfall et al., 1978). Bacteroides and Escherichia coli strains seem to be particularly stimulatory for the development of intestinal IgA immunocytes (Lodinová et al., 1973; Moreau et al., 1978). The large dietary and bacterial antigen load in the gut lumen therefore explains why the greatest density of IgA immunocytes is seen in the intestinal lamina propria, amounting to some 10^{10} cells m^{-1} of adult gut (Brandtzaeg et al., 1999a).

In human lactating mammary glands the immunocyte density is much less, one gland showing an IgA-producing capacity similar to that of only 1 m of intestine (Brandtzaeg, 1983). Thus, the daily output of IgA kg^{-1} wet weight of tissue (minus fat) is no more for lactating mammary glands than for salivary glands. In fact, it remains an enigma how any terminal plasma cell differentiation at all is accomplished in these secretory effector organs, which are at considerable distances from antigen-exposed mucosal surfaces (Brandtzaeg et al., 1999a). Anyhow, the large capacity for storage of pIgA/SIgA in the mammary-gland epithelium and duct system, rather than a high immunocyte density, explains the remarkable output of SIgA during breast-feeding (Brandtzaeg, 1983).

In keeping with an important stimulatory effect of antigens on local B-cell differentiation, defunctioning colostomies in children showed a 50% numerical reduction of mucosal IgA and IgM immunocytes after 2–11 months (Wijesinha and Steer, 1982). Prolonged studies of defunctioned ileal segments in lambs revealed an even more striking scarcity of mucosal immunocytes. This was caused by decreased local proliferation and differentiation of B-cell blasts and perhaps reduced homing from GALT (Reynolds and Morris, 1984). Accordingly, the post-natal establishment of the mucosal IgA system is usually much faster in developing countries than in the industrialized part of the world, a difference that seems to hold true even in undernourished children (Nagao et al., 1993). However, severe vitamin A deficiency has been reported to have an adverse effect on mucosal IgA antibody responses in rodents (Wiedermann et al., 1993), but with no consistent down-regulation of epithelial IgA transport (Stephensen et al., 1996).

It has been reported that undernourished children respond to bacterial overgrowth in the gut with enhanced synthesis, as well as up-regulated external transport, of IgA (Beatty et al., 1983). It is of great clinical importance that detrimental effects of severe malnutrition exerted on the SIgA system can apparently be reversed with nutritional rehabilitation (Watson et al., 1985). In a recent study based on whole gut lavage obtained from healthy adult volunteers in Dhaka, Bangladesh, the intestinal concentration of IgA was found to be almost 50% higher than that of comparable samples collected in Edinburgh, UK; the intestinal IgA antibody titre against lipopolysaccharide (LPS) core types of E. coli was almost seven times higher in the former group of subjects, in contrast to the lower levels of ovalbumin antibodies (Hoque et al., 2000).

In view of the above information, the possibility exists that sub-optimal stimulatory reinforcement of the SIgA-dependent mucosal barrier function might contribute to the increased frequency of certain diseases in industrialized countries, particularly allergies and other inflammatory mucosal disorders. This 'hygiene hypothesis' has been tested in several experimental and clinical studies by evaluating the beneficial effect of probiotic bacterial preparations. In particular, viable strains of the commensal intestinal microflora, such as lactobacilli and bifidobacteria, have been reported to enhance IgA responses, in both humans and experimental animals, apparently in a T-cell-dependent manner (Kaila *et al.*, 1992, 1995; Isolauri *et al.*, 1995; Yasui *et al.*, 1995; Malin *et al.*, 1996; Prokesová *et al.*, 1999). Interestingly, early colonization of infants with a non-enteropathogenic strain of *E. coli* has been reported to have a long-term beneficial effect by reducing both infections and allergies (Lodinová-Zádniková and Cukrowská, 1999). Likewise, a recent double-blind study of infants with a family history of atopic (IgE-mediated) allergy reported the prevalence of atopic eczema to be reduced by 50% at the age of 2 years in those receiving the probiotic *Lactobacillus* GG strain daily for 6 months, compared with those receiving placebo (Kalliomäki *et al.*, 2001a). It remains to be shown whether this striking beneficial effect was mediated via SIgA enhancement or by promotion of oral tolerance, as discussed later.

Individual variations

Post-natal mucosal B-cell development shows large individual variations, even within the same population (Brandtzaeg *et al.*, 1991). This disparity could partly reflect a genetically determined effect on the establishment of the mucosal barrier function. Thus, it has been proposed, on the basis of serum IgA levels, that a hereditary risk of atopy is related to a retarded post-natal development of the IgA system (Taylor *et al.*, 1973; Soothill, 1976). This notion was later supported by a report showing significantly reduced IgA immunocyte numbers (with no compensatory IgM enhancement) in the jejunal mucosa of atopic children (Sloper *et al.*, 1981). Also, an inverse relationship was found between the serum IgE level and the jejunal IgA cell population in children with food-induced atopic eczema (Perkkiö, 1980). It was subsequently reported that infants born to atopic parents showed a significantly higher prevalence of salivary IgA deficiency than age-matched control infants (van Asperen *et al.*, 1985). Interestingly, Kilian *et al.* (1995) found that the throats of 18-month-old infants with presumably IgE-mediated allergic problems contained significantly higher proportions of IgA_1 protease-producing bacteria than age-matched healthy controls, thus supporting a previous report showing much less intact IgA in nasopharyngeal secretions from children with a history of atopic allergy than from controls with episodes of acute otitis (Sørensen and Kilian, 1984). In this context, it is important to note that it takes up to 3 months after birth before the IgA_2-to-IgA_1 immunocyte ratio in salivary glands has increased to the adult value, with approximately 33% IgA_2-producing cells (Thrane *et al.*, 1991).

Altogether, a poorly developed or enzymatically reduced SIgA-dependent mucosal barrier function, combined with a hereditary and/or cytokine-driven hyper-IgE responsiveness (see below), could contribute to the pathogenesis of allergy. This notion accords with the increased frequency not only of infections, but also of atopic allergy and coeliac disease seen in subjects with permanent selective IgA deficiency (Burrows and Cooper, 1997), although compensatory over-production of SIgM may apparently counteract the adverse consequences of their absent mucosal IgA responses, particularly in the gut (Brandtzaeg et al., 1991; Brandtzaeg and Nilssen, 1995).

Mucosal Induction of Tolerance

Suggestive evidence of oral tolerance in humans

The concept of oral tolerance is mainly based on feeding experiments in rodents and has a long history (Brandtzaeg, 1996a). The understanding of this mucosally-induced down-regulatory or suppressive phenomenon has been hampered by an overwhelming mechanistic complexity. Identifiable experimental variables include genetics, age, dose and timing of post-natal feeding, antigenic structure and composition of fed protein, epithelial barrier integrity and the degree of concurrent local immune activation, as reflected by microenvironmental cytokine profiles and the expression of co-stimulatory molecules on mucosal APCs (Brandtzaeg, 1996a; Nagler-Anderson, 2000; Mayer et al., 2001). Also, rodent studies suggest that the commensal microflora is important both for induction of oral tolerance and for reconstitution of this mechanism after its experimental abrogation (Helgeland and Brandtzaeg, 2000). This effect is probably mediated mainly through immune stimulation of GALT, as discussed above.

Although there is little direct evidence that oral tolerance operates in humans, it seems justified to believe that this is the case. Circumstantial evidence is provided by the fact that, in the normal state, the vulnerable gut mucosa, which is separated only by a monolayered epithelium from the enormous intestinal load of live and dead antigenic material, exhibits no substantial IgG response (Brandtzaeg et al., 1987, 1999a) and contains very few T-cells with markers of hyperactivation, such as CD25 (the IL-2 receptor) (Brandtzaeg et al., 1998). Moreover, the systemic IgG response to dietary antigens tends to decrease in humans with increasing age (Rothberg and Farr, 1965; Scott et al., 1985), and direct evidence for a hyporesponsive state in regard to bovine serum albumin has been obtained by intradermal testing with this antigen in adults (Korenblat et al., 1968).

Interestingly, experimental feeding in healthy adults with a protein to which humans are not normally exposed, keyhole limpet haemocyanin (KLH), did result in down-regulation of the peripheral T-cell response, although stimulation of local as well as systemic humoral immunity was observed (Husby et al., 1994). Conversely, intranasal application of KLH tended to suppress both cell-mediated and humoral peripheral immunity to this antigen (Waldo et al., 1994). The mechanisms remain unclear, however, and sequestration of specific immune cells into the antigen-exposed mucosae or regional lymph nodes is an alternative possibility, which may be difficult to refute because local immunity was enhanced in both studies. Such a mechanism has been suggested in untreated coeliac-disease patients whose circulating T-cells show a decreased response to gluten compared with treated patients on a gluten-free diet (Scott *et al.*, 1983). Nevertheless, feeding humans with KLH was recently repeated with parallel systemically immunized controls, and mucosally-induced T-cell tolerance was indeed confirmed in peripheral blood (Mayer *et al.*, 2001, and their unpublished observations). Also notably, feeding low doses of myelin basic protein to patients with multiple sclerosis resulted in a higher frequency of circulating T-cells with a potency for production of the down-regulatory cytokine TGF-β, compared with T-cells from placebo-fed patients (Fukaura *et al.*, 1996).

Putative involvement of lymphoepithelial interactions

A central role of the gut epithelium in oral tolerance is suggested by the observation that its experimental induction depends on the preserved integrity of the mucosal barrier (Nicklin and Miller, 1983; Strobel *et al.*, 1983). Suppressive effects resulting from interactions between the dominating TCRα/β CD8+ IEL subset and a normal epithelium represent one intriguing possibility, and there is some supporting evidence to this effect (Sachdev *et al.*, 1993). It is possible that luminal antigenic peptides are presented by resting enterocytes, with inadequate co-stimulation to IELs or subepithelial CD4+ T-cells (Hoyne *et al.*, 1993). Experiments in CD8 knockout mice have suggested that CD8+ T-cells are crucial for the down-regulation of enterically-elicited mucosal immunity but not for mucosally-induced suppression of systemic antibody responses (Grdic *et al.*, 1998). Moreover, the chief effect obtained when enterocytes have been used as unconventional APCs in various test systems has been stimulation of CD8+ T-cells with a suppressor function (Hershberg and Mayer, 2000; Mayer *et al.*, 2001). Human enterocytes express a ligand (gp180) that, by interaction with the α chain of CD8, may rapidly activate the tyrosine kinase p56[lck] and thereby trigger preferentially CD8+ T-cells (Li *et al.*, 1995). Antigen presentation by MHC or CD1d molecules on enterocytes in this context could theoretically leave cognate IELs and even CD4+ lamina propria Th cells in an unresponsive state or induce an active down-regulatory potential by a deviated cytokine profile (Fig. 14.5). Moreover, basolateral exosomes with MHC class II-dependent antigen-presenting capacity may be released from the gut epithelium and act as 'tolerosomes' (Karlsson *et al.*, 2001), either locally or at distant sites, such as mesenteric lymph nodes or the liver (Fig. 14.5).

The additional involvement of TCRγ/δ+ IELs in oral tolerance is also an intriguing possibility (Fig. 14.5), in view of the suggestion that this subset in the mouse may act as 'contrasuppressor cells', thereby being able to release intestinal IgA responses from T-cell-mediated suppression (Fujihashi *et al.*, 1992). Subsequent studies have shown that this effect can probably be ascribed to IL-10 secreted by CD4+ T-cells, which are controlled by γ/δ T-cells operating through this down-regulatory cytokine in low-dose tolerance (Fujihashi *et al.*, 1999). If this mechanism also operates in humans, the preferential expansion of intraepithelial γ/δ T-cells in the coeliac lesion might contribute to the striking

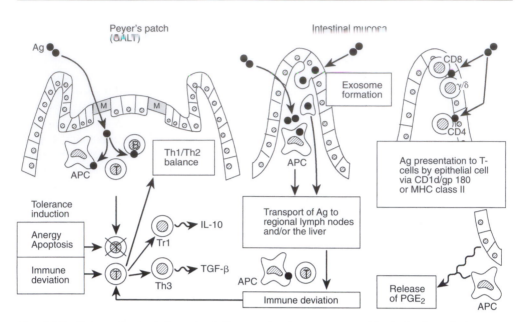

Fig. 14.5. Schematic depiction of putative mechanisms suggested for induction of tolerance via the gut ('oral' tolerance). Hyporesponsiveness to innocuous antigen (Ag) gaining access to immune cells through M cells (M) in gut-associated lymphoid tissue (GALT) or through the intestinal surface epithelium may be explained by T-cell anergy, clonal deletion by apoptosis and cytokine-mediated active suppression (immune deviation), either locally or at distant sites, after dissemination of absorbed Ag or transport of Ag in antigen-presenting cells (APCs) or epithelial exosomes. In the normal state, when only low-grade activation takes place, subepithelial APCs migrate quickly to regional lymph nodes with acquired Ag, thus prohibiting mucosal hyperactivation of T-cells locally. Special regulatory T-cells (Tr1 and Th3), which produce the suppressive cytokines interleukin (IL)-10 and transforming growth factor (TGF)-β, appear to be important for the development of a balanced Th1/Th2 profile. A down-regulatory tone in the gut may also be ascribed to unconventional Ag presentation by epithelial cells (to the right) and the effect of prostaglandin E_2 (PGE_2) released from the epithelium or APCs. Details are discussed in the text. MHC, major histocompatibility complex.

increase of Ig-producing immunocytes and activated lamina propria CD4+ T-cells seen in untreated patients (Scott *et al.*, 1997). However, the increase of TCRγ/δ+ IELs in coeliac disease could instead reflect that they are cytotoxic cells involved in the clearance of microorganisms or damaged epithelium to preserve the surface barrier (Brandtzaeg, 1996a; Groh *et al.*, 1998; Hershberg and Mayer, 2000).

Role of co-stimulation by antigen-presenting cells

Productive T-cell activation with appropriate proliferation and cytokine secre-tion requires two signalling events, one through the TCR and another through a receptor for some co-stimulatory molecule (Fig. 14.6). Without the latter signal, the T-cells mount only a partial response and, more importantly, may be subjected to active tolerance induction (Nagler-Anderson, 2000) or anergy, with no capacity for production of their own growth-factor IL-2 upon restimulation (Janeway and Bottomly, 1994). The required co-stimulation for productive immunity is provided by soluble mediators, such as IL-1, and through cellular interactions, especially ligation of B7 (CD80/CD86) on professional APCs with CD28 on the T-cells (Robey and Allison, 1995). There is particularly great interest in the role of DCs in shaping the phenotypes of naive T-cells during such initial priming. Also, because DCs have migratory properties, they largely determine the tissue site in which primary immune responses will take place (Holt and Stumbles, 2000; Lanzavecchia and Sallusto, 2001).

Immature DC subsets are found both in the circulation and in most peripheral tissues, from which, after endocytosis of antigen, they generally migrate via draining lymphatics into regional lymph nodes to perform antigen presentation (Sallusto and Lanzavecchia, 1999). The actual expression level of various co-stimulatory molecules on the matured and activated DCs during the priming process influences the differentiation of naive T-cells in terms of cytokine

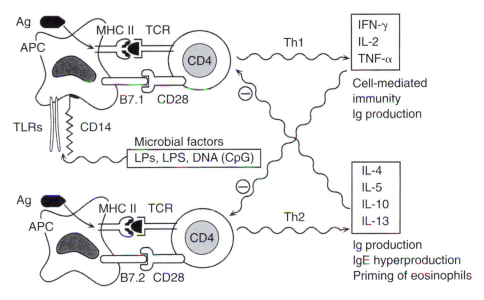

Fig. 14.6. Schematic representation of polarized patterns of cytokines produced by activated T-helper (Th) cells. When naive CD4+ Th cells are primed by a professional antigen-presenting cell (APC) providing adequate co-stimulatory signals, they differentiate into Th1 or Th2 cells. Such skewing of the immune response depends on the presence of microenvironmental factors, such as lipoproteins (LPs), lipopolysaccharide (LPS) and unmethylated CpG nucleotide motifs. Their interaction with APC receptors determine the expression level of various co-stimulatory signals. For simplicity, only the LPS receptor CD14 and Toll-like receptors (TLRs) are indicated, together with the co-stimulatory molecules B7.1 and B7.2. Th1 cells produce predominantly interferon (IFN)-γ, interleukin (IL)-2 and tumour necrosis factor (TNF)-α, while Th2 cells are mainly capable of IL-4, IL-5, IL-10 and IL-13 secretion. Distinct Th1 and Th2 profiles are further promoted by inhibitory feedback loops, as indicated. Ag, antigen; MHC II, major histocompatibility complex class II molecules; TCR, T-cell receptor.

production – that is, a Th1 (IFN-γ, IL-2 and tumour necrosis factor (TNF)-α) versus a Th2 (IL-4, IL-5, IL-10 and IL-13) profile. Interaction of the T-cell CD28 receptor with B7.1 (CD80) appears to favour the former and with B7.2 (CD86) the latter cytokine profile (Kuchroo *et al.*, 1995). This Th1/Th2 paradigm is important in relation to atopic allergy, because IgE production as a basis for type I hypersensitivity is highly dependent on IL-4 and IL-13 (Corry and Kheradmand, 1999). Also, homoeostatic cross-regulation should ideally take place between the Th1 and Th2 responses (Romagnani, 2000).

Considerable information exists about putative aberrant immunoregulatory functions of non-professional APCs, such as keratinocytes, because they lack the appropriate co-stimulatory molecules necessary for productive immunity (Nickoloff and Turka, 1994). As alluded to above, this also applies to enterocytes (Fig. 14.5). Thus, both B7 and intercellular adhesion molecule 1 (CD54) are virtually absent on normal human enterocytes (Bloom *et al.*, 1995). Low levels of B7 might actually engage the high-affinity co-stimulatory molecule cytotoxic T lymphocyte antigen (CTLA)-4 on Th cells (Chambers and Allison, 1999), which could result in a down-regulatory response contributing to oral tolerance (Read *et al.*, 2000).

In the normal state, even the subepithelial professional APCs in human gut mucosa, which have both macrophage and DC properties, show an extremely low level of B7 expression (Rugtveit *et al.*, 1997; Brandtzaeg, 2001) and might therefore ligate CTLA-4 rather than CD28 on T-cells. Also, only B7.2 (CD86) is normally detectable, and this molecule has been shown in animal experiments to be important for low-dose oral tolerance (Liu *et al.*, 1999). Functional characteristics of normal human lamina propria CD4+ T-cells do suggest that they are tightly controlled by suppression. First, they are remarkably unresponsive to signalling via the classical TCR/CD3 pathway alone, whereas anti-CD2 (particularly together with engagement of CD28) induces proliferation and cytokine secretion (Boirivant *et al.*, 1996; Fuss *et al.*, 1996). Second, they appear to be particularly susceptible to Fas (CD95)-mediated apoptosis, which might contribute to the limitation of clonal proliferation in the normal gut (De Maria *et al.*, 1996). Third, they may be kept in check by prostaglandin E_2 released by the gut epithelium or lamina propria macrophages (Newberry *et al.*, 1999).

The fact that resident APCs from normal human gut mucosa are quite inert in terms of immune-productive stimulatory properties (Qiao *et al.*, 1996) supports the notion that they play a central role in the induction of oral tolerance. One possibility is that, in the normal state (i.e. when subjected to only low-grade activation), they carry penetrating dietary and innocuous microbial antigens away from the mucosa, thereby avoiding local hyperactivation of immune cells (Fig. 14.5). Indeed, normal human intestinal mucosa shows only very low expression levels of mRNA for IFN-γ, the key cytokine of activated Th1 cells (Nilsen *et al.*, 1998). The same is true for Th2 cytokines, such as IL-4 and IL-5. Moreover, animal experiments have demonstrated that intestinal APCs can be triggered by pro-inflammatory factors to become mobilized (MacPherson *et al.*, 1995) and even constitutively migrate rapidly with acquired epithelial elements and antigens away from the intestinal mucosa (Gütgemann *et al.*, 1998; Huang *et al.*, 2000). Such successful 'silent' antigen clearance probably depends on relatively low doses of absorbed antigen and may result in systemic T-cell-dependent tolerance induction (Fig. 14.5). Interestingly, *in vivo* expansion of the intestinal APC population enhanced the induction of oral tolerance in mice (Viney *et al.*, 1998), whereas concurrent APC activation by immunization with cholera toxin or treatment of the animals with IL-1 resulted in productive immunity against the fed antigen (Williamson *et al.*, 1999).

Animal studies have suggested differential effects of antigen dose and feeding frequency on the mechanisms of tolerance induction (Brandtzaeg, 1998). At very high doses, both Th1 and Th2 cells were shown to be deleted following initial activation, an event apparently depending on apoptosis in Peyer's patches (Chen *et al.*, 1995). Anergy and clonal deletion would be antigen-specific events, in contrast to active suppression resulting from deviation of cytokine profiles induced by T-cell stimulation locally or in regional lymph nodes or the liver (Knolle *et al.*, 1999; Limmer *et al.*, 2000) after distant transport of antigen in APCs or epithelial exosomes (Fig. 14.5). Experiments performed to induce therapeutic tolerance via the gut in various autoimmune disease models have relied on a bystander effect of stimulated T-cells, which, through immune deviation, have preferentially secreted down-regulatory cytokines, particularly TGF-β (Weiner *et al.*, 1994). It has been suggested that the gut harbours T-cells with a propensity for secretion of TGF-β (so-called Th3 cells), which appear to be particularly resistant to apoptosis (Chen *et al.*, 1995), but this subset has not been clearly identified in humans. Another regulatory T-cell subset (Tr1), with a remarkable propensity for IL-10 production, has been identified in both the murine and the human gut (Groux *et al.*, 1997; Khoo *et al.*, 1997). This subset probably belongs to the activated (CD25+) and CTLA-4-expressing suppressive CD4+ T-cells induced after antigen feeding in mice (Zhang *et al.*, 2001).

Altogether, a complex scenario may be proposed for oral tolerance, depending on apoptosis, when intestinal antigen exposure is excessive, and on anergy, due to lack of co-stimulatory APC molecules, antigen clearance from the mucosa and induction of immune deviation (skewing of T-cell cytokine profile) at lower antigen doses (Fig. 14.5). This scenario is further complicated by the fact that several cytokines contributing to the local profile are produced not only by T-cells, but also by APCs and epithelial cells – for instance, the down-regulatory cytokines TGF-β and IL-10. Furthermore, it remains unclear whether the most important immunoregulatory events for oral tolerance against dietary antigens take place in Peyer's patches, in the lamina propria, in systemic lymphoid organs or in the liver (Chen *et al.*, 2000; Alpan *et al.*, 2001; Fujihashi *et al.*, 2001).

Importance of homoeostatic immune regulation

It may seem paradoxical that mucosal disorders, such as inflammatory bowel disease (IBD) and coeliac disease, appear to depend, at least initially, on putative Th1-cell-driven pathogenic mechanisms (Scott *et al.*, 1997; Brandtzaeg *et al.*, 1999d), while atopic (IgE-mediated) allergy originates from Th2-cell responses (Brandtzaeg, 1997b; Corry and Kheradmand, 1999), which generate the essential cytokines IL-4 and IL-13 (early phase) as well as IL-3, IL-5 and granulocyte–macrophage colony-stimulating factor (GM-CSF) (late phase). According to the 'hygiene hypothesis', the increasing incidence of allergy in Westernized societies may to some extent be explained by a reduced microbial load early in infancy, resulting in too little Th1-cell activity and therefore an insufficient level of IFN-γ to cross-regulate Th2-cell responses optimally (Rook and Stanford, 1998; Erb, 1999; Kirjavainen and Gibson, 1999). In this context, an appropriate composition of the commensal bacterial flora (Isolauri *et al.*, 2000) and exposure to food-borne and orofaecal microbes (Herz *et al.*, 2000; Matricardi *et al.*, 2000) most probably exert an important homoeostatic impact, both by enhancing the SIgA-mediated barrier function (see above) and by promoting oral tolerance through a shift from a predominant Th2-cell activity in the newborn period (Prescott *et al.*, 1998) to a more balanced cytokine profile later on (Fig. 14.5). Thus, the intestinal microflora of young children in Sweden was found to contain a relatively large number of *Clostridium* spp., whereas high levels of *Lactobacillus* spp. and *Eubacterium* spp. were detected in an age-matched population from Estonia (Sepp *et al.*, 1997). Perhaps this difference could explain the lower incidence of allergy in the Baltic countries compared with Scandinavia. Interestingly, the intestinal microflora of children in Estonia was deemed to be somewhat similar to that of Swedish children in the 1960s. Also, the intestinal microflora of Estonian children with allergy appeared to differ from that of their healthy counterparts, particularly by containing fewer lactobacilli (Björkstén *et al.*, 1999). A recent Finnish study likewise reported that atopic infants had more clostridia and tended to have fewer bifidobacteria in their stools than non-atopic controls (Kalliomäki *et al.*, 2001b).

Such observations make a good case for studying the potential clinical benefits of prebiotics and probiotic bacterial strains from the indigenous gut flora (Collins and Gibson, 1999; Kirjavainen and Gibson, 1999; Isolauri *et al.*, 2001). Similarly, there is some hope that immunization with mycobacterial antigens might skew the cytokine profile towards Th1 and thereby, through cross-regulation, dampen Th2-dependent allergic (atopic) symptoms (von Reyn *et al.*, 1997; Hopkin *et al.*, 1998). Newborns are in fact able to mount a Th1-type immune response when appropriately stimulated (Marchant *et al.*, 1999). Also notably, the bacterial endotoxin or LPS receptor CD14, together with the Toll-like receptor (TLR) 4 on APCs, as well as other TLRs that recognize microbial products (e.g. lipoproteins and peptidoglycans) as danger signals or pathogen-associated molecular patterns (PAMPs), are in this respect an important link between innate and specific immunity (Fig. 14.6). This link operates via the nuclear factor kappa B (NFκB) activation pathway to release pro-inflammatory cytokines (Modlin, 2000; Kaisho and Akira, 2001), including the Th1-inducing IL-12 and IL-18 (McInnes *et al.*, 2000; Manigold *et al.*, 2000). Even certain CpG motifs of bacterial DNA have been shown to promote Th1-cell activity through interaction with TLR9 (Klinman *et al.*, 1996; Kadowaki *et al.*, 2001; Peng *et al.*, 2001). Subepithelial intestinal APCs most probably express TLRs, although this has not yet been studied properly in the human gut (MacDonald and Pettersson, 2000). However, low levels of CD14 are normally present on these cells, and its expression is enhanced, together with that of B7.1 and B7.2, by pro-inflammatory factors (Rugtveit *et al.*, 1997; Brandtzaeg, 2001).

Altogether, it appears that the human intestinal immune system preferentially responds with a dominating Th1 profile (Nilsen *et al.*, 1998), even against various food antigens in the seemingly normal state (Nagata *et al.*, 2000). This appears to be true for T-cells also in the duodenal mucosa of children with cow's milk hypersensitivity (Hauer *et al.*, 1997) and might, to some extent, reflect a high expression level of the Th1-promoting cytokine IL-12 observed for putative APCs situated below the FAE of Peyer's patches in children (MacDonald and Monteleone, 2001). The strong bias towards Th1-cell responses in the human gut could thus contribute to the fact that the majority of food-allergic children outgrow their problems (Bischoff *et al.*, 2000). This is in contrast to respiratory atopic allergy, which tends to persist and even increase in severity (Hattevig *et al.*, 1993; Brandtzaeg *et al.*, 1996). Most probably, danger signals from an established intestinal bacterial flora, as well as the environmental microbial exposure, exert an important drive towards an adequate Th1 skewing in the gut, thus counterbalancing excessive Th2 responses (Fig. 14.6). Nevertheless, allergen-specific mucosal Th2 cells have been detected in patients with (presumably) cow's-milk-induced gastroenteritis (Beyer *et al.*, 2001).

Although the immune system in the airways also responds to antigen stimulation in the presence of danger signals (infection or inflammation) with a Th1 profile (Holt and Stumbles, 2000), an increasingly prominent Th2 profile generally develops as the basis for IgE-mediated (atopic) respiratory allergy (Hattevig *et al.*, 1993; Holt *et al.*, 1999) in individuals with a hereditary predisposition (Anderson and Cookson, 1999; Barnes, 2000). This skewing towards Th2-cell responses may be influenced by the so-called 'lymphoid' DC type, recently named plasmacytoid DCs (P-DCs), which can be identified by their high level of IL-3 receptor (CD123) in allergic nasal mucosa (Jahnsen *et al.*, 2000). *In vitro*, P-DCs have been shown to drive naive T-cells towards a Th2 response, with IL-4 and IL-5 production (Rissoan *et al.*, 1999). Interestingly, we have been unable to detect P-DCs in the intestinal lamina propria, even in IBD and coeliac disease (Jahnsen *et al.*, 2000). Therefore, the apparent inability of this DC subset to home to intestinal effector sites might contribute to the Th1 dominance of immune responses in the human gut as a result of little cross-regulation from local Th2 responses. The paucity of human intestinal Th2 responsiveness (MacDonald and Monteleone, 2001) is emphasized by the fact that there is usually no detectable IgE production at this mucosal effector site, even in adult food-allergic individuals with overt atopy (Bengtsson *et al.*, 1991). Hence, there may be several mechanisms other than a local mucosal Th2 response to explain gastrointestinal allergy against dietary antigens (Bruijnzeel-Koomen *et al.*, 1995; Bischoff *et al.*, 2000), including recruitment of mast cells armed with IgE from mesenteric lymph nodes, type III (immune complex)-mediated reactions and type IV (delayed type) hypersensitivity (Brandtzaeg, 1997b).

The feeding and treatment regimen (e.g. antibiotics) to which the newborn is subjected and its nutritional state have a significant impact on the composition of its indigenous microbiota, as well as on its gut integrity, and may hence disturb the balance of its developing mucosal immune system (Zeiger, 2000;

Hoppu *et al.*, 2001; Isolauri *et al.*, 2001). The role of commensal bacteria for mucosal tolerance induction in humans was highlighted in a recent clinical trial with postnatal colonization (for 6 months) of a probiotic lactobacillus strain (Kalliomäki *et al.*, 2001a); after 2 years, a 50% reduction of atopic eczema was observed in these children, compared with placebo controls. Intestinal colonization of lactobacilli and bifidobacteria is promoted by breast milk, because of its large amounts of oligosaccharides, which have prebiotic properties (Hoppu *et al.*, 2001); these microorganisms may directly enhance the Th1 profile in the gut by inducing IL-12, IL-18 and IFN-γ (Miettinen *et al.*, 1998; Hessle *et al.*, 1999). Also notably, *E. coli* is a strong inducer of IL-10 secretion, apparently derived from APCs (Hessle *et al.*, 2000a, b). This has been suggested to be an important suppressive cytokine in the gut (Steidler *et al.*, 2000). Thus, the indigenous microbiota may have an impact on mucosal homoeostasis beyond that of enhancing the SIgA system or promoting a Th1-cytokine profile that counterbalances Th2-cell responsiveness (Holt, 2000).

Immune Exclusion and IgA-mediated Mucosal Homoeostasis

The secretory antibody system and its function

The remarkable magnitude of GALT as an inductive site for B-cells is documented by the fact that more than 80% of all Ig-producing blasts and plasma cells in an adult are located in the intestinal lamina propria (Brandtzaeg *et al.*, 1999a). As mentioned above, most such terminally differentiated mucosal B-cells (immunocytes) produce J-chain-containing dimers and some larger polymers of IgA, collectively called pIgA. These polymers (as well as pentameric IgM with J chain) are efficiently transported externally as SIgA (and SIgM) antibodies by the pIgR (Norderhaug *et al.*, 1999; Johansen *et al.*, 2000), which is constituted by the membrane SC expressed basolaterally on the intestinal crypt cells and other secretory epithelia (Fig. 14.2).

The main purpose of the secretory antibody system is, in cooperation with innate mucosal defence mechanisms, to perform immune exclusion (Fig. 14.7). Most importantly, SIgA inhibits colonization and invasion of pathogens, and pIgR-transported pIgA and pentameric IgM antibodies may even inactivate viruses (e.g. rotavirus and influenza virus) inside secretory epithelial cells and carry the pathogens and their products back to the lumen (Fig. 14.7), thus avoiding cytolytic damage to the epithelium (Norderhaug *et al.*, 1999). Both the agglutinating and the virus-neutralizing antibody effects of pIgA are superior to those of monomeric antibodies (Brandtzaeg *et al.*, 1987), and SIgA antibodies may block microbial invasion quite efficiently. This has been particularly well documented in relation to the human immunodeficiency virus (Mazzoli *et al.*, 1997), and specific SIgA antibodies isolated from human colostrum have been shown to be more efficient in this respect than comparable IgG antibodies (Hocini and Bomsel, 1999).

Induction of SIgA responses has likewise been shown to interfere significantly with mucosal uptake of soluble macromolecules in experimental animals

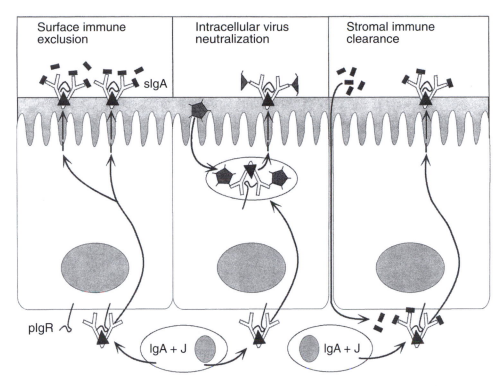

Fig. 14.7. Schematic representation of three levels at which dimeric immunoglobulin (Ig)A or secretory IgA (SIgA) may provide immune protection after being produced with J chain by plasma cells in the mucosal lamina propria. Left: Dimeric IgA is transported by the polymeric Ig receptor (pIgR) across epithelial cells and released into the lumen as SIgA antibodies, which perform immune exclusion by interaction with luminal antigens (black bars). Middle: Dimeric IgA antibodies interact with viral antigens within epithelial cells during pIgR-mediated transport, thereby performing intracellular virus neutralization and removal of viral products. Right: Dimeric IgA antibodies interact with penetrating antigens in the lamina propria and shuttle them back to the lumen by pIgR-mediated transport.

(Brandtzaeg *et al.*, 1987). Collectively, therefore, the function of locally produced pIgA, including antibodies in breast milk, would be to inhibit or modulate the epithelial colonization of microorganisms and to dampen the penetration of soluble antigens; this effect is most probably enhanced by the relatively high levels of polyreactive SIgA antibodies (Quan *et al.*, 1997). In the gut, interaction of SIgA with the endogenous protein Fv (Fv fragment binding protein) may, moreover, build an immune fortress by forming large complexes of intact or degraded antibodies with different specificities, thereby reinforcing immune exclusion (Bouvet and Fischetti, 1999). It has also been claimed that SIgA can enhance the sticking of certain bacteria to mucus, interfere with growth factors (e.g. iron) and enzymes necessary for pathogenic bacteria and parasites (Brandtzaeg *et al.*, 1999a) and exert positive influences on the inductive phase of mucosal immunity, by promoting antigen uptake in GALT via putative IgA receptors on the M cells of FAE (Frey and Neutra, 1997). The latter possibility adds to the importance of breast-feeding in providing a supply of relevant SIgA antibodies for the infant's gut.

Interestingly, free SC released to the lumen (Fig. 14.2) may on its own be able to block epithelial adhesion of *E. coli* (Giugliano *et al.*, 1995) and can bind the potent toxin of *Clostridium difficile* (Dallas and Rolfe, 1998). Also, a pneumococcal surface protein (SpsA) has been shown to interact with both free and bound SC (Hammerschmidt *et al.*, 1997). Such observations suggest that SC has phylogenetically originated from the innate defence system before being exploited by the adaptive secretory immune system to function as pIgR.

Handling of absorbed food antigens

Intact antigens have in several studies been shown to cross the normal gut barrier and enter the bloodstream even in adults, particularly after food intake (Brandtzaeg *et al.*, 1987), although the actual amount reaching the intestinal lamina propria remains uncertain. Work performed in experimental animals with mucosal application of ^{125}I-labelled albumin has been difficult to interpret, due to marker instability; both degradation of the carrier molecule and release of the label can result in considerable overestimation of protein penetrability as determined by scintillation counting, compared with data based on immunological quantification (Brandtzaeg and Tolo, 1977). Intact dietary antigens appear in the circulation of healthy adults 2–5 h after a meal, being partly present in immune complexes. Thus, intake of 1.2 l of bovine milk resulted in some 3 ng ml^{-1} of β-lactoglobulin in peripheral blood (Paganelli and Levinsky, 1980). Ovalbumin up to 10 ng ml^{-1} has likewise been found, corresponding to approximately 10^{-5} of the amount consumed (Husby *et al.*, 1985). Furthermore, both β-lactoglobulin and ovalbumin have been detected in the breast milk of lactating women, but with unexplained large intra- and interindividual variations, the levels ranging from 0.9 to 150 µg l^{-1} (Kilshaw and Cant, 1984; Høst *et al.*, 1990).

Several routes may be visualized for the penetration of intact soluble antigens through the normal intestinal epithelium: paracellular diffusion bypassing the tight junctions; via epithelial discontinuities, such as the cell extrusion zones of the villus tips; translocation through enterocytes by endocytosis and subsequent exocytosis; or transport by M cells in GALT. As discussed elsewhere (Brandtzaeg *et al.*, 1987; Brandtzaeg, 1996a), the relative importance of these mechanisms remains unknown, and the consequences in terms of sensitization or induction of oral tolerance probably depend on the route of uptake, as well as on the nature of the antigen – that is, soluble, lectin-like or particulate (Fig. 14.8). There is likewise no definite knowledge about the effects transmission of food antigens to breast milk might have on the suckling's immune system (Zeiger, 2000; Hoppu *et al.*, 2001), although animal experiments have suggested the possibility of tolerance induction (Johansen *et al.*, 2001).

External transport of pIgA-containing immune complexes by the pIgR has been suggested as an efficient, non-inflammatory antigen clearance mechanism

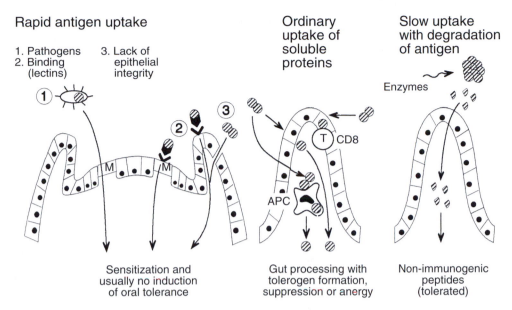

Fig. 14.8. Various theoretical routes of antigen uptake in the gut and putative immunological consequences. Pathogenic microorganisms and dead particulate antigens (1), as well as proteins with special lectin-like properties (2), are rapidly transported through M cells (M) of follicle-associated epithelium covering gut-associated lymphoid tissue (to the left). Breaching of the gut epithelium (3) also allows rapid antigen uptake. Soluble proteins may be taken up by the paracellular route through the villus epithelium and then endocytosed by subepithelial antigen-presenting cells (APCs), or they are transported and presented by enterocytes to intraepithelial (CD8) or subepithelial T-cells (T). The transcellular route through the enterocyte is presumably speeded up by the lectin-like properties of the antigen (2). If the antigen is aggregated, luminal endogenous or bacterial enzymes may degrade it extensively to become non-immunogenic (to the right).

from the gut lamina propria (Fig. 14.7). This notion has recently been supported by experiments performed *in vivo* (Robinson *et al.*, 2001). Pentameric IgM (in contrast to hexameric IgM without J chain) also appears to have little or no complement-activating properties and therefore could probably support the non-inflammatory functions of pIgA in competition with corresponding pro-inflammatory IgG antibodies (Brandtzaeg *et al.*, 1999a, b). Interestingly, monomeric IgA or IgG antibodies, when cross-linked via antigen to pIgA of the same specificity, might contribute to such pIgR-mediated epithelial transcystosis of foreign material (Mazanec *et al.*, 1993). Conversely, complement-activating IgG antibodies against infectious agents and dietary proteins could on its own adversely affect mucosal penetrability for a variety of exogenous proteins while contributing to local protection. This possibility has been suggested by experiments *ex vivo* (Brandtzaeg and Tolo, 1977) and *in vivo* (Lim and Rowley, 1982); IgG antibodies against one antigen were shown to enhance mucosal penetration of bystander molecules. Mucosal integrity was apparently damaged by lysosomal enzymes released from polymorphonuclear granulocytes, which are attracted when immune complexes form locally. Perhaps antigen interaction with maternal IgG antibodies could explain why abrupt introduction of native cow's milk proteins in infants often causes gastrointestinal bleeding (Ziegler et al., 1990).

The pro-inflammatory potential of maternally-derived or locally-produced IgG antibodies is probably less important in the gut of infants who are breast-fed, because milk SIgA antibodies will exert a non-inflammatory blocking effect. Moreover, breast milk contains large amounts of the soluble complement inhibitor protectin, CD59 (Bjørge et al., 1993). Also, this factor and other complement regulatory proteins are expressed by the gastrointestinal epithelium (Berstad and Brandtzaeg, 1998), and these probably counteract immune complex-mediated (type III hypersensitivity) damage of the epithelial barrier.

There is further experimental evidence to suggest that IgA may influence mucosal homoeostasis in various ways through its binding to the Fcα receptor (CD89) when present on lamina propria leucocytes, although in the normal state CD89 expression is extremely low on human intestinal macrophages (Smith et al., 2001). Interestingly, IgA can down-regulate the secretion of the pro-inflammatory cytokine TNF-α from activated monocytes and inhibit activation-dependent generation of reactive oxygen intermediates in neutrophils and monocytes (Wolf et al., 1994a, b). On the other hand, pIgA or aggregated monomeric IgA can trigger monocytes to show increased activity, such as TNF-α secretion (Devière et al., 1991), and also up-regulate B7 on APCs (Geissmann et al., 2001) and induce eosinophil degranulation (Abu-Ghazaleh et al., 1989). This pro-inflammatory potential of IgA probably reflects the need for reinforcement of mucosal antigen elimination mechanisms when immune exclusion fails, such as in intestinal parasitic infestations.

Protective and Immunoregulatory Effects of Breast Milk

Secretory antibodies and free SC

The initial breast milk, or colostrum, is much richer in antibodies than other secretions, because of its remarkably high concentration of SIgA ($\sim$12 g l^{-1}) and SIgM ($\sim$0.6 g l^{-1}). The individual variations are large, however, and the level decreases by a factor of approximately four after 2 weeks and then remains fairly stable throughout lactation (Goldman, 1993; Hanson et al., 1993). Antibodies of these two classes are produced locally by plasma cells as pIgA and pentameric IgM in the lactating breast (Brandtzaeg, 1983). Unoccupied pIgR molecules are also cleaved and released to the lumen as free SC (Fig. 14.2), which is present at a relatively high level in colostrum ($\sim$2 g l^{-1}). Free SC exerts a stabilizing effect on SIgM (Brandtzaeg, 1975) and may by itself contribute to intestinal defence through inhibition of E. coli colonization and C. difficile toxin blocking, as mentioned above. When present in a bound form, SC may activate eosinophils (Lamkhioued et al., 1995), but it may counteract such pro-inflammatory stimulation in its free, soluble form (Motegi and Kita, 1998).

Because the lactating mammary glands are part of the integrated mucosal immune system (Fig.14.4), milk antibodies will reflect antigenic stimulation of MALT in the gut as well as in the airways, as mentioned earlier. The secretory antibodies are thus highly targetted against infectious agents in the mother's environment, which are those likely to be encountered by the baby during its first weeks of life. As mentioned previously, antibodies against various dietary antigens, such as gluten and cow's milk proteins, as well as against other potential allergens (Casas *et al.*, 2000), are also often present in breast milk. The possible role of these IgA antibodies for the clinical presentation of immune-mediated adverse reactions to food in the infant will be discussed below.

Non-specific anti-microbial factors

Numerous constituents of breast milk are thought to exert innate defence functions, and the possible role of free SC was alluded to above. Other factors include lysozyme, lactoferrin, peroxidase, complex oligosaccharides (receptor analogues), fatty acids and mucins (Goldman, 1993; Hoppu *et al.*, 2001). A further discussion of their potential protective effects is beyond the scope of this chapter.

Immune cells and macrophages

A variety of leucocytes occur in colostrum ($\sim 4 \times 10^6$ ml^{-1}) and later in milk ($\sim 10^5$ ml^{-1}). Macrophages (55–60%) and polymorphonuclear granulocytes (30–40%) dominate over lymphocytes (5–10%), the latter being mainly (75–80%) T lymphocytes (Goldman, 1993; Wold and Hanson, 1994). Oral administration of macrophages in newborn mice showed survival of these cells for several hours in the gut and even some mucosal uptake (Hughes *et al.*, 1988). Experiments with milk leucocytes in newborn rats, calves and lambs likewise demonstrated transepithelial migration, lymphocytes apparently being the predominant cell type (Slade and Schwartz, 1987). Also, the distribution of labelled human colostral leucocytes after enteral administration in premature baboons suggested epithelial adherence in the gut, as well as mucosal uptake and persistence for more than 60 h, along with some peripheral migration (Jain *et al.*, 1989). The contribution of milk lymphocytes to the infant's developing intestinal immune system therefore remains an intriguing possibility.

Milk leucocytes generally express markers of previous priming and respond readily to restimulation. The macrophages contain engulfed SIgA that they may release on contact with bacteria in the gut (Slade and Schwartz, 1987). They may also secrete an array of immunologically important cytokines (Wold and Hanson, 1994). It is furthermore of interest that, compared with peripheral blood, breast milk is relatively enriched in T lymphocytes with the alternative TCRγ/δ; this subset mainly employs the Vδ1/Jδ1-encoded receptor, as do intraepithelial γ/δ T-cells in the gut (Bertotto *et al.*, 1991). T lymphocytes of this phenotype with specificity for *Mycobacterium tuberculosis* appear in colostrum of tuberculin-positive nursing mothers (Bertotto *et al.*, 1993). This observation is interesting in view of the direct antimicrobial activity mediated by various T-cell phenotypes upon interaction with microbial targets (Levitz *et al.*, 1995). In this respect, mucosal defence may especially engage γ/δ T-cells. Their supply from breast milk could thus be immunologically important before the baby's IEL population has developed numerically and functionally.

Putative immunoregulatory factors

Glycoproteins from human colostrum have an enhancing effect on T-cell proliferation at low concentrations but an inhibitory effect at high concentrations (Mincheva-Nilsson *et al.*, 1990). The biological significance of this *in vitro* phenomenon is obscure as long as the active factors remain unidentified. One inhibitory mechanism of breast milk was suggested to be down-regulation of IL-2 production (Hooton *et al.*, 1991) and multimeric colostral α-lactalbumin was shown to induce apoptosis in lymphocytes (Håkansson *et al.*, 1995). Conversely, the stimulatory effect of milk on T-cells was tentatively ascribed to lactoferrin (Mincheva-Nilsson *et al.*, 1990), but great confusion exists about the possible immunoregulatory properties of this protein (Brock, 1995).

Several studies have reported that unfractionated supernatants of breast milk cell cultures preferentially stimulate IgA production by peripheral blood lymphocytes (Slade and Schwartz, 1987). An explanation for this effect may be the various cytokines that are secreted by stimulated milk macrophages (Wold and Hanson, 1994). The same soluble cytokines are found in breast milk (Goldman, 1993), and the presence of TGF-β, IL-6 and IL-10 is of particular interest for the development and differentiation of IgA-producing cells (Brandtzaeg *et al.*, 1999a). Evidence to this end has been provided for IL-6 (Saito *et al.*, 1991), as well as for IL-10 and TGF-β (Böttcher *et al.*, 2001), by relating the levels of cytokines in breast milk to salivary IgA concentrations in breast-fed children. Even if these cytokines are unable to survive the passage through the gastrointestinal tract, they may be released locally from milk macrophages in the neonatal gut and promote the development of a balanced mucosal immune system, thus contributing to a subsequent responder phenotype compatible with health. In this context, the balance between the immunosuppressive IL-10 and the Th2-promoting IL-4 in breast milk (Böttcher *et al.*, 2000) might be of particular significance. Also, the high levels of soluble Fas (CD95) could be important, because this protein might protect the intestinal epithelial barrier against apoptosis and favour tolerance induction (Srivastava and Srivastava, 1999).

Effect on productive mucosal immunity development

In addition to the remarkable reinforcement of mucosal defence provided by maternal SIgA (and SIgM) antibodies as a natural immunological 'substitution therapy', it is important to emphasize the positive nutritional effect of breast-feeding on immune development (Brandtzaeg, 1996b). Also, as mentioned above, breast milk contains a number of immune cells, cytokines and growth factors that may exert a significant biological effect in the suckling's gut, apparently enhancing in an indirect way even the long-term health of the individual (Wold and Hanson, 1994; Newman, 1995).

Numerous studies of the effect of breast-feeding on secretory immunity have been performed with salivary IgA measurements as a read-out system. Discrepant observations have been made, probably to some extent reflecting different cytokine levels in the milk as discussed above. The influence of contaminating the saliva sample with milk SIgA, shielding of the suckling's mucosal immune system by maternal SIgA antibodies, and altered growth and composition of the infant's gut flora have been discussed as additional uncontrollable variables (Brandtzaeg *et al.*, 1991). However, the balance of accumulated data suggests that breast-feeding promotes the post-natal development of secretory immunity (Wold and Hanson, 1994; Brandtzaeg, 1998), apparently even in the urinary tract (Newman, 1995); and there are reports of enhanced secretory, as well as systemic, immune responses to oral and parenteral vaccines in breast-fed babies (Hahn-Zoric *et al.*, 1990; Pabst and Spady, 1990).

Nevertheless, several prospective studies have reported that the early physiological increase of salivary IgA (and IgM) is more prominent in formula-fed than in solely breast-fed infants (Gleeson *et al.*, 1986; Stephens, 1986; Brandtzaeg *et al.*, 1991), although this difference seems to disappear after weaning (Tappuni and Challacombe, 1994). It likewise seems that breast-feeding, in comparison with formula-feeding, reduces the salivary IgA antibody titres to cow's milk proteins; this decrease was seen after a nursing period of only 3 weeks and appeared also in infants receiving mixed feeding (Gleeson *et al.*, 1986; Renz *et al.*, 1991). Altogether, therefore, although breast-feeding initially appears to reduce induction of salivary IgA, it will later on in infancy (up to 8 months) boost this response (Avanzini *et al.*, 1992; Fitzsimmons *et al.*, 1994). In a similar manner, experiments in mice have demonstrated that SIgA antibodies from breast milk affect the stimulatory properties of the gut flora in the suckling by retarding bacterial contact with the developing GALT (Cebra *et al.*, 1999). When the host's mucosal immune response subsequently is successfully elicited, GALT will be further shielded by the SIgA antibodies produced in the gut; local immunostimulation is thereby attenuated despite the continued presence of microorganisms (Shroff *et al.*, 1995). This could contribute to the hypo-responsiveness or tolerance that normally exists towards members of the autologous commensal gut bacteria, in both rodents and humans (Helgeland and Brandtzaeg, 2000).

Effect on oral tolerance development

Through avoidance of too early local immune activation – for instance, limiting the intestinal up-regulation of the co-stimulatory B7 molecules (Brandtzaeg, 1998; Chen *et al.*, 2000), the shielding effect exerted by SIgA from breast milk on the suckling's GALT (see above) may contribute to the establishment of oral tolerance not only against the indigenous microflora, but also against dietary antigens, such as gluten. Antibodies to gluten peptides are present in breast milk (Juto and Holm, 1992) and breast-feeding has in fact been shown to protect significantly against the development of coeliac disease in children, an effect that is unrelated to the time of solid food introduction (Brandtzaeg, 1997a). Early exposure to cow's milk has been suggested to be associated with predisposition to type 1 (insulin-dependent) diabetes, and investigations have particularly focused on immune stimulation by bovine serum albumin (Karjalainen et al., 1992), β-lactoglobulin (Dahlquist et al., 1992) and insulin (Vaarala et al., 1999). In a recent study, short-term breast-feeding and early introduction of cow's milk were found to be associated with progressive signs of type 1 diabetes-related autoimmunity (Kimpimäki et al., 2001).

On the basis of such observations, it may be tentatively concluded that mixed feeding, rather than abrupt weaning, appears to promote tolerance to food proteins and thereby also avoidance of potentially harmful cross-reactive autoantibodies. This notion is further supported by reports suggesting that cow's milk allergy is more likely to develop in infants whose mothers have relatively low levels of milk IgA antibodies to bovine proteins (Savilahti et al., 1991; Järvinen et al., 2000). It is also noteworthy in this context that allergic mothers appear to have decreased levels of ovalbumin-specific IgA (Casas et al., 2000) and elevated levels of IL-4 (Böttcher et al., 2000) in their breast milk.

The presence of TGF-β and IL-10 in breast milk might contribute to its tolerogenic properties, because these cytokines exert pronounced immunosuppressive effects in the gut (Ishizaka et al., 1994; Steidler et al., 2000) and TGF-β enhances the epithelial barrier function (Planchon et al., 1994). Although still a somewhat controversial issue (Zeiger, 2000), the balance of epidemiological studies supports the view that breast-feeding protects against atopic allergy and asthma (Saarinen and Kajosaari, 1995; Oddy et al., 1999; Kull et al., 2001). Interestingly, TGF-β has been reported to be present at a higher level in maternal colostrum provided for infants that did not develop atopic eczema during exclusive breast-feeding, compared with those with early-onset symptoms (Kalliomäki et al., 1999). As discussed above, food antigens do appear in breast milk, but dietary restriction during pregnancy and breast-feeding has shown no conclusive effect on the development of atopic diseases in the child (Zeiger, 2000; Hoppu et al., 2001). It remains an open question whether early exposure to small amounts of food antigens may actually have a positive effect on tolerance induction, especially when occurring in its natural context in the gut lumen of a suckling (Johansen et al., 2001).

Conclusions

Several more or less well-defined variables influence the development of productive mucosal immunity and oral tolerance, therefore constituting a complex and rather enigmatic mechanistic basis for adaptive immune defence and adverse immunological reactions to food. An inadequate epithelial barrier against luminal antigens is an important primary or secondary event in the pathogenesis of several mucosal diseases – being influenced by the individual's age (e.g. preterm versus term infant), activation of the epithelium and subepithelial elements, such as APCs and mast cells (e.g. by infection, cytokines or neuropeptides), and the shielding effect of SIgA provided by breast milk or produced by adaptive B-cell responses in the infant's gut. The consequences will depend on how quickly mucosal homoeostasis can be attained or re-established after abrogation.

SIgA is the best-defined effector component of the mucosal immune system, and this first-line specific defence against infectious agents and other harmful substances is of considerable clinical interest. The large capacity for storage of pIgA in the mammary-gland epithelium and duct system explains the remarkable output of SIgA during feeding. Breast milk also contains an array of important immunoregulatory factors and promotes colonization of lactic acid-producing bacteria. These members of the indigenous microbiota are powerful in combating pathogenic intruders that may break oral tolerance (Collins and Gibson, 1999; Isolauri *et al.*, 2001), and they also appear to exert a beneficial effect on the cytokine balance of the host and thereby on the developing immunological responder phenotype (Fig. 14.9). Animal experiments have indeed documented that the commensal bacterial flora is crucial both for the induction of oral tolerance and for its re-establishment after abrogation (Helgeland and Brandtzaeg, 2000). Altogether, this effect might not only be mediated through immune modulation, but could also be explained by the

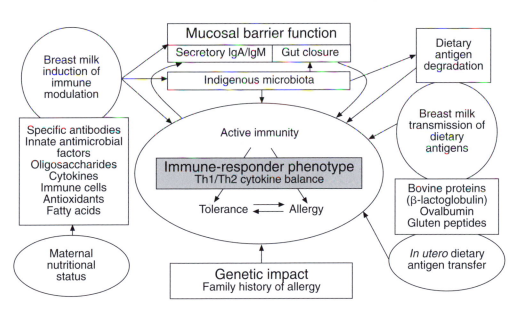

Fig. 14.9. Multiple direct or indirect effects of breast-feeding may be imprinted in the immune-responder phenotype of the infant. Details are discussed in the text. (Modified from Hoppu *et al.*, 2001.)

enzymatic activity of the indigenous flora that degrades food proteins to tolerated peptides (Barone *et al.*, 2000).

Convincing evidence exists for an important role of breast-feeding in the defence against mucosal infections. Its role in oral tolerance and protection against food allergy has been much more difficult to establish conclusively. This is not surprising in view of the complex and poorly understood interface between these two enigmatic biological phenomena, with multiple potential interactions influenced by the numerous bioactive components of breast milk (Fig. 14.9). For ethical reasons, it will not be possible to assign infants to breast- or formula-feeding for long-term follow-up studies. Therefore, perhaps we shall just have to take it on trust that exclusive breast-feeding for several months, followed by mixed feeding, is the natural way to begin life for all mammals, including humans.

Acknowledgements

Studies in the author's laboratory are supported by the Norwegian Cancer Society, the Research Council of Norway, Anders Jahre's Foundation, Rakel and Otto Kr. Bruun's Legacy and the Research Fund for Asthma and Allergy. Hege Eliassen Bryne and Erik K. Hagen are thanked for excellent secretarial assistance.

References

Abu-Ghazaleh, R.I., Fujisawa, T., Mestecky, J., Kyle, R.A. and Gleich, G.J. (1989) IgA-induced eosinophil degranulation. *Journal of Immunology* 142, 2393–2400.

Alpan, O., Rudomen, G. and Matzinger, P. (2001) The role of dendritic cells, B-cells, and M cells in gut-oriented immune responses. *Journal of Immunology* 166, 4843–4852.

Anderson, G.G. and Cookson, W.O. (1999) Recent advances in the genetics of allergy and asthma. *Molecular Medicine Today* 5, 264–273.

Anon. (1994) A warm chain for breastfeeding. *Lancet* 344, 1239–1241.

Avanzini, M.A., Plebani, A., Monafo, V., Pasinetti, G., Teani, M., Colombo, A., Mellander, L., Carlsson, B., Hanson, L.Å., Ugazio, A.G. and Burgio, G.R. (1992) A comparison of secretory antibodies in breast-fed and formula-fed infants over the first six months of life. *Acta Paediatrica* 81, 296–301.

Barnes, K.C. (2000) Atopy and asthma genes – where do we stand? *Allergy* 55, 803–817.

Barone, K.S., Reilly, M.R., Flanagan, M.P. and Michael, J.G. (2000) Abrogation of oral tolerance by feeding encapsulated antigen. *Cellular Immunology* 199, 65–72.

Beatty, D.W., Napier, B., Sinclair-Smith, C.C., McCabe, K. and Hughes, E.J. (1983) Secretory IgA synthesis in kwashiorkor. *Journal of Clinical and Laboratory Immunology* 12, 31–36.

Bengtsson, U., Rognum, T.O., Brandtzaeg, P., Kilander, A., Hansson, G., Ahlstedt, S. and Hanson, L.A. (1991) IgE-positive duodenal mast cells in patients with food-related diarrhea. *International Archives of Allergy and Applied Immunology* 95, 86–91.

Berstad, A.E. and Brandtzaeg, P. (1998) Expression of cell-membrane complement regulatory glycoproteins along the normal and diseased human gastrointestinal tract. *Gut* 42, 522–529.

Bertotto, A., Gerli, R., Castellucci, G., Scalise, F. and Vaccaro, R. (1991) Human milk lymphocytes bearing the γ/δ T-cell receptor are mostly δ TCS1-positive cells. *Immunology* 74, 360–361.

Bertotto, A., Gerli, R., Castellucci, G., Crupi, S., Scalise, F., Spinozzi, F., Fabietti, G., Forenza, N. and Vaccaro, R. (1993) Mycobacteria-reactive γ/δ T-cells are present in human colostrum from tuberculin-positive, but not tuberculin-negative nursing mothers. *American Journal of Reproductive Immunology* 29, 131–134.

Beyer, K., Castro, R., Birnbaum, A., Benkov, K., Pittman, N. and Sampson, H.A. (2001) Human milk-specific mucosal lymphocytes display a Th2 cytokine profile. *Allergy* 56 (Suppl. 68), 95.

Bischoff, S.C., Mayer, J.H. and Manns, M.P. (2000) Allergy and the gut. *International Archives of Allergy and Immunology* 121, 270–283.

Bjørge, L., Jensen, T.S., Vedeler, C.A., Ulvestad, E., Kristoffersen, E.K. and Matre, R. (1993) Soluble CD59 in pregnancy and infancy. *Immunology Letters* 36, 233–234.

Björkstén, B., Naaber, P., Sepp, E. and Mikelsaar, M. (1999) The intestinal microflora in allergic Estonian and Swedish 2-year-old children. *Clinical and Experimental Allergy* 29, 342–346.

Bloom, S., Simmons, D. and Jewell, D.P. (1995) Adhesion molecules intercellular adhesion molecule-1 (ICAM-1), ICAM-3 and B7 are not expressed by epithelium in normal or inflamed colon. *Clinical and Experimental Immunology* 101, 157–163.

Boirivant, M., Fuss, I., Fiocchi, C., Klein, J.S., Strong, S.A. and Strober, W. (1996) Hypoproliferative human lamina propria T-cells retain the capacity to secrete lymphokines when stimulated via CD2/CD28 pathways. *Proceedings of the Association of American Physicians* 108, 55–67.

Børresen, H.C. (1995) Rethinking current recommendations to introduce solid food between four and six months to exclusively breastfeeding infants. *Journal of Human Lactation* 11, 201–204.

Böttcher, M.F., Jenmalm, M.C., Garofalo, R.P. and Björkstén, B. (2000) Cytokines in breast milk from allergic and nonallergic mothers. *Pediatric Research* 47, 157–162.

Böttcher, M.F., Jenmalm, M.C. and Böttcher, B. (2001) Cytokines and chemokines in breast milk in relation to the development of allergy and IgA production in children. *Allergy* 56 (Suppl. 68), 39–40.

Bouvet, J.-P. and Fischetti, V.A. (1999) Diversity of antibody-mediated immunity at the mucosal barrier. *Infection and Immunity* 67, 2687–2691.

Brandtzaeg, P. (1973) Two types of IgA immunocytes in man. *Nature New Biology* 243, 142–143.

Brandtzaeg, P. (1974a) Presence of J chain in human immunocytes containing various immunoglobulin classes. *Nature* 252, 418–420.

Brandtzaeg, P. (1974b) Mucosal and glandular distribution of immunoglobulin components: differential localization of free and bound SC in secretory epithelial cells. *Journal of Immunology* 112, 1553–1559.

Brandtzaeg, P. (1975) Human secretory immunoglobulin M: an immunochemical and immunohistochemical study. *Immunology* 29, 559–570.

Brandtzaeg, P. (1983) The secretory immune system of lactating human mammary glands compared with other exocrine organs. *Annals of the New York Academy of Sciences* 30, 353–382.

Brandtzaeg, P. (1996a) History of oral tolerance and mucosal immunity. *Annals of the New York Academy of Science* 778, 1–27.

Brandtzaeg, P. (1996b) Development of the mucosal immune system in humans. In: Bindels, J.G., Goedhart, A.C. and Visser, H.K.A. (eds) *Recent Developments in Infant Nutrition*. Kluwer Academic Publishers, London, pp. 349–376.

Brandtzaeg, P. (1997a) Development of the intestinal immune system and its relation to coeliac disease. In: Mäki, M., Collin, P. and Visakorpi, J.K. (eds) *Coeliac Disease. Proceedings of the Seventh International Symposium on Coeliac Disease*. Coeliac Disease Study Group, Tampere, pp. 221–244.

Brandtzaeg, P. (1997b) Mechanisms of gastrointestinal reactions to food. *Environmental Toxicology and Pharmacology* 4, 9–24.

Brandtzaeg, P. (1998) Development and basic mechanisms of human gut immunity. *Nutrition Reviews* 56, S5–S18.

Brandtzaeg, P. (1999) Regionalized immune function of tonsils and adenoids. *Immunology Today* 20, 383–384.

Brandtzaeg, P. (2001) Nature and function of gastrointestinal antigen-presenting cells. *Allergy* 56(Suppl. 67), 16–20.

Brandtzaeg, P. and Nilssen, D.E. (1995) Mucosal aspects of primary B-cell deficiency and gastrointestinal infections. *Current Opinion in Gastroenterology* 11, 532–540.

Brandtzaeg, P. and Tolo, K. (1977) Mucosal penetrability enhanced by serum-derived antibodies. *Nature* 266, 262–263.

Brandtzaeg, P., Fjellanger, I. and Gjeruldsen, S.T. (1968) Immunoglobulin M: local synthesis and selective secretion in patients with immunoglobulin A deficiency. *Science* 160, 789–791.

Brandtzaeg, P., Baklien, K., Bjerke, K., Rognum, T.O., Scott, H. and Valnes, K. (1987) Nature and properties of the human gastrointestinal immune system. In: Miller, M. and Nicklin, S. (eds) *Immunology of the Gastrointestinal Tract*. CRC Press, Boca Raton, pp. 1–85.

Brandtzaeg, P., Nilssen, D.E., Rognum, T.O. and Thrane, P.S. (1991) Ontogeny of the mucosal immune system and IgA deficiency. *Gastroenterology Clinics of North America* 20, 397–439.

Brandtzaeg, P., Jahnsen, F.L. and Farstad, I.N. (1996) Immune functions and immunopathology of the mucosa of the upper respiratory pathways. *Acta Otolaryngologica* 116, 149–159.

Brandtzaeg, P., Farstad, I.N. and Helgeland, L. (1998) Phenotypes of T-cells in the gut. *Chemical Immunology* 71, 1–26.

Brandtzaeg, P., Farstad, I.N., Johansen, F.E., Morton, H.C., Norderhaug, I.N. and Yamanaka, T. (1999a) The B-cell system of human mucosae and exocrine glands. *Immunology Reviews* 171, 45–87.

Brandtzaeg, P., Baekkevold, E.S., Farstad, I.N., Jahnsen, F.L., Johansen, F.-E., Nilsen, E.M. and Yamanaka, T. (1999b) Regional specialization in the mucosal immune system: what happens in the microcompartments? *Immunology Today* 20, 141–151.

Brandtzaeg, P., Farstad, I.N. and Haraldsen, G. (1999c) Regional specialization in the mucosal immune system: primed cells do not always home along the same track. *Immunology Today* 20, 267–277.

Brandtzaeg, P., Haraldsen, G., Helgeland, L., Nilsen, E.M. and Rugtveit, J. (1999d) New insights into the immunopathology of human inflammatory bowel disease. *Drugs of Today* 35(Suppl. A), 33–70.

Bridges, R.A., Condie, R.M., Zak, S.J. and Good, R.A. (1959) The morphologic basis of antibody formation: development during the neonatal period. *Journal of Laboratory and Clinical Medicine* 53, 331–357.

Brock, J. (1995) Lactoferrin: a multifunctional immunoregulatory protein? *Immunology Today* 16, 417–419.

Bruijnzeel-Koomen, C., Ortolani, C., Aas, K., Bindslev-Jensen, C., Björkstén, B., Moneret-Vautrin, D. and Wüthrich, B. (1995) Adverse reactions to food: European Academy of Allergology and Clinical Immunology Subcommittee. *Allergy* 50, 623–635.

Burrows, P.D. and Cooper, M.D. (1997) IgA deficiency. *Advances in Immunology* 65, 245–276.

Butcher, E.C., Rouse, R.V., Coffman, R.L., Nottenburg, C.N., Hardy, R.R. and Weissman, I.L. (1982) Surface phenotype of Peyer's patch germinal center cells: implications for the role of germinal centers in B-cell differentiation. *Journal of Immunology* 129, 2698–2707.

Casas, R., Böttcher, M.F., Duchén, K. and Björkstén, B. (2000) Detection of IgA antibodies to cat, β-lactoglobulin, and ovalbumin allergens in human milk. *Journal of Allergy and Clinical Immunology* 105, 1236–1240.

Cebra, J.J., Jiang, H.Q., Strerzl, J. and Tlaskalová-Hogenová, H. (1999) The role of mucosal microbiota in the development and maintenance of the mucosal immune system. In: Ogra, P.L., Mestecky, J., Lamm, M.E., Strober, W., Bienenstock, J. and McGhee, J.R. (eds) *Mucosal Immunology*, 2nd edn. Academic Press, London, pp. 267–280.

Cerf-Bensussan, N. and Guy-Grand, D. (1991) Intestinal intraepithelial lymphocytes. *Gastroenterology Clinics of North America* 20, 549–576.

Chambers, C.A. and Allison, J.P. (1999) Costimulatory regulation of T-cell function. *Current Opinion in Cell Biology* 11, 203–210.

Chen, Y., Inobe, J., Marks, R., Gonnella, P., Kuchroo, V.K. and Weiner, H.L. (1995) Peripheral deletion of antigen-reactive T-cells in oral tolerance. *Nature* 376, 177–180.

Chen, Y., Song, K. and Eck, S.L. (2000) An intra-Peyer's patch gene transfer model for studying mucosal tolerance: distinct roles of B7 and IL-12 in mucosal T-cell tolerance. *Journal of Immunology* 165, 3145–3153.

Collins, M.D. and Gibson, G.R. (1999) Probiotics, prebiotics, and synbiotics: approaches for modulating the microbial ecology of the gut. *American Journal of Clinical Nutrition* 69, 1052S–1057S.

Cornes, J.S. (1965) Number, size, and distribution of Peyer's patches in the human small intestine. *Gut* 6, 225–233.

Corry, D.B. and Kheradmand, F. (1999) Induction and regulation of the IgE response. *Nature* 402, B18–B23.

Crabbé, P.A., Nash, D.R., Bazin, H., Eyssen, H. and Heremans, J.F. (1970) Immunohistochemical observations on lymphoid tissues from conventional and germ-free mice. *Laboratory Investigations* 22, 448–457.

Cuff, C.F., Cebra, C.K., Rubin, D.H. and Cebra, J.J. (1993) Developmental relationship between cytotoxic α/β T-cell receptor-positive intraepithelial lymphocytes and Peyer's patch lymphocytes. *European Journal of Immunology* 23, 1333–1339.

Dahlquist, G., Savilahti, E. and Landin-Olsson, M. (1992) An increased level of antibodies to beta-lactoglobulin is a risk determinant for early-onset type 1 (insulin-dependent) diabetes mellitus independent of islet cell antibodies and early introduction of cow's milk. *Diabetologia* 35, 980–984.

Dallas, S.D. and Rolfe, R.D. (1998) Binding of *Clostridium difficile* toxin A to human milk secretory component. *Journal of Medical Microbiology* 47, 879–888.

De Maria, R., Boirivant, M., Cifone, M.G., Roncaioli, P., Hahne, M., Tschopp, J., Pallone, F., Santoni, A. and Testi, R. (1996) Functional expression of Fas and Fas ligand on human gut lamina propria T lymphocytes: a potential role for the acidic sphingomyelinase pathway in normal immunoregulation. *Journal of Clinical Investigation* 97, 316–322.

Devière, J., Vaerman, J.-P. Content, J., Denys, C., Schandene, L., Vandenbussche, P., Sibille, Y. and Dupont, E. (1991) IgA triggers tumor necrosis factor α secretion by monocytes: a study in normal subjects and patients with alcoholic cirrhosis. *Hepatology* 13, 670–675.

Dickinson, B.L., Badizadegan, K., Wu, Z., Ahouse, J.C., Zhu, X., Simister, N.E., Blumberg, R.S. and Lencer, W.I. (1999) Bidirectional FcRn-dependent IgG transport in a polarized human intestinal epithelial cell line. *Journal of Clinical Investigation* 104, 903–911.

Dickinson, E.C., Gorga, J.C., Garrett, M., Tuncer, R., Boyle, P., Watkins, S.C., Alber, S.M., Parizhskaya, M., Trucco, M., Rowe, M.I. and Ford, H.R. (1998) Immunoglobulin A supplementation abrogates bacterial translocation and preserves the architecture of the intestinal epithelium. *Surgery* 124, 284–290.

Duchmann, R., Neurath, M., Marker-Hermann, E. and Meyer Zum Buschenfelde, K.H. (1997) Immune responses towards intestinal bacteria – current concepts and future perspectives. *Zeitschrift für Gastroenterologie* 35, 337–346.

Dunkley, M.L. and Husband, A.J. (1987) Distribution and functional characteristics of antigen-specific helper T-cells arising after Peyer's patch immunization. *Immunology* 61, 475–482.

Erb, K.J. (1999) Atopic disorders: a default pathway in the absence of infection? *Immunology Today* 20, 317–322.

Fitzsimmons, S.P., Evans, M.K., Pearce, C.L., Sheridan, M.J., Wientzen, R. and Cole, M.F. (1994) Immunoglobulin A subclasses in infants' saliva and in saliva and milk from their mothers. *Journal of Pediatrics* 124, 566–573.

Frey, A. and Neutra, M.R. (1997) Targeting of mucosal vaccines to Peyer's patch M cells. *Behring Institute Mitteilungen* 98, 376–389.

Fujihashi, K., Taguchi, T., Aicher, W.K., McGhee, J.R., Bluestone, J.A., Eldridge, J.H. and Kiyono, H. (1992) Immunoregulatory functions for murine intraepithelial lymphocytes: γ/δ T-cell receptor-positive (TCR+) T-cells abrogate oral tolerance, while α/β TCR+ T-cells provide B-cell help. *Journal of Experimental Medicine* 175, 695–707.

Fujihashi, K., Dohi, T., Kweon, M.N., McGhee, J.R., Koga, T., Cooper, M.D., Tonegawa, S. and Kiyono, H. (1999) γ/δ T-cells regulate mucosally induced tolerance in a dose-dependent fashion. *International Immunology* 11, 1907–1916.

Fujihashi, K., Dohi, T., Rennert, P.D., Yamamoto, M., Koga, T., Kiyono, H. and McGhee, J.R. (2001) Peyer's patches are required for oral tolerance to proteins. *Proceedings of the National Academy of Sciences of the USA* 98, 3310–3315.

Fukaura, H., Kent, S.C., Pietrusewicz, M.J., Khoury, S.J., Weiner, H.L. and Hafler, D.A. (1996) Induction of circulating myelin basic protein and proteolipid protein-specific transforming growth factor-β1-secreting Th3 T-cells by oral administration of myelin in multiple sclerosis patients. *Journal of Clinical Investigation* 98, 70–77.

Fuss, I.J., Neurath, M., Boirivant, M., Klein, J.S., de la Motte, C., Strong, S.A., Fiocchi, C. and Strober, W. (1996) Disparate CD4+ lamina propria (LP) lymphokine secretion profiles in inflammatory bowel disease: Crohn's disease LP cells manifest increased secretion of IFN-γ, whereas ulcerative colitis LP cells manifest increased secretion of IL-5. *Journal of Immunology* 157, 1261–1270.

Gebbers, J.-O. and Laissue, J.A. (1990) Postnatal immunomorphology of the gut. In: Hadziselimovic, F., Herzog, B. and Bürgin-Wolff, A. (eds) *Inflammatory Bowel Disease and Celiac Disease in Children*. Kluwer Academic Publishers, Dordrecht, pp. 3–44.

Geissmann, F., Launay, P., Pasquier, B., Lepelletier, Y., Leborgne, M., Lehuen, A., Brousse, N. and Monteiro, R.C. (2001) A subset of human dendritic cells expresses

IgA Fc receptor (CD89), which mediates internalization and activation upon cross-linking by IgA complexes. *Journal of Immunology* 166, 346–352.

Giugliano, L.G., Ribeiro, S.T., Vainstein, M.H. and Ulhoa, C.J. (1995) Free secretory component and lactoferrin of human milk inhibit the adhesion of enterotoxigenic *Escherichia coli. Journal of Medical Microbiology* 42, 3–9.

Gleeson, M., Cripps, A.W., Clancy, R.L., Hensley, M.J., Dobson, A.J. and Firman, D.W. (1986) Breast feeding conditions a differential developmental pattern of mucosal immunity. *Clinical and Experimental Immunology* 66, 216–222.

Golding, J., Emmett, P.M. and Rogers, I.S. (1997) Does breast feeding protect against non-gastric infections? *Early Human Development* 49(Suppl.), S105–S120.

Goldman, A.S. (1993) The immune system of human milk: antimicrobial, antiinflamma-tory and immunomodulating properties. *Pediatric Infectious Disease Journal* 12, 664–671.

Grdic, D., Hörnquist, E., Kjerrulf, M. and Lycke, N.Y. (1998) Lack of local suppression in orally tolerant CD8-deficient mice reveals a critical regulatory role of CD8$^+$ T-cells in the normal gut mucosa. *Journal of Immunology* 160, 754–762.

Groh, V., Steinle, A., Bauer, S. and Spies, T. (1998) Recognition of stress-induced MHC molecules by intestinal epithelial γδ T-cells. *Science* 279, 1737–1740.

Groux, H., O'Garra, A., Bigler, M., Rouleau, M., Antonenko, S., de Vries, J.E. and Roncarolo, M.G. (1997) A CD4$^+$ T-cell subset inhibits antigen-specific T-cell responses and prevents colitis. *Nature* 389, 737–742.

Gütgemann, I., Fahrer, A.M., Altman, J.D., Davis, M.M. and Chien, Y.H. (1998) Induction of rapid T-cell activation and tolerance by systemic presentation of an orally administered antigen. *Immunity* 8, 667–673.

Guy-Grand, D., Griscelli, C. and Vassalli, P. (1978) The mouse gut T lymphocyte, a novel type of T-cell: nature, origin, and traffic in mice in normal and graft-versus-host conditions. *Journal of Experimental Medicine* 148, 1661–1677.

Hahn-Zoric, M., Fulconis, F., Minoli, I., Moro, G., Carlsson, B., Bottiger, M., Raiha, N. and Hanson, L.A. (1990) Antibody responses to parenteral and oral vaccines are impaired by conventional and low protein formulas as compared to breast-feeding. *Acta Paediatrica Scandinavica* 79, 1137–1142.

Håkansson, A., Zhivotovsky, B., Orrenius, S., Sabharwal, H. and Svanborg, C. (1995) Apoptosis induced by a human milk protein. *Proceedings of the National Academy of Sciences of the USA* 92, 8064–8068.

Hammerschmidt, S., Talay, S.R., Brandtzaeg, P. and Chhatwal, G.S. (1997) SpsA, a novel pneumococcal surface protein with specific binding to secretory immunoglobulin A and secretory component. *Molecular Microbiology* 25, 1113–1124.

Hanson, L.Å., Ashraf, R., Carlsson, B., Jalil, F., Karlberg, J., Lindblad, B.S., Khan, S.R. and Zaman, S. (1993) Child health and the population increase. In: Hanson L.Å. and Köhler, L. (eds) *Peace, Health and Development.* NHV Report 4, University of Göteborg and the Nordic School of Public Health, Gotab, Stockholm, pp.31–38.

Hathaway, L.J. and Kraehenbuhl, J.P. (2000) The role of M cells in mucosal immunity. *Cellular and Molecular Life Sciences* 57, 323–332.

Hattevig, G., Kjellman, B. and Björkstén, B. (1993) Appearance of IgE antibodies to ingested and inhaled allergens during the first 12 years of life in atopic and non-atopic children. *Pediatric Allergy and Immunology* 4, 182–186.

Hauer, A.C., Breese, E.J., Walker-Smith, J.A. and MacDonald, T.T. (1997) The fre-quency of cells secreting interferon-γ and interleukin-4, -5, and -10 in the blood and duodenal mucosa of children with cow's milk hypersensitivity. *Pediatric Research* 42, 629–638.

Helgeland, L. and Brandtzaeg, P. (2000) Development and function of intestinal B and T-cells. *Microbiology and Ecology in Health and Disease* 12(Suppl. 2), 110–127.

Hershberg, R.M. and Mayer, L.F. (2000) Antigen processing and presentation by intestinal epithelial cells – polarity and complexity. *Immunology Today* 21, 123–128.

Herz, U., Lacy, P., Renz, H. and Erb, K. (2000) The influence of infections on the development and severity of allergic disorders. *Current Opinion in Immunology* 12, 632–640.

Hessle, C., Hanson, L.A. and Wold, A.E. (1999) Lactobacilli from human gastrointestinal mucosa are strong stimulators of IL-12 production. *Clinical and Experimental Immunology* 116, 276–282.

Hessle, C., Andersson, B. and Wold, A.E. (2000a) Gram-positive bacteria are potent inducers of monocytic interleukin-12 (IL-12) while Gram-negative bacteria preferentially stimulate IL-10 production. *Infection and Immunity* 68, 3581–3586.

Hessle, C., Hanson, L.A. and Wold, A.E. (2000b) Interleukin-10 produced by the innate immune system masks *in vitro* evidence of acquired T-cell immunity to *E. coli*. *Scandinavian Journal of Immunology* 52, 13–20.

Hocini, H. and Bomsel, M. (1999) Infectious human immunodeficiency virus can rapidly penetrate a tight human epithelial barrier by transcytosis in a process impaired by mucosal immunoglobulins. *Journal of Infectious Disease* 179, S448–S453.

Holt, P.G. (1995) Postnatal maturation of immune competence during infancy and childhood. *Pediatric Allergy and Immunology* 6, 59–70.

Holt, P.G. (2000) Parasites, atopy, and the hygiene hypothesis: resolution of a paradox? *Lancet* 356, 1699–1701.

Holt, P.G. and Jones, C.A. (2000) The development of the immune system during pregnancy and early life. *Allergy* 55, 688–697.

Holt, P.G. and Stumbles, P.A. (2000) Regulation of immunologic homeostasis in peripheral tissues by dendritic cells: the respiratory tract as a paradigm. *Journal of Allergy and Clinical Immunology* 105, 421–429.

Holt, P.G., Clough, J.B., Holt, B.J., Baron-Hay, M.J., Rose, A.H., Robinson, B.W. and Thomas, W.R. (1992) Genetic 'risk' for atopy is associated with delayed postnatal maturation of T-cell competence. *Clinical and Experimental Allergy* 22, 1093–1099.

Holt, P.G., Macaubas, C., Stumbles, P.A. and Sly, P.D. (1999) The role of allergy in the development of asthma. *Nature* 402 (Suppl.), B12–B17.

Hooper, L.V., Wong, M.H., Thelin, A., Hansson, L., Falk, P.G. and Gordon, J.I. (2001) Molecular analysis of commensal host–microbial relationships in the intestine. *Science* 291, 881–884.

Hooton, J.W., Pabst, H.F., Spady, D.W. and Paetkau, V. (1991) Human colostrum contains an activity that inhibits the production of IL-2. *Clinical and Experimental Immunology* 86, 520–524.

Hopkin, J.M., Shaldon, S., Ferry, B., Coull, P., Antrobus, P., Enomoto, T., Yamashita, T., Kurimoto, F., Stanford, J., Shirakawa, T. and Rook, G. (1998) Mycobacterial immunisation in grass pollen asthma and rhinitis. *Thorax* 53(Suppl. 4), S63.

Hoppu, U., Kalliomäki, M., Laiho, K. and Isolauri, E. (2001) Breast milk – immunomodulatory signals against allergic diseases. *Allergy* 56(Suppl. 67), 23–26.

Hoque, S.S., Ghosh, S. and Poxton, I.R. (2000) Differences in intestinal humoral immunity between healthy volunteers from UK and Bangladesh. *European Journal of Gastroenterology and Hepatology* 12, 1185–1193.

Horsfall, D.J., Cooper, J.M. and Rowley, D. (1978) Changes in the immunoglobulin levels of the mouse gut and serum during conventionalisation and following administration of *Salmonella typhimurium*. *Australian Journal of Experimental Biology and Medical Science* 56, 727–735.

Høst, A., Husby, S., Hansen, L.G. and Osterballe, O. (1990) Bovine β-lactoglobulin in human milk from atopic and non-atopic mothers: relationship to maternal intake of homogenized and unhomogenized milk. *Clinical and Experimental Allergy* 20, 383–387.

Hoyne, G.F., Callow, M.G., Kuo, M.-C. and Thomas, W.R. (1993) Presentation of peptides and proteins by intestinal epithelial cells. *Immunology* 80, 204–208.

Huang, F.P., Platt, N., Wykes, M., Major, J.R., Powell, T.J., Jenkins, C.D. and MacPherson, G.G. (2000) A discrete subpopulation of dendritic cells transports apoptotic intestinal epithelial cells to T-cell areas of mesenteric lymph nodes. *Journal of Experimental Medicine* 191, 435–444.

Hughes, A., Brock, J.H., Parrott, D.M. and Cockburn, F. (1988) The interaction of infant formula with macrophages: effect on phagocytic activity, relationship to expression of class II MHC antigen and survival of orally administered macrophages in the neonatal gut. *Immunology* 64, 213–218.

Husband, A.J. and Gleeson, M. (1990) Developmental aspects of gut-associated immunity: a comparative review. In: MacDonald, T.T. (ed.) *Ontogeny of the Immune System of the Gut.* CRC Press, Boca Raton, pp. 83–116.

Husby, S., Jensenius, J.C. and Svehag, S.-E. (1985) Passage of undegraded dietary antigen into the blood of healthy adults: quantification, estimation of size distribution, and relation of uptake to levels of specific antibodies. *Scandinavian Journal of Immunology* 22, 83–92.

Husby, S., Mestecky, J., Moldoveanu, Z., Holland, S. and Elson, C.O. (1994) Oral tolerance in humans. T-cell but not B-cell tolerance after antigen feeding. *Journal of Immunology* 152, 4663–4670.

Hylander, M.A., Strobino, D.M. and Dhanireddy, R. (1998) Human milk feedings and infection among very low birth weight infants. *Pediatrics* 102, E38 (pp. 6, electronic paper).

Ishizaka, S., Kimoto, M., Tsujii, T. and Saito, S. (1994) Antibody production system modulated by oral administration of human milk and TGF-β. *Cellular Immunology* 159, 77–84.

Isolauri, E., Joensuu, J., Suomalainen, H., Luomala, M. and Vesikari, T. (1995) Improved immunogenicity of oral D × RRV reassortant rotavirus vaccine by *Lactobacillus casei* GG. *Vaccine* 13, 310–312.

Isolauri, E., Grönlund, M.M., Salminen, S. and Arvilommi, H. (2000) Why don't we bud? *Journal of Pediatric Gastroenterology and Nutrition* 30, 214–216.

Isolauri, E., Sutas, Y., Kankaanpaa, P., Arvilommi, H. and Salminen, S. (2001) Probiotics: effects on immunity. *American Journal of Clinical Nutrition* 73, 444S–450S.

Israel, E.J., Simister, N., Freiberg, E., Caplan, A. and Walker, W.A. (1993) Immunoglobulin G binding sites on the human fetal intestine: a possible mechanism for the passive transfer of immunity from mother to infant. *Immunology* 79, 77–81.

Jahnsen, F.L., Lund-Johansen, F., Dunne, J.F., Farkas, L., Haye, R. and Brandtzaeg, P. (2000) Experimentally induced recruitment of plasmacytoid (CD123[high]) dendritic cells in human nasal allergy. *Journal of Immunology* 165, 4062–4068.

Jain, L., Vidyasagar, D., Xanthou, M., Ghai, V., Shimada, S. and Blend, M. (1989) *In vivo* distribution of human milk leucocytes after ingestion by newborn baboons. *Archives of Diseases of Childhood* 64, 930–933.

Janeway, C.J. and Bottomly, K. (1994) Signals and signs for lymphocyte responses. *Cell* 76, 275–285.

Janu, P., Li, J., Renegar, K.B. and Kudsk, K.A. (1997) Recovery of gut-associated lymphoid tissue and upper respiratory tract immunity after parenteral nutrition. *Annals of Surgery* 225, 707–715.

Järvinen, K.M., Laine, S.T., Jarvenpaa, A.L. and Suomalainen, H.K. (2000) Does low IgA in human milk predispose the infant to development of cow's milk allergy? *Pediatric Research* 48, 457–462.

Johansen, F.-E., Pekna, M., Norderhaug, I.N., Haneberg, B., Hietala, M.A., Krajci, P., Betsholtz, C. and Brandtzaeg, P. (1999) Absence of epithelial immunoglobulin A transport, with increased mucosal leakiness, in polymeric immunoglobulin receptor/secretory component-deficient mice. *Journal of Experimental Medicine* 190, 915–922.

Johansen, F.-E., Braathen, R. and Brandtzaeg, P. (2000) Role of J chain in secretory immunoglobulin formation. *Scandinavian Journal of Immunology* 52, 240–248.

Johansen, S., Christensen, H.R., Barkholt, V. and Frøkiær, H. (2001) Abolishment of maternally induced oral tolerance to β-lactoglobulin in adult mice by feeding a milk-free diet from weaning. In: *8th International Symposium on Immunological, Chemical and Clinical Problems of Food Allergy*. Venice, p. 23.

Juto, P. and Holm, S. (1992) Gliadin-specific and cow's milk protein-specific IgA in human milk. *Journal of Pediatric Gastroenterology and Nutrition* 15, 159–162.

Kadowaki, N., Antonenko, S. and Liu, Y.J. (2001) Distinct CpG DNA and polyinosinic-polycytidylic acid double-stranded RNA, respectively, stimulate CD11c⁻ type 2 dendritic cell precursors and CD11c⁺ dendritic cells to produce type I IFN. *Journal of Immunology* 166, 2291–2295.

Kaila, M., Isolauri, E., Soppi, E., Virtanen, E., Laine, S. and Arvilommi, H. (1992) Enhancement of the circulating antibody secreting cell response in human diarrhea by a human *Lactobacillus* strain. *Pediatric Research* 32, 141–144.

Kaila, M., Isolauri, E., Saxelin, M., Arvilommi, H. and Vesikari, T. (1995) Viable versus inactivated lactobacillus strain GG in acute rotavirus diarrhoea. *Archives of Diseases of Childhood* 72, 51–53.

Kaisho, T. and Akira, S. (2001) Dendritic-cell function in Toll-like receptor- and MyD88-knockout mice. *Trends in Immunology* 22, 78–83.

Kalliomäki, M., Ouwehand, A., Arvilommi, H., Kero, P. and Isolauri, E. (1999) Transforming growth factor-β in breast milk: a potential regulator of atopic disease at an early age. *Journal of Allergy and Clinical Immunology* 104, 1251–1257.

Kalliomäki, M., Salminen, S., Arvilommi, H., Kero, P., Koskinen, P. and Isolauri, E. (2001a) Probiotics in primary prevention of atopic disease: a randomised placebo-controlled trial. *Lancet* 357, 1076–1079.

Kalliomäki, M., Kirjavainen, P., Eerola, E., Kero, P., Salminen, S. and Isolauri, E. (2001b) Distinct patterns of neonatal gut microflora in infants in whom atopy was and was not developing. *Journal of Allergy and Clinical Immunology* 107, 129–134.

Karjalainen, J., Martin, J.M., Knip, M., Ilonen, J., Robinson, B.H., Savilahti, E., Akerblom, H.K. and Dosch, H.M. (1992) A bovine albumin peptide as a possible trigger of insulin-dependent diabetes mellitus. *New England Journal of Medicine* 327, 302–307.

Karlsson, M.R., Kahu, H., Hanson, L.Å., Telemo, E. and Dahlgren, U.I. (1999) Neonatal colonization of rats induces immunological tolerance to bacterial antigens. *European Journal of Immunology* 29, 109–118.

Karlsson, M.R., Lundin, S., Dahlgren, U.I., Kahu, H., Petterson, I. and Telemo, E. (2001) 'Tolerosomes' are produced by intestinal epithelial cells. *European Journal of Immunology* 31, 2892–2900.

Khoo, U.Y., Proctor, I.E. and Macpherson, A.J. (1997) CD4$^+$ T-cell down-regulation in human intestinal mucosa: evidence for intestinal tolerance to luminal bacterial antigens. *Journal of Immunology* 158, 3626–3634.

Kilian, M., Husby, S., Høst, A. and Halken, S. (1995) Increased proportions of bacteria capable of cleaving IgA1 in the pharynx of infants with atopic disease. *Pediatric Research* 38, 182–186.

Kilshaw, P.J. and Cant, A.J. (1984) The passage of maternal dietary proteins into human breast milk. *International Archives of Allergy and Applied Immunology* 75, 8–15.

Kimpimäki, T., Erkkola, M., Korhonen, S., Kupila, A., Virtanen, S.M., Ilonen, J., Simell, O. and Knip, M. (2001) Short-term exclusive breastfeeding predisposes young children with increased genetic risk of Type I diabetes to progressive beta-cell autoimmunity. *Diabetologia* 44, 63–69.

Kirjavainen, P.V. and Gibson, G.R. (1999) Healthy gut microflora and allergy: factors influencing development of the microbiota. *Annals of Medicine* 31, 288–292.

Klemola, T., Savilahti, E. and Leinikki, P. (1986) Mumps IgA antibodies are not absorbed from human milk. *Acta Pediatrica Scandinavica* 75, 230–232.

Klinman, D.M., Yi, A.K., Beaucage, S.L., Conover, J. and Krieg, A.M. (1996) CpG motifs present in bacteria DNA rapidly induce lymphocytes to secrete interleukin 6, interleukin 12, and interferon γ. *Proceedings of the National Academy of Sciences of the USA* 93, 2879–2883.

Knolle, P.A., Schmitt, E., Jin, S., Germann, T., Duchmann, R., Hegenbarth, S., Gerken, G. and Lohse, A.W. (1999) Induction of cytokine production in naive CD4$^+$ T-cells by antigen-presenting murine liver sinusoidal endothelial cells but failure to induce differentiation toward Th1 cells. *Gastroenterology* 116, 1428–1440.

Knox, W.F. (1986) Restricted feeding and human intestinal plasma cell development. *Archives of Diseases of Childhood* 61, 744–749.

Korenblat, P.E., Rothberg, R.M., Minden, P. and Farr, R.S. (1968) Immune responses of human adults after oral and parenteral exposure to bovine serum albumin. *Journal of Allergy* 41, 226–235.

Kuchroo, V.K., Das, M.P., Brown, J.A., Ranger, A.M., Zamvil, S.S., Sobel, R.A., Weiner, H.L., Nabavi, N. and Glimcher, L.H. (1995) B7–1 and B7–2 costimulatory molecules activate differentially the Th1/Th2 developmental pathways: application to autoimmune disease therapy. *Cell* 80, 707–718.

Kull, I., Nordvall, S.L., Pershagen, G., Tollin, L. and Wickman, M. (2001) Breast-feeding reduces the risk of developing allergic diseases in young children: report from the ongoing Swedish prospective birth cohort study (BAMSE). *Allergy* 56(Suppl. 68), 39.

Lamkhioued, B., Gounni, A.S., Gruart, V., Pierce, A., Capron, A. and Capron, M. (1995) Human eosinophils express a receptor for secretory component: role in secretory IgA-dependent activation. *European Journal of Immunology* 25, 117–125.

Lanzavecchia, A. and Sallusto, F. (2001) The instructive role of dendritic cells on T-cell responses: lineages, plasticity and kinetics. *Current Opinion in Immunology* 13, 291–298.

Levitz, S.M., Mathews, H.L. and Murphy, J.W. (1995) Direct antimicrobial activity of T-cells. *Immunology Today* 16, 387–391.

Lewis, D.B., Yu, C.C., Meyer, J., English, B.K., Kahn, S.J. and Wilson, C.B. (1991) Cellular and molecular mechanisms for reduced interleukin 4 and interferon-γ production by neonatal T-cells. *Journal of Clinical Investigation* 87, 194–202.

Li, J., Kudsk, K.A., Gocinski, B., Dent, D., Glezer, J. and Langkamp-Henken, B.

(1995a) Effects of parenteral and enteral nutrition on gut-associated lymphoid tissue. *Journal of Trauma* 39, 44–51.

Li, J., Kudsk, K.A., Hamidian, M. and Gocinski, B.L. (1995b) Bombesin affects mucosal immunity and gut-associated lymphoid tissue in intravenously fed mice. *Archives of Surgery* 130, 1164–1169.

Li, Y., Yio, X.Y. and Mayer, L. (1995) Human intestinal epithelial cell-induced CD8[+] T-cell activation is mediated through CD8 and the activation of CD8-associated p56[1ck]. *Journal of Experimental Medicine* 182, 1079–1088.

Lim, P.L. and Rowley, D. (1982) The effect of antibody on the intestinal absorption of macromolecules and on intestinal permeability in adult mice. *International Archives of Allergy and Applied Immunology* 68, 41–46.

Limmer, A., Ohl, J., Kurts, C., Ljunggren, H.G., Reiss, Y., Groettrup, M., Momburg, F., Arnold, B. and Knolle, P.A. (2000) Efficient presentation of exogenous antigen by liver endothelial cells to CD8[+] T-cells results in antigen-specific T-cell tolerance. *Nature Medicine* 6, 1348–1354.

Liu, L., Kuchroo, V.K. and Weiner, H.L. (1999) B7.2 (CD86) but not B7.1 (CD80) co-stimulation is required for the induction of low dose oral tolerance. *Journal of Immunology* 163, 2284–2290.

Lodinová, R., Jouja, V. and Wagner, V. (1973) Serum immunoglobulins and coproanti-body formation in infants after artificial intestinal colonization with *Escherichia coli* 083 and oral lysozyme administration. *Pediatric Reseach* 7, 659–669.

Lodinová-Zádniková, R. and Cukrowská, B. (1999) Influence of oral colonization of the intestine with a non-enteropathogenic *E. coli* strain after birth on the frequency of infectious and allergic diseases after 10 and 20 years. *Immunology Letters* 69, 64.

Lu, C.Y., Calamai, E.G. and Unanue, E.R. (1979) A defect in the antigen-presenting function of macrophages from neonatal mice. *Nature* 282, 327–329.

MacDonald, T.T. and Spencer, J. (1993) Development of gastrointestinal immune function and its relationship to intestinal disease. *Current Opinion in Gastroenterology* 9, 946–952.

MacDonald, T.T. and Monteleone, G. (2001) IL-12 and Th1 immune responses in human Peyer's patches. *Trends in Immunology* 22, 244–247.

MacDonald, T.T. and Pettersson, S. (2000) Bacterial regulation of intestinal immune responses. *Inflammatory Bowel Disease* 6, 116–122.

Machado, C.S.M., Rodrigues, M.A.M. and Maffei, H.V.L. (1994) Gut intraepithelial lymphocyte counts in neonates, infants and children. *Acta Paediatrica* 83, 1264–1267.

McInnes, I.B., Gracie, J.A., Leung, B.P., Wei, X.Q. and Liew, F.Y. (2000) Interleukin 18: a pleiotropic participant in chronic inflammation. *Immunology Today* 21, 312–315.

Mackenzie, N.M. (1990) Transport of maternally derived immunoglobulin across the intestinal epithelium. In: MacDonald, T.T. (ed.) *Ontogeny of the Immune System of the Gut*. CRC Press, Boca Raton, Florida, pp. 69–81.

MacPherson, G.G., Jenkins, C.D., Stein, M.J. and Edwards, C. (1995) Endotoxin-mediated dendritic cell release from the intestine: characterization of released dendritic cells and TNF dependence. *Journal of Immunology* 154, 1317–1322.

Malin, M., Suomalainen, H., Saxelin, M. and Isolauri, E. (1996) Promotion of IgA immune response in patients with Crohn's disease by oral bacteriotherapy with *Lactobacillus* GG. *Annals of Nutrition and Metabolism* 40, 137–145.

Manigold, T., Bocker, U., Traber, P., Dong-Si, T., Kurimoto, M., Hanck, C., Singer, M.V. and Rossol, S. (2000) Lipopolysaccharide/endotoxin induces IL-18 via CD14 in human peripheral blood mononuclear cells *in vitro*. *Cytokine* 12, 1788–1792.

Marchant, A., Goetghebuer, T., Ota, M.O., Wolfe, I., Ceesay, S.J., De Groote, D., Corrah, T., Bennett, S., Wheeler, J., Huygen, K., Aaby, P., McAdam, K.P. and

Newport, M.J. (1999) Newborns develop a Th1-type immune response to *Mycobacterium bovis* bacillus Calmette-Guerin vaccination. *Journal of Immunology* 163, 2249–2255.

Matricardi, P.M., Rosmini, F., Riondino, S., Fortini, M., Ferrigno, L., Rapicetta, M. and Bonini, S. (2000) Exposure to foodborne and orofecal microbes versus airborne viruses in relation to atopy and allergic asthma: epidemiological study. *British Medical Journal* 320, 412–417.

Mayer, L., Sperber, K., Chan, L., Child, J. and Toy, L. (2001) Oral tolerance to protein antigens. *Allergy* 56(Suppl. 67), 12–15.

Mazanec, M.B., Nedrud, J.G., Kaetzel, C.S. and Lamm, M.E. (1993) A three-tiered view of the role of IgA in mucosal defence. *Immunology Today* 14, 430–435.

Mazzoli, S., Trabattoni, D., Lo Caputo, S., Piconi, S., Ble, C., Meacci, F., Ruzzante, S., Salvi, A., Semplici, F., Longhi, R., Fusi, M.L., Tofani, N., Biasin, M., Villa, M.L., Mazzotta, F. and Clerici, M. (1997) HIV-specific mucosal and cellular immunity in HIV-seronegative partners of HIV-seropositive individuals. *Nature Medicine* 3, 1250–1257.

Medzhitov, R. and Janeway, C.A. (1997) Innate immunity: impact on the adaptive immune response. *Currrent Opinion in Immunology* 9, 4–9.

Miettinen, M., Matikainen, S., Vuopio-Varkila, J., Pirhonen, J., Varkila, K., Kurimoto, M. and Julkunen, I. (1998) Lactobacilli and streptococci induce interleukin-12 (IL-12), IL-18, and gamma interferon production in human peripheral blood mononuclear cells. *Infection and Immunity* 66, 6058–6062.

Mincheva-Nilsson, L., Hammarström, M.L., Juto, P. and Hammarström, S. (1990) Human milk contains proteins that stimulate and suppress T lymphocyte proliferation. *Clinical and Experimental Immunology* 79, 463–469.

Modlin, R.L. (2000) Immunology: a toll for DNA vaccines. *Nature* 408, 659–660.

Moreau, M.C., Ducluzeau, R., Guy-Grand, D. and Muller, M.C. (1978) Increase in the population of duodenal immunoglobulin A plasmocytes in axenic mice associated with different living or dead bacterial strains of intestinal origin. *Infection and Immunity* 121, 532–539.

Morris, J.F., Hoyer, J.T. and Pierce, S.K. (1992) Antigen presentation for T-cell interleukin-2 secretion is a late acquisition of neonatal B-cells. *European Journal of Immunology* 22, 2923–2928.

Motegi, Y. and Kita, H. (1998) Interaction with secretory component stimulates effector functions of human eosinophils but not of neutrophils. *Journal of Immunology* 161, 4340–4346.

Nagao, A.T., Pilagallo, M.I.D.S. and Pereira, A.B. (1993) Quantitation of salivary, urinary and faecal SIgA in children living in different conditions of antigenic exposure. *Journal of Tropical Pediatrics* 39, 278–283.

Nagata, S., McKenzie, C., Pender, S.L., Bajaj-Elliott, M., Fairclough, P.D., Walker-Smith, J.A., Monteleone, G. and MacDonald, T.T. (2000) Human Peyer's patch T-cells are sensitized to dietary antigen and display a Th cell type 1 cytokine profile. *Journal of Immunology* 165, 5315–5321.

Nagler-Anderson, C. (2000) Tolerance and immunity in the intestinal immune system. *Critical Reviews in Immunology* 20, 103–120.

Nahmias, A., Stoll, B., Hale, E., Ibegbu, C., Keyserling, H., Innis-Whitehouse, W., Holmes, R., Spira, T., Czerkinsky, C. and Lee, F. (1991) IgA-secreting cells in the blood of premature and term infants: normal development and effect of intrauterine infections. *Advances in Experimental Medical Biology* 310, 59–69.

Neish, A.S., Gewirtz, A.T., Zeng, H., Young, A.N., Hobert, M.E., Karmali, V., Rao, A.S. and Madara, J.L. (2000) Prokaryotic regulation of epithelial responses by inhibition of IκB-α ubiquitination. *Science* 289, 1560–1563.

Newberry, R.D., Stenson, W.F. and Lorenz, R.G. (1999) Cyclooxygenase-2-dependent arachidonic acid metabolites are essential modulators of the intestinal immune response to dietary antigen. *Nature Medicine* 5, 900–906.

Newman, J. (1995) How breast milk protects newborns. *Scientific American* 273, 58–61.

Nicklin, S. and Miller, K. (1983) Local and systemic immune responses to intestinally presented antigen. *International Archives of Allergy and Applied Immunology* 72, 87–90.

Nickoloff, B.J. and Turka, L.A. (1994) Immunological functions of non-professional antigen-presenting cells: new insights from studies of T-cell interactions with keratinocytes. *Immunology Today* 15, 464–469.

Nilsen, E.M., Jahnsen, F.L., Lundin, K.E., Johansen, F.E., Fausa, O., Sollid, L.M., Jahnsen, J., Scott, H. and Brandtzaeg, P. (1998) Gluten induces an intestinal cytokine response strongly dominated by interferon gamma in patients with celiac disease. *Gastroenterology* 115, 551–563.

Norderhaug, I.N., Johansen, F.-E., Schjerven, H. and Brandtzaeg, P. (1999) Regulation of the formation and external transport of secretory immunoglobulins. *Critical Reviews in Immunology* 19, 481–508.

Oddy, W.H., Holt, P.G., Sly, P.D., Read, A.W., Landau, L.I., Stanley, F.J., Kendall, G.E. and Burton, P.R. (1999) Association between breast feeding and asthma in 6 year old children: findings of a prospective birth cohort study. *British Medical Journal* 319, 815–819.

Ogra, S.S., Weintraub, D. and Ogra, P.L. (1977) Immunological aspects of human colostrum and milk. III. Fate and absorption of cellular and soluble components in the gastrointestinal tract of the newborn. *Journal of Immunology* 119, 245–248.

O'Leary, A.D. and Sweeney, E.C. (1986) Lymphoglandular complexes of the colon: structure and distribution. *Histopathology* 10, 267–283.

Orlic, D. and Lev, R. (1977) An electron microscopic study of intraepithelial lymphocytes in human fetal small intestine. *Laboratory Investigations* 37, 554–561.

Pabst, H.F. and Spady, D.W. (1990) Effect of breast-feeding on antibody response to conjugate vaccine. *Lancet* 336, 269–270.

Pabst, R. and Gehrke, I. (1990) Is the bronchus-associated lymphoid tissue (BALT) an integral structure of the lung in normal mammals, including humans? *American Journal of Respiratory and Cellular Molecular Biology* 3, 131–135.

Paganelli, R. and Levinsky, R.J. (1980) Solid phase radioimmunoassay for detection of circulating food protein antigens in human serum. *Journal of Immunological Methods* 37, 333–341.

Parrott, D.M.V. (1976) The gut-associated lymphoid tissue and gastrointestinal immunity. In: Ferguson, A. and MacSween, N.R.M. (eds) *Immunological Aspects of the Liver and Gastrointestinal Tract*. MTP Press, Lancaster, pp. 1–32.

Peng, Z., Wang, H., Mao, X., HayGlass, K.T. and Simons, F.E. (2001) CpG oligodeoxynucleotide vaccination suppresses IgE induction but may fail to down-regulate ongoing IgE responses in mice. *International Immunology* 13, 3–11.

Perkkiö, M. (1980) Immunohistochemical study of intestinal biopsies from children with atopic eczema due to food allergy. *Allergy* 35, 573–580.

Pisacane, A., Graziano, L., Zona, G., Granata, G., Dolezalova, H., Cafiero, M., Coppola, A., Scarpellino, B., Ummarino, M. and Mazzarella, G. (1994) Breast feeding and acute lower respiratory infection. *Acta Paediatrica* 83, 714–718.

Planchon, S.M., Martins, C.A., Guerrant, R.L. and Roche, J.K. (1994) Regulation of intestinal epithelial barrier function by TGF-β1: evidence for its role in abrogating the effect of a T-cell cytokine. *Journal of Immunology* 153, 5730–5739.

Prescott, S.L., Macaubas, C., Holt, B.J., Smallacombe, T.B., Loh, R., Sly, P.D. and Holt, P.G. (1998) Transplacental priming of the human immune system to environmental allergens: universal skewing of initial T-cell responses toward the Th2 cytokine profile. *Journal of Immunology* 160, 4730–4737.

Prokesová, L., Ladmanová, P., Cechova, D., Stepánková, R., Kozáková, H., Mlcková, Á., Kuklik, R. and Mára, M. (1999) Stimulatory effects of *Bacillus firmus* on IgA production in human and mice. *Immunology Letters* 69, 55–56.

Qiao, L., Braunstein, J., Golling, M., Schurmann, G., Autschbach, F., Moller, P. and Meuer, S. (1996) Differential regulation of human T-cell responsiveness by mucosal versus blood monocytes. *European Journal of Immunology* 26, 922–927.

Quan, C.P., Berneman, A., Pires, R., Arameas, S. and Bouvet, J.P. (1997) Natural polyreactive secretory immunoglobin A autoantibodies as a possible barrier to infection in humans. *Infection and Immunity* 65, 3997–4004.

Read, S., Malmström, V. and Powrie, F. (2000) Cytotoxic T lymphocyte-associated antigen 4 plays an essential role in the function of $CD25^+CD4^+$ regulatory cells that control intestinal inflammation. *Journal of Experimental Medicine* 192, 295–302.

Renegar, K.B., Johnson, C.D., Dewitt, R.C., King, B.K., Li, J., Fukatsu, K. and Kudsk, K.A. (2001) Impairment of mucosal immunity by total parenteral nutrition: requirement for IgA in murine nasotracheal anti-influenza immunity. *Journal of Immunology* 166, 819–825.

Renz, H., Brehler, C., Petzoldt, S., Prinz, H. and Rieger, C.H. (1991) Breast feeding modifies production of SIgA cow's milk-antibodies in infants. *Acta Paediatrica Scandinavica* 80, 149–154.

Reynolds, J.D. and Morris, B. (1984) The effect of antigen on the development of Peyer's patches in sheep. *European Journal of Immunology* 14, 1–6.

Ridge, J.P., Fuchs, E.J. and Matzinger, P. (1996) Neonatal tolerance revisited: turning on newborn T-cells with dendritic cells. *Science* 271, 1723–1726.

Rissoan, M.C., Soumelis, V., Kadowaki, N., Grouard, G., Briere, F., de Waal Malefyt, R. and Liu, Y.J. (1999) Reciprocal control of T helper cell and dendritic cell differentiation. *Science* 283, 1183–1186.

Roberton, D.M., Forrest, P.J., Frangoulis, E., Jones, C.L. and Mermelstein, N. (1986) Early induction of secretory immunity in infancy: specific antibody in neonatal breast milk. *Archives of Diseases of Childhood* 61, 489–494.

Robey, E. and Allison, J.P. (1995) T-cell activation: integration of signals from the antigen receptor and costimulatory molecules. *Immunology Today* 16, 306–310.

Robinson, J.K., Blanchard, T.G., Levine, A.D., Emancipator, S.N. and Lamm, M.E. (2001) A mucosal IgA-mediated excretory immune system *in vivo*. *Journal of Immunology* 166, 3688–3692.

Romagnani, S. (2000) The role of lymphocytes in allergic disease. *Journal of Allergy and Clinical Immunology* 105, 399–408

Rook, G.A. and Stanford, J.L. (1998) Give us this day our daily germs. *Immunology Today* 19, 113–116.

Rothberg, R.M. and Farr, R.S. (1965) Anti-bovine serum albumine and anti-alpha lactalbumin in the serum of children and adults. *Pediatrics* 35, 571–588.

Rugtveit, J., Bakka, A. and Brandtzaeg, P. (1997) Differential distribution of B7.1 (CD80) and B7.2 (CD86) costimulatory molecules on mucosalmacrophage subsets in human inflammatory bowel disease (IBD). *Clinical and Experimental Immunology* 110, 104–113.

Saarinen, U.M. and Kajosaari, M. (1995) Breastfeeding as prophylaxis against atopic disease: prospective follow-up study until 17 years old. *Lancet* 346, 1065–1069.

Sachdev, G.K., Dalton, H.R., Hoang, P., DiPaolo, M.C., Crotty, B. and Jewell, D.P. (1993) Human colonic intraepithelial lymphocytes suppress *in vitro* immunoglobulin synthesis by autologous peripheral blood lymphocytes and lamina propria lymphocytes. *Gut* 34, 257–263.

Sagie, E., Tarabulus, J., Maeir, D.M. and Freier, S. (1974) Diet and development of intestinal IgA in the mouse. *Israeli Journal of Medical Science* 10, 532–534.

Saito, S., Maruyama, M., Kato, Y., Moriyama, I. and Ichijo, M. (1991) Detection of IL-6 in human milk and its involvement in IgA production. *Journal of Reproductive Immunology* 20, 267–276.

Sanderson, I.R. and Walker, W.A. (1993) Uptake and transport of macromolecules by the intestine: possible role in clinical disorders (an update). *Gastroenterology* 104, 622–639.

Savilahti, E., Tainio, V.-M., Salmenpera, L., Arjomaa, P., Kallio, M., Perheentupa, J. and Siimes, M.A. (1991) Low colostral IgA associated with cow's milk allergy. *Acta Paediatrica Scandinavica* 80, 1207–1213.

Scott, H., Fausa, O. and Thorsby, E. (1983) T-lymphocyte activation by a gluten fraction, glyc-gli: studies of adult celiac patients and healthy controls. *Scandinavian Journal of Immunology* 18, 185–191.

Scott, H., Rognum, T.O., Midtvedt, T. and Brandtzaeg, P. (1985) Age-related changes of human serum antibodies to dietary and colonic bacterial antigens measured by an enzyme-linked immunosorbent assay. *Acta Pathologica, Microbiologica et Immunologica Scandinavica [C]* 93, 65–70.

Scott, H., Nilsen, E., Sollid, L.M., Lundin, K.E., Rugtveit, J., Molberg, O., Thorsby, E. and Brandtzaeg, P. (1997) Immunopathology of gluten-sensitive enteropathy. *Springer Seminars in Immunopathology* 18, 535–553.

Sepp, E., Julge, K., Vasar, M., Naaber, P., Björksten, B. and Mikelsaar, M. (1997) Intestinal microflora of Estonian and Swedish infants. *Acta Paediatrica* 86, 956–961.

Shroff, K.E., Meslin, K. and Cebra, J.J. (1995) Commensal enteric bacteria engender a self-limiting humoral mucosal immune response while permanently colonizing the gut. *Infection and Immunity* 63, 3904–3913.

Simister, N.E. and Mostov, K.E. (1989) An Fc receptor structurally related to MHC class I antigens. *Nature* 337, 184–187.

Slade, H.B. and Schwartz, S.A. (1987) Mucosal immunity: the immunology of breast milk. *Journal of Allergy and Clinical Immunology* 80, 348–358.

Sloper, K.S., Brook, C.G., Kingston, D., Pearson, J.R. and Shiner, M. (1981) Eczema and atopy in early childhood: low IgA plasma cell counts in the jejunal mucosa. *Archives of Diseases of Childhood* 56, 939–942.

Smith, P.D., Smythies, L.E., Mosteller-Barnum, M., Sibley, D.A., Russell, M.W., Merger, M., Sellers, M.T., Orenstein, J.M., Shimada, T., Graham, M.F. and Kubagawa, H. (2001) Intestinal macrophages lack CD14 and CD89 and consequently are downregulated for LPS- and IgA-mediated activities. *Journal of Immunology* 167, 2651–2656.

Soothill, J.F. (1976) Some intrinsic and extrinsic factors predisposing to allergy. *Proceedings of the Royal Society of Medicine* 69, 439–442.

Sørensen, C.H. and Kilian, M. (1984) Bacterium-induced cleavage of IgA in nasopharyngeal secretions from atopic children. *Acta Pathologica, Microbiologica et Immunologica Scandinavica [C]* 92, 85–87.

Spencer, J. and MacDonald, T.T. (1990) Ontogeny of human mucosal immunity. In: MacDonald, T.T (ed.) *Ontogeny of the Immune System of the Gut.* CRC Press, Boca Raton, Florida, pp. 23–50.

Spencer, J., MacDonald, T.T., Finn, T. and Isaacson, P.G. (1986a) The development of gut-associated lymphoid tissue in the terminal ileum of fetal human intestine. *Clinical and Experimental Immunology* 64, 536–543.

Spencer, J., Dillon, S.B., Isaacson, P.G. and MacDonald, T.T. (1986b) T-cell subclasses in fetal human ileum. *Clinical and Experimental Immunology* 65, 553–558.

Splawski, J.B. and Lipsky, P.E. (1991) Cytokine regulation of immunoglobulin secretion by neonatal lymphocytes. *Journal of Clinical Investigation* 88, 967–977.

Srivastava, M.D. and Srivastava, B.I. (1999) Soluble Fas and soluble Fas ligand proteins in human milk: possible significance in the development of immunological tolerance. *Scandinavian Journal of Immunology* 49, 51–54.

Steidler, L., Hans, W., Schotte, L., Neirynck, S., Obermeier, F., Falk, W., Fiers, W. and Remaut, E. (2000) Treatment of murine colitis by *Lactococcus lactis* secreting interleukin-10. *Science* 289, 1352–1355.

Stephens, S. (1986) Development of secretory immunity in breast fed and bottle fed infants. *Archives of Diseases of Childhood* 61, 263–269.

Stephensen, C.B., Moldoveanu, Z. and Gangopadhyay, N.N. (1996) Vitamin A deficiency diminishes the salivary immunoglobulin A response and enhances the serum immunoglobulin G response to influenza A virus infection in BALB/c mice. *Journal of Nutrition* 126, 94–102.

Stoll, B.J., Lee, F.K., Hale, E., Schwartz, D., Holmes, R., Ashby, R., Czerkinsky, C. and Nahmias, A.J. (1993) Immunoglobulin secretion by the normal and the infected newborn infant. *Journal of Pediatrics* 122, 780–786.

Strobel, S., Mowat, A.M., Drummond, H.E., Pickering, M.G. and Ferguson, A. (1983) Immunological responses to fed protein antigens in mice. II. Oral tolerance for CMI is due to activation of cyclophosphamide-sensitive cells by gut-processed antigen. *Immunology* 49, 451–456.

Tappuni, A.R. and Challacombe, S.J. (1994) A comparison of salivary immunoglobulin A (IgA) and IgA subclass concentrations in predentate and dentate children and adults. *Oral Microbiology and Immunology* 9, 142–145.

Taylor, B., Norman, A.P., Orgel, H.A., Stokes, C.R., Turner, M.W. and Soothill, J.F. (1973) Transient IgA deficiency and pathogenesis of infantile atopy. *Lancet* ii, 111–113.

Taylor, S. and Bryson, Y.J. (1985) Impaired production of γ-interferon by newborn cells *in vitro* is due to a functionally immature macrophage. *Journal of Immunology* 134, 1493–1497.

Thrane, P.S., Rognum, T.O. and Brandtzaeg, P. (1991) Ontogenesis of the secretory immune system and innate defence factors in human parotid glands. *Clinical and Experimental Immunology* 86, 342–348.

Tschernig, T., Kleemann, W.J. and Pabst, R. (1995) Bronchus-associated lymphoid tissue (BALT) in the lungs of children who had died from sudden infant death syndrome and other causes. *Thorax* 50, 658–660.

Vaarala, O., Knip, M., Paronen, J., Hamalainen, A.M., Muona, P., Vaatainen, M., Ilonen, J., Simell, O. and Akerblom, H.K. (1999) Cow's milk formula feeding induces primary immunization to insulin in infants at genetic risk for type 1 diabetes. *Diabetes* 48, 1389–1394.

van Asperen, P.P., Gleeson, M., Kemp, A.S., Cripps, A.W., Geraghty, S.B., Mellis, C.M. and Clancy, R.L. (1985) The relationship between atopy and salivary IgA deficiency in infancy. *Clinical and Experimental Immunology* 62, 753–757.

van Elburg, R.M., Uil, J.J., de Monchy, J.G. and Heymans, H.S. (1992) Intestinal permeability in pediatric gastroenterology. *Scandinavian Journal of Gastroenterology* 194(Suppl.), 19–24.

Viney, J.L., Mowat, A.M., O'Malley, J.M., Williamson, E. and Fanger, N.A. (1998) Expanding dendritic cells *in vivo* enhances the induction of oral tolerance. *Journal of Immunology* 160, 5815–5825.

von Reyn, C.F., Arbeit, R.D., Yeaman, G., Waddell, R.D., Marsh, B.J., Morin, P., Modlin, J.F. and Remold, H.G. (1997) Immunization of healthy adult subjects in the United States with inactivated *Mycobacterium vaccae* administered in a three-dose series. *Clinical Infectious Diseases* 24, 843–848.

Waldo, F.B., van den Wall Bake, A.W., Mestecky, J. and Husby, S. (1994) Suppression of the immune response by nasal immunization. *Clinical Immunology and Immunopathology* 72, 30–34.

Watson, R.R., McMurray, D.N., Martin, P. and Reyes, M.A. (1985) Effect of age, malnutrition and renutrition on free secretory component and IgA in secretion. *American Journal of Clinical Nutrition* 42, 281–288.

Weaver, L.T., Wadd, N., Taylor, C.E., Greenwell, J. and Toms, G.L. (1991) The ontogeny of serum IgA in the newborn. *Pediatric Allergy and Immunology* 2, 72–75.

Weiner, H.L., Friedman, A., Miller, A., Khoury, S.J., al-Sabbagh, A., Santos, L., Sayegh, M., Nussenblatt, R.B., Trentham, D.E. and Hafler, D.A. (1994) Oral tolerance: immunologic mechanisms and treatment of animal and human organ-specific autoimmune diseases by oral administration of autoantigens. *Annual Review of Immunology* 12, 809–837.

Wiedermann, U., Hanson, L.A., Holmgren, J., Kahu, H. and Dahlgren, U.I. (1993) Impaired mucosal antibody response to cholera toxin in vitamin A-deficient rats immunized with oral cholera vaccine [published erratum appears in *Infection and Immunity* 61, 5431]. *Infection and Immunity* 61, 3952–3957.

Wijesinha, S.S. and Steer, H.W. (1982) Studies of the immunoglobulin-producing cells of the human intestine: the defunctioned bowel. *Gut* 23, 211–214.

Williamson, E., Westrich, G.M. and Viney, J.L. (1999) Modulating dendritic cells to optimize mucosal immunization protocols. *Journal of Immunology* 163, 3668–3675.

Wold, A.E. and Hanson, L.Å. (1994) Defense factors in human milk. *Current Opinion in Gastroenterology* 10, 652–658.

Wolf, H.M., Fischer, M.B., Pühringer, H., Samstag, A., Vogel, E. and Eibl, M.M. (1994a) Human serum IgA downregulates the release of inflammatory cytokines (tumor necrosis factor-α, interleukin-6) in human monocytes. *Blood* 83, 1278–1288.

Wolf, H.M., Vogel, E., Fischer, M.B., Rengs, H., Schwarz, H.P. and Eibl, M.M. (1994b) Inhibition of receptor-dependent and receptor-independent generation of the respiratory burst in human neutrophils and monocytes by human serum IgA. *Pediatric Research* 36, 235–243.

Wright, A.L., Bauer, M., Naylor, A., Sutcliffe, E. and Clark, L. (1998) Increasing breast-feeding rates to reduce infant illness at the community level. *Pediatrics* 101, 837–844.

Yamanaka, T., Straumfors, A., Morton, H., Fausa, O., Brandtzaeg, P. and Farstad, I. (2001) M cell pockets of human Peyer's patches are specialized extensions of germinal centers. *European Journal of Immunology* 31, 107–117.

Yasui, H., Kiyoshima, J. and Ushijima, H. (1995) Passive protection against rotavirus-induced diarrhea of mouse pups born to and nursed by dams fed *Bifidobacterium breve* YIT4064. *Journal of Infectious Disease* 172, 403–409.

Zeiger, R.S. (2000) Dietary aspects of food allergy prevention in infants and children. *Journal of Pediatric Gastroenterology and Nutrition* 30(Suppl.), S77–S86.

Zhang, X., Izikson, L., Liu, L. and Weiner, H.L. (2001) Activation of CD25$^+$ CD^4 regulatory T-cells by oral antigen administration. *Journal of Immunology* 167, 4245–4253.

Ziegler, E.E., Fomon, S.J., Nelson, S.E., Rebouche, C.J., Edwards, B.B., Rogers, R.R. and Lehman, L.J. (1990) Cow milk feeding in infancy: further observations on blood loss from the gastrointestinal tract. *Journal of Pediatrics* 116, 11–18.

15 Food Allergy

ELIZABETH OPARA

School of Life Sciences, Kingston University and Faculty of Health and Social Care Sciences, St George's Hospital Medical School, Penrhyn Road, Kingston upon Thames, Surrey KT1 2EE, UK

Introduction

Over the past few years, food allergy has become a topical issue, and a question that is commonly asked is why do some foods elicit immune responses in certain individuals? To answer this question requires knowledge of:

- The immune system.
- The reactions that result in the symptoms associated with food allergy.
- How and why such reactions are generated.
- The characteristics and behaviour of allergenic foods and their constituents.

Research in these areas has allowed scientists to provide a gradually expanding picture of food-induced allergic reactions, which, although rare, are increasing in incidence and are, in some instances, life-threatening.

Food Allergy

Definition

In 1995, the European Academy of Allergy and Clinical Immunology (EAACI) prepared a position paper on adverse reactions to food (Bruijnzeel-Koomen *et al.*, 1995). In this paper, the EAACI presented a new classification, which divides adverse reactions to food into toxic and non-toxic reactions and further clearly distinguishes food allergy from food intolerance in the non-toxic category (Fig. 15.1). Based on the classification of the EAACI, food intolerance is defined as a non-immune-mediated adverse reaction to food, while food allergy is defined as an immune-mediated adverse reaction to food.

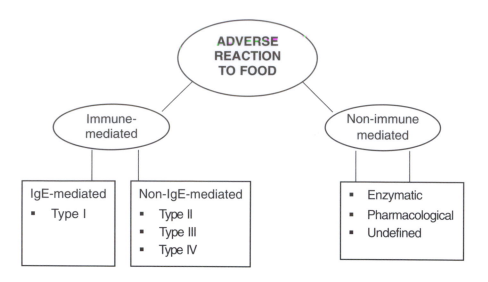

Fig. 15.1. Classification of adverse reactions to food. IgE, immunoglobulin E.

Food intolerance can be further divided into:

1. Enzymatic food intolerance, e.g. lactose intolerance.
2. Pharmacological food intolerance: this may be caused by biogenic amines such as histamine and tyramine, which are found in large amounts in cheese, red wine and tinned food, and which may play a role in migraine. Food additives and histamine-releasing factors present in foods may also be responsible for pharmacological food intolerance.
3. Undefined: adverse reactions to certain food additives for which the mechanisms remain largely unknown.

For further information on food intolerance, see European Commission (1997), Committee on Toxicity (2000) and British Nutrition Foundation (2001).
   Food allergy can be further divided into immunoglobulin E (IgE)-mediated and non-IgE-mediated reactions to food. The IgE-mediated reaction to food, also known as the immediate or type I response, is the most common and frequently reported and its role in food allergy is well established. Thus, unless otherwise stated, food allergy refers to the IgE-mediated type I response. There are three non-IgE-mediated reactions, which will also be discussed, albeit briefly.

Foods that cause allergic reactions

A range of foods are known to trigger type I allergic responses (Table 15.1). These foods contain specific proteins that, in certain individuals, initiate immunological reactions to food. These proteins, called allergens, possess common immunological characteristics that allow them to elicit an allergic, specifically IgE-mediated type I, response. In addition, these proteins (with some exceptions) possess certain common physical and chemical properties that may influence their allergenic potency (see Taylor and Lehrer, 1996; Lehrer *et al.*, 1996; see later section on 'Allergenic Foods and Food Allergens').

Symptoms of food allergy

A range of symptoms result from allergic reactions to food (Table 15.2). These symptoms, which affect different organs, are sometimes mild but some, such as anaphylaxis, can be life-threatening. Symptoms generated by an IgE-mediated response can occur very quickly (within minutes). However, such responses may also give rise to delayed symptoms/reactions. An example of this is food-induced eosinophilic gastroenteritis. Symptoms of this condition include post-prandial nausea, vomiting and diarrhoea and it occurs mainly in infants, children and young adults. This condition appears to involve cellular activity suggestive of the late phase of an IgE-mediated type I allergic reaction (Sampson, 1997).

Other, non-IgE, immune-mediated responses may be responsible for certain food-induced disorders, such as coeliac disease (seen in infants, children and adults) and food protein-induced enterocolitis syndromes, which occur primarily in infants and young children. However, the specific mechanisms that cause these disorders are unknown (see section on 'Other Immunological Reactions to Food').

IgE-mediated (Type I) Allergic Response

There are four allergic reactions, of which the IgE-mediated (type 1) is the most common. The components of the immune system and the ways in which they interact are described by Devereux (Chapter 1, this volume). The IgE-mediated response is a prime example of the interaction and interdependence of innate

Table 15.1. A list of known allergenic foods.

Commonly allergenic foods	Less commonly allergenic foods
Cow's milk	Molluscs:
Egg	• Mussels
Fish:	• Clams
• Cod	• Oysters
Crustacea:	Lupin
• Shrimp	Peas
Peanuts	Rice
Soybeans	Apples
Tree nuts:	Celery
• Brazil nuts	Peach
• Hazelnuts	Tomato
• Pistachio	Melons
Wheat	Cabbage

Table 15.2. Symptoms of allergic reactions to foods.

Reaction	Symptoms	Type of Food Allergy
Oral allergy syndrome (OAS)	Itching and swelling of the lip, tongue and larynx, other symptoms, such as urticaria, rhinitis, asthma, laryngeal oedema and anaphylaxis may also occur (see below)	Type I IgE-mediated
Cutaneous reactions • Urticaria • Angio-oedema • Atopic dermatitis (eczema)	 Wheals Swelling of subcutaneous tissue Itching (pruritus), dry and lined skin	All type I IgE-mediated
Respiratory reactions • Rhinitis • Asthma • Laryngeal oedema	 Inflammation of nasal passages causes runny nose Narrowing of the airways caused by inflammation Wheezing, tightness and breathlessness Constriction of the throat	All type I IgE-mediated
Gastrointestinal reactions or gastro-intestinal anaphylaxis	Abdominal pain, nausea, vomiting, diarrhoea	Type I IgE-mediated
Allergic eosinophilic gastroenteritis	Nausea, vomiting and diarrhoea caused by intestinal immune	Type I IgE-mediated
Gluten-sensitive enteropathy (coeliac disease)	response to gluten (a protein complex in wheat); immune response causes damage to wall of small intestine. This condition is characterized by chronic diarrhoea, weight loss, vomiting and anorexia	Non-IgE-mediated; possibly type III or type IV (see section on 'Other Immunological Reactions to Food')
Systemic reaction • Anaphylaxis	 A severe, generally rapid, reaction, which provokes itching and swelling of the oral cavity, cutaneous, respiratory, gastrointestinal and cardiovasular (chest pain, feeling faint and hypotension) symptoms	Type I IgE-mediated

Ig, immunoglobulin.

and adaptive immunity. However, in this case, the antigen is not a harmful pathogen but a food protein, which contains an IgE epitope recognized by specific T- and B-cells (clonal selection). These cells are thus activated and proliferation (clonal expansion) and antibody (IgE) production occur. These antibodies then interact with cells of innate immunity (mast cells and basophils) and trigger a reaction that results in the symptoms listed in Table 15.2. The IgE-mediated response is divided into two stages: sensitization (which includes the production of IgE antibodies) and the allergic reaction itself.

Sensitization

In allergic individuals, initial exposure to a food allergen (the antigen) causes production of IgE antibodies. The events leading to the production of IgE are:

1. The allergen is processed by antigen-presenting cells and class II major histocompatibility (MHC) proteins present a fragment of the allergen to allergen-specific T-helper (Th) cells.
2. Following binding to the allergen fragment, allergen-specific Th cells proliferate. Sensitization to a food allergen favours a T-helper (Th) 2 rather than a Th1-type response, and leads to the production of interleukin (IL)-4, IL-5, IL-10 and IL-13.
3. Th2-type cytokines promote the differentiation and proliferation of allergen-specific B-cells.
4. B-cells produce allergen-specific IgE antibodies (Fig. 15.2).
5. These allergen-specific IgE antibodies then bind to high-affinity IgE receptors present on mast cells and basophils.
6. Mast cells and basophils are now sensitized (Fig. 15.3).

The allergic reaction

With repeated exposure/ingestion, the food allergen comes into contact with a mast cell/basophil-bound IgE antibody. Since this IgE antibody is specific to the allergen (via the allergen's epitope – an IgE epitope), binding of the allergen to the IgE antibody occurs. This binding causes one IgE antibody to become cross-linked with another IgE antibody. Cross-linking triggers degranulation of the mast cells and basophils, leading to the release of pre-formed mediators, such as histamine, and the synthesis and release of tumour necrosis factor alpha (TNF-α), IL-4, prostaglandins and leucotrienes (Fig. 15.4). Release of these mediators causes an inflammatory reaction, which results in one or more of the symptoms listed in Table 15.2.

Allergenic Foods and Food Allergens

Allergenic foods

The list of foods that have been shown to cause allergic reactions in sensitive individuals is extensive. However, there are a number of foods that are consumed on a regular basis and which account for the majority of IgE-mediated reactions to food. An Expert Consultation of the Food and Agriculture Organization proposed a list of the most common allergenic foods (see Bousquet *et al.*, 1998). This list includes:

- Barley, oats, wheat and products of these (gluten and starch included).
- Crustaceans and other shellfish and products of these.
- Eggs and egg products.

- Fish and fish products.
- Legumes, peas, peanuts, soybeans and products of these.
- Milk and milk products.
- Tree nuts, e.g. Brazil nuts, hazelnuts and walnuts, and products of these.

Antigen is presented by antigen presenting cells to receptors on the surface of a
T-cell. Antibody on the surface of a B-cell also recognizes the antigen and, after
contact with the T-cell, B-cell and its daughter cells are primed to produce IgE.
Interleukin-2 (IL-2), secreted by T-cells, promotes proliferation of B-cells. Interleukin-4
(IL-4), also secreted by T-cells, promotes IgE production.

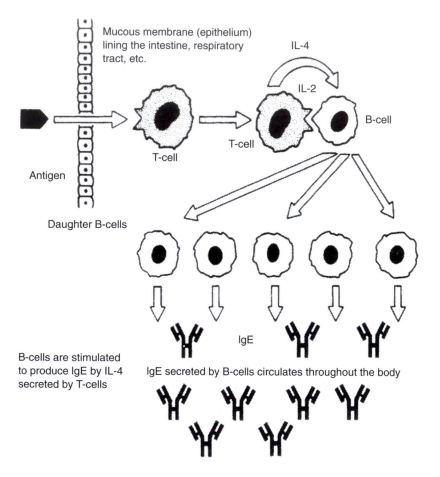

Fig. 15.2. Production of immunoglobulin (Ig)E antibodies. N.B. T-helper cells do not
recognize free antigen but antigen processed and presented by antigen-presenting cells and
class II major histocompatibility complex protein, respectively (see text). (Reprinted with
permission from the International Life Sciences Institute from the ILSI Europe Concise
Monograph on Food Allergy.)

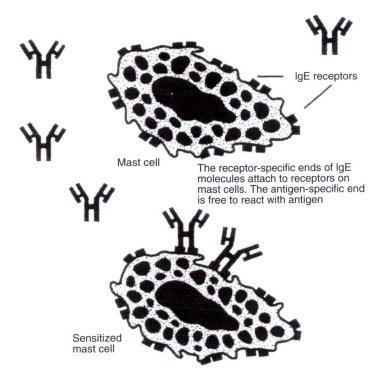

Fig. 15.3. Sensitization of mast cells (reprinted with permission from the International Life Sciences Institute from the ILSI Europe Concise Monograph on Food Allergy). IgE, immunoglobulin E.

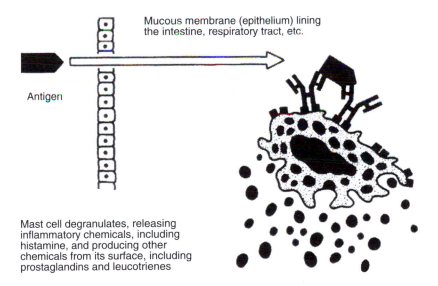

Fig. 15.4. Allergic reaction initiated by mast-cell degranulation (reprinted with permission from the International Life Sciences Institute from the ILSI Europe Concise Monograph on Food Allergy).

Major and minor allergens

Table 15.3 lists the systematic and original names of the allergens present in some allergenic foods. The first three letters of the systematic name come from the genus of the food in which the allergen is found, then follows the first letter of the species, then a number; the number assigned is based on the order of identification. For example, the first allergen described in peanut, *Arachis hypogea*, is designated *Ara h* 1.

Researchers have divided food allergens into major and minor allergens. Major allergens are generally defined as proteins for which 50% or more of the allergic individuals studied have specific IgE. Major allergens are normally abundant in a food. However, there are exceptions, such as *Gad c* 1, which is not abundant in cod but is a major allergen. Minor allergens, although they may have structures similar to major allergens, are unable to cause degranulation of mast cells and basophils because they do not possess the appropriate conformation (see section on 'Biochemical and immunological properties'). However, it has been suggested that minor allergens could be parts of larger major allergens and may therefore have the potential to cause allergic reactions in certain individuals (see Bush and Hefle, 1996).

Why do certain food proteins elicit an allergic response?

Food allergens possess biochemical and immunological characteristics that allow them to elicit an IgE-mediated immune response. In addition, they possess physical and chemical factors that may influence and/or indicate allergenicity (Table 15.4).

Biochemical and immunological properties

For a molecule to 'select'/bind to a T-cell or a B-cell and its antibodies and thus activate an immune response, it must possess an epitope. Thus, an allergen (whether a food, inhalant or venom allergen) must possess an epitope, specifically an epitope that binds IgE (an IgE epitope). To elicit an IgE allergic response, allergens must be able to cross-link one IgE antibody with another

Table 15.3. Some of the major food allergens.

Allergen source	Systematic and original names
Bos domesticus: domestic cattle	
• Cow's milk	• *Bos d* 4; α-lactalbumin
	• *Bos d* 5; β-lactoglobulin
Gallus domesticus: hen	
• Egg	• *Gal d* 1; ovomucoid
	• *Gal d* 2; ovalbumin
Gadus callarias: cod	• *Gad c* 1; allergen M
Metapenaeus ensis: shrimp	• *Met e* 1; tropomyosin
Arachis hypogea: peanut	• *Ara h* 1; vicilin
	• *Ara h* 2; conglutinin

Table 15.4. General properties of food allergens.

Immunological/biochemical
- Possess IgE epitope
- Possess at least two IgE-binding sites to elicit an IgE response

Physical/chemical
- MW between 10 and 70 kDa
- Glycosylated
- Stable at high temperatures ⎤
- Resistant to digestion ⎟ Exception: fruit and
- Resistant to proteolysis ⎬ vegetable allergens
- Resistant to hydrolysis ⎟
- Resistant to acidic environment ⎦

Ig, immunoglobulin; MW, molecular weight.

IgE antibody (both IgE antibodies need to be bound to a mast cell/basophil). Therefore, the allergen needs to be at least bivalent (as far as IgE binding is concerned), with the binding sites appropriately situated (Ishizaka and Ishizaka, 1984). However, it has been observed in mice that some monovalent allergens (e.g. an allergen found in venom, called mellitin) are able to trigger the release of mediators from mast cells or basophils or generate anaphylaxis (see Taylor and Lehrer, 1996). Such allergens can act as haptens (small molecules that elicit an immune response when bound to large molecules, such as bovine serum albumin), and thus are able to achieve cross-linking of IgE antibodies when part of a large complex. The significance of this mode of cross-linking in allergic disease has yet to be determined.

With the gradual elucidation of the biochemical structure of some common food allergens, comparisons between structures have been made in an attempt to identify common features. However, there does not appear to be any pattern of consistency between structures. For example, comparison of linear amino acid sequences and secondary and tertiary structures of these allergens has not revealed any general features. Such observations do not necessarily mean that general biochemical features between food allergens are not present, but that such features, which may cause food allergens to differ from other food proteins, have yet to be identified. Research on the biochemical and immunochemical characteristics of food allergens, specifically the properties of IgE epitopes – both B-cell epitopes and T-cell epitopes – in an attempt to identify unique features is ongoing (see Taylor and Lehrer, 1996; Bush and Hefle, 1996; Shin *et al.*, 1998).

Allergen cross-reactivity

Different allergens may share the same or similar IgE epitope structure, which may result in cross-reactivity. A well-documented example is that of individuals with pollen allergies – for example, birch, oak and mugwort – who may also suffer from adverse reactions to certain fruits and vegetables, including apple, pear, hazelnuts, kiwi, carrots and celery (Bruijzeel-Koomen *et al.*, 1995; Kazemi-Shirazi *et al.*, 2000). Another example of allergen cross-reactivity is latex and banana (see Perkin, 2000). Cross-reactivity also exists between food allergens. For example, cross-reactivity between allergens present in foods that belong to the legume family and between different fish species has been documented (see Bush and Hefle, 1996). The magnitude of the clinical manifestation of cross-reactivity does vary between individuals. For example, not all individuals with pollen allergies present symptoms following the ingestion of certain fruits and vegetables. This variation in clinical symptoms has also been observed between proteins in related foods – for example, the legume family – that cross-react. In general, the manifestation of symptoms is rare, but very severe reactions have been reported (See Bush and Hefle, 1996).

Physical and chemical properties

MOLECULAR WEIGHT AND CARBOHYDRATE MOIETIES. Most known food allergens have a molecular weight of between 10 and 70 kDa. However, smaller molecules may be able to elicit an allergic response and some food allergens, such as some of the peanut allergens, are very large (200–300 kDa) in their native form. In addition, most food allergens are glycosylated and have acidic isoelectric points. However, many proteins that are not allergens possess these properties, and thus molecular weight, glycosylation and isoelectric point are not useful indicators of allergenicity (see Taylor and Lehrer, 1996).

HEAT STABILITY. Most, but not all, food allergens are resistant to high temperatures. Heat causes denaturation of allergenic proteins and the loss of conformational IgE epitopes. However, some food allergens still retain their allergenicity, indicating that epitope conformation is not always essential for IgE binding to certain allergens (although appropriate epitope conformation is essential for cross-linking). Cow's milk, fish, soybean and peanut allergens have all been shown to be resistant to heat. However, these food allergens are not always 100% resistant to high temperatures. For example, the IgE-binding capacity of β-lactoglobulin, a cow's-milk allergen, is diminished but not completely eliminated by heating at 80–100°C. The IgE-binding capacity of the peanut allergen *Ara h 1* is unaffected by temperatures as high as 100°C (see Taylor and Lehrer, 1996).

RESISTANCE TO DIGESTION, PROTEOLYSIS, HYDROLYSIS AND LOW-PH ENVIRONMENT. Digestion, proteolysis and hydrolysis may destroy both conformational and linear epitopes. However, a number of common food allergens, including cow's milk, egg, peanut, fish and soybean allergen, have been shown to be resistant to:

- Specific enzymes that are involved in gastric and intestinal digestion of proteins, such as pepsin and trypsin.
- Simulated gastric and intestinal fluids over time *in vitro*.
- Chemicals, such as cyanogen bromide and hydrochloric acid, that hydrolyse proteins (see Taylor and Lehrer, 1996).

Generally, the allergenicity of the above, assessed by IgE-binding capacity, was fully retained or diminished but not eliminated. However, the resistance to digestion may not be consistent: a study on the effects of pepsin digestion on the allergenicity of peanut showed that pepsin eliminated its IgE-binding capacity (Hong *et al.*, 1999).

A few studies have indicated that digestion may enhance the allergenicity of food proteins, since digestion may unravel hidden epitopes. One such study reported that IgE from the serum of some patients with cow's-milk allergy is more reactive with digests of β-lactoglobulin than with the undigested form (see Taylor and Lehrer, 1996).

Fruit and vegetable allergens are completely heat-labile and are more sensitive to digestion, proteolysis and hydrolysis than the allergens discussed above. Reactions to fruit and vegetable allergens occur primarily in the mouth and cause oral allergy syndrome (see Table 15.2).

Effects of food processing

Since certain food allergens are resistant to high temperatures and proteolysis, food-processing techniques (such as thermal processing and enzymatic proteolysis) have, in general, very little effect on their allergenicity. However, a recent study reported that the binding of roasted peanut to IgE from individuals with peanut allergy was approximately 90-fold higher than that of raw peanut to IgE (Maleki *et al.*, 2000). The study also reported that two major peanut allergens (*Ara h* 1 and *Ara h* 2) bound higher levels of IgE and were more resistant to heat and digestive enzymes once they had undergone the Maillard reaction. The Maillard reaction is a reaction between amino acids in protein and reducing sugars – glucose, fructose, lactose and maltose – which causes browning of food and the production of compounds that impart a burnt and caramel-like flavour. The impact of roasting on the allergenicity of peanut proteins is further supported by an investigation by Beyer *et al.* (2001) of the effect of cooking methods on peanut allergenicity. This study showed that, in contrast to frying and boiling, the roasting of peanuts increased the allergenic properties of *Ara h* 1 and *Ara h* 2, indicated by IgE binding. Thus, thermal processing (i.e. roasting) may play a role in the enhancement of the allergenic properties of peanut protein.

Some food processes, specifically phenolic browning and lyophilization, have been shown to diminish IgE-binding capacities of apple and fish allergens, respectively. However, such effects are said to be rare (see Taylor and Lehrer, 1996).

Over the past several years, the effect of novel food techniques, such as genetic modification and protein microparticulation (the heating and shearing of food proteins to cause coagulation) on the allergenicity of food proteins has become a major food-safety issue. However, assessing the impact of such techniques on allergenicity is not always straightforward. One reason for this is that some novel techniques, specifically genetic modification, utilize proteins for which the allergenic history is unknown and thus the determination of IgE-binding capacities is difficult because IgE antibodies with an appropriate specificity are unavailable. For further information on assessing the potential allergenicity of novel foods, see Lehrer *et al.* (1996), Metcalfe *et al.* (1996),

Nestle (1996), Nordlee *et al.* (1996), Opara *et al.* (1998, 1999), Bucchini (2001) and Taylor and Hefle (2001a, b).

Development of Food Allergy

There are a number of factors that may contribute to susceptibility to IgE-mediated food allergies:

* A genetic predisposition.
* Early exposure to foods when the gut mucosal barrier is immature.
* The high consumption of certain foods.
* The introduction of new foods to the diet.

Genetic predisposition

The development of food allergy may be influenced by a familial history of atopy. Atopy is a genetic predisposition towards mounting IgE antibody responses. Thus, atopic individuals make IgE constantly and have unusually high levels of IgE in their serum (unlike non-atopic individuals, in which an IgE response can only be elicited via the mechanism described above). Atopy is associated with allergic diseases, such as asthma, rhinitis, atopic dermatitis (eczema) and also food allergies. Atopic individuals are commonly defined, in practice, as those who exhibit sensitization to two allergens or more.

Studies on children have shown that the risk of developing an IgE-mediated food allergy ranges from 13.5 to 58% when one parent is atopic (uniparental history of atopy) and up to 100% when both parents are atopic (biparental history of atopy) (see European Commission, 1997).

Overall, work in the area of the genetics of food allergy is limited. A study carried out in the UK suggests that the MHC genes that code for class II human leucocyte antigen (HLA) proteins may play a role in determining susceptibility to peanut allergy (Howell *et al.*, 1998). The same study also suggests that there is a higher rate of peanut allergy among siblings compared with the general population of the UK. A study from the USA (Sicherer *et al.*, 2000) investigated the role of genetic and environmental factors in the development of peanut allergy by looking at twins – identical and non-identical – in whom one or both siblings had peanut allergy (not all their parents were peanut-allergic). The study reported a significantly higher concordance rate of peanut allergy among identical twins than among non-identical twins. In addition, common (e.g. parental style and eating habits) and specific (e.g. separate peer groups) environmental factors were shown not to influence the development of peanut allergy. Thus, in this study, the genetic influence on the development of peanut allergy is seen to be significant. Whether this genetic influence is conferred via the action of genes that code for HLA II proteins was not investigated. However, the authors of this study highlighted the need for further work to identify the genes that are likely to influence food allergy. However, given that the prevalence of allergic disorders has increased over the recent past, it is considered that environmental factors are also highly significant (Warner *et al.*, 2000; Wills-Karp *et al.*, 2001).

Early exposure to foods

Early exposure to foods is believed to be a major influence on the development of food allergy in young children. One of the main reasons for this is the immaturity of the gut mucosal barrier in young children (see Brandtzaeg, Chapter 14, this volume). The gut mucosal barrier does not mature fully until the age of approximately 9–10 years. The gut mucosa of young children exhibits a greater permeability than that of older children and adults, and thus allows more protein, including food allergens, through. As a result, systemic exposure of the ingested allergen to the child's immune system occurs. Thus, due to mucosal-barrier immaturity, early exposure of new foods may influence the development of IgE-mediated food allergy in infants and children. With maturation, the mucosal barrier becomes less permeable and more efficient as a barrier and studies have shown that with this maturation many cases of allergic reactions to certain foods (e.g. egg and milk) cease (Dannaeus and Inganaes, 1981; Høst and Halken, 1990).

An immature mucosal barrier may also be linked to the duration of peanut allergy. A study on the resolution of peanut allergy suggests that peanut allergy in a small proportion of young children who were sensitized to peanut early in life resolves in a similar way to egg and milk allergies (Hourihane *et al.*, 1998). However, peanut allergy rarely resolves in older children and adults, in whom severe peanut allergy is common. One possible explanation for the resolution of peanut allergy focuses on epitope structure, IgE binding and gut-mucosa maturity. Studies suggest that children who develop a tolerance to peanut may possess IgE that binds more to conformational epitopes than to linear epitopes; children who do not develop tolerance to peanuts possess IgE that binds mostly to linear epitopes. Conformational epitopes are generally more labile, whereas linear epitopes are more stable. Thus, as the gut mucosal barrier matures more linear than conformational epitopes pass through the mucosal barrier and elicit an IgE-mediated response (Berger, 1998).

Early exposure of young children in the USA and Scandinavia to peanuts and fish, respectively, has been attributed to the development of both allergies (Aas, 1966; Sampson, 1996). Whether this is due to gut mucosal immaturity is unclear. However, the development of peanut allergy in young children following early exposure may be linked to atopy. The Department of Health (1998) report on peanut allergy advises that, in an attempt to reduce the risk of developing peanut allergy, the introduction of peanuts and products containing peanuts into the diets of infants from families with a history of atopy should be avoided.

Early exposure to foods and therefore food allergens may also occur via the maternal diet. Studies have shown that cow's milk allergen, β-lactoglobulin and egg allergen, ovalbumin, can be transmitted to infants via breast milk in variable amounts (1–1000 µg l^{-1}) (Department of Health, 1998). In addition, Vadas *et al.* (2001) reported the presence of two peanut allergens (*Ara h* 1 and

Ara h 2) in the breast milk of lactating women following the ingestion of 50 g of roasted peanuts. Collectively, these studies demonstrate the potential for sensitization of at-risk infants via breast milk. Sensitization may also occur *in utero*. Fetal blood mononuclear cells responded to allergens following exposure to house-dust mite, birch pollen, milk and egg allergens during pregnancy (Jones *et al.*, 1996; Warner *et al.*, 2000). In addition, mothers from atopic families who consumed peanuts more than once a week during pregnancy have been shown to be more likely to have a child who is allergic to peanut than mothers who consumed peanuts less than once a week (Marian *et al.*, 1999) (see also section on 'Prevention, Management and Treatment of Food Allergy').

The high consumption of certain foods

Persistent exposure to foods that are allergenic may also play a role in the development of IgE-mediated food allergy. Peanut and fish allergy are more common in the USA and Scandinavia, respectively (Aas, 1966; Sampson, 1996). The frequent consumption of these foods may to some extent determine the likelihood of the development of their respective allergies. On the other hand, the high consumption of these foods may only be linked to the prevalence of their respective food allergies and not to development (see section on 'Prevalence of Allergic Reactions to Food').

Introduction of new food into the diet

The introduction of soybean to the French diet in the mid-1980s led to an increase in the incidence of soybean allergy (Moneret-Vautrin, 1986). In addition, the introduction of kiwi fruit into the USA in the 1980s was followed by reports of allergic reactions to kiwi in the literature (Fine, 1981).

In light of the association between the introduction of new foods into a diet and the development of food allergy, the possibility that the introduction of foods generated using novel techniques, such as genetically modified foods, may influence the development of new food allergies is real. One prime example of this is the transgenic soybean that contained a gene (which expressed the protein 2S albumin) isolated from Brazil nut, a known allergenic food. Tests on this transgenic soybean revealed that individuals allergic to Brazil nut, but not to soybean, were allergic to transgenic soybean (Nordlee *et al.*, 1996). This finding highlights the importance of assessing potentially allergenic new foods. However, as stated earlier, the difficulty in attempting to broach this area of food allergy is that many genetically modified foods contain proteins of unknown allergenic history. In addition, such foods may contain proteins that are not recognized as allergenic in their modified form or may become allergenic due to the modification that the food has undergone. Research is ongoing to develop new approaches to tackle the potential problem of allergenicity and genetically modified foods.

Prevalence of Allergic Reactions to Food

The prevalence of food allergy is unclear. One reason for this lack of clarity is that many food allergies are perceived and not real. As many as 20–30% of the UK population think they have a food allergy. However, the prevalence of true food allergy in the UK is estimated to be between 1 and 3% and possibly less (Department of Health, 1998; Committee on Toxicity, 2000; British Nutrition Foundation, 2001).

A number of factors influence the prevalence of food allergy. These include:

- Geography. A number of studies on cow's milk allergy carried out in the USA, Sweden, Canada, England, Denmark and Holland estimate prevalence to range from 0.1 to 7.5% (Høst, 1994). The prevalence of peanut allergy also appears to vary based on location: peanut allergy affects 0.6% of the US population and 0.4% of US children (Sicherer *et al.*, 1999). However, estimation of the prevalence of peanut allergy in Australian children is reported to be 1.9% (Hill *et al.*, 1997) (to the author's knowledge, no data are available for prevalence of peanut allergy in Australian adults). In Asian and African countries, peanut allergy is reported to be rare; however, few data on the incidence of peanut allergy in these countries are available (Department of Health, 1998).
- Cross-reactivity. Similarities in the IgE epitope structures between food allergens and between pollen and food allergens can influence prevalence. For example, in areas where allergy to birch and mugwort pollen is prevalent, 30–50% of individuals with these allergies present with symptoms following the ingestion of fruits and vegetables that share the same or similar IgE epitope structures with those of both pollens (De Blay *et al.*, 1991). However, as stated previously, the magnitude of the clinical manifestation of cross-reactivity between food allergens can vary between individuals.
- Genetic predisposition.
- Resolution of food allergy over time.
- Exposure to new and novel foods.
- The high consumption of allergenic foods. Generally, in countries where the consumption of a commonly allergenic food (such as peanuts and fish) is high, the incidence of allergic reactions to that food is more common. For example, as stated earlier, a high rate of peanut consumption has been linked to peanut allergy being more common in the USA. However, the rate of peanut consumption in China is also high, but the prevalence of peanut allergy in China is much lower than that in the USA. This difference in prevalence may be linked to the methods used in the cooking of peanuts. The methods of boiling and frying peanuts are common practices in China and both boiling and frying have been reported to decrease the allergenicity of peanut protein (Beyer *et al.*, 2001). In contrast, roasting, which is the main way in which peanuts are cooked in the USA, has been reported to increase the allergenicity of peanut proteins (Maleki *et al.*, 2000; Beyer *et al.*, 2001). Thus, modes of cooking may also have an impact on prevalence.

In addition to the factors listed above, differences in the approaches utilized in the study of food-allergy prevalence might be important (Høst, 1994).

Diagnosis of Food Allergy

Since many food allergies are perceived and not real, any study on food allergy using humans requires confirmation of the allergy. There are a number of techniques available for the diagnosis of food allergy:

- Clinical history and physical examination.
- Elimination diets.
- Double-blind, placebo-controlled food challenge (DBPCFC): an *in vivo* test.
- Skin-prick test: an *in vivo* test.
- Radioallergosorbent test (RAST): an *in vitro* test.

Clinical history and physical examination

The clinical history of an individual who has reported suffering from a food allergy is taken to identify the suspect food(s) and thus to determine whether the food(s) is(are) the likely cause(s) of allergic symptoms (Committee on Toxicity, 2000). A clinical history includes:

- A description of the symptoms caused by the food.
- The time between ingestion of the food(s) and the onset of symptoms.
- The quantity of food that generates a response.
- The consistency of symptoms.
- The presence of other factors that generate the same symptoms – for example, exercise (see section on 'Other Immunological Reactions to Food').
- The length of time of the reaction.

A standard physical examination can be used to support a clinical history. In addition to the above, a review of family history for atopic individuals (particularly when diagnosing food allergy in children) may help identify individuals at risk of developing food allergies.

Elimination diets

Verification of the suspect food can be achieved by eliminating the food from the diet, since then symptoms caused by the food would no longer occur. For such diets to be successful:

- One needs to be aware of any other foods that may have an adverse effect.

- The diets need to be based on thorough and accurate dietary history and knowledge of foods and their components.

Double blind, placebo controlled food challenge

If a clinical history indicates that an individual is suffering from a food allergy, a DBPCFC can be carried out to confirm the food allergy (see Bruijnzeel-Koomen *et al.*, 1995; European Commission, 1997; Committee on Toxicity, 2000; British Nutrition Foundation, 2001). This test is considered to be the 'gold standard' for diagnosing food allergy and involves giving an individual the suspect food. To prevent a subjective response, the smell and taste of the food are masked, although this can sometimes be difficult due to the quantity of food needed for the challenge and/or the strong flavours and odours that the food of interest may possess. This test is not always practical, since severe reactions to the food can arise, and it must therefore be carried out under medical control. In addition, interpretation of results from DBPCFC is not always straightforward, since a positive response to a food challenge indicates a cause-and-effect relationship but will not provide information about the underlying mechanism that caused the response (Watson, 1995). Such information may be obtained from the results of other diagnostic techniques, which are discussed below.

Skin-prick test

This test involves pricking an extract of the suspect food on to an individual's skin (normally on the back of the forearm; sometimes on the back); positive control substances (e.g. histamine) and negative control substances are also tested. The appearance of a wheal-and-flare reaction peaking in 15–25 min and disappearing in 1–2 h is a positive response. Late reactions with skin-prick tests are rare. Although a skin-prick test can demonstrate sensitization to food allergens, a positive skin-prick test cannot be used to determine whether the suspect food gives rise to clinical symptoms and only indicates that the food and the individual's symptoms (wheal and flare) are related. To determine whether the predictive value of the skin-prick test is high, a DBPCFC would need to be carried out.

   Although the skin-prick test is practical and commonly used to screen for food allergy, the use of different forms of the same food can generate varied responses. For example, commercial extracts of the same food allergen from different manufacturers have been shown to have varied allergenic activities. One possible reason for this is that the process of extraction may alter the activity of the allergen. For example, labile allergens from fruit and vegetables are unlikely to resist the extraction. Thus, skin-prick tests with commercial extracts of fruit and vegetable allergens are variable and probably unreliable. Fresh food can be used instead of commercial extracts and its use in skin-prick tests has been shown to be more sensitive and reproducible than using commercially available extracts. In addition, skin prick tests using fresh foods have shown greater concordance with DBPCFC than those using commercial extracts (see Bruijnzeel-Koomen *et al.*, 1995; European Commission, 1997; Committee on Toxicity, 2000).

Radioallergosorbent test

RAST is the most common *in vitro* diagnostic test for food allergy and may be used as an alternative to the skin-prick test. RAST involves measuring the levels of allergen-specific IgE in the sera of allergic individuals. However, as with the skin-prick test, RAST cannot provide a definitive diagnosis of food allergy and thus a DBPCFC would need to be carried out to ascertain its predictive power. RAST is generally believed to be less sensitive than the skin-prick test and is more expensive. In addition, the results of RAST are not immediately available. There are also problems relating to the quality of the food allergens used for this test (see Bruijnzeel-Koomen *et al.*, 1995; European Commission, 1997; Committee on Toxicology, 2000).

Despite the drawbacks associated with measuring allergen-specific IgE, investigations have indicated that quantifying the levels of allergen-specific IgE may be a viable alternative to the DBPCFC. Using children and adolescents (most (90%) with a family history of atopic disease), Sampson and Ho (1997) and Sampson (2001) demonstrated that the concentrations of IgE specific to cow's milk, egg, peanut and fish, measured using an enzyme-linked immunosorbent assay, could be used to predict the likelihood of a clinical response to these foods and thus eliminate the need for DBPCFC.

Other diagnostic tests

Another *in vitro* test involves measuring the release of mediators from mast cells or basophils following exposure to the suspected food. These tests vary in sensitivity and specificity, and they show varying degrees of concordance with other tests. However, since such tests require the preparation and use of serum and mast cells/basophils, they are time-consuming and cannot be used routinely for the diagnosis of food allergy.

A number of other methods have been used in the diagnosis of food allergy. However, there is no scientific evidence to suggest that such tests are in any way useful (Committee on Toxicity, 2000; British Nutrition Foundation, 2001). These tests include:

1. Electroacupuncture, in which the electrical activity of the skin is determined at points considered appropriate for the detection of food allergy.
2. Applied kinesiology, which is based on muscle strength.
3. Autologous urine injections, in which urine from a sensitive individual is said to cause a positive skin reaction in another individual with the same sensitivity.

Prevention, Management and Treatment of Food Allergy

Prevention

Based on research on the impact of early nutrition on the immune system of infants, advice on the prevention of food allergy is focused on reducing risk of development in infants and young children, particularly those who are related to atopic individuals. Much of this preventive advice is linked to reducing or eliminating the presence of common allergenic foods from the diets of atopic mothers/mothers-to-be and their children.

Dietary modification (i.e. eliminating common allergenic foods from their diets) by pregnant women with a history of allergy in the family has been shown to be beneficial in terms of allergy outcome in the infant (see Hampton, 1999; Chandra, 2000). However, studies indicate that, for these elimination diets to be useful, they (the diets) must begin before week 22 of pregnancy, since sensitization may occur as early as the second trimester (Jones *et al.*, 1996) and that these diets should continue until the end of lactation. Such diets may put stress on the mother, which may be detrimental to the fetus and thus any gain in respect of preventing the development of atopic disease and allergy may be lost (Hampton, 1999).

Research has also shown that the early introduction of weaning foods and the greater diversity of these foods, particularly those that are highly allergenic, such as milk, eggs, soybean, fish and nuts, may result in an increased incidence of food allergy in infants from atopic families (Hampton, 1999; Chandra, 2000).

Based on these studies, recommendations to reduce the risk of development of food allergies highlight the need for mothers with a history of atopy to:

- Avoid allergenic food during pregnancy and lactation.
- Delay introduction of solid foods, particularly those that are highly allergenic, such as milk, dairy products, eggs, fish, soybean, nuts and peanuts, until after 4 months, limiting variety until at least 6 months.
- Breast-feed exclusively and for a prolonged period. Breast-feeding may provide partial protection against the development of food allergy (Chandra, 2000). Reasons for this include reduced exposure to food proteins that would be present in formulas, improved maturation of the gut mucosal barrier, reduced infection and the presence of anti-inflammatory and immunological factors in human breast milk (Peat *et al.*, 1999; see also Brandtzaeg, Chapter 14, this volume).

In its report on peanut allergy, the advice of the Department of Health (1998) on reducing the risk of developing peanut allergy is directed at pregnant mothers 'who are themselves atopic, or those for whom the father or any sibling of the unborn child has an atopic disease'. These individuals are advised to avoid eating peanuts, peanut products and foods containing peanuts. The same advice is directed at atopic breast-feeding mothers. The report goes on to advise that infants with a parent or sibling with atopic disease should be breast-fed for 4–6 months and that, during weaning and until at least 3 years of age, their diets should not include peanuts, peanut products and foods containing peanuts. However, in spite of the above recommendations/advice, it must be stressed that not all studies support maternal avoidance of highly allergenic foods during pregnancy and/or during lactation (Hattevig *et al.*, 1999; Zeiger, 2000; British Nutrition Foundation, 2001). Thus, researchers have highlighted the need for further studies to facilitate a clearer understanding of the role of maternal diet in the occurrence of atopic diseases and sensitization to allergenic foods (Zeiger, 2000; British Nutrition Foundation, 2001).

Maternal avoidance of peanuts and other highly allergenic foods during pregnancy and lactation also raises the issue of tolerance. In its report on peanut allergy, the Department of Health (1998) states that the rarity of peanut allergy in African and Asian countries may be due to peanut allergy going unrecognized, genetic differences or the development of tolerance to peanut. Differences in cooking practices may also be a factor. Concerning tolerance, it may be that exposure of infants to peanut allergens – for example, via breast milk – may allow the child to build up a tolerance to peanut. However, until data on the consumption and prevalence of peanut and peanut allergy, respectively, in African and Asian countries are obtained, such a possibility cannot begin to be confirmed.

The use of hydrolysed milk formulas to prevent the development of cow's milk allergy has also been investigated. Hydrolysed milk formulas, which are nutritionally adequate, vary in their degree of hypoallergenicity; however, they are not completely non-allergenic, since some can still cause allergic reactions in individuals with cow's milk allergy. Studies have shown that such formulas reduce the incidence of cow's milk allergy, atopic dermatitis and specific cow's milk IgE in infants. Furthermore, studies note that these effects are specific for cow's milk allergy and are limited to infants when given before 6 months of age (Zeiger, 2000). However, since many of these studies had technical and methodological limitations, such as inadequate sample size, further work is needed.

Alternative formulas, specifically soya formula, have also been investigated. Although soybean is itself allergenic, studies have reported that in infants of atopic parents fed soya formula from birth or early in life, the incidence of soya allergy is very low. In these studies, soya allergy was diagnosed using DBPCFC. However, in studies where DBPCFC was not used, the results do not suggest a low soya allergy in such infants. Soya formulas may be used as a safe alternative for children with IgE-mediated cow's milk allergy (Zeiger, 2000; see section on 'Other Immunological Reactions to Food'). However, concerns have been raised about the bioavailability of nutrients, specifically the micronutrients calcium, zinc and iron, in soya drinks and soya-based infant formulas, due to the presence of phytates in these products (Sandstrom *et al.*, 1983; Lonnerdal *et al.*, 1984; Hurrell *et al.*, 1992; Reddy *et al.*, 1996; Couzy *et al.*, 1998; Heaney *et al.*, 2000).

Management and treatment

Exclusion diets

Currently, the only way to manage food allergy is by exclusion of the offending food/s. Expert dietary advice on exclusion diets is essential to ensure (Baker and David, 1996):

1. Dietary compliance – complete avoidance of the offending food/s.
2. That the nutritional requirements of the patient are being met.
3. That the patient has knowledge of how to read and interpret food labels (although food labels do not always contain the information required to make decisions about the suitability of foods).
4. That patients are able to lead as near as possible to a normal life in spite of the obstacles placed by dietary compliance and are aware of whole foods that are hidden sources of the offending food.

Novel approaches to the management and treatment of food allergy

PROBIOTICS. One of the recent novel approaches involves the use of probiotics (microbial cell preparations or components of microbes that are reported to maintain health via their action on gut flora (see Gill and Cross, Chapter 13, this volume)). Studies have linked the development of atopy and subsequent atopic disease with the composition of gut flora (Björksten *et al.*, 2001; Kalliomäki *et al.*, 2001; Ouwehand *et al.*, 2001). In addition, studies focusing on the therapeutic role of probiotics have provided clinical evidence for their potential use in the management of food allergy. Trapp *et al.* (1993) reported that volunteers given yoghurt had decreased concentrations of IgE in their serum and a lower frequency of allergies. Matsuzaki *et al.* (1998) showed that oral feeding of the probiotic bacterium *Lactobacillus casei* inhibited ovalbumin-induced IgE production in mice. Furthermore, Majamaa and Isolauri (1997) showed that probiotics significantly improved the clinical symptoms associated with food allergy in infants with atopic eczema and cow's milk allergy. However, information on the efficacy of probiotics in the treatment of food allergy is limited and thus more research is needed (Isolauri *et al.*, 1999; Kirjavainen *et al.*, 1999).

GENE THERAPY. Another novel approach, which is in its infancy, is gene therapy. A report by Roy *et al.* (1999) described the use of gene therapy in the treatment of peanut allergy. The study involved cloning the major peanut allergen *Ara h 2* and administering it in a murine model of peanut allergy and anaphylaxis. Subsequent dosing with *Ara h 2* was associated with a decrease in IgE levels and also reduced the severity of anaphylaxis, indicating that the mice had built up a degree of tolerance. However, this approach is far from being used clinically and further studies are required on the efficacy of this therapy in mice that are already sensitized to peanuts, as is the case in humans.

Other Immunological Reactions to Food

Non-IgE-mediated allergic reactions

There are three non-IgE-mediated allergic reactions:

1. Type II. Antibody-dependent cytotoxic hypersensitivity reactions involve the binding of antibodies (IgG or IgM) to cell-bound antigen/allergen and the subsequent destruction of the cell-bound antigen by complement proteins, macrophages or killer cells.

2. Type III. Immune-complex-mediated hypersensitivity reactions involve the generation of large insoluble antibody (IgG or IgM) antigen/allergen complexes. Their presence activates complement proteins, which leads to cellular (neutrophil, mast cell, basophil and eosinophil) infiltration and activation and ultimately tissue damage.

3. Type IV. Delayed T-cell-mediated hypersensitivity reactions are not antibody-mediated but T-cell-mediated and involve the proliferation of antigen/allergen-specific T-cells, which normally results in a delayed (after 24 h) inflammatory response.

There is very little information on the role of non-IgE-mediated reactions to food (British Nutrition Foundation, 2001). Some foods do give rise to non-IgE mediated reactions, but the specific mechanisms are not generally known. However, both type III and type IV reactions have been associated with gluten, cow's milk and soybean allergies and are associated with the manifestation of gastrointestinal and cutaneous symptoms (Høst, 1994).

Exercise-induced anaphylaxis

Cases of anaphylaxis induced by exercise following the ingestion of food have been reported in the literature. The first case involved an individual who developed anaphylactic reactions (cutaneous and respiratory reactions, including urticaria and airway obstruction) when running 12 h after ingesting shellfish; each time the individual went for a run following the earlier ingestion of shellfish, anaphylactic reactions ensued. The relationship between exercise-induced anaphylaxis and the earlier ingestion of food remains controversial and the immunology behind it is unclear, since it may or may not be mediated by IgE (Tilles and Schocket, 1997).

Conclusion

Food allergy is believed to be on the increase and its symptoms can sometimes be life-threatening. Why the immune system reacts to certain foodstuffs as if they were pathogens is still unclear. However, research into this area of nutrition and immunity has provided an increased understanding of the immune mechanisms that are generated in response to food and the proteins that cause them. Continuing research into the properties that confer allergenicity on to food proteins and into the development of food allergy, in particular the role that genes may play in predisposing to adverse responses to some foods, may bring us closer to finding out why these reactions occur.

References

Aas, K. (1966) Studies of hypersensitivity to fish: a clinical study. *International Archives of Allergy* 29, 346–363.

Baker, H.B. and David, T.J. (1996) The dietetic and nutritional management of food allergy. *Journal of the Royal Society of Medicine* 90(Suppl. 30), 45–50.

Berger, A. (1998) Science commentary: why do some children grow out of peanut allergy? *British Medical Journal* 316, 1275.

Beyer, K., Morrow, E., Li, X.-M., Bardina, L., Bannon, G.A., Burks, A.W. and Sampson, H.A. (2001) Effects of cooking methods on peanut allergenicity. *Journal of Allergy and Clinical Immunology* 107, 1077–1081.

Björksten, B., Sepp, E., Julge, K., Voor, T. and Mikelsaar, M. (2001) Allergy development and the intestinal microflora during the first year of life. *Journal of Allergy and Clinical Immunology* 108, 516–520.

Bousquet, J., Björkstén, B., Bruijnzeel-Koomen, C., Hugget, A., Ortolani, C., Warner, J.O. and Smith, M. (1998) Scientific criteria and the selection of allergenic foods for product labelling. *Allergy* 53, 3–21.

British Nutrition Foundation (2001) Buttriss, J. (ed.) *Adverse Reactions to Foods – the Report of the British Nutrition Foundation Task Force*. Blackwell Science, Oxford.

Bruijnzeel-Koomen, C., Ortolani, C., Aas, K., Bindslev-Jensen, C., Björksten, B., Moneret-Vautrin, D. and Wüthrich, B. (1995) Adverse reactions to food. *Allergy* 50, 623–635.

Bucchini, L. (2001) Allergenic risk from novel plants is very important and difficult to predict. *Journal of Allergy and Clinical Immunology* 108, 654.

Bush, R.K. and Hefle, S.L. (1996) Food allergens. *Critical Reviews in Food Science and Nutrition* 36, S119–S163.

Chandra, R.K. (2000) Food allergy and nutrition in early life: implications for later health. *Proceedings of the Nutrition Society* 59, 273–277.

Committee on Toxicity (2000) *Adverse Reactions to Food and Food Ingredients*. Food Standards Agency, London.

Couzy, F., Mansourian, R., Labate, A., Guinchard, S., Montagne, D.H. and Dirren, H. (1998) Effect of dietary phytic acid on zinc absorption in the healthy elderly, as assessed by serum concentration curve tests. *British Journal of Nutrition* 80, 177–182.

Dannaeus, A. and Inganaes, M. (1981) A follow up study of children with food allergy: clinical course in relation to serum IgE and IgG antibody levels to milk, egg and fish. *Clinical Allergy* 11, 533–539.

De Blay, F., Pauli, G. and Bessot, J.C. (1991) Cross reactions bewteen respiratory and food allergens. *Allergy Proceedings* 12, 313–317.

Department of Health (1998) *Peanut Allergy – Report of the Committee on Toxicity of Chemicals in Food, Consumer Products and the Environment*. Department of Health, London.

European Commission (1997) *Study of Nutritional Factors in Food Allergies and Food Intolerances*. European Commission, Luxembourg.

Fine, A.J. (1981) Hypersensitivity reaction to kiwi fruit (Chinese gooseberry, *Actinidia chinensis*). *Journal of Allergy and Clinical Immunology* 6, 235–237.

Hampton, S.M. (1999) Prematurity, immune function and infant feeding practices. *Proceedings of the Nutrition Society* 58, 75–78.

Hattevig, G., Sigurs, N. and Kjellman, B. (1999) Effects of maternal dietary avoidance during lactation on allergy in children at 10 years of age. *Acta Paediatrica* 88, 7–12.

Heaney, R.P., Dowell, M.S., Rafferty, K. and Bierman, J. (2000) Bioavailability of the calcium in fortified soy imitation milk, with some observations on method. *American Journal of Clinical Nutrition* 71, 1166–1169.

Hill, D.J., Hosking, C.S., Zhie, C.Y., Leung, R., Barawidjaja, K., Iikura, Y., Iyngkaran, N., Gonzalez-Andaya, A., Wah, L.B. and Hsieh, K.H. (1997) The frequency of food allergy in Australia and Asia. *Environmental Toxicology and Pharmacology* 4, 101–110.

Hong, S.-J., Michael, J.G., Fehringer, A. and Leung, D.Y.M. (1999) Pepsin digested peanut contains T-cell epitopes but no IgE epitopes. *Journal of Allergy and Clinical Immunology* 104, 473–477.

Høst, A. (1994) Cow's milk protein allergy and intolerance in infancy. *Pediatric Allergy and Immunology* 5(Suppl. 5), 5–36.

Høst, A. and Halken, S. (1990) A prospective study of cow's milk allergy in Danish infants during the first 3 years of life: clinical course in relation to clinical and immunological type of hypersensitivity reaction. *Allergy* 45, 587–596.

Hourihane, J.O., Roberts, S.A. and Warner, J.O. (1998) Resolution of peanut allergy: case–control study. *British Medical Journal* 316, 1271–1275.

Howell, W.M., Turner, S.J., Hourihane, J.O., Dean, T.P. and Warner, J.O. (1998) HLA class II DRB 1 and DPB 1 genotypic associations with peanut allergy: evidence from a family based and case-control study. *Clinical and Experimental Allergy* 28, 156–162.

Hurrell, R.F., Juillerat, M.A., Reddy, M.B., Lynch, S.R., Dassenko, S.A. and Cook, J.D. (1992) Soy protein, phytate and iron absorption in humans. *American Journal of Clinical Nutrition* 56, 573–578.

Ishizaka, T. and Ishizaka, K. (1984) Activation of mast cells for mediator release through IgE receptors. *Progress in Allergy* 34, 188–235.

Isolauri, E., Salminen, S. and Mattila-Sandholm, T. (1999) New functional foods in the treatment of food allergy. *Annals of Medicine* 31, 299–302.

Jones, A.C., Miles, E.A., Warner, J.O., Colwell, B.M., Bryant, T.N. and Warner, J.A. (1996) Fetal peripheral blood mononuclear cell proliferative responses to mitogenic and allergenic stimuli during gestation. *Pediatric Allergy and Immunology* 7, 109–116.

Kalliomäki, M., Kirjavainen, P., Eerola, E., Kero, P., Salminen, S. and Isolauri, E. (2001) Distinct patterns of neonatal gut microflora in infant in whom atopy was and was not developing. *Journal of Allergy and Clinical Immunology* 107, 129–134.

Kazemi-Shirazi, L., Pauli, G., Purohit, A., Spitzauer, S., Fröschi, R., Hoffmann-Sommergruber, K., Breiteneder, H., Scheiner, O., Kraft, D. and Valenta, R. (2000) Quantitative IgE inhibition experiments with purified recombinant allergens indicate pollen derived allergens as the sensitizing agents responsible for many forms of plant food allergy. *Journal of Allergy and Clinical Immunology* 105, 116–125.

Kirjavainen P.V., Apostolou, E., Salminen, S.J. and Isolauri, E. (1999) New aspects of probiotics – a novel approach in the management of food allergy. *Allergy* 54, 909–915.

Lehrer, S.B., Horner, W.E. and Reese, G. (1996) Why are some proteins allergenic? Implications for biotechnology. *Critical Reviews in Food Science and Nutrition* 36, 553–564.

Lonnerdal, B., Cederblad, A., Davidsson, L. and Sandstrom, B. (1984) The effect of individual components of soy formula and cows' milk formula on zinc bioavailability. *American Journal of Clinical Nutrition* 40, 1064–1070.

Majamaa, H. and Isolauri, E. (1997) Probiotics: a novel approach in the management of food allergy. *Journal of Allergy and Clinical Immunology* 99, 179–185.

Maleki, S.J., Chung, S.-Y., Champagne, E.T. and Raufman, J.-P. (2000) The effects of roasting on the allergenic properties of peanut proteins. *Journal of Allergy and Clinical Immunology* 106, 763–768.

Marian, F.L., Visser, M., Weinberg, E. and Potter, P.C. (1999) Exposure to peanuts *in utero* and in infancy and the development of sensitization to peanut allergens in young children. *Pediatric Allergy and Immunology* 10, 27–32.

Matsuzaki, T., Yamazaki, R., Hashimoto, S. and Yokokura, T. (1998) The effect of oral feeding of *Lactobacillus casei* strain Shirota on immunoglobulin E production in mice. *Journal of Dairy Science* 81, 48–53.

Metcalfe, D.D., Astwood, J.D., Townsend, R., Sampson, H.A., Taylor, S.L. and Fuchs, R.L. (1996) Assessment of the allergenic potential of foods derived from genetically engineered crop plants. *Critical Reviews in Food Science and Nutrition* 36, S165–S186.

Moneret-Vautrin, D. (1986) Food antigens and additives. *Journal of Allergy and Clinical Immunology* 78, 1039–1045.

Nestle, M. (1996) Allergies to transgenic foods: questions of policy. *New England Journal of Medicine* 334, 726–727.

Nordlee, J.A., Taylor, S.L., Townsend, J.A., Thomas, L.A. and Bush, R.K. (1996) Identification of a Brazil nut allergen in transgenic soybeans. *New England Journal of Medicine* 334, 688–692.

Opara, E.I., Oehlschlager, S.L. and Hanley, A.B. (1998) Immunoglobulin E mediated food allergy: modelling and application of diagnostic and predictive tests for existing and novel foods. *Biomarkers* 3, 1–19.

Opara, E.I., Oehlschlager, S.L., Day, L., Ridley, S.A., Vaughan, R. and Hanley, A.B. (1999) An *in vitro* cell based model for assessing the potential of allergens to release mediators through the cross-linking of IgE. *Toxicology In Vitro* 13, 811–815.

Ouwehand, A.C., Isolauri, E., He, F., Hashimoto, H., Benno, Y. and Salminen, S. (2001) Differences in *Bifidobacterium* flora composition in allergic and healthy infants. *Journal of Allergy and Clinical Immunology* 108, 144–145.

Peat, J.K., Allen, J. and Oddy, W. (1999) Beyond breast-feeding. *Journal of Allergy and Clinical Immunology* 104, 526–530.

Perkin, J.E. (2000) The latex and food allergy connection. *Journal of the American Dietetics Association* 100, 1381–1384.

Reddy, M.B., Hurrell, R.F., Juillerat, M.A. and Cook, J.D. (1996) The influence of different protein sources on phytate inhibition of nonheme-iron absorption in humans. *American Journal of Clinical Nutrition* 63, 203–207.

Roy, K., Mao, H.-Q., Huang, S.-K. and Leong, K.W. (1999) Oral gene delivery with chitosan-DNA nanoparticles generates immunogenic protection in a murine model of peanut allergy. *Nature Medicine* 5, 387–391.

Sampson, H.A. (1996) Managing peanut allergy. *British Medical Journal* 312, 1050–1051.

Sampson, H.A. (1997) Immediate reactions to foods in infants and children. In: Metcalf, D.D., Sampson, H.A. and Simon, R.A. (eds) *Food Allergy: Adverse Reactions to Foods and Food Additives*, 2nd edn. Blackwell Science, Oxford, pp. 169–182.

Sampson, H.A. (2001) Utility of food-specific IgE concentrations in predicting symptomatic food allergy. *Journal of Allergy and Clinical Immunology* 107, 891–896

Sampson, H.A. and Ho, D.G. (1997) Relationship between food-specific concentrations and the risk of positive food challenges in children and adolescents. *Journal of Allergy and Clinical Immunology* 100, 444–451.

Sandstrom, B., Cederblad, A. and Lonnerdal, B. (1983) Zinc absorption from human milk, cow's milk and infant formulas. *American Journal of Diseases of Childhood* 137, 726–729.

Shin, D.S., Compadre, C.M., Malek, S.J., Kopper, R.A., Sampson, H.A., Huang, S.K., Burks, A.W. and Bannon, G.A. (1998) Biochemical and structural analysis of IgE binding sites on *Ara h* 1, an abundant and highly allergenic peanut protein. *Journal of Biological Chemistry* 273, 13753–13759.

Sicherer, S.H., Muñoz-Furlong, A., Burks, A.W. and Sampson, H.A. (1999) Prevalence of peanut and tree nut allergy in the United States of America determined by a random digit dial telephone survey. *Journal of Allergy and Clinical Immunology* 103, 559–562.

Sicherer, S.H., Furlong, T.J., Maes, H.H., Desnick, R.J., Sampson, H.A. and Gelb, B.D. (2000) Genetics of peanut allergy: a twin study. *Journal of Allergy and Clinical Immunology* 106, 53–56.

Taylor, S.L. and Hefle, S.L. (2001a) Will genetically modified food be allergenic? *Journal of Allergy and Clinical Immunology* 107, 756–771.

Taylor, S.L. and Hefle, S.L. (2001b) Allergenic risk from novel plants is very important and difficult to predict: reply. *Journal of Allergy and Clinical Immunology* 108, 654.

Taylor, S.L. and Lehrer, S.B. (1996) Principles and characteristics of food allergens. *Critical Reviews in Food Science and Nutrition* 36, S91–S118.

Tilles, S.A. and Schocket, A.L. (1997) Exercise- and pressure-induced syndromes. In: Metcalf, D.D., Sampson, H.A. and Simon, R.A. (eds) *Food Allergy: Adverse Reactions to Foods and Food Additives*, 2nd edn. Blackwell Science, Oxford, pp. 303–310.

Trapp, C.L., Chang, C.C., Halpern, G.M., Keen, C.L. and Gerschwin, M.E. (1993) The influence of chronic yoghurt consumption on populations of young and elderly adults. *International Journal of Immunotherapy* 9, 53–64.

Vadas, P., Wai, Y., Burks, W. and Perelman, B. (2001) Detection of peanut allergens in breast milk of lactating women. *Journal of the American Medical Association* 285, 1746–1748

Warner, J.A., Jones, C.A., Jones, A.C. and Warner, J.O. (2000) Prenatal origins of allergic disease. *Journal of Allergy and Clinical Immunology* 105, S493–S496.

Watson, W.T.A. (1995) Food allergy in children: diagnostic strategies. *Clinical Reviews in Allergy and Immunology* 13, 347–359.

Wills-Karp, M., Santeliz, J. and Karp, C.L. (2001) The germless theory of allergic disease: revisiting the hygiene hypothesis. *Nature Reviews: Immunology* 1, 69–75.

Zeiger, R.S. (2000) Dietary aspects of food allergy prevention in infants and children. *Journal of Pediatric Gastroenterology and Nutrition* 30, S77–S86.

16 Exercise and Immune Function – Effect of Nutrition

EMIL WOLSK PETERSEN AND BENTE KLARLUND PEDERSEN

Copenhagen Muscle Research Centre and Department of Infectious Diseases, Rigshospitalet, University of Copenhagen, Tagensvej 20, 2200 Copenhagen N, Denmark

Introduction

Regular recreational exercise is generally understood to be beneficial to health, whereas total inactivity is detrimental. Regular exercise may increase resistance to infections such as the common cold, whereas hard training is associated with increased respiratory-tract infections (Brines *et al.*, 1996). Indeed, as early as 1902, the Boston marathon was used as an experiment in violent exercise to demonstrate post-exercise leucocytosis, and, in more recent years, it has been shown that élite athletes may become more immune-suppressed through over-training (see Hoffman-Goetz and Pedersen, 1994). The physiological basis of altered resistance to infections is not well understood, but exercise-induced changes in the cellular immune system are among the possible explanations. The relationship between nutritional factors and resistance to infections has generated considerable interest over the past several decades. It is possible that the exercise-induced immunological changes can be modulated by nutritional factors and that dietary factors influence resting levels of immune activity in athletes (Pedersen *et al.*, 1998, 1999).

Exercise and Immune Function

Effects of acute exercise

Acute exercise induces dramatic changes in the immune system (for an extensive review, see Pedersen and Hoffman-Goetz, 2000). The neutrophil concentration in the bloodstream increases during exercise and continues to increase post-exercise. The lymphocyte concentration increases during exercise but falls below pre-exercise values following intense long-duration exercise, although not after moderate exercise.

© CAB *International* 2002. *Nutrition and Immune Function*
(eds P.C. Calder, C.J. Field and H.S. Gill)

Several reports describe exercise-induced changes in subsets of blood lymphocytes (for references, see Pedersen and Hoffman-Goetz, 2000). Increased lymphocyte concentration is probably due to the recruitment of all lymphocyte subpopulations (CD4+ T-cells, CD8+ T-cells, B-cells and natural killer (NK) cells) to the vascular compartment. During exercise, the CD4/CD8 ratio of circulating lymphocytes decreases, reflecting the greater increase in CD8+ lymphocytes than in CD4+ lymphocytes. CD4+ and CD8+ T-cells contain both CD45RO+ (memory) and CD45RA+ (naive) cells. It has been shown that it is mainly memory cells that are mobilized to the circulation in response to acute physical exercise (Bruunsgaard et al., 1999). It has also been shown that the lymphocytes recruited to the blood have short telomere lengths (Bruunsgaard et al., 1999), which strongly indicates that 'old' lymphocytes with a long replicative history are recruited to the blood. Thus, the initial increase in CD4+ and CD8+ cells after exercise is not due to repopulation by newly generated cells but may be a redistribution of activated cells. It is therefore likely that the cells are mobilized from peripheral compartments, such as the spleen, and it has indeed been demonstrated that splenectomized patients are not able to mount a normal lymphocyte response to exercise (Nielsen et al., 1997).

Following intense long-duration exercise the functions of NK, T- and B-cells are suppressed (for references, see Pedersen and Hoffman-Goetz, 2000). Thus, NK-cell activity (the ability to kill target tumour cells) and lymphocyte proliferation are inhibited. Furthermore, B-cell function is inhibited and the local production of secretory immunoglobulin (Ig)A in saliva decreases (Gleeson and Pyne, 2000).

There are few studies that document immune function in vivo in relation to exercise. However, impairment of in vivo cell-mediated immunity, but not specific antibody production, could be demonstrated after intense exercise of long duration (triathlon race) (Bruunsgaard et al., 1997). The cellular immune system was evaluated as a delayed-type hypersensitivity (DTH) 'skin'-test response to seven recall antigens. The response was significantly lower in subjects who performed a triathlon race compared with triathletes and untrained controls who did not participate in the triathlon. However, no differences in specific antibody titres to pneumococcal, diphtheria or tetanus vaccines were found between the groups (Bruunsgaard et al., 1997).

In summary, during moderate as well as intense exercise, lymphocytes are mobilized to the circulation. However, following intense exercise, the lymphocyte concentration declines, T-cell proliferation is impaired, NK-cell function is decreased and the level of IgA in saliva is suppressed. During the post-exercise immune impairment, also called 'the open window' in the immune system, it has been suggested that microorganisms may invade the host and establish infections (Fig. 16.1).

Strenuous exercise also induces increased circulating levels of several cytokines in the blood (for a review, see Pedersen, 2000). Interleukin (IL)-6 has been found to be markedly enhanced in several studies. Thus, after a marathon, the concentration of IL-6 in the bloodstream has been shown to increase 100-fold (Ostrowski et al., 1999). Recent studies demonstrate that IL-6 is produced locally in contracting skeletal muscles and that the net-IL-6 release

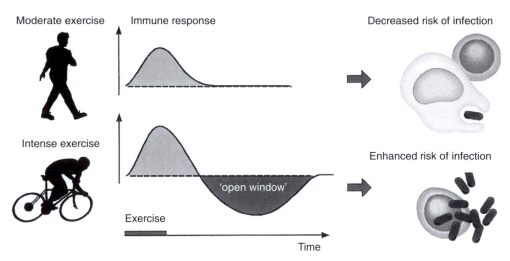

Fig. 16.1. Generalized scheme of the effects of moderate and intense exercise on immune function and susceptibility to infection. During moderate and intense exercise, the immune system is enhanced (as shown by mobilization of lymphocytes to the circulation), but intense exercise is followed by a period of immune impairment (decreased natural killer cell activity, lymphocyte proliferation and levels of salivary immunoglobulin A), during which there is an 'open window' of opportunity for pathogens.

from skeletal muscles can solely account for the exercise-induced increase in arterial plasma IL-6 (Steensberg *et al.*, 2000). It is likely that IL-6 mediates some of the exercise-related metabolic responses (Steensberg *et al.*, 2001). A full cytokine cascade develops in response to exercise, including tumour necrosis factor (TNF)-α, IL-1β, IL-1 receptor antagonist (IL-1ra), IL-8, IL-10, TNF-receptors (TNF-R) and macrophage inhibitory proteins (MIP)-1 (Pedersen *et al.*, 2001; Fig. 16.2).

Effects of chronic exercise

Although exercise has an acute effect on circulating lymphocyte numbers, on immune cell functions and on plasma cytokine concentrations (see above), many immune functions are similar in resting athletes and non-athletes (see Nieman, 2000). Components of the adaptive immune system (measured in resting athletes) seem to be largely unaffected by intensive and prolonged exercise training. The innate immune system appears to respond differentially to the chronic stress of intensive exercise, with NK-cell activity tending to be enhanced, while neutrophil function is suppressed.

Based on epidemiological studies a relationship between exercise and upper respiratory-tract infections (URTI) has been modelled in the form of a 'J-shaped' curve. This model suggests that while the risk of URTI may decrease below that of a sedentary individual when one engages in moderate exercise training, the risk may rise above average during periods of excessive amounts

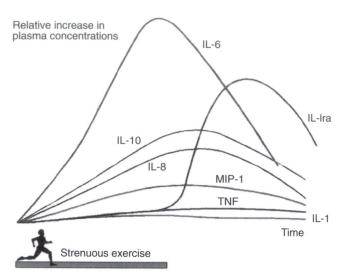

Fig. 16.2. Changes in plasma cytokine concentrations in relation to strenuous exercise. TNF, tumour necrosis factor; IL, interleukin; IL-1ra, IL-1 receptor antagonist; MIP, macrophage inhibitory protein.

of high-intensity exercise. The link between exercise-associated immune changes and sensitivity to infections may be explained by the so-called 'open window' of altered immunity. It is hypothesized that viruses and bacteria may gain a foothold, increasing the risk of sub-clinical and clinical infection. However, it remains to be demonstrated if athletes showing the most extreme immunosuppression following heavy exertion are those that contract an infection within the following 1–2 weeks.

Exercise, Nutrition and Immune Function

The mechanisms underlying exercise-associated immune changes are multifactorial and include neuroendocrinological factors, such as adrenalin, noradrenalin, growth hormone, cortisol and beta-endorphin (see Pedersen and Hoffman-Goetz, 2000; Fig. 16.3). It has been suggested that altered protein metabolism, such as decreased glutamine concentration in the plasma, influences lymphocyte function and that decreased plasma glucose concentration increases stress-hormone levels and thereby reduces immune function. Furthermore, as a consequence of the catecholamine- and growth-hormone-induced immediate changes in leucocyte subsets, the relative proportions of these subsets change and activated leucocyte subpopulations may be mobilized to the blood. Free radicals and prostaglandins (PG) released by the elevated number of neutrophils and monocytes may influence the function of lymphocytes and contribute to the impaired function of the latter cells. Thus, nutritional supplementation with glutamine, carbohydrate, antioxidants or PG inhibitors may, in principle, influence exercise-associated changes in immune function.

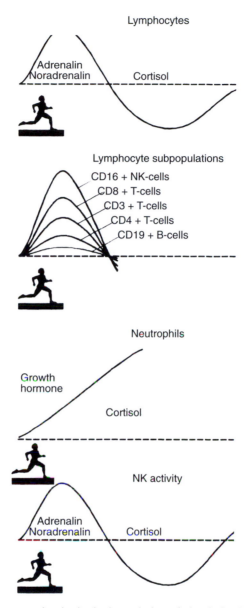

Fig. 16.3. A model of the neuroendocrinological regulation of circulating leucocyte subpopulations and natural killer (NK) cell activity in response to exercise.

Glutamine

Skeletal muscle is the major tissue involved in glutamine production and is known to release glutamine into the bloodstream at a high rate (see Calder and Newsholme, Chapter 6, this volume). It has been suggested that the skeletal muscle plays a vital role in maintenance of the key process of glutamine utilization in the immune cells. Consequently, the activity of the skeletal muscle may directly influence the immune system. It has been hypothesized that during intense physical exercise, or in relation to surgery, trauma, burn and sepsis, the demand on muscle and other organs for glutamine is such that the immune system may be forced into a glutamine debt, which temporarily affects its function (see Calder and Newsholme, Chapter 6, this volume). Thus, factors that directly or indirectly influence glutamine synthesis or release could theoretically influence the function of immune cells (see Calder and Newsholme, Chapter 6, this volume). Following intense long-term exercise and other physical stress disorders, the glutamine concentration in plasma declines (Rohde *et al.*, 1998a). In four placebo-controlled glutamine intervention studies (Rohde *et al.*, 1998b, c; Krzywkowski *et al.*, 2001a, b), it was found that glutamine supplementation abolished the post-exercise decline in plasma glutamine without influencing post-exercise impairment in immune function. Thus, these studies do not support the hypothesis that the post-exercise decline in immune function is caused by a decrease in the plasma glutamine concentration.

Carbohydrate

Earlier research has established that a reduction in blood glucose levels is linked to hypothalamic–pituitary–adrenal activation, increased release of adrenocorticotrophic hormone and cortisol, increased plasma growth hormone, decreased insulin and a variable effect on blood adrenalin level. Given the link between stress hormones and immune responses to prolonged and intensive exercise, increased availability of carbohydrate should maintain plasma glucose concentrations and attenuate increases in stress hormones and thereby diminish changes in immunity. This hypothesis has been tested in a number of studies, using double-blind, placebo-controlled randomized designs. Carbohydrate beverage ingestion before, during and after 2.5 h of exercise was associated with higher plasma glucose levels, an attenuated cortisol and growth-hormone response, fewer perturbations in blood immune cell counts, lower granulocyte and monocyte phagocytosis and oxidative-burst activity and a diminished pro- and anti-inflammatory cytokine response (for a review, see Nieman, 1998). Overall, the hormonal and immune responses in the subjects taking carbohydrate were less affected by exercise than in subjects in the placebo groups. Some immune variables were affected slightly by carbohydrate ingestion (e.g. granulocyte and monocyte function), while others were strongly influenced (e.g. plasma cytokine concentrations, blood immune cell numbers) (see Nieman, 1998). The clinical significance of these carbohydrate-induced effects on the endocrine and immune systems awaits further research. At this point, the data indicate that athletes ingesting carbohydrate beverages before, during and after prolonged and intensive exercise should experience lowered physiological stress. Research to determine whether carbohydrate ingestion will improve host protection against viruses in endurance athletes during periods of intensified training or following competitive endurance events is warranted.

Lipids

There are two principal classes of polyunsaturated fatty acids (PUFA): the n-6 and the n-3 families (see Calder and Field, Chapter 4, this volume). The precursor of the n-6 family is linoleic acid, which is converted to arachidonic acid, the precursor of PG and leucotrienes (LT), which have potent pro-inflammatory and immunoregulatory properties (see Calder and Field, Chapter 4, this volume). The precursor of the n-3 family of PUFA is α-linolenic acid. If the ratio of n-6 to n-3 PUFA in the diet is decreased by administration of a diet rich in n-3 fatty acids, PGE_2-mediated immunosuppression may be abolished (see Calder and Field, Chapter 4, this volume).

The possible interaction between intense acute exercise, immune function and PUFA was examined in inbred female C57Bl/6 mice. The animals received either a natural ingredient diet or a diet supplemented with various fats, such as beef tallow, safflower oil (rich in the n-6 PUFA linoleic acid), fish oil (rich in long-chain n-3 PUFA) or linseed oil (rich in the n-3 PUFA α-linolenic acid) for an 8-week period. Linseed oil abolished post-exercise suppression of the IgM plaque-forming cell response (Benquet et al., 1994). Although some experiments show that the increase in IL-1 and TNF following administration of endotoxin is reduced when the animals are pretreated with n-3 PUFA as fish oil (see Calder and Field, Chapter 4, this volume), a recent study showed that n-3 PUFA did not influence the exercise-induced elevation of pro- or anti-inflammatory cytokines (Toft et al., 2000).

Antioxidants

During exercise, the enhanced oxygen utilization leads to production of reactive oxygen species, as indicated by the blood glutathione redox status. Antioxidants may in theory neutralize the reactive species that are produced by neutrophilic leucocytes during phagocytosis (see Hughes, Chapter 9, this volume). The effect of vitamin C supplementation on lymphocyte function and stress-hormone levels after exercise has been studied. Supplementation with vitamin C did not influence circulating leucocyte subsets, NK-cell activity, lymphocyte proliferative responses, granulocyte phagocytosis or activated burst or circulating concentrations of catecholamines and cortisol (Nieman et al., 1997; Petersen et al., 2001).

Conclusion

There is recruitment of lymphocytes to the circulation during exercise. Following strenuous exercise, the lymphocyte count declines, natural immunity and T-cell proliferation are impaired and the level of secretory IgA in saliva is low. Few studies have addressed the potential protective role of dietary supplementation in exercise-induced immunosuppression. Exercise-related immunosuppression in animals was prevented by a diet rich in n-3 fatty acids, but there is a lack of human studies. Antioxidant supplementation has no effect on exercise induced changes in NK and T-cell functions, but vitamin C supplementation has been shown to decrease the incidence of post-race URTI symptoms in some studies. Glutamine supplementation has not been effective in abolishing post-exercise suppression of the immune system, whereas carbohydrate loading diminishes the hormonal and immune responses to exercise. The clinical consequences of carbohydrate loading remain to be determined. At this point in time, it is premature to make recommendations regarding nutritional supplementation to avoid exercise-induced immune changes.

Acknowledgement

The authors' work was supported by the National Research Foundation grant no. 504–14.

References

Benquet, C., Krzystyniak, K., Savard, R. and Guertin, F. (1994) Modulation of exercise-induced immunosuppression by dietary polyunsaturated fatty acids in mice. *Journal of Toxicology and Environmental Health* 43, 225–227.

Brines, R., Hoffman-Goetz, L. and Pedersen B.K. (1996) Can your exercise make your immune system fitter? *Immunology Today* 17, 252–254.

Bruunsgaard, H., Hartkopp, A., Mohr, T., Konradsen, H., Heron, I., Mordhorst, C.H. and Pedersen, B.K. (1997) *In vivo* cell-mediated immunity and vaccination response following prolonged, intense, exercise. *Medicine and Science in Sports and Exercise* 29, 1176–1181.

Bruunsgaard, H., Jensen, M.S., Schjerling, P., Halkjær-Kristensen, J., Ogawa, K., Skinhøj, P. and Pedersen, B.K. (1999) Exercise induces recruitment of lymphocytes with an activated phenotype and short telomere lengths in young and elderly humans. *Life Sciences* 65, 2623–2633.

Gleeson, M. and Pyne, D.B. (2000) Exercise effects on mucosal immunity. *Immunology and Cell Biology* 78, 536–544.

Hoffman-Goetz, L. and Pedersen, B.K. (1994) Exercise and the immune system: a model of the stress response? *Immunology Today* 15, 345–392.

Krzywkowski, K., Petersen, E.W., Ostrowski, K., Boza, J., Halkjaer-Kristensen, J. and Pedersen, B.K. (2001a) Effect of glutamine supplementation on exercise-induced changes in lymphocyte function. *American Journal of Physiology* 281, C1259-C1265.

Krzywkowski, K., Petersen, E.W., Ostrowski, K., Link-Amster, H., Boza, J., Halkjaer-Kristensen, J. and Pedersen, B.K. (2001b) Effect of glutamine and protein supplementation on exercise-induced decrease in saliva secretory IgA in athletes. *Journal of Applied Physiology* 91, 832–838.

Nielsen, H.B., Halkjær-Kristensen, J., Christensen, N.J. and Pedersen, B.K. (1997) Splenectomy impairs lymphocytosis during maximal exercise. *American Journal of Physiology* 272, R1847–R1852.

Nieman, D.C. (1998) Influence of carbohydrate on the immune responses to intensive, prolonged exercise. *Exercise Immunology Review* 4, 64–76.

Nieman, D.C. (2000) Is infection risk linked to exercise work load? *Medicine and Science in Sports and Exercise* 32, S406–S411.

Nieman, D.C., Henson, D.A., Butterworth, D.E., Warren, B.J., Davis, J.M., Fagoaga, O.R. and Nehlsen-Canarella, S.L. (1997) Vitamin C supplementation does not alter the immune response to 2.5 hours of running. *International Journal of Sports Nutrition* 7, 173–184.

Ostrowski, K., Rohde, T., Asp, S., Schjerling, P. and Pedersen, B.K. (1999) Pro- and anti-inflammatory cytokine balance in strenuous exercise in humans. *Journal of Physiology* 515, 287–291.

Pedersen, B.K. (2000) Exercise and cytokines. *Immunology and Cell Biology* 78, 532–535.

Pedersen, B.K. and Hoffman-Goetz, L. (2000) Exercise and the immune system: regulation, integration and adaptation. *Physiological Reviews* 80, 1055–1081.

Pedersen, B.K., Ostrowski, K., Rohde, T. and Bruunsgaard, H. (1998) Nutrition, exercise and the immune system. *Proceedings of the Nutrition Society* 57, 43–47.

Pedersen, B.K., Bruunsgaard, H., Jensen, M., Krzywkowski, K. and Ostrowski, K. (1999) Exercise and immune function: effect of ageing and nutrition. *Proceedings of the Nutrition Society* 58, 733–742.

Pedersen, B.K., Steensberg, A. and Schjerling, P. (2001) Muscle-derived interleukin – possible metabolic effects: topical review. *Journal of Physiology* 536, 329–337.

Petersen, E.W., Ostrowski, K., Ibfelt, T., Richelle, M., Offord, E., Halkjær-Kristensen, J. and Pedersen, B.K. (2001) Effect of vitamin supplementation on the cytokine response and on muscle damage following strenuous exercise. *American Journal of Physiology* 280, C1570–C1575.

Rohde, T., Krzywkowski, K. and Pedersen, B.K. (1998a) Glutamine, exercise and the immune system: is there a link? *Exercise Immunology Review* 4, 49–63.

Rohde, T., MacLean, D.A. and Pedersen, B.K. (1998b) Effect of glutamine supplementation on changes in the immune system induced by repeated exercise. *Medicine and Science in Sports and Exercise* 30, 856–862.

Rohde, T., Asp, S., MacLean, D.A. and Pedersen, B.K. (1998c) Competitive sustained exercise in humans, lymphokine activated killer cell activity, and glutamine – an intervention study. *European Journal of Applied Physiology* 78, 448–453.

Steensberg, A., van Hall, G., Osada, T., Sachetti, M., Saltin, B. and Pedersen, B.K. (2000) Production of IL-6 in contracting human skeletal muscles can account for the exercise-induced increase in plasma IL-6. *Journal of Physiology* 529, 237–242.

Steensberg, A., Febbraio, M.A., Osada, T., Schjerling, P., van Hall, G., Saltin, B. and Pedersen, B.K. (2001) Low glycogen content increases interleukin-6 production in contracting human skeletal muscle. *Journal of Physiology* 537, 633–639.

Toft, A.D., Ostrowski, K., Asp, S., Møller, K., Iversen, S., Hermann, C., Søndergaard, S.R. and Pedersen, B.K. (2000) The effects of n-3 PUFA on the cytokine response to strenuous exercise. *Journal of Applied Physiology* 89, 2401–2405.

17 Nutrition and Ageing of the Immune System

BRUNO LESOURD*, AGATHE RAYNAUD-SIMON AND LYNDA MAZARI

Département de Gérontologie Clinique, Hôpital Nord du CHU de Clermont-Ferrand, BP 56, 63118 Cébazat, France

Introduction

Many experimental and clinical data gathered over a number of years have demonstrated a marked decline in many immune responses with the ageing process (Makinodan and Kay, 1980; Lesourd, 1990a; Miller, 1992). In contrast, in recent years it has emerged that some immune responses do not decline, and can even increase, with age (Kubo and Cinader, 1990, Ershler *et al.*, 1993; Barrat *et al.*, 1997). As a consequence, the influence of ageing on the immune system is generally described nowadays as a progressive occurrence of dysregulation, rather than as a general decline in function (Weksler, 1995; Cakman *et al.*, 1996). In addition, it has also been shown that many decreased immune responses described as age-related are actually linked to other factors, such as poor nutritional status (Lesourd, 1990a, 1999; Lesourd and Mazari, 1999). In fact, in carefully selected, very healthy subjects, decreased immune responses are observed only in the very oldest (> 90 years of age) (Mazari and Lesourd, 1998).

Most investigations into ageing in human subjects rely on data from apparently healthy aged individuals without checking for the possibility of underlying factors, such as ongoing disease, which is not clinically apparent, or poor nutritional status. However, some studies have attempted to identify such confounding factors. The first was the use of the Senieur protocol (Ligthart *et al.*, 1984), but later studies added additional factors for the selection of very healthy elderly subjects (Reibnegger *et al.*, 1988; Lesourd *et al.*, 1994; Lesourd and Mazari, 1999). In such very carefully selected aged individuals, the immune changes observed are due to the ageing process alone, and not to environmental (including nutritional) influences. In fact, we reported that changes due to

*Corresponding author.

© CAB *International* 2002. *Nutrition and Immune Function*
(eds P.C. Calder, C.J. Field and H.S. Gill)

nutritional factors in aged subjects are similar to what was previously described as immune ageing (Lesourd and Meaume, 1994; Lesourd *et al.*, 1994). Furthermore, the changes of immune responses in aged individuals are proportional to the intensity of the observed nutritional deficits (Lesourd *et al.*, 1992).

This chapter will describe:

1. The primary ageing immune deficiency. This is observed in the very carefully selected healthy elderly (VCSH elderly), in whom all known influence of external factors has been eliminated. We focus here on studies comparing VCSH elderly persons of different ages, referred to as 'young elderly' (60–80 years of age) and 'old elderly' (> 90 years of age), with young adults. These subjects fit the Senieur criteria for healthiness and, in addition, have 'normal' nutritional status (as defined by the EURONUT/SENECA European study (Haller *et al.*, 1996)) and a serum albumin concentration > 39 g l^{-1}.
2. The secondary nutritionally induced immune deficiency in the elderly. This can be observed in VCSH elderly persons with poor nutritional status but without any detectable acute and/or chronic disease. These subjects are referred to as 'apparently healthy elderly'. These subjects fit the same criteria as the VCSH elderly except that they have a serum albumin concentration of 30–39 g l^{-1}.
3. The tertiary immune deficiency in the elderly. This corresponds to the immune responses measured in diseased elderly subjects, in whom not only nutrient deficiencies, but also diseases, induce changes in immune responses.

Primary (Ageing) Immune Deficiency

Decreases in T-cell generation and maturation

Stem cells are generated in bone marrow and mature as T lymphocytes in the thymus. Although stem cell generation does not appear to decline with age, the ability of stem cells to undergo clonal proliferation declines with age (Tyan, 1981), as does thymocyte maturation in relation to thymus involution (Steinmann *et al.*, 1985; Hirokawa *et al.*, 1994). Such involution starts relatively early in life (at puberty) and the major changes are mostly related to the end of the maturation period and to early adulthood, rather than to ageing. Thymic function is almost lost by the age of 60 years.

Changes in peripheral T-cell subsets and functions

Circulating lymphocyte numbers are decreased in aged persons (Lesourd *et al.*, 1994; Huppert *et al.*, 1998), but the decline is usually quite small (10–15%), even in the 'old elderly' when they are very healthy (Mazari and Lesourd, 1998), and indeed the decline is not always observed in 'young elderly' (Wick and Grubeck-Loewenstein, 1997). Although T-cell numbers show little change with ageing, T-cell subsets do change: there are decreases in the number of fully mature T-cells (CD3+) and parallel increases in the number of 'immature' T-cells (CD2+ CD3–) (Lesourd *et al.*, 1994; Table 17.1). Equivalent changes are observed in both 'young elderly' and 'old elderly', indicating that they mainly occur earlier in life, probably at middle age (Mazari and Lesourd, 1998). It appears that this change is simply a marker of the end of the T-cell maturation period, rather than a phenomenon linked to old age. As a consequence, peripheral T lymphocytes from aged subjects exhibit lower proliferative ability, since the CD2+ CD3– subset has a lower proliferative response than the CD3+ subset (Alès-Martinez *et al.*, 1988). The inability of the thymus to generate new T lymphocytes is partly compensated, in aged animals (Abo, 1992) and in humans (Lesourd *et al.*, 1994), by the occurrence of new T-cells, which are not fully mature, in other primary immune organs, such as the liver (Nakayama *et al.*, 1994). As a result, aged individuals have difficulty in generating fully mature T lymphocytes, and this becomes most apparent when there is an increased need for this. For example, lung infections induce killing of peripheral T lymphocytes and, as a consequence, cause lymphopenia in the elderly (Proust *et al.*, 1986), since the elderly are unable to rapidly generate new T-cells.

Two other changes in T-cell subsets occur with ageing. There is a decrease in naive T-cell (CD45RA+) numbers, with a parallel increase in memory T-cell (CD45RO+) numbers (Cossarizza *et al.*, 1992) and a decrease in cytotoxic T-cell (CD8+) numbers (Lesourd and Meaume, 1994; Lesourd *et al.*, 1994; Wick and Grubeck-Loewenstein, 1997). The switch from CD45RA to CD45RO occurs mainly within the first three decades of life, when the individual is inducing new immune responses to antigens not previously encountered. Within the third decade, about 65% of peripheral T lymphocytes bear CD45RO (Cossarizza *et al.*, 1992; Mazari and Lesourd, 1998; Table 17.1). Later in life, the switch towards CD45RO continues, but at a far slower rate (10% increase from 30 to 80 years of age). Therefore, this important change is not an ageing phenomenon but rather a component of the maturation of the immune system (Lesourd, 2000).

The change in CD8+ T-cell numbers mainly occurs during adulthood (20–25% decrease from age 20 to 70) and is associated with decreases in the subset exhibiting the highest level of expression of CD8 molecules on the cell surface (Lesourd *et al.*, 1994). This is probably related to changes in T-helper (Th) cells (see below) and is partly compensated for by an increase in the CD8+ subset exhibiting a low level of expression of CD8 (Lesourd *et al.*, 1994; Mazari and Lesourd, 1998), probably generated within the liver. Both changes result in lower cell-mediated immune functions. CD45RO memory cells are poor interleukin (IL)-2 secretors and therefore exhibit lower proliferative levels (Nagelkerken *et al.*, 1991; Hobbs and Ernst, 1997). Thus, the change in the naive/memory ratio with ageing will result in lower lymphocyte proliferative responses. Nevertheless, these changes are probably not of very great influence on the immune system, since it has recently been shown that 'young elderly' have comparable proliferative responses and similar IL-2 secretion to those of young adults (Mazari and Lesourd, 1998; Myslinska *et al.*, 1998; Table 17.1). The decline in IL-2 production and proliferation occurs only in the very old (Lesourd and Mazari, 1999). The decrease in the number of CD8+ cells is

Table 17.1. Subsets and functions of peripheral blood T lymphocytes from healthy elderly subjects. All subjects were recruited using the Senieur criteria (Ligthart et al., 1984) and additional criteria previously reported (Mazari and Lesourd, 1998).

	Very healthy young adults (25–34 years) (n = 57)		Very healthy 'young elderly' (65–85 years) (n = 41)		Very healthy 'old elderly' (> 90 years) (n = 19)		Apparently healthy 'young elderly' (70–85 years) (n = 51)	
	Mean	Standard deviation	Mean	Standard deviation	Mean	Standard deviation	Mean	Standard deviation
Age (years)	29.1	3.2	79.6	5.3	94.3	3.2	78.9	6.2
Albumin (g l^{-1})	43.5	2.8	42.4	4.1	41.7	3.7	37.2	3.9
Lymphocytes (number μl^{-1})	2248	456	1993	568	1817*	598	1705**	434
CD2+ cells (number μl^{-1})	2014	321	1794**	397	1586**	434	1511***†	427
CD3+ cells (number μl^{-1})	1897	264	1565**	311	1323**†	356	1207***†	299
CD2+ CD3− cells (number μl^{-1})	117	105	214*	224	254*	242	283**	241
CD4+ cells (number μl^{-1})	1267	209	1136*	243	997*	264	812***††	271
CD8+ cells (number μl^{-1})	672	144	437***	174	378***	211	387***	196
CD45RA cells (number μl^{-1})	1234	314	658***	228	404***††	197	464***†	213
CD45R0 cells (number μl^{-1})	846	201	1222***	365	1192***	462	1057*	497
IL-2 production‡ (ng l^{-1})	2.01	0.35	1.84	0.34	1.21***†	0.44	1.11***††	0.38
IL-6 production (ng l^{-1})	1.37	0.16	1.82*	0.22	1.99***	0.34	1.48	0.40
Lymphocyte proliferation§ (10^3 cpm 10^6 cells^{-1})	152	40	114	35	75**	32	54**†	34

IL, interleukin.
Significant differences from very healthy young adult controls: * $P < 0.05$, ** $P < 0.01$, *** $P < 0.001$.
Significant differences from very healthy 'young elderly': † $P < 0.05$, †† $P < 0.01$.
‡Determined using 5 μg mitogen 10^6 cells^{-1}.
§Determined using 1 μg mitogen 10^6 cells^{-1}.

associated with decreased cytotoxic T-cell function (Bruley-Rosset and Payelle, 1987; Mbawuike *et al.*, 1997). This may be because the cells bearing a low level of CD8 on their surface have poor cytotoxic function.

Since the early 1990s immune ageing has also been described as a change in the ratio of the Th1 to the Th2 phenotype (see Devereux, Chapter 1, this volume). There is a progressive decrease in Th1 function and a relative preservation and/or increase in Th2 function with age (Cakman *et al.*, 1996; Shearer, 1997). Decreased IL-2 secretion, a Th1 function, with age was described some time ago (Rabinowich *et al.*, 1985; Nagel *et al.*, 1988). Nevertheless, such a decline is not observed in all mouse strains (Engwerda *et al.*, 1996). More recently, it was shown that lymphocytes from 'young elderly' subjects produce similar amounts of IL-2 to those from young adults (Mazari and Lesourd, 1998; Myslinska *et al.*, 1998; Lesourd and Mazari, 1999; Table 17.1).

Another Th1 function, interferon-γ (IFN)-γ secretion, has been described as declining with ageing (Chen *et al.*, 1987). This was considered to be a major phenomenon of the ageing immune system, although it could be reversed by exogenous IL-12 supply in a cell-culture setting (Mbawuike *et al.*, 1997), suggesting that decreased IFN-γ production was due to the absence of a stimulating factor rather than to an inability of Th1 cells to respond. Indeed, other reports have shown than IFN-γ production does not decline with age and might even increase (Sindermann *et al.*, 1993; Barrat *et al.*, 1997). IFN-γ is secreted by memory T-cells, as well as Th1 cells (Sanders *et al.*, 1998), which may explain these contradictory reports. In summary, it is not obvious that Th1 functions decline in all aged persons. The influence of ageing on Th1 function may be very different between individuals, linked to differences in genetic background (Proust *et al.*, 1982; Yong-Xing *et al.*, 1997).

Most reports show increases in the release of Th2 cytokines (IL-4, IL-5, IL-6, IL-10) with ageing (Kubo and Cinader, 1990; Daynes *et al.*, 1993; Ershler *et al.*, 1993; Barrat *et al.*, 1997; James *et al.*, 1997). This change starts in middle adulthood (Myslinska *et al.*, 1998) and continues progressively thereafter. Thus, ageing is characterized by a progressive switch towards Th2-type responses. Antigenic pressures throughout life may be responsible for this change. Indeed, it has been reported that a similar change occurs during the evolution of human immunodeficiency virus (HIV) infection and that, when Th2 becomes the dominant response, significant immune deficiency occurs and then the clinical signs of the disease, such as opportunistic infections, start to occur (Clerici *et al.*, 1992).

In summary, if cell-mediated immunity declines with age, this probably occurs at a very old age in very healthy persons, but may occur sooner in some individuals, due to intense and accumulative antigenic pressures throughout life.

Changes in humoral immune responses

Humoral immune responses are less severely affected by the ageing process than cell-mediated immune responses are (Lesourd, 1990a). There are reports of an age-related increase in Immunoglobulins G and A (Batory *et al.*, 1984; Moulias *et al.*, 1984), a change that has been linked to the relative increase in Th2 function (Lesourd, 1997). In contrast, primary antibody responses to vaccine are decreased with ageing, while booster responses are comparable to those seen in earlier adulthood (Moulias *et al.*, 1985). The decreased antibody responses have been associated with age-related decreases in Th-cell function (Miller, 1996) and to the increased production (or accumulation) of anti-idiotype antibodies (Arreaza *et al.*, 1993), which leads to synthesis of antibodies with lower antigen affinities (Muller *et al.*, 1986). The lower affinity of the antibodies produced after vaccination also results from a dysregulation of B-cell subsets with ageing: decreases in the CD5– subset, which produces antibody against foreign antigens, and relative increases in the CD5+ subset, which produces autoantibodies, are observed (Weksler, 1995). Therefore, even though the secondary responses produce similar levels of antibodies (Huang *et al.*, 1992), the antibodies produced exhibit lower antigen specificity and antibody responses are less adapted to the stimulus (Lesourd, 1997).

Changes in monocyte–macrophage functions

The functions of monocytes and macrophages are preserved, or even enhanced, with the ageing process (Lesourd, 1999; Table 17.2). Antigen processing and presentation are comparable in young and old mice (Goidl, 1987; Doria, 1988). IL-1 release is sustained in old mice (Goldberg *et al.*, 1991) and in elderly humans (Nafziger *et al.*, 1993; Mazari and Lesourd, 1998). IL-6 release is increased by cells from 'young elderly' compared with those from young adults (Mazari and Lesourd, 1998; Table 17.2). Macrophages from aged animals and humans exhibit greater production of prostaglandin (PG)E_2 and free radicals (Meydani *et al.*, 1986, 1995; Hayek *et al.*, 1997). There may be a continuous activation of these cells. This is certainly of great importance, since PGE_2 induces suppression of T-cell functions and since lymphocytes from aged individuals are more susceptible to PGE_2 than those from younger individuals (Goodwin, 1992). Therefore, ageing may be characterized by a continuous ongoing monocyte activation, which induces a permanent suppression of T-cell functions. This represents another age-related dysregulation of the immune system.

Secondary Immunodeficiency in the Elderly: Role of Nutritional Factors

This section will review the immune responses of the healthy and apparently healthy elderly (i.e. those without ongoing disease), in whom immune responses reflect both the ageing process and nutritional status.

Lower nutritional status, indicated by lower albumin levels or by low folate status (although still within the normal range), is associated with lower lymphocyte proliferation (Lesourd and Meaume, 1994; Lesourd *et al.*, 1994; Mazari

Table 17.2. Functions of peripheral blood monocytes from elderly subjects. Groups were selected, using previously described criteria (Mazari and Lesourd, 1998), as being very healthy, self-sufficient home-living apparently healthy (frail and/or undernourished) or profoundly undernourished old subjects with undernourishment due only to insufficient nutrient intakes (with mild inflammatory process: CRP < 30 mg l⁻¹).

	Very healthy 'young elderly' (65–85 years) (n = 41)		Apparently healthy frail 'young elderly' (70–85 years) (n = 51)		Undernourished, self-sufficient 'young elderly' (70–85 years) (n = 25)		Very undernourished hospitalized 'young elderly' (70–85 years) (n = 17)	
	Mean	Standard deviation	Mean	Standard deviation	Mean	Standard deviation	Mean	Standard deviation
Age (years)	79.6	5.3	78.9	6.2	78.7	5.9	79.6	6.4
Albumin (g l⁻¹)	42.4	4.1	37.2	3.9	29.4***†	3.2	22.3***††	2.8
CRP (mg l⁻¹)	< 6		7.1	4.2	16.8*†	12.6	26.4***†††	9.6
IL-1 production (ng ml⁻¹)								
Spontaneous release	ND		ND		1.4	1.5	0.5	1.1
Using 25 µg LPS 10⁶ cells⁻¹	2.6	2.2	2.4	2.1	1.2*†	1.6	0.7***††	1.0
IL-6 production (ng ml⁻¹)								
Spontaneous release	ND		0.1	0.1	0.35	0.18	0.24	0.26
Using 25 µg LPS 10⁶ cells⁻¹	1.7	0.3	1.9	0.4	0.98***†††	0.41	0.31***†††	0.25

CRP, c-reactive protein; IL, interleukin; LPS, lipopolysaccharide.
Significant differences from very healthy 'young elderly': * $P < 0.05$, ** $P < 0.01$, *** $P < 0.001$.
Significant differences from apparently healthy 'young elderly': † $P < 0.05$, †† $P < 0.01$, ††† $P < 0.001$.
ND, not detectable.

and Lesourd, 1998). In addition, the changes in T-cell subsets related to ageing (decreased numbers of CD3+ cells with a parallel increase in numbers of CD2+ CD3– cells; decreased numbers of CD8+ cells) are greater in such apparently healthy elderly subjects than in those with better nutritional status. Treatment of such elderly individuals with folic acid induces an increase in immune responses to levels similar to those seen in young adults, without a change in T-cell subsets (B. Lesourd unpublished data). Therefore, even in the apparently healthy elderly, low nutritional status (although still within the 'normal' range) is associated with lower immune responses. Interestingly, the effects of lower nutritional status on immune functions in the apparently healthy elderly were not observed in young adults (Mazari and Lesourd, 1998), indicating that the immune system of the elderly may be more sensitive to nutritional status than that of young adults.

The association between lower nutritional status and lower immune responses in apparently healthy elderly subjects has been the basis of a number of studies aimed at improving immune function with nutritional intervention. Talbott *et al.* (1987) showed that decreased immune responses in the elderly are linked to lower vitamin B_6 status and that supplementation with vitamin B_6 induces an increase in lymphocyte proliferation, but only in individuals with low vitamin B_6 status. Subsequently, other studies, using either a single micronutrient (e.g. zinc (Boubaïka *et al.*, 1993; Prasad *et al.*, 1993), vitamin E (Meydani *et al.*, 1990, 1997), vitamin B_6 (Meydani *et al.*, 1991)), a few antioxidant micronutrients (Penn *et al.*, 1991; Fortes *et al.*, 1993) or several micronutrients (Bogden *et al.*, 1990, 1994; Chandra, 1992a; Pike and Chandra, 1995), have shown increased immune responses with supplementation. Such increases in immune responses with micronutrient supplementation have also been observed in institutionalized elderly subjects (Galan *et al.*, 1997). These effects are related to correction of micronutrient deficiencies (Bogden *et al.*, 1990; Chandra, 1992a; Galan *et al.*, 1997). Micronutrient deficiencies are quite common in the elderly: half of apparently healthy elderly subjects have low intakes of at least one micronutrient (Amorin-Cruz *et al.*, 1996) and a third have low status of at least one micronutrient (Haller *et al.*, 1996; Lesourd and Mazari, 1999). Some of the lowest intakes or the lowest status, quantified in apparently healthy elderly subjects are reported for micronutrients known to influence the activity of the immune system: vitamin B_6 (6–26% of subjects deficient), folic acid (9–16%), vitamin C (5–10%) (Haller *et al.*, 1996; Lesourd *et al.*, 1998). All supplementation studies concern micronutrients for which nutritional deficit is linked to immune deficit: zinc (Keen and Gershwin 1990; Cunningham-Rundles *et al.*, 1991; see also Prased, Chapter 10, this volume), vitamin B_6 (Chandra and Sudhakaran, 1990; Rall and Meydani, 1993), antioxidants (Meydani *et al.*, 1995; see also Hughes, Chapter 9, this volume). In some reports, it has been shown that long-term (1 year) supplementation may reduce infection rate and/or length of infections in independent (Chandra, 1992a) and institutionalized (Girodon *et al.*, 1997) elderly subjects. These findings demonstrate that nutritional deficiency may be of great significance to the health and well-being of elderly persons, even if they are apparently healthy. They also show the close association between nutritional status, immune responses and clinical state in such elderly subjects.

In addition to enhanced immune responses upon supplementation in apparently healthy self-sufficient elderly who exhibit decreased micronutrient status, vitamin E supplements improved immune responses of healthy elderly subjects who apparently did not have vitamin E deficiency (Meydani *et al.*, 1990, 1997; see also Hughes, Chapter 9, this volume). Vitamin E deficiency is uncommon, affecting less than 1% of such elderly subjects (Amorin-Cruz *et al.*, 1996; Lesourd *et al.*, 1998). The effect of vitamin E was obtained using a high dose (50–800 mg α-tocopherol acetate day^{-1}), four to 80 times the recommended intake in many Western countries (e.g. Cynober *et al.*, 2000). Vitamin E supplementation increased lymphocyte proliferation, IL-2 production, delayed-type hypersensitivity and antibody responses to some vaccines (Meydani *et al.*, 1990, 1997). Furthermore, vitamin E decreased PGE$_2$ and free-radical production by macrophages (Meydani *et al.*, 1986, 1997). These are two changes that are considered part of 'normal' ageing (Lang *et al.*, 1992). Thus, the effect of vitamin E may be important in slowing the effect of ageing. If some ageing phenomena, such as permanent macrophage activation and decreased T-cell responses, can be reversed by high-dose micronutrient supplementation (e.g. with vitamin E), then the recommended intakes for such micronutrients may be too low.

The findings from these studies are of great importance. First, they show that micronutrient deficiencies are deleterious for immune responses. Second, they indicate that recommended micronutrient intakes are probably too low for the elderly, at least for some micronutrients with antioxidant properties. Therefore, they point to a new direction for slowing the ageing process: higher recommendations for intakes of some micronutrients. Since these nutrients influence the immune system, the measurement of T-cell and macrophage functions is probably a sensitive functional marker to quantify the consequences of nutrient deficiencies and the ageing process.

However, before recommending nutritional supplementation for the elderly, it should be noted that there are reports of high doses of some micronutrients (e.g. zinc) having deleterious effects on immune responses. For example, one study showed that immune recovery occurs faster when a supplement does not contain zinc (Bogden *et al.*, 1990), while Chandra (1984) showed a deleterious immunological effect of high zinc supplements (300 mg d^{-1}) in young adults. This indicates that the use of such supplements should be approached cautiously and adapted properly to the micronutrient status of the individual concerned.

Tertiary Immunodeficiency in the Elderly: Role of Protein-Energy Malnutrition

Protein–energy malnutrition (PEM) exerts a strong influence on immune responses, particularly at the extremes of life (Chandra, 1989, 1992b; Lesourd, 1990a, b, 1995, 2000; see also Chandra, Chapter 3, this volume). PEM affects all types of immune responses in elderly subjects leading to decreased cell-mediated immunity (Chandra, 1989; Lesourd, 1990b, 1995, 2000), decreased humoral immunity (Chandra *et al.*, 1984) and decreased innate immunity (Rudd and Banerjee, 1989; Lesourd and Mazari 1997, 1999). PEM accentuates the age-related decline of immune responses so that undernourished elderly subjects have further changes in peripheral blood lymphocyte counts, and further decreases in CD3+ cell nunbers, in lymphocyte proliferation and in cytokine release (Lesourd and Meaume, 1994; Lesourd *et al.*, 1994; Lesourd and Mazari, 1999; Table 17.3). PEM and ageing exert cumulative effects on T-cell responses, so that the degree of the immunodeficiency in the elderly patient is linked to the degree of PEM (Chandra, 1989; Lesourd *et al.*, 1992). Besides this cumulative effect, PEM induces other changes in immune responses of the elderly: in aged persons with PEM, the number of CD4+ cells is decreased (Lesourd and Meuame, 1994; Lesourd *et al.*, 1994; Table 17.3) in line with the degree of the nutritional deficit (Lesourd, 1995). PEM is also associated with decreased humoral responses, measured as lower antibody responses to vaccine (Chandra *et al.*, 1984; Lesourd 1995) and by decreased non-specific immunity either of polymorphonuclear (Lipschitz and Udupa, 1986) or macrophage functions (Rudd and Banerjee, 1989; Lesourd and Mazari, 1997; Table 17.2). Undernutrition and ageing exert cumulative effects on non-specific immune responses in animals (Lipschitz and Udupa, 1986) and in humans (Lesourd and Mazari, 1997).

The influence of nutritional status on macrophage functions is of great importance for elderly subjects. Indeed, ageing induces a disequilibrium between macrophage functions, which are preserved in the apparently healthy elderly, while T-cell functions start to decline. If any disease occurs, the disequilibrium leads macrophages to release more cytokines in order to stimulate an efficient T-cell response. This can have detrimental effects on the host (Lesourd, 1996; Lesourd *et al.*, 1996). Macrophage-derived cytokines are responsible for the mobilization of body nutritional reserves in order to provide activated cells with the nutrients they need for their high metabolic activity (Klasing, 1988; Lesourd, 1992). In the elderly, nutritional reserves are lost at a similar rate to that in younger adults, but they are not fully restored after recovery from disease (Lesourd, 1996; Lesourd *et al.*, 1996). This is due to the age-related disequilibrium between muscle catabolism, which is preserved with ageing (Fereday *et al.*, 1997), and muscle anabolism, which declines in aged individuals (Welle *et al.*, 1993; Yarasheski *et al.*, 1993). Therefore, during any disease, the rate of muscle catabolism exceeds that of muscle anabolism (Fereday *et al.*, 1997), so that aged persons recover after the disease with muscle and bone deficits that are never fully rebuilt (Lesourd, 1996; Lesourd *et al.*, 1996). Therefore, any disease process pushes the elderly to a more frail state and this is a common situation in elderly patients who exhibit continuous increases in monocyte/macrophage cytokines (Cederholm *et al.*, 1997).

If such disease occurs in combination with PEM in the elderly, cytokine release from macrophages is lower and then the stimulation of defence mechanisms is less effective (Nafziger *et al.*, 1993). Hypercatabolism lasts longer and is quite permanent (Cederholm *et al.*, 1997) and the decline in body nutritional reserves is more pronounced (Fereday *et al.*, 1997). Therefore, undernutrition is a factor that pushes the elderly to a more frail state (Lesourd, 2000).

Table 17.3. Subsets and functions of peripheral blood T lymphocytes from elderly subjects with different nutritional and health status. Groups were selected, using previously described criteria (Mazari and Lesourd, 1998), as being very healthy, self-sufficient home-living apparently healthy (frail and/or undernourished) or profoundly undernourished old subjects with undernourishment due only to insufficient nutrient intakes (with mild inflammatory process: CRP < 30 mg l⁻¹).

	Very healthy 'young elderly' (65–85 years) (n = 41)		Apparently healthy 'young elderly' (70–85 years) (n = 51)		Undernourished, self-sufficient 'young elderly' (70–85 years) (n = 25)		Very undernourished hospitalized 'young elderly' (70–85 years) (n = 17)	
	Mean	Standard deviation	Mean	Standard deviation	Mean	Standard deviation	Mean	Standard deviation
Age (years)	79.6	5.3	78.9	6.2	78.7	5.9	79.6	6.4
Albumin (g l⁻¹)	42.4	4.1	37.2	3.9	29.4***†	3.2	22.3***††	2.8
Lymphocytes (number μl⁻¹)	1993	568	1705**	434	1356**	287	859**	214
CD2+ cells (number μl⁻¹)	1794**	397	1511***†	427	1264***†	336	864***†	217
CD3+ cells (number μl⁻¹)	1565**	311	1207***†	299	935***†	221	517***††	167
CD2+CD3– cells (number μl⁻¹)	214*	224	283**	241	335*	148	356*†	203
CD4+ cells (number μl⁻¹)	1136*	243	812***††	271	461***††	188	354***†††	271
CD8+ cells (number μl⁻¹)	437***	174	387***	196	395	165	256*†	178
CD45RA cells (number μl⁻¹)	658***	228	464***†	213	517*	245	549	276
CD45R0 cells (number μl⁻¹)	1222***	365	1057***	497	831**	497	372***†††	349
IL-2 production‡ (ng l⁻¹)	1.84	0.34	1.11***†	0.38	0.77***††	0.28	0.45***†††	0.33
IL-6 production‡ (ng l⁻¹)	1.82*	0.22	1.48	0.40	1.10***†	0.44	0.77***†††	0.31
Lymphocyte proliferation§ (10³ cpm 10⁶ cells⁻¹)	114	35	54**†	34	43***	29	21***††	32

CRP, C-reactive protein; IL, interleukin.
Significant differences from very healthy 'young elderly': * $P < 0.05$, ** $P < 0.01$, *** $P < 0.001$.
Significant differences from apparently healthy 'young elderly': † $P < 0.05$, †† $P < 0.01$, ††† $P < 0.001$.
‡Determined using 5 μg mitogen 10⁶ cells⁻¹.
§Determined using 1 μg mitogen 10⁶ cells⁻¹.

Conclusion

There is now strong evidence that ageing exerts less influence on the immune system than environmental factors. In VCSH elderly subjects, ageing induces changes in T-cell and B-cell subsets, but most immune functions are preserved until very old age. Furthermore, it appears that non-specific immunity is even increased, perhaps in relation to a continuous activation of macrophages. Undernutrition, irrespective of the nutrient concerned, induces immunodeficiency even in apparently self-sufficient, non-diseased elderly subjects. Indeed, chronic low intakes of some nutrients, even though they are within the normal range, induce lower cell-mediated immune responses. As chronic low intakes are quite common in the apparently healthy elderly population, it is possible that many immune changes that were previously reported to be age-related are, in fact, due to the influence of undernutrition. Treatment of such nutritional deficits with supplements enhances immune responses in relation to the correction of the deficit. Vitamin E supplements also enhance immune responses, even though the elderly do not exhibit vitamin E deficiency, as defined by current recommendations. Such vitamin E supplementation induces immune changes that partly reverse immune ageing. Thus, it is possible that current recommendations for intakes of some micronutrients are insufficient to prevent or to slow the ageing process.

Nutritional influences on immune responses seem greater in elderly subjects with disease. PEM lowers non-specific and specific immune mechanisms, induces longer hypercatabolic responses and then, in combination with the age-related changes in protein metabolism, pushes the elderly towards a more frail state. Nutrition, through its action on such process, is an efficient way to slow the ageing process, even in diseased aged patients.

References

Abo, T. (1992) Extrathymic differentiation of T lymphocytes and its biological function. *Biological and Medical Research* 13, 1–39.

Alès-Martinez, J.E., Alvarez-Mon, M., Merino, F., Boniilla, F., Martinez-Alés, C., Durantez, A. and De La Hera, A. (1988) Decreased TcR–CD3–T-cell numbers in healthy aged humans: evidence that T-cell defects are masked by a reciprocal increase of TcR–CD3– CD2+ natural killer cells. *European Journal of Immunology* 18, 1827–1830.

Amorin-Cruz, J.A., Moreiras, O. and Brzozowska, A. (1996) Longitudinal changes in the intakes of vitamins and minerals of elderly Europeans. *European Journal of Clinical Nutrition* 50(Suppl. 2), S77–S85.

Arreaza, E.E., Gibbons, J.J., Sisking, G.W. and Weksler, M.E. (1993) Lower antibody response to tetanus toxoid associated with higher auto-anti-idiotype antibody in old compared with young humans. *Clinical and Experimental Immunology* 92, 169–176.

Barrat, F., Lesourd, B.M., Louise, A., Boulouis, H.J., Vincent-Naulleau, S., Thibault, D., Neway, T., Sanaa, M. and Pilet, C. (1997) Surface antigens expression in spleen cells of C57 BL/6 mice during ageing: influence of sex and breeding. *Clinical and Experimental Immunology* 107, 593–600.

Batory, G., Janeso, A., Puskas, E., Redei, A. and Lengyei, E. (1984) Antibody and immunoglobulin levels in aged humans. *Archives of Gerontology and Geriatrics* 3, 175–188.

Bogden, J.D., Oleske, J.M., Lavenhar, M.A., Munves, E.M., Kemp, F.W., Bruening, K.S., Holding, K.J., Denny, T.N., Guarino, M.A. and Holland, B.K. (1990) Effects of one year of supplementation with zinc and other micronutrients on cellular immunity in the elderly. *Journal of the American College of Nutrition* 59, 214–225.

Bogden, J.D., Bendich, A., Kemp, F.W., Bruening, K.S., Shurrick, J.H., Denny, T., Baker, H. and Louria, D.B. (1994) Daily micronutrient supplements enhanced delayed-hypersensitivity skin test responses in the older people. *Journal of the American College of Nutrition* 60, 437–447.

Boubaïka, N., Flament, C., Acher, S., Chappuis, Ph., Pian, A., Fusselier, M., Dardenne, M. and Lemonnier, D. (1993) A physiological amount of zinc supplementation: effects on nutritional, lipid, and thymic status in an elderly population. *American Journal of Clinical Nutrition* 57, 566–572.

Bruley-Rosset, M. and Payelle, B. (1987) Deficient tumor specific immunity in old mice: *in vivo* mediation by suppressor cells, and correction of the defect by inter-leukin 2 supplementation *in vitro* but not *in vivo*. *Journal of Immunology* 17, 307–312.

Cakman, I., Rohwer, J., Schûtz, R.M., Kirchner, H. and Rink, L. (1996) Dysregulation betwen TH1 and TH2 cell sub-populations in the elderly. *Mechanisms of Ageing and Development* 87, 197–209.

Cederholm, T., Wretling, B., Hellstrom, K., Andersson B., Engstrom, L., Brismark, K., Scheynius, A., Faslid, J. and Palmblad, J. (1997) Enhanced generation of inter-leukins 1β and 6 may contribute to the cachexia of chronic disease. *American Journal of Clinical Nutrition* 65, 876–882.

Chandra, R.K. (1984) Excessive intake of zinc impairs immune responses. *Journal of the American Medical Association* 252, 1443–1446.

Chandra, R.K. (1989) Nutrition, regulation of immunity and risk of infection on old age. *Immunology* 67, 141–147.

Chandra, R.K. (1992a) Effect of vitamin and trace-element supplementation on immune responses and infection in elderly subjects. *Lancet* 340, 1124–1127.

Chandra, R.K. (1992b) Nutrition and immunobiology: experience of an old traveller and recent observations. In: Chandra, R.K. (ed.) *Nutrition and Immunology*. ARTS Biomedical, St John's, pp. 9–43.

Chandra, R.K. and Sudhakaran, L. (1990) Regulation of immune responses by vitamin B$_6$. *Annals of the New York Academy of Sciences* 585, 404–423.

Chandra, R.K., Chandra, S. and Gupta, S. (1984) Antibody affinity and immune complexes after immunization with tetanus toxoid in protein–energy malnutrition. *American Journal of Clinical Nutrition* 40, 131–134.

Chen, W.F., Liu, S.L., Gao, X.M. and Pang, X.I. (1987) The capacity of lymphokine production by peripheral blood lymphocytes from aged humans. *Immunological Investigations* 15, 575–583.

Clerici, M., Wynn, T.A. and Berkovsky, J.A. (1992) Role of interleukin-10 in T-helper cell dysfunction in asymptomatic individuals infected with the immunodeficiency virus. *Metabolism* 75, 1125–1132.

Cossarizza, A., Ortolani, C., Paganelli, R., Monti, D., Barbieri, D., Sansoni, P., Fafiolo, U., Forti, E., Londei, M. and Carter, D.M. (1992) Age-related imbalance of virgin (CD45RA+) and memory (CD45RO+) cells between CD4+ and CD8+ T lymphocytes in humans: study from newborns to centenarians. *Journal of Immunological Research* 4, 117–126.

Cunningham-Rundles, S., Bockam, R.S., Lin, A., Giardana, P.V., Hilgratner, M.W., Caldell-Brown, D. and Carter, D.M. (1991) Physiological and pharmacological effects of zinc on immune response. *Annals of the New York Academy of Sciences* 590, 113–122.

Cynober, L., Alix, E., Arnaud-Battandier, F., Bonnefry, M., Brocher, P., Cals, M.J., Chubat, C., Copplo, C., Feny, M., Ghisolfi-Marque, A., Kratcheno, T., Lesourd, B., Mignot, C. and Partineau, P.L. (2000) Apports nutritionnels conseillés chez la personne âgée. *Nutrition Clinique et Métabolisme* 14(Suppl. 1), 1s–64s.

Daynes, R.A., Areanéo, B.A., Ershler, W.B., Maloney, C., Li, G.Z. and Ryu, S.Y. (1993) Altered regulation of IL-6 production with normal ageing. *Journal of Immunology* 150, 5219–5230.

Doria, G. (1988) Immunoregulation in ageing. *Italian Journal of Medicine* 4, 83–85.

Engwerda, C.R., Fox, B.S. and Handwerger, B.S. (1996) Cytokine production by T lymphocytes from young and old mice. *Journal of Immunology* 156, 3621–3630.

Ershler, W.B., Sun, W.H., Binkley, N., Gravenstein, S., Volk, M.J., Kamoske, G., Kloop, R.G., Roecker, E.B., Daynes, R.A. and Weindruch, R. (1993) Interleukin-6 and ageing: blood levels and mononuclear cell production increase with advancing age and *in vitro* production modifiable by dietary restriction. *Lymphokine and Cytokine Research* 12, 225–230.

Fereday, A., Gibson, N.R., Cox, M., Pacy, P.J. and Millward, D.J. (1997) Protein requirements and ageing: metabolic demand and efficiency of utilization. *British Journal of Nutrition* 77, 685–702.

Fortes, C., Forastiere, F., Agabiti, N., Fano, V., Pacifici, R., Virgili, F., Piras, G., Guidi, L., Bartonoli, C., Tricerri, A., Ziccaro, P., Ebrahim, S. and Perucci, C.A. (1993) The effects of zinc and vitamin A supplementation on immune response in an older population. *Journal of the American Geriatrics Society* 46, 19–26.

Galan, P., Preziosi, P., Richard, M.J., Monget, A.L., Arnaud, J., Lesourd, B., Favier, A., Girodon, F., Laisney, C., Bourgeois, C.F., Keller, H., Hercberg, S. et le réseau gériatrie/MIN.VIT.AOX. (1997) Biological and immunological effects of trace element and/or vitamin supplementation in the elderly. In: *Proceedings of the 4th International Conference on Trace-elements in Medicine and Biology.* Paris, France, pp. 197–210.

Girodon, F., Lombard, M., Galan, P., Brunet-Lecomte, P., Monget, A.L., Arnaud, J., Preziosi, P. and Hercberg, S. (1997) Effect of micronutrient supplementation on infection in institutionalized elderly subjects: a controlled trial. *Annals of Nutrition and Metabolism* 41, 98–107.

Goidl, E.A. (1987) Aging and autoimmunity. In: Goidl, E.A. (ed.) *Aging and the Immune Response.* Raven Press, New York, pp. 345–358.

Goldberg, T.H., Baker, D.G. and Shumacher, H.R. (1991) Interleukin-1 and the immunology of ageing and disease. *Aging, Immunology and Infecious Diseases* 3, 81–86.

Goodwin, J.S. (1992) Changes in lymphocyte sensitivity to prostaglandin E_2, histamine, hydrocortosone, and X irradiation with age: studies in a healthy elderly population. *Clinical and Experimental Immunology and Immunopathology* 25, 243–251.

Haller, J., Weggemans, R.M., Lammi-Keefe, C.J. and Ferry, M. (1996) Changes in the vitamin status of elderly Europeans: plasma vitamins A, E, B-6, B-12, folic acid and carotenoids. *European Journal of Clinical Nutrition* 50(Suppl. 2), S32–S46.

Hayek, G.M., Mura, C., Wu, D., Beharka, A.A., Han S.N., Paulson, E., Hwang, D. and Meydani, S.N. (1997) Enhanced expression of inducible cyclooxygenase with age in murine macrophages. *Journal of Immunology* 159, 2445–2451.

Hirokawa, K., Utsuyama, M., Kasai, M., Kurishima, C., Ishijima, S. and Zong, Y.X.

(1994) Understanding the mechanisms of the age changes of thymic function to promote T-cell differentiation. *Immunology Letters* 40, 269–277.

Hobbs, M.V. and Ernst, D.N. (1997) T-cell differentiation and cytokine expression in late life. *Developmental and Comparative Immunology* 21, 464–470.

Huang, Y.P., Gauthey, L., Michel, J.P., Loveto, M., Paccaud, M., Pechere, J.C. and Michel, J.P. (1992) The relationship between influenza vaccine-induced specific antibody responses and vaccine-induced non specific autoantibody responses in healthy older women. *Journal of Gerontology* 47, M50–M55.

Huppert, F.A., Solomou, W., O'Connor, S., Morgan, K., Sussams, P. and Brayne, C. (1998) Aging and lymphocyte subpopulations: whole-blood analysis of immune markers in a large population sample of healthy elderly individuals. *Experimental Immunology* 33, 593–600.

James, K., Premchand, N., Skibinska, A., Skibinski, G., Nicol, M. and Mason, J.I. (1997) IL-6, DHEA and the ageing process. *Mechanisms of Ageing and Development* 93, 15–24.

Keen, C.L. and Gershwin, M.E. (1990) Zinc deficiency and immune function. *Annual Review in Nutrition* 10, 415–431.

Klasing, K.C. (1988). Nutritional aspects of leucocyte cytokines: critical review. *Journal of Nutrition* 11, 1436–1446.

Kubo, M. and Cinader, B. (1990) Polymorphism of age-related changes in interleukin (IL) production: differential changes of T helper subpopulation, synthesizing IL-2, IL-3, and IL-4. *European Journal of Immunology* 24, 133–136.

Lang, G.A., Naryshkin, S., Schneider, D.L., Mills, B.J. and Lindeman, R.D. (1992) Low blood glutathione levels in healthy ageing adults. *Journal of Laboratory and Clinical Medicine* 120, 720–725.

Lesourd, B. (1990a) Le vieillissement immunologique: influence de la dénutrition. *Annales de Biologie Clinique* 48, 309–318.

Lesourd, B. (1990b) La dénutrition protéique: principale cause de déficit immunitaire chez le sujet âgé. *Age and Nutrition* 3, 132–138.

Lesourd, B. (1992) Conséquences nutritionnelles des cytokines: facteur de gravité des hypercatabolismes chez le sujet âgé. *Age and Nutrition* 3, 100–109.

Lesourd, B.M. (1995) Protein undernutrition as the major cause of decreased immune function in the elderly: clinical and functional implications. *Nutrition Reviews* 53, S86–S94.

Lesourd, B.M. (1996) Hypermetabolism: a frightening symptom that push elderly to enter a vicious circle. In: Viidik, A. and Hofecker, G. (eds) *Vitality Mortality and Ageing*. Vienna Ageing Series, Facultas Universitats Verlag, Vienna, pp. 363–376.

Lesourd, B. (1997) Le vieillissement du sytème immunitaire: un facteur favorisant la survenue et la gravité des infections chez les sujets âgés. In: Veyssier, P. (ed.) *Infection Chez les Sujets Âgés*. Ellipses, Paris, pp. 60–70.

Lesourd, B. (1999) Immune response during disease and recovery in the elderly. *Proceedings of the Nutrition Society* 58, 1–14.

Lesourd, B. (2000) Undernutrition: a factor of accelerated ageing in healthy and diseased aged persons. In: Watson, R.R. (ed.) *Handbook of Nutrition in the Aged*. CRC Press, New York, pp. 145–158.

Lesourd, B.M. and Mazari, L. (1997) Immune responses during recovery from protein–energy malnutrition. *Clinical Nutrition* 16(Suppl. 1), 37–46.

Lesourd, B. and Mazari, M. (1998) Monocyte cytokines in elderly: a reflect of aged persons to react in adapted way. *The Immunologist* (Suppl. 1), 448.

Lesourd, B. and Mazari, L. (1999) Nutrition and immunity in the elderly. *Proceedings of the Nutrition Society* 58, 685–695.

Lesourd, B. and Meaume, S. (1994) Cell-mediated immunity changes in ageing: relative importance of cell subpopulation switches and of nutritional factors. *Immunology Letters* 40, 235–242.

Lesourd, B.M., Moulias, R., Favre-Berrone, M. and Rapin, C.H. (1992) Nutritional influences on immune responses in elderly. In: Chandra, R.K. (ed.) *Nutrition and Immunology*. ARTS Biomedical, St John's, pp. 211–223.

Lesourd, B., Laisney, C., Salvatore, R., Meaume, S. and Moulias, R. (1994) Decreased maturation of T-cell population factors on the appearance of double negative CD4–, CD8–, CD2+ cells. *Archives of Gerontology and Geriatrics* 4(Suppl.), 139–154.

Lesourd, B.M., Salvatore, R. and Weil-Engerer, S. (1996) Undernutrition: a common symptom of hospitalized elderly which needs urgent treatment. In: Viidik, A. and Hofecker, G. (eds) *Vitality, Mortality and Ageing*. Vienna Ageing Series, Facultas Universitats Verlag, Vienna, pp. 377–386.

Lesourd, B., Mazari, L. and Ferry, M. (1998) The role of nutrition in immunity in the aged. *Nutrition Reviews* 56, S113–S125.

Ligthart, G.J., Corberand, J.X., Fournier, C., Galanaud, P., Hijmans, W., Kennes, B., Muller-Hermelink, H.K. and Steinmann, G.G. (1984) Admission criteria for immunogerontological studies in man: the Senieur protocol. *Mechanisms of Ageing and Development* 28, 47–55.

Lipschitz, D.A. and Udupa, K.B. (1986) Infuence of ageing and protein deficiency on neutrophil function. *Journal of Gerontology* 41, 281–288.

Makinodan, T. and Kay, M.M.B. (1980) Age influence on the immune system. *Advances in Immunology* 29, 287–330.

Mazari, L. and Lesourd, B. (1998) Nutritional influences on immune response in healthy aged persons. *Mechanisms of Ageing and Development* 104, 25–40.

Mbawuike, I.N., Acuna, C.L., Walz, K.C., Atmar, R.L., Greenberg, S.B. and Couch, R.B. (1997) Cytokines and impaired CD8+ CTL activity among elderly persons and the enhancing effect of IL-12. *Mechanisms of Ageing and Development* 94, 25–39.

Meydani, S.N., Meydani, M., Verdon, C.P., Shapiro, A.C., Blumberg, J.B. and Hayes, K.C. (1986) Vitamin E supplementation suppresses prostaglandin E2 synthesis and enhances the immune response of aged mice. *Mechanisms of Ageing and Development* 34, 191–201.

Meydani, S.N., Barklund, M.P., Lui, S., Meydani, M. and Miller, R.A. (1990) Vitamin E supplementation enhances cell-mediated immunity in healthy elderly. *American Journal of Clinical Nutrition* 52, 557–563.

Meydani, S.N., Ribaya-Mercado, J.D., Russell, R.B., Sahyoun, N., Morrow, F.D. and Gershoff, S.N. (1991) Vitamin B-6 deficiency impairs interleukin 2 production and lymphocyte proliferation in elderly adults. *American Journal of Clinical Nutrition* 53, 1275–1280.

Meydani, S.N., Wu, D., Santos, M.S. and Hayek, M.G. (1995) Antioxidants and immune response in aged persons: overview of the present evidence. *American Journal of Clinical Nutrition* 62, 1462S–1476S.

Meydani, S.N., Meydani, M., Blumberg, J.B., Lekal, S., Siber, G., Loszewski, R., Thompson, C., Pedrosa, C., Diamond, R.D. and Stollar, B.D. (1997) Vitamin E supplementation and *in vivo* immune response in healthy elderly subjects. *Journal of the American Medical Association* 277, 1380–1386.

Miller, R.A. (1992) Aging and immune function. *International Cytokine Reviews* 124, 187–214.

Miller, R.A. (1996) The ageing immune system: primer and prospectus. *Science* 273, 70–74.

Moulias, R., Proust, J., Wang, A., Congy, F., Marescot, M., Devillechabrolle, A., Paris-

Hamelin, A. and Lesourd, B. (1984) Age related increase in autoantibodies *Lancet* i, 1128–1129.

Moulias, R., Devillechabrolle, A., Lesourd, B., Proust, J., Marescot, M.R., Doumerc, S., Favre-Berrone, M., Congy, F. and Wang, A. (1985) Respective roles of immune and nutritional factors in the priming of the immune responses in the elderly. *Mechanisms of Ageing and Development* 31, 123–137.

Muller, S., Chang, H.C., Ward, M.M., Huang, J.H. and Kölher, H. (1986) Idiotype shifts. In: Goidl, E. (ed.) *Aging and the Immune Responses: Cellular and Humoral Aspects.* Marcel Dekker, New York, pp. 309–327.

Myslinska, J., Bryl, E., Foerster, J. and Myslinski, A. (1998) Increase of interleukin 6 and decrease of interleukin 2 production during the ageing process are influenced by the health status. *Mechanisms of Ageing and Development* 100, 313–328.

Nafziger, J., Bessege, J.P., Guillosson, J.J., Damais, C. and Lesourd, B. (1993) Decreased capacity of IL-1 production by monocytes of infected elderly patients. *Aging, Immunology and Infectious Disease* 4, 25–34.

Nagel, J.E., Chopra, R.K., Chrest, F.J., McCoy, M.T., Schneider, E.L., Holbrook, N.J. and Adler, W.H. (1988) Decreased proliferation interleukin 2 synthesis and interleukin 2 receptor expression are accompanied by decreased mRNA expression, in phytohemagglutinin-stimulated cells from elderly donors. *Journal of Clinical Investigation* 81, 1096–1102.

Nagelkerken, L., Hertogh-Huijbregts, A., Dobber, R. and Dräger, A. (1991) Age-related changes in lymphokine production related to a decreased number of CD45Rbohi CD4+ T-cells. *European Journal of Immunology* 21, 273–281.

Nakayama, K.I., Nakayama, K., Negishi, I., Kuids, K., Louie, M.C., Kamagawa, D., Nakauchi, H. and Loh, D.Y. (1994) Requirement for DC8 beta chain in positive selection of CD8 lineage T-cells. *Science* 263, 1131–1133.

Penn, N.D., Purkins, L., Kelleher, J., Heartley, R.V., Masie-Taylor, B.H. and Belfield, P.W. (1991) The effect of dietary supplementation with vitamins A, C and E on cell-mediated immune function in elderly long-stay patients: a randomized, controlled trial. *Age and Aging* 20, 169–174.

Pike, J. and Chandra, R.K. (1995) Effect of vitamin and trace element supplementation on immune indices in healthy elderly. *International Journal of Vitaminology and Nutrition Research* 65, 117–121.

Prasad, A.S., Fitzgerald, J.T., Hess, J.W., Kaplan J., Pelen, F. and Dardenne, M. (1993) Zinc deficiency in elderly patients. *Nutrition* 9, 218–224.

Proust, J., Moulias, R., Mumeron, F., Beckkhoucha, F., Bussone, M., Schmid, M. and Hors, J. (1982) HLA and longevity. *Tissue Antigens* 19, 168–173.

Proust, J., Rosenzweig, P., Debouzy, C. and Moulias, R. (1986) Lymphopenia induced by acute bacterial infections in the elderly: a sign of age-related immune dysfunction of major prognostic significance. *Gerontology* 31, 178–185.

Rabinowich, H., Goses, Y., Reshef, T. and Klajman A. (1985). Interleukin 2 production and activity in aged humans. *Mechanisms of Ageing and Development* 32, 213–226.

Rall, L.C. and Meydani, S.N. (1993) Vitamin B6 and immune competence. *Nutrition Reviews* 51, 217–225.

Reibnegger, G., Hubber, L.A., Jurgens, G., Schrönitzer, D., Werner, E.R., Watcher, H., Wick, G. and Traill, K.N. (1988) Approach to define 'normal ageing' in man: immune function, serum lipids, lipoproteins and neopterin. *Mechanisms of Ageing and Development* 46, 67–82.

Rudd, A.G. and Banerjee, D.K. (1989) Interleukin-1 production by human monocytes in ageing and disease. *Age and Ageing* 18, 43–46.

Sanders, M.E., Maggoba, M.W., Sharrow, S.E., Olephany D., Spriger A., Young, H.A. and Shaw, S. (1998) Human memory T lymphocytes express increased level of three cell adhesion molecules (LFA3, CD2, and LFA1) and three other molecules (UCHL-1, CDw29, and Pgp-1) and have enhanced IFN-γ production. *Journal of Immunology* 140, 1401–1407.

Shearer, G.M. (1997) Th1/Th2 changes in ageing. *Mechanisms of Ageing and Development* 94, 1–5.

Sindermann, J., Kruse, A., Frercks, H.J., Schutz, R.M. and Kirchner, H. (1993) Investigations of the lymphokine system in elderly individuals. *Mechanisms of Ageing and Development* 70, 149–159.

Steinmann, G.G., Klaus, B. and Muller-Hermelink, H.K. (1985) The involution of the ageing human thymic epithelium is independent of puberty. *Scandinavian Journal of Immunology* 22, 563–575.

Talbott, M.C., Miller, L.T. and Kerkvliet, N.I. (1987) Pyridoxine supplementation: effect on lymphocyte responses in elderly person. *American Journal of Clinical Nutrition* 46, 659–664.

Tyan, M.L. (1981) Marrow stem cells during development and ageing. In: Kay, M.M.B. and Makinodan, T. (eds) *Handbook of Immunology and Ageing*. CRC Press, New York, pp. 87–102.

Weksler, M.E. (1995) Immune senescence: deficiency or dysregulation. *Nutrition Reviews* 53, S3–S7.

Welle, S., Thornton, C. and Jozefowicz, R. (1993) Myofibrillar protein synthesis in young and old men. *American Journal of Physiology* 264, E693–E698.

Wick, G. and Grubek-Loewenstein, B. (1997) Primary and secondary alterations of immune reactivity in the elderly: impact of dietary factors and disease. *Immunology Reviews* 160, 171–184.

Yarasheski, K.E., Zachwieja, J.J. and Bier, D.M. (1993) Acute effects of resistance exercice on muscle protein synthesis rat in young and elderly men and women. *American Journal of Physiology* 265, E210–E214.

Yong-Xing, M., Yue, Z., Zan-Shun, W., Chuan-Fu, W., Su-Ying, C., Mao-Tong, Z., Gong-Liang, Z., Su-Qin, Z., Jian-Gang, Z., Qi, G. and Lin, H. (1997) HLA and longevity or ageing among Shanghai Chinese. *Mechanisms of Ageing and Development* 94, 191–198.

18 Nutrition, Infection and Immunity: Public Health Implications

ANDREW TOMKINS

Centre for International Child Health, Institute of Child Health, 30 Guilford Street, London WC1N 1EH, UK

Introduction

Infection accounts for the deaths of millions of children and contributes to the deaths of nearly a million mothers each year globally. With new strains of pathogens emerging and antibiotic resistance developing, there is an urgent need to look for new strategies for infection control. There is now solid evidence for a role for nutrition interventions to achieve reduction of child and maternal mortality and morbidity. Nutrition policies need developing and implementing. Nutrition researchers and practitioners can play a major role if they apply their science to the various stages of the policy process used by ministries of health, agriculture and community development. Evidence for a nutritional impact needs to be assembled using biological plausibility, clinical studies, randomized controlled trials, effectiveness studies and a review of what promotes the sustenance of nutrition intervention. The process of establishing an evidence base that is sufficiently robust to stimulate the development of new nutrition interventions that are sustainable even in poor populations is examined. This chapter examines several nutritional deficiency syndromes and focuses on the particular roles of vitamin A, zinc and selenium and examines the issues around iron supplementation in malarious populations.

General Overview

The importance of preventing and treating malnutrition as a strategy to reduce the prevalence, severity and mortality associated with infectious disease is now well recognized. Around 13 million children worldwide die every year, mostly from infectious diseases, including pneumonia, diarrhoea, malaria, measles, meningitis and septicaemia. In a high proportion of these cases, malnutrition is a major contributing factor; the World Health Organization (WHO) and the United Nations Children's Fund (UNICEF) estimate that almost 60% of child deaths are malnutrition-associated (Pelletier *et al.*, 1995). As a result, training in the early recognition and treatment of malnutrition has been incorporated into the Integrated Management of Childhood Illness (IMCI) Programme of WHO/UNICEF, which is being implemented globally among less developed countries (World Health Organization, 2001). Over 600,000 women die every year from pregnancy-related causes (Tomkins, 2001a). A recent landmark study showing an almost 50% reduction in maternal mortality in Nepal as a result of vitamin A or β-carotene supplements (West *et al.*, 1999) emphasizes the importance of nutritional strategies to prevent mortality. Nutritional interventions now need to be included more actively within the Safe Motherhood programmes of WHO/UNICEF, which have been introduced in most less developed countries, as this is where nearly all the maternal mortality occurs. With increasing longevity in many industrialized countries, there is greater interest in the role of micronutrients in preventing infection among the elderly (e.g. see Hughes, Chapter 9, this volume). With increasing sophistication of intensive care, after surgical interventions in particular, there is more awareness of the importance of improving nutrition as a means of improving surgical outcome (e.g. see Duff and Daly, Chapter 5 and Calder and Newsholine, Chapter 6, this volume).

Despite the strong evidence base for nutrition interventions, they are less often included in policies for public health or clinical management by national and international agencies than are vaccines, anti-microbial therapy, anti-retroviral therapy, impregnated mosquito-nets, improved sanitation, clean water and better personal hygiene. There are various reasons for the omission of nutrition interventions from health strategies. First, there has been a tendency to focus on dietary interventions as the key means of improving nutrition – often to the exclusion of other means, such as food fortification or supplements. The result is an assumption by many that improving nutrition can only be achieved by improving household food security and this depends on improving economic status, often a slow process. Second, nutrition has not been 'marketed' as aggressively as other interventions, such as antibiotics, which have been strongly promoted by pharmaceutical companies with the skills and resources to ensure that their products are made widely available. Third, until recently, there have been few examples of clear nutritional management regimes; without their inclusion within the curriculum of training programmes for health or community workers, nutritional interventions have not been taken seriously. The challenge is to review and present the benefits of nutritional interventions more effectively. This is even more important now that new microbial pathogens are emerging and anti-microbial resistance is more prevalent. It is extremely unlikely that new effective anti-microbials will be sufficiently available in poor communities, even if they are developed by pharmaceutical companies. Nutritional interventions could come to occupy the key position that anti-microbials occupied until they failed.

There is now strong evidence for cost-effective nutrition interventions to prevent and manage infectious disease in both industrialized and less developed countries. The recent studies have focused on three areas. First, there is susceptibility to infection – this includes studies on different components of the host immune system, the pathogenicity of individual organisms and the replication rates of the organisms at different stages of disease. In addition there is new information on genetic susceptibility, which makes certain individuals more susceptible to micronutrient deficiency during infection (Delanghe *et al.*, 1998). Second, there is severity of disease – this includes data on the degree of tissue invasion, clinical indicators of disease severity and speed of recovery, which may relate to a combination of the speed of elimination of the infection causing the organism and/or the immune response by the host to the organism. Important studies show how nutritional interventions also reduce mortality. Third, there is disease prevention – there is new information on the ways in which interventions influence the epidemiology of infection, indicating that improved nutrition may have just as much impact as traditional public health measures, if not more.

Despite the strong evidence for a preventive or therapeutic role for nutrition interventions, there are key operational issues that have delayed the introduction and maintenance of nutritional interventions. If a reduction in the prevalence of infection is to be achieved through the introduction of nutritional interventions, several hurdles need to be overcome more efficiently.

First, which government agency should be responsible for championing nutrition as an infection control strategy? Intersectoral collaboration is difficult to achieve, but this is improving. Officials in ministries of health often see nutrition as being the responsibility of the ministry of agriculture. They in turn see their role as increasing national household food security, but hope that nutrition will increase as a result of improving economic purchasing power and see nutrition as the responsibility of the ministry of economic affairs or planning. There have been strong pressures by proponents for the 'food-based approaches are good; supplement-based approaches are bad' philosophy. The artificial polarization towards either/or for the choice of which nutrition interventions to use has created confusion among health and agriculture professionals alike. The lack of clarity among nutrition experts who have taken 'polar positions' has not been helped by Western donors, who failed to include nutrition as an intervention within the health sector. Many donors, often in concert with the large international banks, argued that improved nutrition would only result from economic improvement, which was supposed to accompany structural adjustment, fiscal reforms and free-market economies (World Bank, 2001). There are now welcome recent signs of change. For example, the latest policy of the UK's Department for International Development places a key importance on specific, focused nutrition interventions, especially with micronutrients, as a strategy for improving child health, survival and development (Department for International Development, 2001). There have been considerable efforts to clarify the nature of nutritional interventions during such international activities as the country case-studies following the United Nations World Summit for Children in 1990 (UNICEF, 2001), the Micronutrient Conference on Ending Hidden Hunger in 1991 and the International Conference on Nutrition in 1992 (World Health Organization, 2001). The results of improved collaboration between partner organizations over the last 10 years have been encouraging.

There are now many more opportunities for collaboration between different ministries, each recognizing and respecting the crucial role of the other's activities. Programmes such as the Prevention of Low Birth Weight of UNICEF now include ministries of health, agriculture and community development.

Second, how do nutritional interventions fit within the 'life-cycle' approach that is increasingly espoused by international agencies (Tomkins, 2001b)? There is now greater emphasis on public health and societal interventions from 'conception to the grave'. The new data on the benefits of nutrition interventions at critical phases of the life cycle, such as pregnancy, the early neonatal period and among infants, school-age children and adolescents, make it possible to identify specific activities that have a short- and long-term impact on infection. For instance, strategies that improve the height and nutritional status of primiparous women are likely to lead to improved pregnancy outcome and birth weight, resulting in improved immune status of the fetus, now recognized to be so important for immunological programming (Moore et al., 1999). The benefits of improved birth weight for subsequent immunity have been recognized for years, but other aspects of fetal malnutrition are now increasingly recognized as contributing towards immunity in childhood and possibly even adult life (Barker, 1997). The life-cycle approach provides an opportunity for nutritional interventions to be planned that will have an immediate impact, for example, on the developing fetus in present pregnancies (e.g. through malarial prophylaxis, deworming, infection control and multiple micronutrient supplements) and pregnancies in future generations (e.g. through interventions that will enhance the weight, height and micronutrient status of girls/women at their first pregnancy).

Third, how widespread does malnutrition have to be across the community before public health interventions should be implemented for all the population? Ideally, policy-makers need to know what the benefits are before they can divert scarce resources towards nutrition interventions. Calculations of the cost of nutrition interventions have been most persuasively made for vitamin A supplementation, results of which have been used to estimate the cost of saving lives or preventing serious infections (Murray and Lopez, 1994). However, there is increasing interest in other micronutrients, such as zinc, iron and selenium (see also Prasad, Chapter 10, Kuvibidila and Baliga, Chapter 11, and McKenzie et al., Chapter 12, this volume). Precise cost–benefit calculations cannot yet be made because the precise impact of interventions with these and other nutrients has not yet been fully evaluated. In the meantime, it is valuable to review the types of information that governments need before they implement nutrition interventions.

Establishing biological plausibility is vital. A case can be made by compiling data from apparently disparate studies and synthesizing the responses in different parts of the immune system during experimental malnutrition in human volunteers or animals. The strength of such data may be enhanced by an analysis of the impact of nutritional interventions on immune function or susceptibility to infection. One of the difficulties facing investigators seeking to identify the significance, in terms of susceptibility to infection, is the widespread finding that an acute or chronic infection may decrease serum levels of micronutrients. This leads to an incorrect assumption of a causal relationship where a low serum level of a particular nutrient predisposes towards increased risk of becoming infected or developing a more rapid progression of disease. This is a particular problem in human studies, where infection often coexists with nutritional deficiencies. Similarly, individuals with low serum levels of micronutrients may well be deficient because of poverty; the poor physical and social environment that such people live in may be a key factor explaining their susceptibility to infection. Thus, however strong the evidence is for biological plausibility, a case for intervention can only really be made if a randomized controlled clinical trial can be established. These are invaluable and have been pivotal in identifying the impact of vitamin A supplementation, for example (see also Semba, Chapter 8, this volume). However, such a trial is not always easy to establish. There may be technical issues as to what the 'placebo' should contain and doubts over whether it is possible to prepare a nutritional intervention that is really a 'placebo'. Sometimes there are additional logistical and political issues, where it is felt that a 'placebo' is not acceptable. In such circumstances, where it is desirable, but impossible, to perform a randomized controlled trial, a careful analysis of changes as a result of interventions introduced in a phased manner may be performed. The impact of phased dietary supplementation on birth weight and perinatal mortality was carefully assessed in communities in the Gambia (Ceesay *et al.*, 1997), where provision of additional food for some but not all communities would have been unacceptable. However strong the design of the epidemiological study and however rigorous the peer review process, it needs more than one or more published papers to promote the development and implementation of a new policy.

International working groups and agencies play a vital role by publicizing and synthesizing data from all studies available. The use of meta-analysis allows a stronger conclusion than is possible from individual studies. From these, expert working groups can produce generic policies that are applicable for countries with a reasonably defined level of deficiency, using community-based clinical and biochemical surveys, even if no specific research on the nutrition intervention in question has been performed in the country concerned. Unlike many health interventions, such as vaccinations, where it is assumed that most citizens are at risk, nutritional deficiencies may not be nationwide. Governments need to decide what proportion of the population is deficient and whether there are enough citizens at risk to merit regional or national interventions.

Even if some form of national nutrition survey is performed, information on nutritional status alone is not enough to make a case for a nutrition intervention, especially when there are competing demands for resources. This requires a careful analysis of what benefits a nutritional intervention will bring over and above or even instead of other public health interventions. While almost all nations are signatories to the Convention on the Rights of the Child, which contains a strong commitment to the provision of an adequate diet, many less developed countries have to make painful decisions about what can be afforded and what cannot. This needs a critical review of how nutrition fits into national or regional health policies – information on costs, resources, training and community acceptability is necessary. Arguing an evidence-based case for nutrition interventions may seem perfectly logical, but there are competing demands for resources and sometimes considerable difficulties in establishing change, however logical that may appear.

In many less developed countries, the provision of resources for the introduction or maintenance of primary health care/public health programmes is often 'kick-started' by supplies and training provided by bilateral or multilateral donors. Indeed, such activities may sometimes antedate the development of a national policy. Once the donor supply ceases, a government needs to decide whether to continue with the intervention or not. This can create problems if sufficient resources have not been allocated from government funds in the first place. There are many reasons for the continuation or discontinuation of nutrition programmes; they are often influenced by central and local politics. As many governments now tend to decentralize their planning and delivery of health services, allowing regional authorities to decide on priorities for expenditure, it is quite possible for regions to have different priorities for nutrition interventions. It is difficult for senior health staff to make judgements on these comparative issues. They have a difficult task in deciding what to focus on. The availability of well-argued policy documents in which the benefits of nutrition interventions are clearly displayed and 'marketed' can be very influential.

Finally, no strategy for improving nutritional status will succeed unless there is a strong sense of conviction among the communities that the intervention proposed is worth the additional effort. Case studies are needed to document whether there has been sufficient 'social marketing' of nutritional interventions. This is particularly important where changes in food-production practices are being promoted or where supplements need to be bought, however cheaply. Research-funding agencies tend not to be interested in such 'applied' knowledge. Yet all the biochemical arguments in the world may be of less importance than what citizens think about the significance of a nutritional deficiency and what is suggested that they and their government might do about it.

How then can governments or international agencies make evidence-based reviews of the importance of nutritional interventions as an infection-control strategy in their own situation? Despite the value of meta-analyses and expert working groups, it is not always possible to extrapolate from one environment to another. For instance, the very favourable effects of micronutrient supplementation in Nepal need to be examined among women in sub-Saharan Africa, where human immunodeficiency virus (HIV) and malaria are endemic. There may need to be different infant-feeding policies for different communities. For instance, similar rates of post-natal transmission of HIV from mothers to children in South Africa are found among exclusively breast-feeding women and women who use infant formulas (Coutsoudis *et al.*, 1999). These results are particularly important in areas where feeding infant formulas is associated with higher mortality (UNICEF, 1998a). Thus, infant-feeding policies that have been developed for HIV-positive mothers in Europe and North America (where breast-feeding is always discouraged) are not appropriate for women living in poor environments.

There are ethical issues facing researchers and policy-makers as they conduct studies and analyse published data in seeking to develop their own country-specific nutrition policies. The design of such interventions needs to take account of current changes in ethical climates and considerations, such as in the Helsinki declaration. However, many of the principles developed by modern ethics committees relate to the problems of performing clinical trials among individuals with a disease who are allocated to a standard compared with a novel treatment. There is a deficiency of ethical guidelines suitable for research in public health nutrition.

The development of the evidence base for the design and implementation of public health nutrition interventions is a complex process. It needs to take account of biological plausibility, the cost-effectiveness of the impact in comparison with other interventions and an analysis of the social factors affecting the sustenance of a programme. This chapter seeks to provide an analytical approach to enable policy-makers to reach informed conclusions. It uses the above framework to examine particular nutritional deficiencies.

The difference between the effects of a large dose of a micronutrient, the regular consumption of a better diet or smaller doses of supplements needs clarification. Some micronutrients appear to have a particularly profound effect on immunity – vitamin A, selenium and zinc (see Semba, Chapter 8, Prasad, Chapter 10, and McKenzie *et al.*, Chapter 12, this volume). Their impact is so striking that pharmaconutrient immunological responses may well be the cause for a change in immunity rather than repletion of a deficiency state. Furthermore, there are differences in the effect of micronutrients on different diseases. For instance, vitamin A benefits pneumonia associated with measles (Hussey and Klein, 1990), but not other types of pneumonia (Fawzi *et al.*, 2000). Zinc supplements seem effective against the prevalence and severity of both diarrhoea and respiratory infection (Bhutta *et al.*, 1999a; see also Prasad, Chapter 10, this volume). This information is sufficient to generate global programmes of vitamin A supplementation and some interesting possibilities for supplementation programmes for zinc. Selenium has an increasingly recognized anti-infective property, but data on its role in public health are lacking. Now that the immunological benefits of individual micronutrients are recognized, it seems intuitively sensible to combine these into a multiple micronutrient preparation. Interestingly, there has been almost no regulatory control on multiple micronutrients. Any company can produce or market micronutrients and their advertising claims have rarely been subjected to any form of evaluation. A rare but notable exception has been the recommendations to avoid toxic levels of vitamin A during pregnancy. Despite the widespread lack of published evaluation of their efficacy, many people in industrialized countries consume multiple micronutrients on a daily basis. The finding of deficient serum levels of antioxidants in apparently well-nourished subjects who smoke has increased concerns in smokers, who are increasingly taking antioxidants to 'protect' themselves against the toxic effects of tobacco smoking. There are widespread public concerns that 'modern' diets are not adequate nutritionally and the shelves of pharmacies in many industrialized countries are stocked with single and multimicronutrient supplements. Many pregnant and lactating women take them. Parents frequently give them to their children. However, there are almost no data on their efficacy.

The interaction of individual micronutrients on the absorption and metabolism of other micronutrients is well recognized. For that reason, most preparations contain up to two times the recommended intake. It is at present uncertain as to whether there is an additive or interactive effect of micronutrients that individually have been shown to have profound immunological effects. Will a multiple micronutrient capsule containing vitamin A, zinc and selenium produce the same immunological and anti-infective benefit as when these have been given individually?

New analytical approaches are necessary if the potential benefits of micronutrient interventions in particular are to be achieved. With the escalating costs of the development of new antibiotics and anti-retrovirals, giving very high patient costs for treatment of an infection, the relative cheapness of nutritional interventions is becoming increasingly attractive, especially as they are not associated with the development of disease-resistant strains and are rarely associated with patient toxicity.

Malnutrition and Infection

There are clear descriptions of the criteria for classifying individuals as underweight, thin or short (World Health Organization, 2001). However, such individuals may also be micronutrient-deficient independently of their anthropometric status.

Many studies have identified the impaired immunity and high infection rates among children with severe malnutrition (Waterlow *et al.*, 1992). Undoubtedly, the high rates of mortality among such children were attributable to the high rates of infections, such as septicaemia, pneumonia, diarrhoea and meningitis. It is often difficult to know which came first – the infection or the malnutrition – in the severely malnourished, heavily infected child. However, comparison of the low rates of mortality during nutrition rehabilitation of children in the Caribbean, where malaria, measles and tuberculosis were uncommon (Waterlow *et al.*, 1992), and the high rates of mortality among malnourished children in sub-Saharan Africa (Kessler *et al.*, 2000), even when similar nutrition rehabilitation rates were used (Prudhon *et al.*, 1997), indicates the importance of the additional burden of infection on the mortality. Rates as low as 1 or 2% mortality or less are commonly achieved in the management of severe malnutrition, such as children with kwashiorkor or marasmus, in Jamaica. Rates of mortality among severely malnourished children in Africa may be as high as 50%. Intermediate results are obtained in Asia (Khanum *et al.*, 1998). Ashworth and Khanum (1997) identified key nutritional and infection-control interventions, demonstrating that it is possible to bring down mortality to around 10% or even less, even in difficult circumstances in Africa, showing the importance of improving nutritional and infection management together (Schofield and Ashworth, 1996).

The interactions between immunity and the presence of severe metabolic disturbances associated with systemic and intestinal infection have been reviewed (Waterlow *et al.*, 1992; Tomkins, 2000). Despite the importance of severe malnutrition as a challenge for health care professionals and community workers alike, it should be recognized that, for every one severely malnourished child, there are at least another 20 with moderate malnutrition. It is estimated that around 150 million children are underweight, with particularly large numbers in South Asia (over 85 million) and sub-Saharan Africa (over 30 million) (UNICEF, 2001). Using prospective observational studies, in which measurements of weight and height are accompanied by environmental and socio-economic assessments, it has been possible to assess the significance of mild to moderate malnutrition on subsequent risk of infection or mortality. These studies have controlled for the differences in physical, socio-economic and caring environments that malnourished children often live in. A study of almost 5000 preschool children in Uganda showed that there was an increasing mortality risk according to decreasing nutritional status, allowing for socio-economic factors that also increased the risk of mortality (Vella *et al.*, 1994). A study of malnutrition and risk for infection, as assessed by regular home visits, showed an increase in the prevalence of several types of infection; the greatest impact, however, was on the duration of illness (Pickering *et al.*, 1987). The use of the mid upper arm circumference as an indicator of malnutrition has been promoted over the years (UNICEF, 2001) and data from Uganda demonstrate the mortality risk for individual infections, such as respiratory and diarrhoeal disease, against mid upper arm circumference (Vella *et al.*, 1992, 1993). Moreover, the data demonstrate that different cut-off levels may be selected for identifying individuals at high risk of mortality. The precise cut-off chosen is a trade-off between a high sensitivity or prediction (resulting in a high proportion of children needing to be seen by a health/nutrition professional) with a lower sensitivity but a smaller number of individuals being selected as being below the cut-off for referral. The importance that nutrition within infection-control strategies has been given in recent years is best seen in the programme for IMCI by WHO/UNICEF. In this programme, careful guidelines are provided for basically trained health workers for the recognition and management of malnutrition (WHO/UNICEF, 1997). There are specific opportunities for the introduction of micronutrient interventions, such as vitamin A, within the under-5 child health programme, seeing the visit to a clinic by a sick child as an opportunity for ensuring that prophylactic micronutrient administration is up to date.

The overall conclusion is that severely malnourished subjects are at great risk of infection, such that infective diseases are probably a more common cause of death than metabolic failure. Many studies have demonstrated that micronutrient deficiency is common among severely malnourished children, but there is very little published evidence of the benefit of supplementation in terms of infection outcome. Interestingly, despite the widespread notion that vitamin A should be given to all children with severe malnutrition, there have not been randomized controlled trials investigating the benefits in terms of mortality, though the benefits in terms of the prevention of xerophthalmia are well established (Sommer, 1993). Similarly although zinc is now known to prevent infection and reduce the severity of infection, there have been few randomized clinical trials investigating the precise impact of zinc in severe malnutrition (see also Prasad, Chapter 10, this volume).

Vitamin A and Infection

Vitamin A and childhood morbidity and mortality

Early studies showed a high risk of mortality among children with clinical and biochemical evidence of vitamin A deficiency (Humphrey et al., 1992). Data on the effects of vitamin A on immunity are now available through preventive and therapeutic studies (see also Semba, Chapter 8, this volume). Several randomized controlled clinical trials showed that regular administration of vitamin A (in capsules) reduces mortality by over 20% among infants and young children in vitamin-A-deficient areas (Sommer, 1997). There was also a reduction in morbidity, though not necessarily mortality, in the neonatal and early infant periods if vitamin A was given in the post-natal period (West et al., 1995; Humphrey et al., 1996). In Ghana, regular supplementation with vitamin A reduced by around 15% the prevalence of episodes of infection that were severe enough to require a clinic attendance (Ghana VAST, 1993). This was particularly noticeable for children presenting with severe, dehydrating episodes of diarrhoea. Regular supplementation with vitamin A also has an impact on malaria, according to a recent study in Papua New Guinea (Shankar et al., 1999). There was a 30% decrease in the number of febrile episodes with a high parasite count. Parasite density was also reduced. In the Ghana study of vitamin A supplementation and child survival, there was no evidence of a decrease in morbidity or mortality from malaria, as assessed by reports of febrile episodes, but there was a 20–30% reduction in the prevalence of malaria slide-positive episodes in the vitamin-A-supplemented group (Ghana VAST, 1993). The sample size was not large enough to know whether there was any impact on malaria-related mortality in the Ghana or Papua New Guinea studies.

The impact of vitamin A as a treatment has been evaluated, with a special focus on the clinical outcome of diarrhoea and pneumonia in children (Semba, 1999a). There has been a variable response to the use of high-dose vitamin A in the treatment of diarrhoea. In Dhaka, Bangladesh, a randomized controlled trial with factorial design compared the use of vitamin A and/or zinc with placebo in children with diarrhoea of > 3 days' duration (Faruque et al., 1999). A dose of 4500 IU of vitamin A daily for 15 days had no effect on the mean duration of diarrhoea. However, there was a trend towards a reduction in the risk of prolonged diarrhoea (> 7 days in this group). A study from New Delhi, India, analysed the effect of 60 mg vitamin A on the mean duration of diarrhoea and stool frequency (Bhan and Bhandari, 1998). There were no differences between intervention and control groups as a whole, although there was a significant lower risk of persistent diarrhoea in the vitamin A-treated group. However, in a subgroup analysis of children who were not breast-fed, there was a significant reduction in all the main outcome measures of the study among the children receiving vitamin A. This included a 16% reduction in the length of the average diarrhoeal episode, 27% reduction in the mean stool frequency and 60% reduction in the proportion of children who passed watery stools. These benefits were not seen in breast-fed children. Another study from New Delhi evaluated the role of vitamin A supplementation (100,000 or

200,000 IU, according to age) on the clinical outcome of acute diarrhoea of < 3 days' duration (Dewan *et al.*, 1995). There was no effect of vitamin A on the group as a whole, but in those children who had pre-existing vitamin A deficiency, as defined by abnormal conjunctival impression cytology, there was a significant reduction in the duration of diarrhoea. A further study from Bangladesh (Henning *et al.*, 1992) found no effect of vitamin A on the duration of acute watery diarrhoea and no reduction in the subsequent number of episodes with persistent diarrhoea. A study of children with acute shigellosis in Bangladesh given 200,000 IU as a single dose showed an increased proportion of children who were clinically cured at 5 days, even though there was no difference in the bacteriological cure rate (Faruque *et al.*, 1999). A study in South Africa comparing early and late administration of a large dose of vitamin A showed no impact on clinical outcome or the extent of intestinal damage as assessed by lactulose and mannitol excretion in the urine after an oral dose; vitamin A levels assessed by relative dose response and plasma retinol levels were the same 8 weeks later (Rollins *et al.*, 2000). Overall, it seems that, with the exception of dysentery, vitamin A does not have a therapeutic role in acute diarrhoea, although there are insufficient data to enable conclusions on its role in persistent diarrhoea.

Stephensen *et al.* (1998) gave vitamin A to children with pneumonia in Peru. Those receiving vitamin A had a longer duration of clinical signs and a greater need for supplemental oxygen. These adverse effects were not so severe as to require longer hospitalization. Among children hospitalized with pneumonia in Mozambique, there was no benefit overall in giving vitamin A, but there was a reduction in the number of children still requiring hospitalization after day 5 from those given vitamin A if they were < 1 year of age (Julien *et al.*, 1999). Overall, therefore, it seems as though vitamin A treatment in non-measles-associated pneumonia is not beneficial and may even have some side-effects.

Vitamin A treatment has been evaluated in measles-associated pneumonia. The evidence for a role of vitamin A in the treatment of measles is strong. A study from Tanzania showed a mortality of 7% in the vitamin A-supplemented group, compared with 13% in the placebo group (Barclay *et al.*, 1987). The largest decrease in mortality was seen in the under-2-year-olds and in those children who had measles-related complications, especially croup. A similar study in South Africa showed significant reductions in mean duration of stay, rates of admission to the intensive care unit and mortality in children > 15 months old (Klein and Hussey, 1990). A further study, also in South Africa, of measles-associated pneumonia showed a significant improvement in recovery and in morbidity assessed by a local integrated score system (Hanekom *et al.*, 1997). In a study of Zambian children with measles-associated pneumonia who were insufficiently ill to require hospital admission, there was no benefit from prescribing vitamin A during the acute stage of the illness (Gernaat *et al.*, 1998). However, when analysed at 4 weeks, there was a significant reduction in cough and pneumonia in the vitamin A group. Overall, there seems to be a very strong effect of vitamin A in measles-associated pneumonia. The reasons for the difference between the effect in measles-associated pneumonia and non-measles-associated pneumonia have not been clarified, but the profound immune suppression in measles may be a factor that is amenable to response to vitamin A supplementation.

Vitamin A and HIV-associated infection in children

A study in Tanzania showed that vitamin A supplementation reduced acquired immune deficiency syndrome (AIDS)-specific mortality in Tanzanian children (Fawzi et al., 1999). A South Africa study has similarly shown a reduction in morbidity among HIV-positive children with pneumonia and given vitamin A (Bobat et al., 1999). A recent study showed that antenatal vitamin A has an effect on the intestinal tract of HIV-positive, but not HIV-negative, infants in the first few weeks of life (Filteau et al., 2001). These studies suggest that vitamin A has a selective response, exerting a strong preventive activity against infection and mortality in childhood if the infections are associated with measles or HIV. This compares with the somewhat less striking effect in HIV-negative children reviewed above.

Vitamin A and clinical outcome in adults

In view of the well-recognized effect of vitamin A deficiency on epithelial surfaces, it is interesting that shedding of HIV from the reproductive tract is greater among women with low serum retinols in Kenya (Mostad et al., 1997). There is also an association between low levels of vitamin A and high rates of transmission of HIV from mothers to their infants in Malawi (Semba et al., 1994). It is difficult to know whether these relationships between low serum retinol and pathological change are causal, as low levels of plasma retinol are often indicative of an acute-phase response. Thus, the women with the highest viral load and clinical manifestations of HIV-related disease, and therefore more likely to shed or transmit the virus, are also likely to have low serum retinols. It was hoped that intervention with vitamin A in pregnant HIV-positive women would reduce the prevalence of mother-to-child transmission of the virus (Nduati et al., 1995). Unfortunately, preliminary results of such studies have failed to show such a beneficial effect of vitamin A supplementation among pregnant women in South Africa (Coutsoudis et al., 1997). Results of studies in other countries are awaited.

Vitamin A and maternal morbidity and mortality

A recent review outlines some aspects of the interaction between vitamin A and causes of maternal mortality, emphasizing biological plausibility (Faisel and Pittrof, 2000). Women who had low serum vitamin A levels during the second trimester of pregnancy and throughout the post-partum period had an increased risk of puerperal infection (West et al., 1999). This study also showed that pregnant women with night blindness were twice as likely to develop genitourinary infections as women without night blindness (Christian *et al.*, 2000). However, the impact of systemic infection and metabolic stress on vitamin A is well documented and it is almost impossible to know which came first – the metabolic/infective stress or the low serum vitamin A status. The Nepal study also showed a remarkable reduction in maternal mortality as a result of supplementation with β-carotene or vitamin A (West *et al.*, 1999): 44,646 married women, of whom 20,119 became pregnant 22,189 times, were included in the study. The women were randomized to receive weekly a single oral supplement of placebo, vitamin A (7000 μg retinol equivalents) or β-carotene (42 mg or 7000 retinol equivalents) for over 3.5 years. All causes of mortality in women during pregnancy and up to 12 weeks post-partum (pregnancy-related mortality) and mortality during pregnancy to 6 weeks post-partum, excluding deaths apparently related to injury (maternal mortality), were used as the main outcome measures. Mortality related to pregnancy in the placebo, vitamin A and β-carotene groups was 704, 426 and 361 deaths per 100,000 pregnancies, respectively. Combined, vitamin A or β-carotene lowered mortality by 44% and reduced the maternal mortality-rate ratio from 645 to 385 deaths per 100,000 live births. Important causes of maternal mortality, in order of frequency, were obstetric-related causes, eclampsia, haemorrhage, sepsis and injury. There was not sufficient statistical power to ascribe the mortality impact of vitamin A or β-carotene to their effect on one cause of mortality rather than another. However, an analysis of the impact of the supplements on symptoms of illness was performed (Christian *et al.*, 1998). There was no impact of either supplement on morbidity rates reported up to 28 week of gestation. However, in late pregnancy (> 28 weeks), symptoms of nausea, faintness and night blindness were reduced with vitamin A, but not β-carotene, supplementation. Vitamin A supplementation shortened the length of labour by 1.5 h and 50 min among nulliparous and multiparous women, respectively. Both interventions reduced the post-partum prevalence of diarrhoea (at least four loose stools) and night blindness. β-Carotene supplementation also reduced symptoms of high fever post-partum. The mean number of days of any reported illness symptoms was 3–4 per week throughout pregnancy. Among women receiving vitamin A, the total number of days of illness symptoms accrued over the last 12 weeks of pregnancy was lower by 5 days compared with the placebo recipients. There are very few publications on rates of morbidity among pregnant women and the above study is the only one published to date describing the impact of a micronutrient supplementation on morbidity.

A study of 1075 HIV-positive women in Dar es Salaam, Tanzania, examined the impact of vitamin A, with or without micronutrients (20 mg vitamin B_1, 20 mg vitamin B_2, 25 mg vitamin B_6, 100 mg niacin, 50 mg vitamin B_{12}, 500 mg vitamin C, 30 mg vitamin E and 0.8 mg folic acid), on pregnancy outcome (Fawzi *et al.*, 1998). Women were recruited at between 12 and 27 weeks' gestation and received their regular supply of ante-natal iron and folic acid. They were randomized to receive placebo, vitamin A, a mixture of multivitamins without vitamin A or a mixture of multivitamins, including vitamin A. There were 30 fetal deaths in the women receiving multivitamins compared with 49 among those not receiving multivitamins. The prevalence of low birth weight (< 2500 g) was 15.8% in those receiving placebo and 8.8% in those receiving the multivitamins. The prevalence of *severe prematurity* (< 37 weeks) was 10.2% in those receiving placebo and 6.2% in those receiving multiple micronutrients. Interestingly, vitamin A did not affect any of these variables, and multivitamins, but not vitamin A, resulted in an increase in the number of CD4, CD8 and CD3 cells in the bloodstream. This is the only published study on the effect of multivitamins on such outcomes to date.

A review of the impact of vitamin A supplements as 'anti-infective' interventions (Semba, 1999b) describes the earlier work of supplementation with cod liver oil as a protection against puerperal sepsis in the UK. Using various criteria for puerperal sepsis, there was a lower incidence among women receiving cod liver oil than among those who did not. In view of the recent interest in the immunological effect of vitamin D (Wilkinson *et al.*, 2000), the high concentration of vitamin D in cod liver oil may also have been important; it would be interesting to explore this in future studies.

An extensive review of nutritional interventions for the prevention of maternal morbidity concluded that there is an urgent need for trials such as the above with sufficient statistical power in order to determine what micronutrients could usefully achieve in terms of improved immune function and morbidity (Kulier *et al.*, 1998). The benefits of regular doses of vitamin A should not overshadow the many opportunities there are for increasing intake of dietary vitamin A and integrating supplementation with improved dietary intake (Filteau and Tomkins, 1999). However, the problems in achieving satisfactory improvement in vitamin A status using fruits and vegetables have been highlighted recently (de Pee *et al.*, 1999). The development of the new data on the effects of vitamin A and its incorporation into policies and programmes has been a very good 'model' for evidence-based public health nutrition policy.

Selenium and Infection

There is increasing interest in the role of selenium deficiency in infection (see also McKenzie *et al.*, Chapter 12, this volume). Initially, the interest came because of the recognized value of selenium as an antioxidant. More recently, there seems to be increasing evidence for a role in cellular immunity (see McKenzie *et al.*, Chapter 12, this volume). The presence of selenium is important within the enzyme glutathione peroxidase, which catalyses the reduction of peroxides as part of an antioxidant response to infection.

A dietary supplementation study in young volunteers using 200 μg day^{-1} of sodium selenite for 8 weeks showed a 118% increase in cytotoxic lymphocyte-mediated tumour toxicity and an 82.3% increase in natural killer cell activity, as compared with baseline values (Kiremidjian-Schumacher *et al.*, 1994). There was also a significant augmentation of the ability of peripheral blood lymphocytes to respond to stimulation with mitogen and to express the high-affinity interleukin (IL)-2 receptor on their surface (Roy *et al.*, 1994). These changes occurred despite the failure of the supplementation regime to increase plasma selenium levels. A study of elderly Italian subjects showed an association between the percentage of natural killer cells in the circulation and serum selenium concentrations (Ravaglia *et al.*, 2000). Overall, there seems to be a good case for including selenium within supplements for improving immunity.

Keshan disease, an epidemic form of myocarditis occurring in certain parts of China, is particularly prevalent in areas with a low selenium content of soil and food and is associated with low plasma selenium levels (Ge and Yang, 1993). Sodium selenite, given as an oral dose once a week, reduced the prevalence and mortality from this cardiac disease, which seemed extremely likely to be precipitated by a virus in view of its epidemiology (Blot *et al.*, 1993). The pathophysiology of Coxsackie virus and selenium deficiency has been investigated in great detail by an elegant series of experiments, which demonstrated that certain strains of this virus induced more severe pathological damage in the myocardium of selenium-deficient animals (Beck and Levander, 1998). There was an interaction with vitamin E deficiency, which increased the severity of the disease (Beck *et al.*, 1994; Beck, 1999). Of great interest was the demonstration that passage of the virus through certain strains of selenium-deficient animals resulted in change in the viral RNA genome (Beck, 1997). This demonstration that host malnutrition might actually change the structure of a viral genome has major public health nutrition implications for infectious disease.

The interaction between selenium and viral infection has been explored in other infections in China. It was noted that hepatitis B virus was more common in populations with selenium deficiency (Yu *et al.*, 1989); regular selenium supplementation resulted in a decrease in its carriage rate. Interestingly, subjects with HIV have decreased plasma selenium levels (Cirelli *et al.*, 1991); these are associated with increased indicators of lipid peroxidation, such as plasma lipid peroxides and breath pentane and ethane output (Aghdassi and Allard, 2000). However, there are also low plasma levels of other antioxidants, including vitamin E, β-carotene and zinc, in HIV-infected subjects. There is an association between selenium concentrations and severity of HIV, as measured by erythrocyte sedimentation rate and haemoglobin concentration (Cirelli *et al.*, 1991), indicating that low plasma selenium levels may be part of the impact of an inflammatory response on plasma micronutrient levels. Low serum selenium was a good predictor of clinical deterioration. Among children with HIV, a low serum selenium had a particularly strong predictive power for risk of mortality (Baum *et al.*, 1997). Daily supplements of 100 μg selenium alone failed to show an impact on CD4 count or incidence of opportunistic infections in the supplemented group, even though the serum selenium was maintained, whereas the placebo group experienced a decrease in serum selenium (Constans *et al.*, 1995, 1999). When comparing micronutrient levels and risk of mortality among HIV-infected drug users, serum selenium was more predictive than vitamin A (Baum and Shor-Posner, 1997). The only other published result of selenium supplementation describes a combination of selenium (500 μg day^{-1}) and N-acetylcysteine in HIV-positive subjects. There was an effect on the CD4–CD8 ratio but no impact on viral load; no clinical impact was reported (Look *et al.*, 1998). Overall, there is strong biological plausibility for a role of selenium in immunity but, so far, there is insufficient evidence that selenium supplements influence the severity or outcome of infection.

Zinc and Infection

Zinc has many effects on immunity and the host response to infection (see Prasad, Chapter 10, this volume). It plays a pivotal role in many hundreds of enzymes, stabilizes cell membranes, modulates humoral and cell-mediated immunity and is increasingly recognized to be responsible for the control of apoptosis and oxidative capacity.

Studies of experimental zinc deficiency in humans showed that the functions of T-helper (Th) 1 cells, as evidenced by production of interferon-γ, IL-2 and tumour necrosis factor alpha, were decreased (Beck et al., 1997). Functions of Th2 cells (as evidenced by production of IL-4, IL-6 and IL-10) were unaffected by zinc deficiency. This imbalance between Th1 and Th2 cells and the decreased percentage of cytotoxic T-cells may account for the decreased cell-mediated immune functions in zinc-deficient subjects. Antibody titres measured after elderly subjects had been vaccinated with influenza vaccine were higher in apparently healthy subjects who received a mixture of zinc and selenium (Turk et al., 1998). Zinc supplementation has been studied in patients with sickle-cell disease, who are often zinc-deficient due to increased requirements resulting from haemolysis: zinc supplements resulted in an increase in B lymphocyte and granulocyte zinc levels and in IL-2 production (Prasad et al., 1999). This was accompanied by a decreased incidence of documented bacteriologically positive infections and a decreased number of hospitalizations. The authors concluded that zinc deficiency results in decreased production of IL-2, as a result of decreased activation of nuclear factor kappa B and subsequent decreased expression of IL-2 and IL-2 receptor genes (Prasad, 2000). In a placebo-controlled study, preschool children in India were supplemented with zinc gluconate, providing 10 mg of elemental zinc daily unless they had diarrhoea, in which case they were given 20 mg. Zinc supplementation resulted in a decrease in the percentage of children who were anergic or hypoergic (using the induration score after a Mantoux test) (Sazawal et al., 1997). The zinc-supplemented group had a significantly higher increase in the numbers of CD3 and CD4 cells and in the CD4-to-CD8 ratio, but there was no difference in the numbers of CD8 or CD20 cells. These data show clearly that zinc supplements have wide-ranging effects on the immune system, even in apparently well-nourished subjects. This emphasizes the fact that zinc deficiency may occur independently of malnutrition assessed by anthropometric indices.

The effects of zinc deficiency on the infection, growth and survival of children with severe malnutrition are well described (Golden and Golden, 1979). Zinc supplements are now recommended for the routine management of children with severe malnutrition. Zinc supplementation improves tissue function and integrity. Experimental studies of zinc deficiency show a marked effect on intestinal morphology and function, producing villous atrophy and a heightened secretory response to diarrhoeal pathogens, such as the toxin from *Vibrio cholerae* (Tomkins, 2000). Studies of the effect of zinc supplementation among malnourished children in Bangladesh showed a reduction in loss of intestinal fluid among children with acute diarrhoea and a shortening of the duration of diarrhoea (Roy *et al.*, 1997). Similarly, among malnourished Bangladeshi children with persistent diarrhoea syndrome, there was a beneficial effect of zinc supplementation on the duration and severity of diarrhoea (Roy *et al.*, 1998); there was also a lower mortality among the zinc-supplemented group, but the sample size was small. Improvement in the intestinal barrier, as assessed by urinary excretion of lactulose and mannitol after an oral test dose, occurred following zinc supplementation in both studies (Roy *et al.*, 1992). Regular follow-up to the homes of these children showed that the zinc-supplemented children had fewer episodes of diarrhoea and respiratory infection. More recent studies have examined the effect of daily doses of zinc syrup among malnourished children in an urban slum in India. Children who received daily doses of zinc experienced a decrease (around 45%) in the incidence of respiratory infection (Sazawal *et al.*, 1998). Among low-birth-weight full-term infants in Brazil, there was a 28% decrease in the prevalence of diarrhoea and a 33% decrease in the prevalence of cough in a zinc-supplemented group (Lira *et al.*, 1998). A cohort of children aged 12–59 months and recovering from acute diarrhoea was studied in India. Children with a low initial plasma zinc concentration ($\leq$ 8.4 μM) had significantly more episodes of diarrhoea and severe diarrhoea than did children with a normal plasma zinc. The mean prevalence rate of diarrhoea was four times higher in the zinc-deficient group and the mean prevalence rate of acute lower respiratory-tract infections was 3.5 times higher in children with low plasma zinc (Bahl *et al.*, 1998). A study of preschool children in Mexico showed that those supplemented with 20 mg of zinc had fewer episodes of disease overall and, in particular, had fewer episodes of diarrhoea (Rosado *et al.*, 1997). A study among malnourished children in Bangladesh examined the long-term effects of giving a 2-week course of elemental zinc (20 mg day^{-1}) on morbidity episodes over the following 8 weeks (Roy *et al.*, 1999). Zinc-supplemented children had significantly fewer episodes of diarrhoea and acute lower respiratory-tract infections compared with the control group. The impact of zinc supplementation on underweight children (< 71% weight for age) on diarrhoeal episodes was even more striking. Among preschool children in Guatemala, those receiving a zinc supplement for 7 months (given as 10 mg elemental zinc day^{-1}) had a 20% lower median incidence of diarrhoea, with an even more marked reduction among those who had low weight-for-length at baseline (Ruel *et al.*, 1997). Zinc supplementation also produced a 67% reduction in the percentage of children who had one or more episodes of persistent diarrhoea. Interestingly, in this study, zinc did not change the incidence of respiratory infections. This contrasted with the experience in India, where, using zinc gluconate (10 mg day^{-1} unless the children had diarrhoea, in which case they were given 20 mg day^{-1}), a significant reduction (45%) in the number of respiratory infections among zinc-supplemented children was observed (Sazawal *et al.*, 1998).

Many of these studies have been subject to a pooled analysis of randomized controlled trials for the effect of zinc on acute and persistent diarrhoea

(Bhutta *et al.*, 1999a). Overall, zinc-supplemented children had a 15% lower probability of continuing diarrhoea on a given day in the acute diarrhoea trials, a 24% lower probability of continuing diarrhoea and a 42% lower rate of treatment failure or death in the persistent diarrhoea trials. In none of the subgroup analyses were the two subgroups of each pair significantly different from each other. However, in persistent diarrhoea, there tended to be a greater effect of zinc in subjects aged < 12 months who were male or who had wasting or lower baseline plasma zinc concentrations (Bhutta *et al.*, 2000). Zinc-supplemented children had a 41% lower probability of developing pneumonia. Despite a large number of trials investigating the effect of zinc on the clinical outcome of the common cold, a careful meta-analysis performed recently showed that the data are inconclusive for a therapeutic role for zinc (Marshall, 2000). Overall, there is a very strong case for improvement in zinc status as a means of preventing diarrhoea and pneumonia.

Zinc deficiency may also contribute to decreased immunity and increased morbidity and mortality during pregnancy. There are several reviews of the association of zinc deficiency and a series of complications in pregnancy and their contribution to maternal mortality (Caulfield *et al.*, 1998). Rather few supplementation studies have been performed and most of the published data have been from studies among women with marginal zinc deficiency. Several studies show an improvement in birth weight following zinc supplementation. Other studies show an association between zinc deficiency and increased risk of pregnancy-related morbidity, such as prolonged labour, toxaemia and blood loss (Goldenberg *et al.*, 1995), but there are no solid data on the impact of zinc supplementation on these aspects of maternal health and morbidity. How much of the pathophysiology is due to immune change is uncertain. The importance of including an adequate dietary zinc intake for pregnant and lactating women is recognized, but studies from Malawi show the considerable problem in obtaining zinc from high-phytate cereals (Gibson *et al.*, 1998; Huddle *et al.*, 1998). There are many theoretical possibilities for a key role for zinc in HIV by its effect on the immune system, viral replication and clinical responsiveness. A study of adults with HIV/AIDS in Zambia failed to show an effect of a combination of micronutrients, including zinc, on clinical outcomes, but these patients were studied late in their disease (Kelly *et al.*, 1999). A study of late-stage HIV patients receiving antiretroviral therapy in Italy showed that the provision of 45 mg of elemental zinc daily for 30 days resulted in decreased incidents of infection with *Pneumocystis* and *Candida* (Mocchegiani and Muzzioli, 2000). In a study examining the rate of progression from HIV to AIDS and mortality in adults in the USA, the consumption of high doses of zinc supplements was associated with an increased rate of progression to clinical AIDS and mortality during the follow-up of the study (Tang *et al.*, 1993). This study did not, however, conform to standard practice for conducting randomized controlled trials. A recent study of adults with HIV showed low serum zinc levels in 23% of HIV subjects (Wellinghausen *et al.*, 2000). This was associated with a low CD4 count, a high viral load and increased neopterin and immunoglobulin A levels. The mean serum zinc level was highest in stage C and lowest in stage A, suggesting that, even if anti-retroviral triple therapy is available, zinc deficiency may well be of clinical importance.

There has been rather little focus on the impact of zinc deficiency in relation to susceptibility to nematode parasitic infections, but experimental and some clinical studies suggest that zinc deficiency may produce profound effects on the gut mucosal immune system (Scott and Koski, 2000). However, it is important to recognize that not all studies of zinc supplementation show benefit. A study of severely malnourished Pakistani children who were receiving a rehabilitation diet of lentils, rice and milk did not show any benefit in terms of diarrhoea morbidity or weight gain if zinc supplements were also given (Bhutta et al., 1999b). It may be that the addition of zinc salts to the local high-phytate diet impairs their bioavailability or that the zinc content of the rehabilitation diet might have been sufficient anyway. Severely malnourished children in a nutrition rehabilitation centre in Bangladesh showed an increased mortality when given large doses of oral zinc (Doherty et al., 1998). Several explanations are possible. Copper deficiency is recognized during large-dose zinc supplementation – zinc impairs copper absorption. Copper deficiency may cause a severe leucopenia, with a consequent decrease in immune function (Percival, 1998).

Overall, there is a strong case for improving zinc status as a means of preventing diarrhoea and pneumonia. Its impact on other infections has not been sufficiently evaluated. Its impact on established disease is well demonstrated for diarrhoea, but there has been no evaluation of it in pneumonia, septicaemia or malaria. Its potential role in HIV is intriguing but unproved. A key challenge facing those who wish to improve zinc status is the need to provide small quantities on a regular basis; in this regard, it has a disadvantage when compared with vitamin A. However, the administration of zinc on a daily basis is quite possible – many citizens in industrialized countries do it regularly without any scientific basis. It seems very important to examine the effect of such doses among deficient subjects in environments with a high risk of infection.

Iron and Infection

Iron deficiency is frequently present in subjects with immune deficiency and high loads of infection. Severe iron deficiency causes suppression of several aspects of the immune system (Bhaskaram and Reddy, 1975; see also Kuvibidila and Baliga, Chapter 11, this volume), but the level of immune suppression is less than that experienced in zinc deficiency. Experimental studies on iron deficiency have shown some effect on immunity, but this is mild, certainly in comparison with the effects of zinc or vitamin A. Periodontal disease, due to Actinobacillus, is associated with low levels of mucin MG2 (Groenink et al., 1999). Subjects with periodontal disease were noted to have a low level of lactoferrin in the bloodstream, suggesting that this predisposed the subjects to the infection. The significance of low levels of lactoferrin in iron-deficient children in developing countries, in whom periodontal disease is common, has not been explored. There are associations between indicators of iron status, such as ferritin levels, and infection. High levels of ferritin and intense iron stores in bone-marrow macrophages have been associated with shorter survival times in patients with HIV, and studies of anaemia in pregnancy in Malawi have shown high mortality among HIV-infected women who have high levels of iron in their bone-marrow examinations (van den Broek and Letsky, 2000). Non-transferrin-bound iron is increased in the lower respiratory tract of patients with *Pneumocystis* pneumonia, who show eight to ten times higher levels in bronchoalveolar lavage fluid, compared with controls (Mateos *et al.*, 1999). The authors suggested the use of iron-chelating agents as a rationale for improved management, but the high levels may reflect the chronic inflammatory response rather than a form of iron metabolism that is contributing to the pathology. A study of apparently healthy residents in Lagos, Nigeria, showed an association between high ferritin levels and parasitaemia (Odunukwe *et al.*, 2000). The authors point out the difficulty of assessing iron status using ferritin levels in malaria-endemic regions. Ferritin is certainly very labile in infection and cannot be used as an indicator of iron status. The measurement of transferrin receptors may be more useful, as they are less affected by inflammation (Beesley *et al.*, 2000). HIV-infected patients carrying the haptoglobin 2–2 phenotype show a worse prognosis with a more rapid rate of viral replication and higher mortality (Delanghe *et al.*, 1998; Gordeuk *et al.*, 2001). These patients had higher serum iron, transferrin saturation and ferritin levels and a low vitamin C concentration, suggesting that less efficient protection against haemoglobin/iron-driven oxidative stress may be a direct mechanism for stimulating viral replication. Further evidence of a toxic effect of iron comes from studies of neutrophil dysfunction in haemosiderosis (Cantinieaux *et al.*, 1999). Serum samples from such patients induced a defect in neutrophil function, which was prevented by coincubation with desferrioxamine. The transferrin–albumin fraction of serum had no effect on neutrophils, whereas the ferritin fraction of normal serum was deleterious to neutrophils and the same fraction from thalassaemic serum decreased neutrophil function even further (Cantinieaux *et al.*, 1999). Overall, there is rather little evidence that iron deficiency impairs the immune response and quite strong evidence that iron overload is damaging.

There are two characteristics of iron that are especially important in infection. First, iron induces oxidative stress (Walker and Walker, 2000). This has been demonstrated in volunteers taking low doses of oral iron and it is particularly marked in subjects receiving large doses of iron by intramuscular or intravenous routes (Oppenheimer, 1998). Second, iron is a stimulant for microbial growth, both for free-living bacteria in the blood, such as *Salmonella* and coliforms, and for intracellular organisms, including parasites, such as malaria. There are considerable advantages in improving iron status with regard to features of child development, such as improved growth and cognitive development. However, in communities where infection loads are high, the desire to improve iron status may enhance the risk of infection. There has been considerable interest in iron status in relation to hepatitis C. Several studies indicate that high-dose iron may actually enhance the infection (Bassett *et al.*, 1999). Iron supplementation increases growth of the hepatitis C virus in culture (Kakizaki *et al.*, 2000). However, there was no improved liver function following iron depletion of subjects with hepatitis C (Herrera, 1999). These studies certainly indicate that there is a risk from iron therapy in terms of oxidative damage or stimulation of microbial growth. There seems to be some form of dose relationship, with lower doses being non-toxic and higher doses being toxic, especially if injected. This has led to the proposal for iron chelation during certain infections (Thuma *et al.*, 1998). A particularly extensive review of this complex relationship between iron and infection has been produced by Oppenheimer (2001).

The increased mortality associated with severe anaemia is well established among children and pregnant women (Brabin *et al.*, 1990). Many public health programmes include iron supplementation of pregnant women, but very few provide iron supplementation for infants and children. There have been several theoretical or empirical reasons why iron has not been advised in populations where infections are endemic. First, experimental studies show an increased bacterial growth when iron is added to the culture medium (Andrews, 1998; Brochu *et al.*, 1998). Second, there were initial reports of increased intestinal parasitic infection during refeeding of refugees, though these were observational studies and there were confounding variables (Murray *et al.*, 1978). Third, there was increased respiratory morbidity and mortality when iron was given intramuscularly to anaemic infants in Papua New Guinea (Oppenheimer *et al.*, 1986). Fourth, there have been reports that iron supplementation increased susceptibility of infants and children to malaria (see Oppenheimer, 2001). Thus, iron deficiency has often been portrayed as a 'protective mechanism'.

However, there is conflicting evidence and several recent studies show no deleterious effects of iron supplementation, even in malarious areas. A rigorous study of supplementation of Tanzanian infants in an area that is endemic for malaria has compared different prophylactic regimes (Menendez *et al.*, 1997). Those subjects who received daily iron supplements had a lower rate of anaemia than those who received malarial prophylaxis alone. The data showed a protective efficacy for iron of 28.8%, compared with the control population that did not receive iron. The attack rate for anaemia, as assessed by regular anaemia surveillance, was 0.62 cases per child year^{-1}, compared with 1.00 case per child year^{-1} in the controls. The groups did not experience different attack rates of clinical malaria. The frequency of malaria episodes in unsupplemented vs. supplemented children was 0.87 vs. 1.00 cases per child year^{-1}. A study of Tanzanian children aged 5 months to 3 years examined the impact of providing a low-dose micronutrient supplement, including iron, three times per week (Ekvall *et al.*, 2000). The mean haemoglobin level was 8 g l^{-1} higher among supplemented children during the 5-month period of the study. In a group of supplemented children who also received sulphadoxine-pyrimethamine, the mean level of haemoglobin increased by 22 g l^{-1}. Supplementation with iron did not affect malaria incidence. Supplementation of older children with a mixture of several micronutrients, including iron, improved biochemical status but did not increase the frequency or severity of clinical episodes of malaria (Bates *et al.*, 1987; Fuller *et al.*, 1988). A study of the effect of weekly iron supplements in adolescent girls in Tanzania showed benefits of supplementation in terms of raised ferritin levels and growth (Beasley *et al.*, 2000). There was slightly increased malaria parasitaemia, but there were no adverse clinical effects. These recent studies indicate that the provision of regular oral iron supplements contributes to the prevention of anaemia, with little or no increased risk of malaria. Although there are dangers if parenteral iron is given to children in malarious communities, as reviewed above, the benefits of improving iron status in anaemic communities appears to outweigh the risk of enhancing infection in children. The effects of iron on HIV infection and associated opportunistic infection are not yet clarified.

Mixed Micronutrients and Infection

In view of the evidence that individual micronutrients have quite marked effects on morbidity and mortality from infectious disease, there is increasing interest in combining micronutrients. There are important interactions between micronutrients, such that large doses of one may inhibit the absorption of another, and these need to be considered in interpreting the results of multiple micronutrient intervention. Mixtures of micronutrients have been investigated in many studies where the focus has been on nutritional outcomes (Ndossi and Taylor, 1999). Variable responses in haemoglobin, plasma zinc and retinol, with increases in linear growth, have been observed in Vietnam (Thu *et al.*, 1999), though effects on morbidity were not recorded. Indeed, at present, there are remarkably few studies on the effect of multiple micronutrient interventions on immunity or morbidity in women and children. One of the most recent is an evaluation of the impact of multiple micronutrients on the pregnancy outcome of HIV-positive women in Tanzania (Fawzi *et al.*, 1998). Mothers received either a placebo, vitamin A alone or vitamin A with a range of additional micronutrients. These consisted of vitamins B_1, B_2, B_6, B_{12}, C and E, niacin and folic acid. There were several important findings. First, there was an increase in numbers of circulating CD3, CD4 and CD8 lymphocytes among the mothers receiving mixed micronutrients, whereas supplementation with vitamin A had no effect. Similarly, there was no effect of vitamin A supplementation on pregnancy outcome. In contrast, multiple micronutrient supplementation was associated with a significant reduction in the percentage of women who had fetal deaths (9.6 vs. 5.9%), stillbirths (6.1 vs. 3.5%), low birth weight (15.8 vs. 8.8%), a composite of preterm birth or low birth weight (8.8 vs. 3.8%) or an infant who was small for gestation age (17.6 vs. 10.0%). These rather striking findings are important for HIV-positive women, but there is no evidence yet that such improvements occur in women who are HIV-negative.

Breast-feeding and Infection

The benefits of breast-feeding with regard to infection in the neonate and older infant are extensive and well documented (Victoria *et al.*, 1989). The benefits have mostly focused on the reduction in incidence, severity, duration and mortality from diarrhoea, especially among malnourished children (Brown *et al.*, 1989). Several studies have also emphasized the protective effect of breast-feeding against pneumonia, which is fast becoming the most important global cause of death among children under 5 years of age. A recent study from Brazil showed that infants who were not being breast-fed were 17 times more likely to be admitted to hospital for pneumonia (Cesar *et al.*, 1999). The benefits of breast-feeding were considerably reduced if infant formula was used as well as breast milk. Rates of pneumonia were much higher in those receiving solids, fluid supplements and/or formula milk. The excess risk was particularly pronounced in infants less than 3 months of age but was still present among older infants. These data support the promotion of exclusive breast-feeding, especially during the first 3 months of life.

The demonstration of transmission of HIV from mother to infant presents a tragic dilemma. Millions of children have now been infected with HIV; most of them live in sub-Saharan Africa (Newell, 1999). Transmission can be attributed in about equal proportions to infection *in utero*, during delivery or from breast milk, though the relative contribution to each of the opportunities for infection varies considerably (Dunn *et al.*, 1992; Bertolli *et al.*, 1996).

Whereas in industrialized countries mother-to-child transmission of HIV has been dramatically reduced by the use of anti-retroviral agents during pregnancy, appropriate obstetric care and exclusive formula feeding after delivery, these options are usually not available or feasible for women in less developed countries. The cost of anti-retroviral therapy, such as AZT, in pregnancy is still so high and its availability so low that only a minute fraction of the population will be able to have access to it. Some of the alternative options have been reviewed (Kuhn and Stein, 1997). Recent data on the use of nevirapine, a much cheaper drug, given as two single doses – one in labour and the other to the infant – show a striking reduction in transmission (UNICEF, 1998b). However, even with nevirapine, transmission by breast milk is still significant. Unfortunately from the perspective of transmission, the cost and safety of infant formula in poor socio-economic conditions are such that the potential benefit of preventing post-natal transmission of HIV by using formula may result in increased mortality from infectious disease as a result of the lack of breast-feeding. An added dilemma is caused by the lack of diagnostic facilities. Currently, the only tests widely available are for HIV antibodies rather than virus; it is not possible to know whether an infant is truly HIV-positive or negative until at least 12 months, and feeding advice based on knowledge of infectious status is not possible on an individual basis.

Although it is estimated that about a third of cases of paediatric HIV globally contract their infection from breast milk, these figures vary considerably from country to country. A meta-analysis showed that transmission was much higher (29%) if the HIV infection was acquired by the mother during lactation than if the mother was already HIV-positive during pregnancy (15%) (Dabis *et al.*, 1993). An important factor is the duration of breast-feeding (Coovadia and Coutsoudis, 2000). If transmission is more common in early lactation, these data would tend to overestimate the proportion of infants with HIV who acquire their infection from breast milk. Recent calculations using pooled data from African children who were known to be HIV-negative at 3 months post-partum indicate a risk of transmission of 3.2 cases per 100 child years of breast-feeding (Leroy *et al.*, 1998).

The HIV load is highest in colostrum (Markham *et al.*, 1994) and in early lactation (Van de Perre, 1999), but breast milk immune factors are also higher at these times. The relationship between viral load in breast milk and transmission via this route needs further study. Other risk factors are likely to be important in the post-natal transmission of HIV. These include deficiency of some of the many immunologically active components of breast milk. The presence of sulphated glycosaminoglycans is of potential importance, because of their inhibition of binding of CD4 cells to the HIV envelope glycoprotein (Newburg *et al.*, 1992). Impaired immunity in the mother, assessed by clinical staging of HIV/AIDS and CD4 and CD8 counts as a result of HIV itself, breast abscess or cracked nipples, systemic maternal infection (from pelvic inflammation or malaria) or increased viral shedding in vitamin A deficiency have each been proposed. There may also be altered immune function and viral uptake by the intestinal mucosa of the infant. This could be influenced by dietary antigen stimulation and malnutrition (including zinc and vitamin A deficiency, which are known to affect immunological competence and mucosal structure and function). Other factors that could enable increased viral uptake include candidal lesions of the buccal mucosa and intestinal damage from infections.

An additional, novel hypothesis has been put forward during studies of breast milk immunology among women in Bangladesh, Tanzania and South Africa (Georgeson and Filteau, 2000; Willumsen *et al.*, 2000). It was noted that around 20% of women in these countries have subclinical mastitis, as assessed by a high ratio of sodium (Na) to potassium (K) and high IL-8 levels in breast milk. This is especially important within the HIV context, because of the association between high numbers of HIV particles and subclinical mastitis (Filteau *et al.*, 1999a). The veterinary literature has recognized subclinical mastitis for several decades. It is known to be associated with a high load of a range of bacteria and is especially common among cattle being fed on antioxidant-deficient pastures. Subclinical mastitis has been noted to be associated with poor milk volume and growth faltering in farm animals and was also present in the study of infant growth in relation to subclinical mastitis in Bangladesh (Filteau *et al.*, 1999b). A recent study in South Africa shows that there are certain patterns of occurrence of subclinical mastitis (Willumsen *et al.*, 2000). Bilateral subclinical mastitis is of a typical mild form, with low Na/K ratios, whereas unilateral subclinical mastitis is more common and is often more severe, with high Na/K ratios and elevated levels of IL-8; there are higher viral loads in samples from women with subclinical mastitis in Durban. The association between subclinical mastitis, viral load and mother-to-child transmission of HIV has been demonstrated in Malawi, though no information on the pattern of subclinical mastitis was provided (Semba and Neville, 1999).

The demonstration that HIV viral load is increased among women with subclinical mastitis has enormous implications for the transmission of HIV in breast milk. It puts great emphasis on the reduction of the prevalence and severity of subclinical mastitis by whatever means possible. A recent study among women in Tanzania shows that the prevalence of subclinical mastitis is lower among women who received dietary supplements with sunflower-seed oil during pregnancy and lactation (Filteau *et al.*, 1999a). Sunflower-seed oil has a high level of vitamin E; the potential antioxidant capacity of this may be extremely relevant to the decrease in levels of mastitis. Interestingly, the role of deficiency of selenium and vitamin E in the development of mastitis in cattle is well recognized (Hogan et al., 1993).

Among the women studied in South Africa, those who fed their infants with breast milk exclusively had a lower prevalence of subclinical mastitis than those who used mixed feeding. It is postulated that milk stasis, attributable to the introduction of mixed feeding, might contribute to the establishment of sub-clinical mastitis. Thus, a combination of infection, micronutrient deficiency and mechanical issues, such as placement, may be important in the development of subclinical mastitis (Willumsen et al., 2001).

Rates of mother-to-child transmission of HIV in relation to type of infant feeding have been studied in an urban community in Durban, South Africa (Coutsoudis et al., 1999). Transmission was 18.8% among never-breast-fed children (i.e. those who received infant formula alone). This compared with 14.6% among exclusively breast-fed infants and 24.1% among infants receiving mixed feeding. Even after allowance for potential confounders, such as maternal CD4/CD8 cell ratio, syphilis-screening results and premature delivery, there was a significantly lower risk of HIV transmission (hazard ratio of 0.52) among exclusively breast-fed infants compared with those receiving mixed feeding. There are several possible explanations. First, the protective effect of exclusive breast-feeding may be due to lower levels of subclinical mastitis and therefore a decrease in the accompanying viral load in breast milk (Willumsen et al., 2000). Second, the delay in introduction of dietary antigens may cause less immunological response in the intestinal mucosa; this may decrease the uptake of virus from the gut into the circulation. Third, the addition of microbes in a mixed diet may damage the intestinal mucosa; indeed, this is suggested by previous studies of intestinal permeability in different dietary groups (Udall et al., 1981).

The findings from Durban suggest that the risk of transmission is relatively low if infants are breast-fed exclusively for 3 months. However, the infection rates thereafter, not yet available from the Durban study, are quite high in other studies and, in the absence of more data, it seems that, after 3 months, breast milk should not be given if accompanied by other foods. It is hoped that, with more widespread availability and effectiveness of new anti-retroviral drugs, the mother-to-child transmission rates are likely to fall. Even so, it will still be necessary to promote the reduction of transmission of HIV by dietary means. At present, it seems that the appropriate advice in poor communities is to reinforce existing messages promoting the exclusive use of breast-feeding until 3–4 months of age. Thereafter, the message is not so clear. In the absence of carefully controlled studies examining the post-natal transmission of HIV using different regimes of stopping breast milk, it is not possible to calculate the additional risk of mother-to-child transmission if breast milk is continued after 4–6 months. If early cessation of breast-feeding is promoted, there may be considerable deficiencies of iron, zinc and other micronutrients. Growth faltering, anaemia, impaired immune responses and an increase in the prevalence of severe infection are all possible in the non-breast-fed child. In addition, the loss of the contraceptive benefits of breast-feeding increases the risk of early, further pregnancies, with associated detriment to maternal health.

Other infections are also transmitted through breast milk; these include hepatitis B, hepatitis C and cytomegalovirus. It is estimated that 58–76% of cytomegalovirus-positive mothers transmit the infection to their children (Georgeson and Filteau, 2000). Premature babies are at special risk of developing cytomegalovirus, HIV and other infections. It seems advisable that a range of lactation interventions should be tested, including the role of the promotion of exclusive breast-feeding and the correct positioning and attachment of the child to minimize breast trauma, the promotion of antioxidant micronutrient status and improved control of opportunistic infection.

Policy Implications

National governments and international agencies have several options. They can improve dietary intake, fortify certain foods with particular micronutrients or provide supplements. They obviously need to keep their 'eyes on the ball' as regards the essential first option, but providing the second and third options is also essential. Government commitments to provide an adequate diet are enshrined within many important international agreements, such as the Convention on the Rights of the Child and the International Conference on Nutrition in Rome. There is further opportunity to rededicate themselves to this goal as a result of the World Summit for Children in 2001.

The demonstration that improved nutritional status has a profound effect on immunity, disease susceptibility, illness severity and mortality should drive governments and civil society to improve dietary intake from all perspectives – 'human rights' and a 'right to the best health status that is possible' and pragmatic concerns to enhance human development.

The second option – food fortification – is technically possible and logistically feasible. Objections have in the past been raised that those populations eating centrally processed food, such as vitamin A-fortified sugar, iodine-fortified salt or folic acid-fortified wheat, would be predominantly in the better-off urban areas, leaving the rural areas untouched by such strategies. With increasing urbanization globally and the presence of many millions of individuals in very-low-income areas of cities, micronutrient deficiencies will definitely occur in subjects who purchase food rather than growing their own and, for this reason, there are immense benefits available from fortification.

Whether either of the above forms of micronutrient provision enhances dietary intake sufficiently to increase micronutrient status and improve immunity and resistance to infection is uncertain. Whereas a small number of studies have examined the impact of fortified-food provision on nutritional indicators, such as haemoglobin concentrations, there have been no studies on the impact of the provision of fortified food on infection. There is an urgent need to establish such studies, particularly now that reliable and robust technologies exist for fortifying foods with a range of micronutrients.

It will be particularly important to perform efficacy and effectiveness studies. It is one thing to show that nutritional status and disease prevalence change as a result of the administration of fortified food in controlled circumstances; it is another to see what happens in the free-market situation in which the food industry and malnourished populations interact. New programmes for nutritional supplementation require consideration of what the extra manpower and other necessary resources are in relation to the existing activities in ministries of health and community development; they are already busy with established programmes that were promoted by evidence-based proposals and the 'champions' who promoted them. Governments can be persuaded to 'invest in nutrition'.

Within the health sector, a strong case has been made for providing regular vitamin A capsules, and this has now been adopted as UNICEF/WHO policy globally and increasingly countries are implementing this at national and district level. It is clear that the impressive mortality and morbidity benefits from regular doses of vitamin A are so striking that the supplementation programme for deficient populations should be regarded as essential under any circumstances.

Supplementation with iron is an effective way of improving haemoglobin in malnourished populations. Many studies have shown the benefit of weekly, as opposed to daily, iron. Certain target populations such as school children can be assisted by school-based or parent–teacher-based distribution systems. Among young children, where malarious morbidity and mortality are of greatest risk, the results indicate that the provision of low-dose iron supplements improves haemoglobin without increasing malarious risk. High-dose oral preparations or any intramuscular preparations are not advisable because of the direct toxicity of iron and the possibility of increasing infection.

The benefits of providing daily doses of zinc during carefully controlled field trials are impressive, with well-documented impacts on morbidity reduction. Unfortunately, because of limited body stores of zinc, it is not possible to give infrequent large doses, as it is for vitamin A. Whereas vitamin A given three times a year has profound effects on mortality, daily administration of zinc is necessary if an impact is to be achieved. There are, to date, no data on the effectiveness of encouraging the daily administration of zinc by child carers in a less intensive manner than that of a field trial. Such studies are, however, under way and will provide important data on effectiveness (where an intervention is given in a strongly promoted manner but not intensively supervised), as opposed to efficacy (where the provision of the intervention is closely supervised). Similarly, while there are individual studies showing the benefits of closely supervised supplementation with selenium or vitamin E, there are very few data on the impact of community-based provision of these micronutrients on a regular basis.

Should single micronutrient programmes be continued? In the light of the clear evidence for a benefit in regard to immunity and infection of vitamin A, zinc and possibly selenium, it seems logical to provide these as a multiple micronutrient preparation. There are now many preparations available for adults and some for children. The recently prepared WHO/UNICEF preparation provides about the recommended daily amount for an adult subject. There are currently several studies examining the nutritional, immunological and health benefits of regular provision of these to women in pregnancy and to young children. When these studies are completed, it will be possible to provide specific information on the degree by which immunity and health indicators are enhanced. Given the remarkable success of the promotion of vitamin A supplementation, largely as a result of data that show an impressive reduction in morbidity and mortality, there is great interest in knowing how much a multiple micronutrient supplementation will change these indicators in children and adults. Nutrition interventions now provide one of the most effective ways of preventing illness, reducing mortality and promoting child development and human capital. The challenge now is whether science can be presented in ways that will persuade governments and civil leaders to take active steps to make a major attack on infectious disease using nutrition interventions.

Acknowledgements

The author acknowledges the support of the following funding agencies: the Wellcome Trust, the Department for International Development, UNICEF and WHO.

References

Aghdassi, E. and Allard, J.P. (2000) Breath alkanes as a marker of oxidative stress in different clinical conditions. *Free Radicals in Biology and Medicine* 28, 880–886.

Andrews, S.C. (1998) Iron storage in bacteria. *Advances in Microbial Physiology* 40, 281–351.

Ashworth, A. and Khanum, S. (1997) Cost-effective treatment for severely malnourished children: what is the best approach? *Health Policy and Planning* 12, 115–121.

Bahl, R., Bhandari, N., Hambidge, K.M. and Bhan, M.K. (1998) Plasma zinc as a predictor of diarrheal and respiratory morbidity in children in an urban slum setting. *American Journal of Clinical Nutrition* 68, 414S–417S.

Barclay, A.J., Foster, A. and Sommer, A. (1987) Vitamin A supplements and mortality related to measles: a randomised clinical trial. *British Medical Journal* 294(6567), 294–296.

Barker, D.J. (1997) Intrauterine programming of coronary heart disease and stroke. *Acta Paediatrica* 423(Suppl.), 178–182.

Bassett, S.E., Di Bisceglie, A.M., Bacon, B.R., Sharp, R.M., Govindarajan, S., Hubbard, G.B., Brasky, K.M. and Lanford, R.E. (1999) Effects of iron loading on pathogenicity in hepatitis C virus-infected chimpanzees. *Hepatology* 29, 1884–1892.

Bates, C.J., Powers, H.J., Lamb, W.H., Gelman, W. and Webb, E. (1987) Effect of supplementary vitamins and iron on malaria indices in rural Gambian children. *Transactions of the Royal Society of Tropical Medicine and Hygiene* 81, 286–291.

Baum, M.K. and Shor-Posner, G. (1997) Nutritional status and survival in HIV-1 disease. *AIDS* 11, 689–690.

Baum, M.K., Shor-Posner, G., Lai, S., Zhang, G., Lai, H., Fletcher, M.A., Sauberlich, H. and Page, J.B. (1997) High risk of HIV-related mortality is associated with selenium deficiency. *Journal of Acquired Immune Deficiency Syndromes and Human Retrovirology* 15, 370–374.

Beasley, N.M., Tomkins, A.M., Hall, A., Lorri, W., Kihamia, C.M. and Bundy, D.A. (2000) The impact of weekly iron supplementation on the iron status and growth of adolescent girls in Tanzania. *Tropical Medicine and International Health* 5, 794–799.

Beck, F.W., Prasad, A.S., Kaplan, J., Fitzgerald, J.T. and Brewer, G.J. (1997) Changes in cytokine production and T-cell subpopulations in experimentally induced zinc-deficient humans. *American Journal of Physiology* 272, E1002–E1007.

Beck, M.A. (1997) Rapid genomic evolution of a non-virulent coxsackievirus B3 in selenium-deficient mice. *Biomedical and Environmental Sciences* 10, 307–315.

Beck, M.A. (1999) Selenium and host defence towards viruses. *Proceedings of the Nutrition Society* 58, 707–711.

Beck, M.A. and Levander, O.A. (1998) Dietary oxidative stress and the potentiation of viral infection. *Annual Review of Nutrition* 18, 93–116.

Beck, M.A., Kolbeck, P.C., Shi, Q., Rohr, L.H., Morris, V.C. and Levander, O.A. (1994) Increased virulence of a human enterovirus (coxsackievirus B3) in selenium-deficient mice. *Journal of Infectious Diseases* 170, 351–357.

Beesley, R., Filteau, S., Tomkins, A., Doherty, T., Ayles, H., Reid, A., Ellman, T. and Parton, S. (2000) Impact of acute malaria on plasma concentrations of transferrin receptors. *Transactions of the Royal Society of Tropical Medicine and Hygiene* 94, 295–298.

Bertolli, J., St-Louis, M.E., Simonds, R.J., Nieburg, P., Kamenga, M., Brown, C., Tarande, M., Quinn, T. and Ou, C.Y. (1996) Estimating the timing of mother-to-child transmission of human immunodeficiency virus in a breast-feeding population in Kinshasa, Zaire. *Journal of Infectious Diseases* 174, 722–726.

Bhan, M.K. and Bhandari, N. (1998) The role of zinc and vitamin A in persistent diarrhea among infants and young children. *Journal of Pediatric Gastroenterology and Nutrition* 26, 446–453.

Bhaskaram, C. and Reddy, V. (1975) Cell-mediated immunity in iron- and vitamin-deficient children. *British Medical Journal* 3(5982), 522.

Bhutta, Z.A., Black, R.E., Brown, K.H., Gardner, J.M., Gore, S., Hidayat, A., Khatun, F., Martorell, R., Ninh, N.X., Penny, M.E., Rosado, J.L., Roy, S.K., Ruel, M., Sazawal, S. and Shankar, A. (1999a) Prevention of diarrhea and pneumonia by zinc supplementation in children in developing countries: pooled analysis of randomized controlled trials. *Journal of Pediatrics* 135, 689–697.

Bhutta, Z.A., Nizami, S.Q. and Isani, Z. (1999b) Zinc supplementation in malnourished children with persistent diarrhea in Pakistan. *Pediatrics* 103, e42.

Bhutta, Z.A., Bird, S.M., Black, R.E., Brown, K.H., Gardner, J.M., Hidayat, A., Khatun, F., Martorell, R., Ninh, N.X., Penny, M.E., Rosado, J.L., Roy, S.K., Ruel, M., Sazawal, S. and Shankar, A. (2000) Therapeutic effects of oral zinc in acute and persistent diarrhea in children in developing countries: pooled analysis of randomized controlled trials. *American Journal of Clinical Nutrition* 72, 1516–1522.

Blot, W.J., Li, J.Y., Taylor, P.R., Guo, W., Dawsey, S., Wang, G.Q., Yang, C.S., Zheng, S.F., Gail, M., Li, G.Y., Yu, Y., Liu, B.Q., Tangrea, J., Sun, Y.H., Liu, F.S., Fraumeni, J.F., Zhang, Y.H. and Li, B. (1993) Nutrition intervention trials in Linxian, China: supplementation with specific vitamin/mineral combinations, cancer incidence, and disease- specific mortality in the general population. *Journal of the National Cancer Institute* 85, 1483–1492.

Bobat, R., Coovadia, H., Moodley, D. and Coutsoudis, A. (1999) Mortality in a cohort of children born to HIV-1 infected women from Durban, South Africa. *South African Medical Journal* 89, 646–648.

Brabin, B.J., Ginny, M., Sapau, J., Galme, K. and Paino, J. (1990) Consequences of maternal anaemia on outcome of pregnancy in a malaria endemic area in Papua New Guinea. *Annals of Tropical Medicine and Parasitology* 84, 11–24.

Brochu, V., Greinier, D. and Mayrand, D. (1998) Human transferrin as a source of iron for *Streptococcus intermedius. FEMS Microbiology Letters* 166, 127–133.

Brown, K.H., Black, R.E., Lopez, D.R. and Creed. D.K. (1989) Infant-feeding practices and their relationship with diarrheal and other diseases in Huascar (Lima), Peru. *Pediatrics* 83, 31–40.

Cantinieaux, B., Janssens, A., Boelaert, J.R., Lejeune, M., Vermylen, C., Kerrels, V., Comu, G., Winand, J. and Fondu, P. (1999) Ferritin-associated iron induces neutrophil dysfunction in hemosiderosis. *Journal of Laboratory and Clinical Medicine* 133, 353–361.

Caulfield, L.E., Zavaleta, N., Shankar, A.H. and Merialdi, M. (1998) Potential contribution of maternal zinc supplementation during pregnancy to maternal and child survival. *American Journal of Clinical Nutrition* 68, 499S–508S.

Ceesay, S.M., Prentice, A.M., Cole, T.J., Foord, F., Weaver, L.T., Poskitt, E.M. and Whitehead, R.G. (1997) Effects on birth weight and perinatal mortality of maternal dietary supplements in rural Gambia: 5 year randomised controlled trial. *British Medical Journal* 315(7111), 786–790.

Cesar, J.A., Victora, C.G., Barros, F.C., Santos, I.S. and Flores, J.A. (1999) Impact of breast feeding on admission for pneumonia during postneonatal period in Brazil: nested case–control study. *British Medical Journal* 318(7194), 1316–1320.

Christian, P., Schulze, K., Stoltzfus, R.J. and West, K.P., Jr (1998) Hyporetinolemia, illness symptoms, and acute phase protein response in pregnant women with and without night blindness. *American Journal of Clinical Nutrition* 67, 1237–1243.

Christian, P., West, K.P., Jr, Khatry, S.K., Kimbrough-Pradhan, E., LeClerq, S.C, Katz, J., Shrestha, S.R., Dali, S.M. and Sommer, A. (2000) Night blindness during pregnancy and subsequent mortality among women in Nepal: effects of vitamin A and beta-carotene supplementation. *American Journal of Epidemiology* 152, 542–547.

Cirelli, A., Ciardi, M., de Simone, C., Sorice, F., Giordano, R., Ciaralli, L. and Costantini, S. (1991) Serum selenium concentration and disease progress in patients with HIV infection. *Clinical Biochemistry* 24, 211–214.

Constans, J., Pellegrin, J.L., Sergeant, C., Simonoff, M., Pellegrin, I., Fleury, H., Leng, B. and Conri, C. (1995) Serum selenium predicts outcome in HIV infection. *Journal of Acquired Immune Deficiency Syndromes and Human Retrovirology* 10, 392.

Constans, J., Conri, C. and Sergeant, C. (1999) Selenium and HIV infection. *Nutrition* 15, 719–720.

Coovadia, H.M. and Coutsoudis, A. (2000) HIV in pregnancy: strategies for management. *Seminars in Neonatology* 5, 181–188.

Coutsoudis, A., Moodley, D., Pillay, K., Harrigan, R., Stone, C., Moodley, J. and Coovadia, H.M. (1997) Effects of vitamin A supplementation on viral load in HIV-1-infected pregnant women [letter]. *Journal of Acquired Immune Deficiency Syndromes and Human Retrovirology* 15, 86–87.

Coutsoudis, A., Pillay, K., Spooner, E., Kuhn, L. and Coovadia, H.M. (1999) Influence of infant-feeding patterns on early mother-to-child transmission of HIV-1 in Durban, South Africa: a prospective cohort study. *Lancet* 354, 471–476.

Dabis, F., Msellati, P., Dunn, D., Lepage, P., Newell, M.L., Peckham, C., van der Perre, P., Fransen, L., Msellati, P., Nkowane, B., Peckham, C., Andiman, W., Bhat, G., Blanche, S., Boulos, R., Bulterys, M., Chiphangwi, J., Datta, P., Embree, J., Giaquinto, C., Halsey, N., Hitimana, G., Hom, D., Karita, E., Lallemant, M., Malanda, N., Mayaux, M.J., Mitchell, C., Miotti, P., Mmiro, F., Nzingoula, S.,

Omenaca, F., Ryder, R., Shaffer, N., Commenges, D., Adjorlolo, G., Butzler, J.P., Casanova, J., Delaporte, E., Fumbi, J., Heyward, W., Lapointe, N., Piot, P., Stevens, A.M., Tardieu, M. and Temmerman, M. (1993) Estimating the rate of mother-to-child transmission of HIV: report of a workshop on methodological issues Ghent (Belgium), 17–20 February 1992. *AIDS* 7, 1139–1148.

Delanghe, J.R., Langlois, M.R., Boelaert, J.R., Van Acker, J., Van Wanzeele, F., van der Groen, G., Hemmer, R., Verhofstede, C., De Buyzere, M., De Bacquer, D., Arendt, V. and Plum, J. (1998) Haptoglobin polymorphism, iron metabolism and mortality in HIV infection. *AIDS* 12, 1027–1032.

Department for International Development (2001) www.dfid.gov.uk

de Pee, S., Bloem, M.W., Tjiong, R., Martini, E., Satoto, Gorstein, J., Shrimpton, R. and Muhilal (1999) Who has a high vitamin A intake from plant foods, but a low serum retinol concentration? Data from women in Indonesia. *European Journal of Clinical Nutrition* 53, 288–297.

Dewan, V., Patwari, A.K., Jain, M. and Dewan, N. (1995) A randomized controlled trial of vitamin A supplementation in acute diarrhea. *Indian Pediatrics* 32, 21–25.

Doherty, C.P., Sarkar, M.A., Shakur, M.S., Ling, S.C., Elton, R.A. and Cutting, W.A. (1998) Zinc and rehabilitation from severe protein-energy malnutrition: higher-dose regimens are associated with increased mortality. *American Journal of Clinical Nutrition* 68, 742–748.

Dunn, D.T., Newell, M.L., Ades, A.E. and Peckham, C.S. (1992) Risk of human immuno-deficiency virus type 1 transmission through breastfeeding. *Lancet* 340, 585–588.

Ekvall, H., Premji, Z. and Bjorkman, A. (2000) Micronutrient and iron supplementation and effective antimalarial treatment synergistically improve childhood anaemia. *Tropical Medicine and International Health* 5, 696–705.

Faisel, H. and Pittrof, R. (2000) Vitamin A and causes of maternal mortality: association and biological plausibility. *Public Health Nutrition* 3, 321–327.

Faruque, A.S., Mahalanabis, D., Haque, S.S., Fuchs, G.J. and Habte, D. (1999) Double-blind, randomized, controlled trial of zinc or vitamin A supplementation in young children with acute diarrhoea. *Acta Paediatrica* 88, 154–160.

Fawzi, W.W., Msamanga, G.I., Spiegelman, D., Urassa, E.J., McGrath, N., Mwakagile, D., Antelman, G., Mbise, R., Herrara, G., Kapiga, S., Willett, W. and Hunter, D.J. (1998) Randomised trial of effects of vitamin supplements on pregnancy outcomes and T-cell counts in HIV-1-infected women in Tanzania. *Lancet* 351, 1477–1482.

Fawzi, W.W., Mbise, R.L., Hertzmark, E., Fataki, M.R., Herrera, M.G., Ndossi, G. and Spiegelman, D. (1999) A randomized trial of vitamin A supplements in relation to mortality among human immunodeficiency virus-infected and uninfected children in Tanzania. *Pediatric Infectious Disease Journal* 18, 127–133.

Fawzi, W.W., Mbise, R., Spiegelman, D., Fataki, M., Hertzmark, E. and Ndossi, G. (2000) Vitamin A supplements and diarrheal and respiratory tract infections among children in Dar es Salaam, Tanzania. *Journal of Pediatrics* 137, 660–667.

Filteau, S.M. and Tomkins, A.M. (1999) Promoting vitamin A status in low-income countries. *Lancet* 353, 1458–1459.

Filteau, S.M., Lietz, G., Mulokozi, G., Bilotta, S., Henry, C.J. and Tomkins, A.M. (1999a) Milk cytokines and subclinical breast inflammation in Tanzanian women: effects of dietary red palm oil or sunflower oil supplementation. *Immunology* 97, 595–600.

Filteau, S.M., Rice, A.L., Ball, J.J., Chakraborty, J., Stoltzfus, R., de Francisco, A. and Willumsen, J.F. (1999b) Breast milk immune factors in Bangladeshi women supplemented postpartum with retinol or beta-carotene. *American Journal of Clinical Nutrition* 69, 953–958.

Filteau, S.M., Rollins, N.C., Coutsoudis, A., Sullivan, K.R., Willumsen, J.F. and Tomkins, A.M. (2001) The effect of antenatal vitamin A and beta-carotene supplementation on gut integrity of infants of HIV-infected South African women. *Journal of Pediatric Gastroenterology and Nutrition* 32, 464–470.

Fuller, N.J., Bates, C.J., Hayes, R.J., Bradley, A.K., Greenwood, A.M., Tulloch, S. and Greenwood, B.M. (1988) The effects of antimalarials and folate supplements on haematological indices and red cell folate levels in Gambian children. *Annals of Tropical Paediatrics* 8, 61–67.

Ge, K. and Yang, G. (1993) The epidemiology of selenium deficiency in the etiological study of endemic diseases in China. *American Journal of Clinical Nutrition* 57, 259S–263S.

Georgeson, J.C. and Filteau, S.M. (2000) Physiology, immunology, and disease transmission in human breast milk. *AIDS Patient Care and Standards* 14, 533–539.

Gernaat, H.B., Dechering, W.H. and Voorhoeve, H.W. (1998) Mortality in severe protein–energy malnutrition at Nchelenge, Zambia. *Journal of Tropical Pediatrics* 44, 211–217.

Ghana VAST (1993) Vitamin A supplementation in northern Ghana: effects on clinic attendances, hospital admissions, and child mortality: Ghana VAST Study Team. *Lancet* 342, 7–12.

Gibson, R.S., Ferguson, E.L. and Lehrfeld, J. (1998) Complementary foods for infant feeding in developing countries: their nutrient adequacy and improvement. *European Journal of Clinical Nutrition* 52, 764–770.

Golden, B.E. and Golden, M.H. (1979) Plasma zinc and the clinical features of malnutrition. *American Journal of Clinical Nutrition* 32, 2490–2494.

Goldenberg, R.L., Tamura, T., Neggers, Y., Copper, R.L., Johnston, K.E., DuBard, M.B. and Hauth, J.C. (1995) The effect of zinc supplementation on pregnancy outcome. *Journal of the American Medical Association* 274, 463–468.

Gordeuk, V.R., Delanghe, J.R., Langlois, M.R. and Boelaert, J.R. (2001) Iron status and the outcome of HIV infection: an overview. *Journal of Clinical Virology* 20, 111–115.

Groenink, J., Walgreen-Weterings, E., Nazmi, K., Bolscher, J.G., Veerman, E.C., van Winkelhoff, A.J. and Amerongen, A.V.H. (1999) Salivary lactoferrin and low-Mr mucin MG2 in *Actinobacillus actinomycetemcomitans*-associated periodontitis. *Journal of Clinical Periodontology* 26, 269–275.

Hanekom, W.A., Potgieter, S., Hughes, E.J., Malan, H., Kessow, G. and Hussey, G.D. (1997) Vitamin A status and therapy in childhood pulmonary tuberculosis. *Journal of Pediatrics* 131, 925–927.

Henning, B., Stewart, K., Zaman, K., Alam, A.N., Brown, K.H. and Black, R.E. (1992) Lack of therapeutic efficacy of vitamin A for non-cholera, watery diarrhoea in Bangladeshi children. *European Journal of Clinical Nutrition* 46, 437–443.

Herrera, J.L. (1999) Iron depletion is not effective in inducing a virologic response in patients with chronic hepatitis C who failed to respond to interferon therapy. *American Journal of Gastroenterology* 94, 3571–3575.

Hogan, J.S., Weiss, W.P. and Smith, K.L. (1993) Role of vitamin E and selenium in host defence against mastitis. *Journal of Dairy Science* 76, 2795–2803.

Huddle, J.M., Gibson, R.S. and Cullinan, T.R. (1998) Is zinc a limiting nutrient in the diets of rural pregnant Malawian women? *British Journal of Nutrition* 79, 257–265.

Humphrey, J.H., West, K.P., Jr and Sommer, A. (1992) Vitamin A deficiency and attributable mortality among under-5-year-olds. *Bulletin of the World Health Organisation* 70, 225–232.

Humphrey, J.H., Agoestina, T., Wu, L., Usman, A., Nurachim, M., Subardja, D.,

Hidayat, S., Tielsch, J., West, K.P. and Sommer, A. (1996) Impact of neonatal vitamin A supplementation on infant morbidity and mortality. *Journal of Pediatrics* 128, 489–496.

Hussey, G.D. and Klein, M. (1990) A randomized, controlled trial of vitamin A in children with severe measles. *New England Journal of Medicine* 323, 160–164.

Julien, M.R., Gomes, A., Varandas, L., Rodrigues, P., Malveiro, F., Aguiar, P., Kolsteren, P., van der Stuyft, P., Hildebrand, K., Labadarios, D. and Ferrinho, P. (1999) A randomized, double-blind, placebo-controlled clinical trial of vitamin A in Mozambican children hospitalized with nonmeasles acute lower respiratory tract infections. *Tropical Medicine and International Health* 4, 794–800.

Kakizaki, S., Takagi, H., Horiguchi, N., Toyoda, M., Takayama, H., Nagamine, T., Mori, M. and Kato, N. (2000) Iron enhances hepatitis C virus replication in cultured human hepatocytes. *Liver* 20, 125–128.

Kelly, P., Musonda, R., Kafwembe, E., Kaetano, L., Keane, E. and Farthing, M. (1999) Micronutrient supplementation in the AIDS diarrhoea-wasting syndrome in Zambia: a randomized controlled trial. *AIDS* 13, 495–500.

Kessler, L., Daley, H., Malenga, G. and Graham, S. (2000) The impact of the human immunodeficiency virus type 1 on the management of severe malnutrition in Malawi. *Annals of Tropical Paediatrics* 20, 50–56.

Khanum, S., Ashworth, A. and Huttly, S.R. (1998) Growth, morbidity, and mortality of children in Dhaka after treatment for severe malnutrition: a prospective study. *American Journal of Clinical Nutrition* 67, 940–945.

Kiremidjian-Schumacher, L., Roy, M., Wishe, H.I., Cohen, M.W. and Stotzky, G. (1994) Supplementation with selenium and human immune cell functions. II. Effect on cytotoxic lymphocytes and natural killer cells. *Biological Trace Element Research* 41, 115–127.

Klein, M. and Hussey, G.D. (1990) Vitamin A reduces morbidity and mortality in measles. *South African Medical Journal* 78, 56–58.

Kuhn, L. and Stein, Z. (1997) Infant survival, HIV infection, and feeding alternatives in less-developed countries. *American Journal of Public Health* 87, 926–931.

Kulier, R., de Onis, M., Gulmezoglu, A.M. and Villar, J. (1998) Nutritional interventions for the prevention of maternal morbidity. *International Journal of Gynaecology and Obstetrics* 63, 231–246.

Leroy, V., Newell, M.L., Dabis, F., Peckham, C., Van de Perre, P., Bulterys, M., Kind, C., Simonds, R.J., Wiktor, S. and Sellati, M. (1998) International multicentre pooled analysis of late postnatal mother-to-child transmission of HIV-1 infection. *Lancet* 352, 597–600.

Lira, P.I., Ashworth, A. and Morris, S.S. (1998) Effect of zinc supplementation on the morbidity, immune function, and growth of low-birth-weight, full-term infants in northeast Brazil. *American Journal of Clinical Nutrition* 68, 418S–424S.

Look, M.P., Rockstroh, J.K., Rao, G.S., Barton, S., Lemoch, H., Kaiser, R., Kupfer, B., Sudhop, T., Spengler, U. and Sauerbruch, T. (1998) Sodium selenite and *N*-acetylcysteine in antiretroviral-naive HIV-1-infected patients: a randomized, controlled pilot study. *European Journal of Clinical Investigation* 28, 389–397.

Markham, R.B., Coberly, J., Ruff, A.J., Hoover, D., Gomez, J., Holt, E., Desormeaux, J., Boulos, R., Quinn, T.C. and Halsey, N.A. (1994) Maternal IgG1 and IgA antibody to V3 loop consensus sequence and maternal-infant HIV-1 transmission. *Lancet* 343, 390–391.

Marshall, I. (2000) Zinc for the common cold. *Cochrane Database Systematic Reviews* CD001364.

Mateos, F., Gonzalez, C., Dominguez, C., Losa, J.E., Jimenez, A. and Perez-Arellano,

J.L. (1999) Elevated non-transferrin bound iron in the lungs of patients with *Pneumocystis carinii* pneumonia. *Journal of Infection* 38, 18–21.

Menendez, C., Kahigwa, E., Hirt, R., Vounatsou, P., Aponte, J.J., Font, F., Acosta, C.J., Schellenberg, D.M., Galindo, C.M., Kimario, J., Urassa, H., Brabin, B., Smith, T.A., Kitua, A.Y., Tanner, M. and Alonso, P.L. (1997) Randomised placebo-controlled trial of iron supplementation and malaria chemoprophylaxis for prevention of severe anaemia and malaria in Tanzanian infants. *Lancet* 350, 844–850.

Mocchegiani, E. and Muzzioli, M. (2000) Therapeutic application of zinc in human immunodeficiency virus against opportunistic infections. *Journal of Nutrition* 130, 1424S–1431S.

Moore, S.E., Cole, T.J., Collinson, A.C., Poskitt, E.M., McGregor, I.A. and Prentice, A.M. (1999) Prenatal or early postnatal events predict infectious deaths in young adulthood in rural Africa. *International Journal of Epidemiology* 28, 1088–1095.

Mostad, S.B., Overbaugh, J., DeVange, D.M., Welch, M.J., Chohan, B., Mandaliya, K., Nyange, P., Martin, H.L., Ndinya Achola, J., Bwayo, J.J. and Kreiss, J.K. (1997) Hormonal contraception, vitamin A deficiency, and other risk factors for shedding of HIV-1 infected cells from the cervix and vagina. *Lancet* 350, 922–927.

Murray, C.J. and Lopez, A.D. (1994) Global and regional cause-of-death patterns in 1990. *Bulletin of the World Health Organisation* 72, 447–480.

Murray, M.J., Murray, A.B., Murray, M.B. and Murray, C.J. (1978) The adverse effect of iron repletion on the course of certain infections. *British Medical Journal* 2(6145), 1113–1115.

Ndossi, G. and Taylor, A.M. (1999) *Multiple Micronutrient Supplementation in Tanzania – a Literature and Policy Review by UNICEF*. UNICEF, Dar es Salaam, Tanzania.

Nduati, R.W., John, G.C., Richardson, B.A., Overbaugh, J., Welch, M., Ndinya, A.J., Moses, S., Holmes, K., Onyango, F. and Kreiss, J.K. (1995) Human immunodeficiency virus type 1-infected cells in breast milk: association with immunosuppression and vitamin A deficiency. *Journal of Infectious Diseases* 172, 1461–1468.

Newburg, D.S., Viscidi, R.P., Ruff, A. and Yolken, R.H. (1992) A human milk factor inhibits binding of human immunodeficiency virus to the CD4 receptor. *Pediatric Research* 31, 22–28.

Newell, M.L. (1999) Infant feeding and HIV-1 transmission. *Lancet* 354, 442–443.

Odunukwe, N.N., Salako, L.A., Okany, C. and Ibrahim, M.M. (2000) Serum ferritin and other haematological measurements in apparently healthy adults with malaria parasitaemia in Lagos, Nigeria. *Tropical Medicine and International Health* 5, 582–586.

Oppenheimer, S.J. (1998) Iron and infection in the tropics: paediatric clinical correlates. *Annals of Tropical Paediatrics* 18, S81–S87.

Oppenheimer, S.J. (2001) Iron and its relation to immunity and infectious disease. *Journal of Nutrition* 131, 616S–636S.

Oppenheimer, S.J., Gibson, F.D., Macfarlane, S.B., Moody, J.B., Harrison, C., Spencer, A. and Bunari, O. (1986) Iron supplementation increases prevalence and effects of malaria: report on clinical studies in Papua New Guinea. *Transactions of the Royal Society of Tropical Medicine and Hygiene* 80, 603–612.

Pelletier, D.L., Frongillo, E.A.J., Schroeder, D.G. and Habicht, J.P. (1995) The effects of malnutrition on child mortality in developing countries. *Bulletin of the World Health Organisation* 73, 443–448.

Percival, S.S. (1998) Copper and immunity. *American Journal of Clinical Nutrition* 67, 1064S–1068S.

Pickering, H., Hayes, R.J., Tomkins, A.M., Carson, D. and Dunn, D.T. (1987) Alternative measures of diarrhoeal morbidity and their association with social and environmental factors in urban children in The Gambia. *Transactions of the Royal Society of Tropical Medicine and Hygiene* 81, 853–859.

Prasad, A.S. (2000) Effects of zinc deficiency on Th1 and Th2 cytokine shifts. *Journal of Infectious Diseases* 182, S62–S68.

Prasad, A.S., Beck, F.W., Kaplan, J., Chandrasekar, P.H., Ortega, J., Fitzgerald, J.T. and Swerdlow, P. (1999) Effect of zinc supplementation on incidence of infections and hospital admissions in sickle cell disease (SCD). *American Journal of Hematology* 61, 194–202.

Prudhon, C., Golden, M.H., Briend, A. and Mary, J.Y. (1997) A model to standardise mortality of severely malnourished children using nutritional status on admission to therapeutic feeding centres. *European Journal of Clinical Nutrition* 51, 771–777.

Ravaglia, G., Forti, P., Maioli, F., Bastagli, L., Facchini, A., Mariani, E., Savarino, L., Sassi, S., Cucinotta, D. and Lenaz, G. (2000) Effect of micronutrient status on natural killer cell immune function in healthy free-living subjects aged ≥ 90 y. *American Journal of Clinical Nutrition* 71, 590–598.

Rollins, N.C., Filteau, S.M., Elson, I. and Tomkins, A.M. (2000) Vitamin A supplementation of South African children with severe diarrhea: optimum timing for improving biochemical and clinical recovery and subsequent vitamin A status. *Pediatric Infectious Disease Journal* 19, 284–289.

Rosado, J.L., Lopez, P., Munoz, E., Martinez, H. and Allen, L.H. (1997) Zinc supplementation reduced morbidity, but neither zinc nor iron supplementation affected growth or body composition of Mexican preschoolers. *American Journal of Clinical Nutrition* 65, 13–19.

Roy, M., Kiremidjian-Schumacher, L., Wishe, H.I., Cohen, M.W. and Stotzky, G. (1994) Supplementation with selenium and human immune cell functions. I. Effect on lymphocyte proliferation and interleukin 2 receptor expression. *Biological Trace Element Research* 41, 103–114.

Roy, S.K., Behrens, R.H., Haider, R., Akramuzzaman, S.M., Mahalanabis, D., Wahed, M.A. and Tomkins, A.M. (1992) Impact of zinc supplementation on intestinal permeability in Bangladeshi children with acute diarrhoea and persistent diarrhoea syndrome. *Journal of Pediatric Gastroenterology and Nutrition* 15, 289–296.

Roy, S.K., Tomkins, A.M., Akramuzzaman, S.M., Behrens, R.H., Haider, R., Mahalanabis, D. and Fuchs, G. (1997) Randomised controlled trial of zinc supplementation in malnourished Bangladeshi children with acute diarrhoea. *Archives of Diseases of Childhood* 77, 196–200.

Roy, S.K., Tomkins, A.M., Mahalanabis, D., Akramuzzaman, S.M., Haider, R., Behrens, R.H. and Fuchs, G. (1998) Impact of zinc supplementation on persistent diarrhoea in malnourished Bangladeshi children. *Acta Paediatrica* 87, 1235–1239.

Roy, S.K., Tomkins, A.M., Haider, R., Behren, R.H., Akramuzzaman, S.M., Mahalanabis, D. and Fuchs, G.J. (1999) Impact of zinc supplementation on subsequent growth and morbidity in Bangladeshi children with acute diarrhoea. *European Journal of Clinical Nutrition* 53, 529–534.

Ruel, M.T., Rivera, J.A., Santizo, M.C., Lonnerdal, B. and Brown, K.H. (1997) Impact of zinc supplementation on morbidity from diarrhea and respiratory infections among rural Guatemalan children. *Pediatrics* 99, 808–813.

Sazawal, S., Jalla, S., Mazumder, S., Sinha, A., Black, R.E. and Bhan, M.K. (1997) Effect of zinc supplementation on cell-mediated immunity and lymphocyte subsets in preschool children. *Indian Pediatrics* 34, 589–597.

Sazawal, S., Black, R.E., Jalla, S., Mazumdar, S., Sinha, A. and Bhan, M.K. (1998) Zinc supplementation reduces the incidence of acute lower respiratory infections in infants and preschool children: a double-blind, controlled trial. *Pediatrics* 102, 1–5.

Schofield, C. and Ashworth, A. (1996) Why have mortality rates for severe malnutrition remained so high? *Bulletin of the World Health Organisation* 74, 223–229.

Scott, M.E. and Koski, K.G. (2000) Zinc deficiency impairs immune responses against parasitic nematode infections at intestinal and systemic sites. *Journal of Nutrition* 130, 1412S–1420S.

Semba, R.D. (1999a) Vitamin A and immunity to viral, bacterial and protozoan infections. *Proceedings of the Nutrition Society* 58, 719–727.

Semba, R.D. (1999b) Vitamin A as 'anti-infective' therapy, 1920–1940. *Journal of Nutrition* 129, 783–791.

Semba, R.D. and Neville, M.C. (1999) Breast-feeding, mastitis, and HIV transmission: nutritional implications. *Nutrition Reviews* 57, 146–153.

Semba, R.D., Miotti, P.G., Chiphangwi, J.D., Saah, A.J., Canner, J.K., Dallabetta, G.A. and Hoover, D.R. (1994) Maternal vitamin A deficiency and mother-to-child transmission of HIV-1. *Lancet* 343, 1593–1597.

Shankar, A.H., Genton, B., Semba, R.D., Baisor, M., Paino, J., Tamja, S., Adiguma, T., Wu, L., Rare, L., Tielsch, J.M., Alpers, M.P. and West, K.P. (1999) Effect of vitamin A supplementation on morbidity due to *Plasmodium falciparum* in young children in Papua New Guinea: a randomised trial. *Lancet* 354, 203–209.

Sommer, A. (1993) Vitamin A, infectious disease, and childhood mortality: a 2-cent solution? *Journal of Infectious Diseases* 167, 1003–1007.

Sommer, A. (1997) Vitamin A prophylaxis. *Archives of Diseases of Childhood* 77, 191–194.

Stephensen, C.B., Franchi, L.M., Hernandez, H., Campos, M., Gilman, R.H. and Alvarez, J.O. (1998) Adverse effects of high-dose vitamin A supplements in children hospitalized with pneumonia. *Pediatrics* 101, E3.

Tang, A.M., Graham, N.M., Kirby, A.J., McCall, L.D., Willett, W.C. and Saah, A.J. (1993) Dietary micronutrient intake and risk of progression to acquired immunodeficiency syndrome (AIDS) in human immunodeficiency virus type 1 (HIV-1)-infected homosexual men. *American Journal of Epidemiology* 138, 937–951.

Thu, B.D., Schultink, W., Dillon, D., Gross, R., Leswara, N.D. and Khoi, H.H. (1999) Effect of daily and weekly micronutrient supplementation on micronutrient deficiencies and growth in young Vietnamese children. *American Journal of Clinical Nutrition* 69, 80–86.

Thuma, P.E., Mabeza, G.F., Biemba, G., Bhat, G.J., McLaren, C.E., Moyo, V.M., Zulu, S., Khumalo, H., Mabeza, P., M'Hango, A., Parry, D., Poltera, A.A., Brittenham, G.M. and Gordeuk, V.R. (1998) Effect of iron chelation therapy on mortality in Zambian children with cerebral malaria. *Transactions of the Royal Society of Tropical Medicine and Hygiene* 92, 214–218.

Tomkins, A. (2000) Malnutrition, morbidity and mortality in children and their mothers. *Proceedings of the Nutrition Society* 59, 135–146.

Tomkins, A. (2001a) Nutrition and maternal morbidity and mortality. *British Journal of Nutrition* 85, S93–S99.

Tomkins, A. (2001b) Vitamin and mineral nutrition for the health and development of the children of Europe. *Public Health Nutrition* 4, 91–99.

Turk, S., Bozfakioglu, S., Ecder, S.T., Kahraman, T., Gurel, N., Erkoc, R., Aysura, N., Turkman, A., Bekiroglu, N. and Arrk, E. (1998) Effects of zinc supplementation on the immune system and on antibody response to multivalent influenza vaccine in hemodialysis patients. *International Journal of Artificial Organs* 21, 274–278.

Udall, J.N., Pang, K., Fritze, L., Kleinman, R. and Walker, W.A. (1981) Development of gastrointestinal mucosal barrier. I. The effect of age on intestinal permeability to macromolecules. *Pediatric Research* 15, 241–244.

UNICEF (1998a) *HIV and Infant Feeding – a Review of HIV Transmission through Breast Feeding.* www.unicef.org

UNICEF (1998b) *HIV and Infant Feeding – Guidelines for Decision Makers.* www.unicef.org

UNICEF (2001) www.unicef.org

van den Broek, N.R. and Letsky, E.A. (2000) Etiology of anemia in pregnancy in south Malawi. *American Journal of Clinical Nutrition* 72, 247S–256S.

Van de Perre, P. (1999) Transmission of human immunodeficiency virus type 1 through breast-feeding: how can it be prevented? *Journal of Infectious Diseases* 179, S405–S407.

Vella, V., Tomkins, A., Nidku, J. and Marshall, T. (1992) Determinants of child mortality in south-west Uganda. *Journal of Biosocial Science* 24, 103–112.

Vella, V., Tomkins, A., Borghesi, A., Migliori, G.B., Ndiku, J. and Adriko, B.C. (1993) Anthropometry and childhood mortality in northwest and southwest Uganda. *American Journal of Public Health* 83, 1616–1618.

Vella, V., Tomkins, A., Ndiku, J., Marshal, T. and Cortinovis, I. (1994) Anthropometry as a predictor for mortality among Ugandan children, allowing for socio-economic variables. *European Journal of Clinical Nutrition* 48, 189–197.

Victora, C.G., Smith, P.G., Vaughan, J.P., Nobre, L.C., Lombardi, C., Teixeira, A.M., Fuchs, S.C., Moreira, L.B., Grigante, L.P. and Barros, F. (1989) Infant feeding and deaths due to diarrhea: a case-control study. *American Journal of Epidemiology* 129, 1032–1041.

Walker, E.M., Jr and Walker, S.M. (2000) Effects of iron overload on the immune system. *Annals of Clinical and Laboratory Science* 30, 354–365.

Waterlow, J.C., Tomkins, A.M. and Grantham-Mcgregor, S.M. (1992) *Protein Energy Malnutrition.* Edward Arnold, London.

Wellinghausen, N., Kern, W.V., Jochle, W. and Kern, P. (2000) Zinc serum level in human immunodeficiency virus-infected patients in relation to immunological status. *Biological Trace Element Research* 73, 139–149.

West, K.P.J., Katz, J., Shrestha, S.R., LeClerq, S.C., Khatry, S.K., Pradhan, E.K., Adhikiri, R., Wu, L.S.F., Pokhrel, R.P. and Sommer, A. (1995) Mortality of infants < 6 mo of age supplemented with vitamin A: a randomized, double-masked trial in Nepal. *American Journal of Clinical Nutrition* 62, 143–148.

West, K.P.J., Katz, J., Khatry, S.K., LeClerq, S.C., Pradhan, E.K., Shrestha, S.R., Conner, P.B., Dali, S.R., Christian, P., Pokhrel, R.P. and Sommer, A. (1999) Double blind, cluster randomised trial of low dose supplementation with vitamin A or beta carotene on mortality related to pregnancy in Nepal: the NNIPS–2 Study Group. *British Medical Journal* 318, 570–575.

WHO/UNICEF (1997) Integrated management of childhood illness: a WHO/UNICEF initiative. *Bulletin of the World Health Organization* 75 (Suppl. 1), 1–128.

Wilkinson, R.J., Llewelyn, M., Toossi, Z., Patel, P., Pasvol, G., Lalvani, A., Wright, D. Latif, M. and Davidson, R.N. (2000) Influence of vitamin D deficiency and vitamin D receptor polymorphisms on tuberculosis among Gujarati Asians in west London: a case–control study. *Lancet* 355, 618–621.

Willumsen, J.F., Filteau, S.M., Coutsoudis, A., Uebel, K.E., Newell, M.L. and Tomkins, A.M. (2000) Subclinical mastitis as a risk factor for mother–infant HIV transmission. *Advances in Experimental Medicine and Biology* 478, 211–223.

Willumsen, J.F., Newell, M.L., Filteau, S.M., Coutsoudis, A., Dwarika, S., York, D., Tomkins, A.M. and Coovadia, H.M. (2001) Variation in breastmilk HIV-1 viral load in left and right breasts during the first 3 months of lactation. *AIDS* 15, 1896–1898.

World Bank (2001) www.worldbank.org

World Health Organization (2001) www.who.org

Yu, S.Y., Li, W.O., Zhu, Y.J., Yu, W.P. and Hou, C. (1989) Chemoprevention trial of human hepatitis with selenium supplementation in China. *Biology and Trace Element Research* 20, 15–22.

Index

Page numbers in **bold** refer to figures and tables

Browse Read and Buy

www.cabi.org/bookshop

ANIMAL & VETERINARY SCIENCES
BIODIVERSITY   CROP PROTECTION
HUMAN HEALTH   NATURAL RESOURCES
ENVIRONMENT   PLANT SCIENCES
SOCIAL SCIENCES

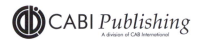 CABI *Publishing*
A division of CAB International

Online **BOOK** SHOP

Subjects

Search

Reading Room

Bargains

New Titles

Forthcoming

Order & Pay Online!

 MasterCard

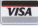 VISA

AMERICAN EXPRESS

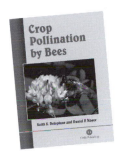 Crop Pollination by Bees
Keith S. Delaplane and Daniel F. Mayer

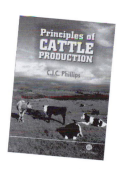 A DICTIONARY OF Entomology
G Gordh and D H Headrick

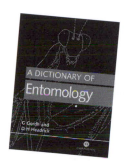 Principles of CATTLE PRODUCTION
C.J.C. Phillips

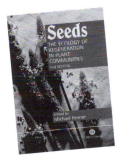 Seeds
THE ECOLOGY OF REGENERATION IN PLANT COMMUNITIES
2nd EDITION
Edited by Michael Fenner

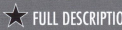 FULL DESCRIPTION   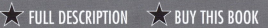 BUY THIS BOOK   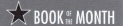 BOOK OF THE MONTH

Tel: +44 (0)1491 832111 Fax: +44 (0)1491 829292